Evaluation and Treatment of the Aging Face

Melvin L. Elson
Editor

Evaluation and Treatment of the Aging Face

With a Foreword by John M. Yarborough, Jr.

With 286 Illustrations in 345 Parts
83 Pieces in Color

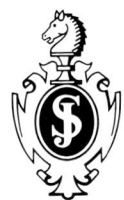

Springer-Verlag
New York Berlin Heidelberg London Paris
Tokyo Hong Kong Barcelona Budapest

Melvin L. Elson
The Dermatology Center, Inc.
4535 Harding Road
Nashville, TN 37205-2120, USA

Library of Congress Cataloging-in-Publication Data
Evaluation and treatment of the aging face / [edited by] Melvin L.
Elson.
   p. cm.
  Includes bibliographical references and index.
  ISBN 0-387-94237-8. — ISBN 3-540-94237-8 :
  1. Facelift. 2. Skin—Surgery. 3. Face—Surgery. I. Elson,
Melvin L.
  [DNLM: 1. Face—surgery. 2. Surgery, Plastic—in old age.
3. Surgery, Plastic—methods. WE 705 E916 1994]
RD119.5.F33E93 1994
617.5′20592—dc20
DNLM/DLC
                                                            94-14223

Printed on acid-free paper.

© 1995 Springer-Verlag New York Inc.
All rights reserved. This work may not be translated or copied in whole or in part without the written permission of the publisher (Springer-Verlag New York, Inc., 175 Fifth Avenue, New York, NY 10010, USA), except for brief excerpts in connection with reviews or scholarly analysis. Use in connection with any form of information and retrieval, electronic adaptation, computer software, or by similar or dissimilar methodology now known or hereafter developed is forbidden.
The use of general descriptive names, trade names, trademarks, etc., in this publication, even if the former are not especially identified, is not to be taken as a sign that such names, as understood by the Trade Marks and Merchandise Marks Act, may accordingly be used freely by anyone.
While the advice and information in this book are believed to be true and accurate at the date of going to press, neither the authors nor the editors nor the publisher can accept any legal responsibility for any errors or omissions that may be made. The publisher makes no warranty, express or implied, with respect to the material contained herein.

Production coordinated by Chernow Editorial Services, Inc., and managed by Natalie Johnson; manufacturing supervised by Jacqui Ashri.
Typeset by TechType Inc., Upper Saddle River, NJ, USA.
Printed and bound by Walsworth Publishing Co. Inc., Marceline, MO, USA.
Printed in the United States of America.

9 8 7 6 5 4 3 2 1

ISBN 0-387-94237-8 Springer-Verlag New York Berlin Heidelberg
ISBN 3-540-94237-8 Springer-Verlag Berlin Heidelberg New York

To the memory of J. Lamar Callaway, M.D., James B. Duke Professor of Dermatology and Chairman of the Dermatology Division at Duke University Medical Center from its inception until June 30, 1986, who taught me not only to look but to see, and to my dear wife Betty, who has shown me what true beauty—both inside and out—is really all about.

Foreword

There are individuals a tad past the full bloom of maturity who verily venerate the stigmata and effluvia of aging. These are folk who loftily display a needlepoint pillow whose legend trumpets "I've earned every wrinkle." Most of us, however, exert some effort to maintain or to reclaim vitalization of our torpid bodies and impercipiate minds. Hard-won gains in mental and physical revivification lead many of us to consider synchronous rejuvenation of our tracked faces.

Evaluation and Treatment of the Aging Face is a text for physicians who practice the art of facial refinement. Presented by international experts in dermatologic surgery from such disparate parts of the globe as Rome, Hamamatsu, and Nashville, the text provides instructional and practicable insights into optional surgical techniques, as well as information from the experienced vanguard regarding appropriate use of sunscreens, retinoids, alphahydroxy acids, and dermal fillers.

Although dermatologic surgery has occupied only a brief span in the history of medicine, its accelerated evolution during the last decade has challenged dermatologic surgeons to master these stimulating advances. *Evaluation and Treatment of the Aging Face* is a source that can enhance the skills of all physicians who refine skin of the aging face. This advanced text, however, should not intimidate the novice as it incorporates much basic information about technique, appropriate anesthetics, design of office-based surgery centers, psychosocial aspects of cosmetic surgery, and the esthetician's role in care of the skin. Adequate information is provided to assist the physician with decisions about personal mastery of individual techniques or the need for referral. Particularly relevant is the precaution to perform only those procedures for which one is trained and with which one feels comfortable.

As dermatologists, care of the skin is our right and responsibility. Expanding understanding of the biology and physiology of aging has afforded us more control of retardation as well as rejuvenation. The contributors, all dermatologists, have compiled a near global reference that should be useful for all physicians who treat the aging face. It is hoped that this effort also will encourage conscientious interspeciality cooperation so that all physicians who care for the aging face will do so skillfully and harmoniously.

> John M. Yarborough, Jr., M.D.
> Clinical Professor of Dermatology
> Tulane University School of Medicine
> New Orleans, LA

Preface

Dermatology has always been a specialty full of changes. As general practitioners of the skin, dermatologists have had the opportunity to observe a vast array of disorders in both sexes and in all age groups from the cradle to the grave. As the population has become increasingly older, it falls to the dermatologist and the dermatologic surgeon to treat the most common of all skin diseases—aging. Dr. John M. Yarborough, Jr., the president of the American Society for Dermatologic Surgery, sets the tone for the text in the foreword.

This text presents an overall picture of the aging face, the factors that comprise it, and how these factors are treated. To begin to treat a problem, one must have a comprehensive understanding of its characteristics, as well as the dynamic factors that comprise the continually changing picture of the aging face. The successful interaction of the various factors and the available procedures is crucially important in treating the aging face. Treatment may begin only after the evaluation is made and the precise plan for a particular patient has been determined.

All patients should use a sunscreen daily. Only a generation ago, most individuals believed that sun exposure was either beneficial or not so harmful that they should miss the warmth and "healthy glow" afforded by sun exposure. We now know, of course, the damaging effects of the sun not only in regard to the production of basal cell carcinoma, but in the development of malignant melanoma and photoaging. Dr. Rigel's chapter on sunscreens is an up-to-date compendium of what is available, what to avoid, and what to recommend. The controversies regarding appropriate levels of SPF, the determination of SPF as to UVA and UVB, government guidelines, and many other issues are clearly and concisely addressed.

No one is more qualified to discuss the use of retinoids in the treatment of photoaging than Dr. Al Kligman. As the inventor of Retin A, as well as the first to discover its ability to treat photoaging, he is also the foremost expert on all aspects of skin aging and has led dermatology into this field almost singlehandedly. We all owe a great debt to him and I feel most privileged to have his contribution in the textbook.

Dr. David Harris is well known for his innovative ideas, especially with regard to treating the aging face. His contribution on the use of glycolic acid in the treatment of aging is one of the most timely chapters, as the popularity of the AHAs continues to soar in both dermatology and cosmetics.

Dr. Paul Collins has lectured worldwide on the process of chemical peeling, and his chapter is complete and up-to-the-minute from the history of peeling to the future.

Dr. Bruce Katz is representative of the shining stars on the horizon of dermatologic surgery. His keen mind and innovative ideas come through in his chapter on dermabrasion.

Dr. Rhoda Narins and Dr. Bill Coleman team up to produce all the necessary information on liposuction and lipotransfer for the aging face in concise, practical chapters.

Dr. Tom Alt is one of the most respected cosmetic surgeons in the world today, and his practical presentation of rhytidectomy provides the necessary introduction to the procedure as well as pointers for the accomplished surgeon.

Dr. Larry David and Dr. Sterling Baker present an up-to-date picture of one of the most elegant of the cosmetic procedures—upper and lower lid blepharoplasties. Many dermatologists are now performing this increasingly common procedure, but even those who are not should have a working knowledge of it.

Dr. Bill Hanke, a triprofessor at Indiana University and president-elect of the International Society for Dermatologic Surgery, reminds us that not all lumps and bumps are due to the sun and that the patient seeks treatment from the dermatologic surgeon to improve the appearance in many ways.

An internationally respected surgeon, Dr. Bluford (Blu) Stough, discusses how to make certain that the frame around the picture of the aging face presents the best possible appearance.

Almost everyone speaks with both the muscles of the face and the hands. Dr. Bob Clark's chapter on the aging hand is particularly important to prevent a mismatch from occurring, as when the face is treated and the hands are not.

The next two chapters discuss new directions in dermatologic surgery. Dr. Jeff Klein's personal look at the establishment of a cosmetic surgery center gives a great deal of insight into the many ramifications of taking such a step, with practical sensible advice.

More and more, paramedical personnel are alleviating the load on the dermatologist and dermatologic surgeon. Dr. Mark Lees and Dianne Young graciously accepted the assignment of discussing how the roles are meshing. They are two of the most outstanding aestheticians in the world and highly respected both within their field and outside of it.

The last full chapter puts all this together. What are we about? How does aging affect our patients and what happens when we intervene? Dr. Judith Waters and George Ellis put it in perspective. What we are doing in treatment of the aging face is by no means frivolous. Looking at the psychosocial impact of our procedures is one way to grasp the importance. Another way is to look at our patient's eyes—the sparkle after the procedure.

The final chapter combines the knowledge of many of the leaders in dermatologic surgery and dermatology from around the world. From innovative techniques, new devices, and new material for soft tissue augmentation, to the role of the dermatologic surgeon, this chapter leads us into the future.

We are really only beginning to understand aging and the treatments that can be provided to our patients. Certainly, with the surgical advances on the horizon as well as new materials for soft tissue augmentation, topical agents to reverse aging, and better and more elegant sunscreens, we are poised to make tremendous advances. In addition, research into aging of the skin may very well provide insight into what aging really is, and how it can be treated and reversed.

Melvin L. Elson

Acknowledgments

A textbook of this magnitude requires the concerted and sincere efforts of a great number of people. There would have been no way to dedicate the amount of time required for this task without the support of my family and office staff. My two secretaries, Ruth Norfleet and Kathy Fullerton, worked many hours typing, correcting, calling, and cajoling all the authors. Esther Gumpert and her very capable staff at Springer-Verlag have always been available and open to my ideas.

A great deal of thanks must be given to my patients without whom there would be no textbook. I learn from them every day. Finally, I am very fortunate to have the contributions from so many of the world's best dermatologic surgeons and dermatologists, whom I am also fortunate to be able to count as my friends. They made this monumental task a pleasure.

There are, of course, many dermatologists who, over the years, have taken our specialty forward. As the specialty continues to change and grow, many more step forward to lead us into the next era. Hopefully, this textbook will inspire the next generation to excel, improve, and stretch the limits of current knowledge.

Contents

Foreword vii
Preface ix
Acknowledgments xiii
Contributors xix

1. Evaluation and Treatment of the Aging Face 1
   Melvin L. Elson

2. Sunscreen: Prevention of Aging and Skin Cancer 9
   Darrell S. Rigel

3. Topical Tretinoin Can Correct the Structural
   Abnormalities of Human Photoaged Skin 16
   Albert M. Kligman

4. Treatment of the Aging Skin with Glycolic Acid 22
   David R. Harris

5. Chemical Face Peeling 34
   Paul S. Collins

6. Dermabrasion 68
   Bruce E. Katz

7. Soft Tissue Augmentation 79
   Melvin L. Elson

8. Liposuction Surgery of the Face and Neck 93
   Rhoda S. Narins

9. Lipotransfer 101
   William P. Coleman III

10. Facelift Surgery 110
    Thomas H. Alt

11. Blepharoplasty.. 169
    Laurence M. David and *Sterling S. Baker*

12. Skin Lesions of Aging... 187
    C. William Hanke and *Lisa A. Francis*

13. Hair Restoration... 212
    D. Bluford Stough and *Craig S. Schauder*

14. Treatment of the Aging Hands 243
    Robert E. Clark and *Susan C. Carson*

15. Establishing a Dermatologic Surgicenter 255
    Jeffrey Alan Klein

16. The Esthetician's Role in Skin Care 261
    Mark Lees and *Diane Young*

17. The Psychosocial Aspects of Cosmetic Surgery................. 272
    Judith Waters and *George Ellis*

18. Surgical Vignettes.. 283

    Manual Dermasanding and Low Strength Trichloroacetic
    Acid Peeling: A Simple Technique to Improve
    Photodamaged Skin.. 283
    David R. Harris

    Cosmetics vs. Cosmeceuticals: A New
    Rational Science 292
    Nia K. Terezakis

    Cryosurgery 293
    Gloria F. Graham

    Evaluation and Treatment of the Aging Face..................... 294
    Richard G. Glogau

    The Ligmaject 295
    Arnold William Klein

    The Dermatologist's Role in Treating the Aging Skin........ 296
    Sheldon V. Pollack

    Microsurgical Treatment of the Aging Face 296
    Toshio Kobayashi

    Vitamins: Therapy for Aging? 300
    Wilma F. Bergfeld and *Thomas N. Helm*

    European View of Evaluation and Treatment
    of the Aging Face 301
    Eckart Hancke

The "How Did This Happen to Me?" Syndrome.............. 301
Daniel A. Gross

The Use of Gore-Tex Combined with Other Fillers 302
Alejandro Camps-Fresneda

The "Sandwich Technique" for Filling the
Nasolabial Fold 304
António Picoto

Crosslinked Hyaluronic Acid (Hylan Gel)
as a Soft Tissue Augmentation Material:
A Preliminary Assessment.. 304
Daniel Piacquadio

Surgical Correction of Neck Flaccidity
in the Older Male... 308
Arthur K. Balin

Index... 315

Contributors

Thomas H. Alt, M.D., Department of Dermatology, University of Minneapolis Medical School, Minneapolis, MN 55455, and Alt Cosmetic Surgery Center, 4920 Lincoln Drive, Minneapolis, MN 55436-1701, USA

Sterling S. Baker, M.D., Department of Ophthalmology, University of Oklahoma Health Sciences Center, Oklahoma City, OK 73104, USA

Arthur K. Balin, M.D., 2129 Providence Avenue, Chester, PA 19013-5506, USA

Wilma F. Bergfeld, M.D., Department of Dermatology, Case Western Reserve University School of Medicine, Cleveland, OH 44106-4915, and Department of Dermatology, The Cleveland Clinic Foundation, 9500 Euclid Avenue, Cleveland, OH 44195-0001, USA

Alejandro Camps-Fresneda, M.D., Department of Dermatology, Hospital General de Catalunya, San Cugat Del Valles, 08790 Barcelona, Spain, and c/Balmes 347, 08006 Barcelona, Spain

Susan C. Carson, M.D., 335 Penny Lane, Concord, NC 28025, USA

Robert E. Clark, M.D., Department of Medicine, Division of Dermatology, Duke University School of Medicine, Durham, NC 27710, and Dermatologic Surgery and Cutaneous Oncology Unit, Duke University Medical Center, Durham, NC 27710-0001, USA

William P. Coleman III, M.D., Department of Dermatology, Tulane University School of Medicine, New Orleans, LA 7012, and Coleman Clinic, 4425 Conlin Street, Metairie, LA 70006, USA

Paul S. Collins, M.D., Department of Dermatology, Stanford University School of Medicine, Stanford, CA 94305, and 84 Santa Rosa Street, San Luis Obispo, CA 93405-1812, USA

Laurence M. David, M.D., Department of Dermatologic Surgery, Institute of Laser Cosmetic Surgery, 415 Pier Avenue, Hermosa Beach, CA 90254, USA

George Ellis, M.A., Department of Psychology, Fairleigh Dickinson University, Madison, NJ 07940, USA

Melvin L. Elson, M.D., The Dermatology Center, Inc., 4535 Harding Road, Nashville, TN 37205-2120, USA

Lisa A. Francis, Department of Dermatology, Pathology and Otolaryngology, Indiana University School of Medicine, Indianapolis, IN 46202-5267, USA

Richard G. Glogau, M.D., Department of Dermatology, University of California San Francisco, San Francisco, CA 94116, USA

Gloria G. Graham, M.D., 12949 Caminito Pointe Del Mar, Del Mar, CA 92014, USA

Daniel A. Gross, M.D., Department of Medicine, Division of Dermatology, UCLA School of Medicine, Los Angeles, CA 90033, and Valley Dermatology Medical Group, Inc., 18364 Clark Street, Tarzana, CA 91356, USA

Eckart Hancke, Prof. Dr. med., Dr. med. habil., Department of Dermatology, Ferdinand-Sauerbruch-Klinikum, Arrenbergerstrasse 20-56, 1 Wuppertal 42117, Germany

C. William Hanke, M.D., Departments of Dermatology, Pathology and Otolaryngology, Indiana University School of Medicine, Indianapolis, IN 46202-5267, USA

David R. Harris, M.D., Department of Dermatology, Stanford University School of Medicine, Campbell, CA 95008, USA

Thomas N. Helm, M.D., Department of Dermatology, State University of New York at Buffalo, Buffalo, NY 14203, USA

Bruce E. Katz, M.D., Department of Dermatology, College of Physicians and Surgeons of Columbia University, New York, NY 10032, and 14 East 82 Street, New York, NY 10028, USA

Arnold William Klein, M.D., Department of Medicine, Division of Dermatology, UCLA School of Medicine, Los Angeles, CA 90033, and 435 North Roxbury Drive, Beverly Hills, CA 90210, USA

Jeffrey Alan Klein, M.D., Department of Dermatology, University of California at Irvine, College of Medicine, Irvine, CA 92717, and 30280 Rancho Viejo Road, San Juan Capistrano, CA 92675, USA

Albert M. Kligman, M.D., Ph.D., Department of Dermatology, University of Pennsylvania, Philadelphia, PA 19104, USA

Toshio Kobayashi, M.D., Hamamatsu Clinic of Dermatologic Surgery, 11-1 Asahicho, Hamamatsu 430, Japan

Mark Lees, Ph.D., Mark Lees Skincare Inc., 4400 Bayou Boulevard, Pensacola, FL 32503, USA

Rhoda S. Narins, M.D., Department of Dermatology, New York University School of Medicine, New York, NY 10016, and 33 Davis Avenue, White Plains, NY 10605, USA

Daniel Piacquadio, M.D., Department of Dermatology, University of San Diego, San Diego, CA 92103-8420, USA

António Picoto, M.D., Av. General Carmona No. 17, Estoril 2765, Portugal

Sheldon V. Pollack, M.D., Department of Medicine, Division of Dermatology, Faculty of Medicine, University of Toronto, Toronto, Ontario M5S 1A8, Canada, and 200 St. Clair Avenue West, Toronto, Ontario M4V 1R1, Canada

Darrell S. Rigel, M.D., Department of Dermatology, New York University Medical Center, New York, NY 10016, and 213 Madison Avenue, New York, NY 10016-3814, USA

Craig S. Schauder, M.D., One Mercy Lane, Hot Springs, AR 71913, USA

D. Bluford Stough, M.D., Department of Dermatology, University of Arkansas for Medical Sciences, Hot Springs, AR 71913, USA

Nia K. Terezakis, M.D., Department of Dermatology, Tulane University School of Medicine, New Orleans, LA 70112, and 2633 Napoleon Avenue, New Orleans, LA 70115, USA

Judith Waters, Ph.D., Department of Psychology, Fairleigh-Dickinson University, Madison, NJ 07940, USA

Diane Young, Diane Young Anti-Aging Salon, 38 East 57th Street, New York, NY 10022, USA

John M. Yarborough, Jr., M.D., Department of Dermatology, Tulane University School of Medicine, New Orleans, LA 70112, USA

1
Evaluation and Treatment of the Aging Face

Melvin L. Elson

Introduction

In order effectively to treat the patient who presents for rejuvenation of the aging face, it is necessary to be able to evaluate the face and the various factors that go into producing this dynamic picture at any given time.

Basically, two methods have been used to determine how the face is influenced and, therefore, which treatment is most appropriate as the aging process manifests itself: one method examines the individual factors that go into producing the picture of the aging face,[1] while the other relies upon a division of the face into areas that interact with one another over time and are influenced differently to produce the picture at any given time.[2]

In addition an objective method of assessing the face would certainly be helpful to determine both the benefits obtained from treatment and surgery as well as a method to be able to compare results scientifically from physician to physician in order to discuss treatment in a less subjective manner than is currently used.

Factors in the Aging Face

The aging face, regardless of its place in chronological years, is composed of five interacting factors: intrinsic aging, sleep lines, gravity, expression lines, and photoaging.

Figures 1.1 and 1.2 are photographs of a patient who presented with all five of the factors of the aging face. A computer image was made of the lateral view of her face; then the aging factors were eliminated from the computer image. Figure 1.3 shows the result of this process: a computer image approximating what the patient may have looked like at age 20.[3]

Figures 1.4 through 1.8 represent what would have occurred to the patient's face had only a single specific factor been present as the patient aged. Figure 1.4 represents intrinsic aging; Figure 1.5, sleep lines; Figure 1.6, gravity; Figure 1.7, expression lines; and Figure 1.8, photoaging. Figure 1.9 puts all these factors back into the face to represent the aged picture.

Intrinsic aging refers to a true loss of tissue, an atrophy of both dermal and subcutaneous tissue, primarily manifested in the triangle formed by the zygomatic arch, the nasolabial fold, and the mandibular line (the submalar triangle). As true aging occurs—usually manifested in the seventh decade or later, this area thins and gives the gaunt appearance that is characteristic of true old age.[4] The face is thin, as there is actual loss of the roundness characteristic of a young face as the buccal fat pad is lost. In addition, there is atrophy of the temporal area and the upper malar eminence.[5]

Even though intrinsic aging does not play a significant role in most patients who present to the cosmetic dermatologic surgeon for treatment for aging (they are usually 35–55 years of age) some do present from this older age group, and certainly intrinsic aging may occur in some individuals at a younger age than is the norm.

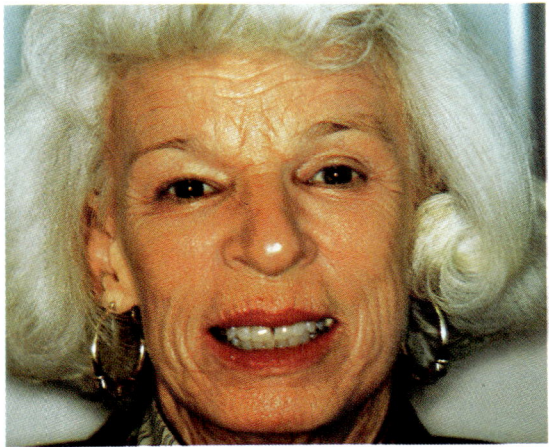

FIGURE 1.1. A frontal view of a patient presenting with all five factors of the aging face: intrinsic aging, sleep lines, gravity, expression lines, and photoaging.

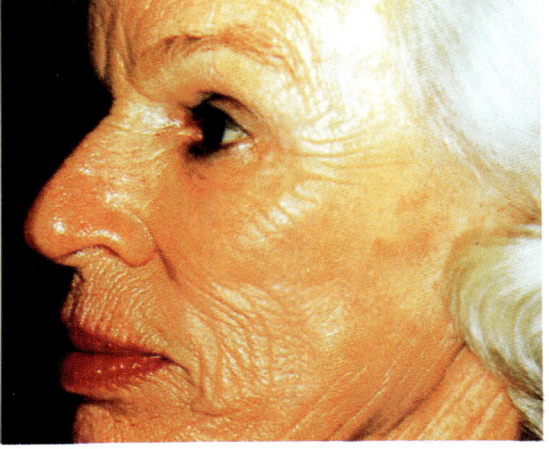

FIGURE 1.2. A side view of the patient presenting with all the factors of the aging face.

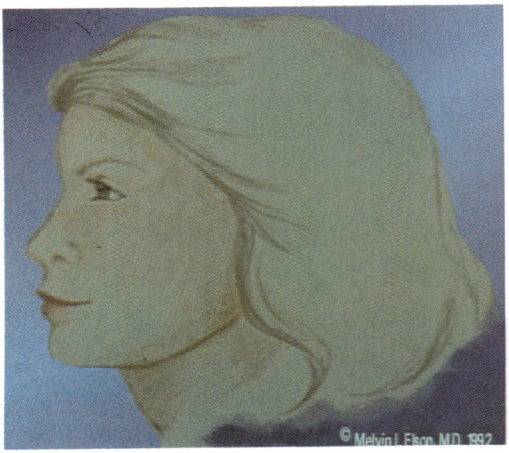

FIGURE 1.3. A computer image suggesting what the patient photographed in Figures 1.1 and 1.2 may have looked like at age 20.

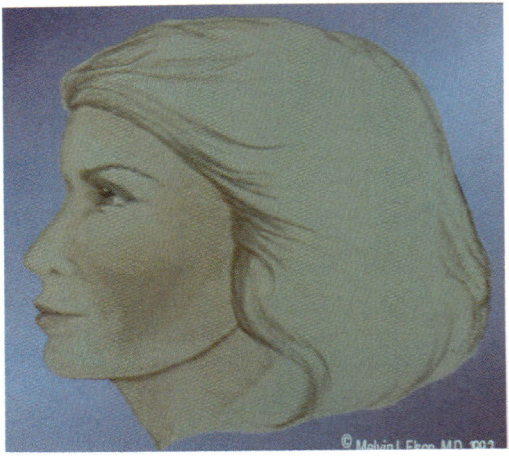

FIGURE 1.4. A computer image representing the intrinsic aging factor in the aging face.

Treatment for these individuals must be aimed at replacing the tissue that has been lost and, therefore, this is the area in which fat transplantation and solid implants play a significant role in the treatment of the aging face.[6]

Sleep lines etch the surface of the skin. They tend to be unilateral and cross other lines. Sleep lines occur from putting the face into the pillow or sheet in the same position every night, creating a crease, much as a crease occurs in a napkin laying in a drawer. Sleep lines tend to occur on the forehead in men and on the cheeks of women. As chronological age progresses, the lines, which are temporary in youth, become permanently ingrained, so that they do not recede during the day and are always present in older individuals.[7]

Treatment can be quite difficult, as attempts to change the sleep pattern are generally ineffective. "Sleep pillows," available from a number of sources, hold the patient's head in the position perpendicular to the bed, not allowing movement. This option obviously can make sleep quite difficult. The lines can be filled

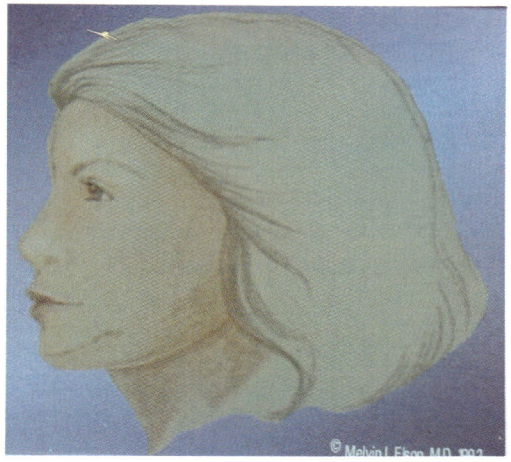

FIGURE 1.5. A computer image representing the sleep lines factor.

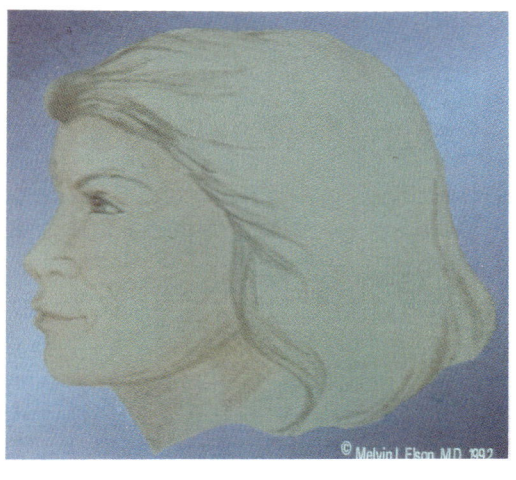

FIGURE 1.7. A computer image representing the expression lines factor.

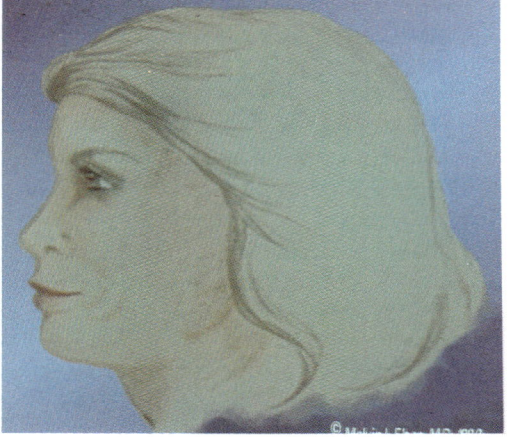

FIGURE 1.6. A computer image representing the gravity factor.

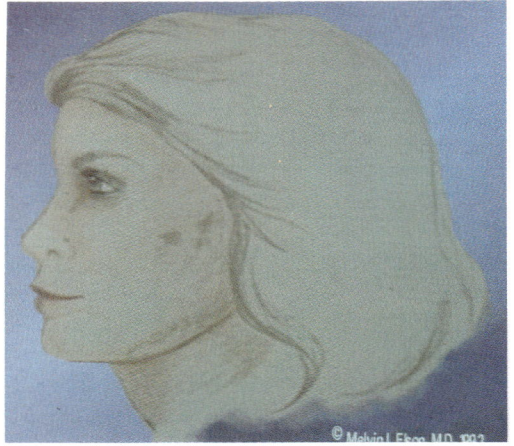

FIGURE 1.8. A computer image representing the photoaging factor.

with collagen injectable material or other fillers for temporary relief of the problem.

Gravity is a major factor in the production of what we call the aged face. It begins slowly to manifest itself as soon as an individual begins to stand and continues throughout life. One of the earliest visible manifestations is the downward turn of the angle of the mouth that occurs as early as age 7 or 8. The eyelids then begin to fall—both upper and lower—with the upper lids falling over the iris and pupil, to the point that vision may eventually be obstructed, especially in the lateral one-third of the visual fields.[8] The fat pads under the eyes move downward onto the cheeks, forming a hollow appearance and thinning the skin under the eyes. On occasion the opposite will occur in this area—that is, a puffiness may occur due to a decrease in the fascial and muscular support of the fatty deposits just under the eyes, allowing them to bulge and produce the puffiness.[9] In the area around the nose, a number of complicated interacting processes occur to decrease the support of the cartilage itself, allowing the tip of the nose to point downward.[10] Lateral to the nose, the nasolabial fold forms and the overhang of tissue occurs as the facial muscles move downward and centrally along with overlying subcutaneous fat and skin.

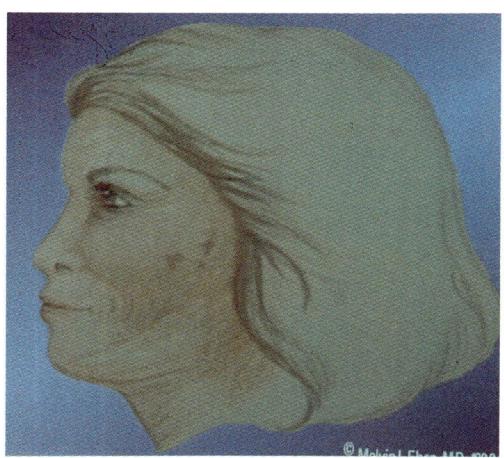

FIGURE 1.9. A computer image representing the presence of all five factors of the aging face.

The upper lip becomes smaller and loses its shape, flattening out and receding into the mouth.[11] The oral commissure beginning at the lateral edges of the lips and continuing down the chin is partially due to the pull of gravity and may have a significant overhang. With time and the pull of gravity, a groove forms in the midchin area as the mental process shifts and begins to point downward.[12] The mandibular line becomes obliterated as the skin and subcutaneous tissue hang over the mandible. The skin in this area continues to move downward and eventually forms the "turkey-neck" deformity, with loose, hanging skin. In addition, the ears elongate and become somewhat thinner over a period of time.[13]

Although many modalities of treatment may influence the gravity factor, this factor classically is treated by surgical methods—rhytidectomy, rhinoplasty, solid implants in the chin and upper cheek areas, upper and lower lid blepharoplasty, and otoplasty.

Injectable collagen may be used to lift the corners of the lip and decrease the harshness of the oral commissure.[14] This is certainly the treatment of choice to reshape and bring the upper lip back to its youthful shape and position.[15] Procedures have also recently been developed that allow augmentation around and under the eyes with collagen injectable material,[16] so this is another area where a modality other than surgery may influence the gravity factor.

Dermabrasion and medium to deep chemical peels, although not so effective for the gravity factor as for other factors, may have somewhat of a lifting effect in some patients.[17]

Expression lines occur because muscles pull on the collagen fibers of the skin in the same direction day after day, particularly around orifices of the face where muscle groups encircle—orbicularis oculi and orbicularis oris groups. In addition, the action of the frontalis muscle over the forehead produces horizontal lines and the procerus produces the glabellar fold.

The nasolabial fold is a complex structure where a number of muscular interactions occur from the masseter, to the orbicularis oris, to the other facial muscles. As mentioned previously, there is also a gravity component contributing to a deepening of the fold in the overhang.[18]

Accessory lines occur over the cheeks, running parallel to the nasolabial fold as more collagen fibers over the face are influenced by underlying muscle groups.

Lines extending from circular muscle groups—"crow's feet" around the orbicularis oculi and lip lines around the orbicularis oris—are particularly disconcerting, especially to female patients when lipstick "runs."

Although dermabrasion and chemical peeling may afford some benefit for this factor and rhytidectomy may temporarily improve the appearance, classically this factor is best treated with filling materials such as injectable collagen. Soft tissue augmentation is the treatment of choice for expression lines.[19]

A final factor accounts for most of what is referred to and is perceived as aging; this is, of course, *photoaging*. In addition to the effects of ultraviolet radiation to induce abnormal epidermal turnover, leading to actinic keratosis and squamous cell and basal cell carcinoma, there are a myriad of other effects on the epidermis, dermis, adnexal structures, and subcutaneous tissue related to the aging face.

Ultraviolet light, both UVA and UVB has certain effects on the skin to produce aging. These effects must be communicated to patients if any preventive program with regard to aging is to be effective. Ultraviolet light causes the disruption of the normal progression of epidermal cells from the basal layer to the stratum corneum.[20] In addition to the malignant potential, this creates an unevenness to the surface of the skin and contributes to the coarse dryness of the face as well as many of the benign overgrowths of the skin that appear with age.[21]

Cutaneous vessels break and collagen support for the vessels is decreased, leading to telangiectasia as well as spider veins. The collagen and elastic fibers are damaged, and there is decreased fibroblast activity, leading to fine wrinkling. In addition, melanocytes are overstimulated and, in some instances, obliterated, leading to a play on color over the face, with both increased and decreased color.[22]

There is also a decrease in the vascular network in the dermis and subcutaneous tissue, resulting in a yellow color to the skin as opposed to the pink glow of youthful skin.[23]

All these manifestations of photoaging—dryness, coarseness, fine wrinkling, broken vessels, overgrowths of the surface, play on color and texture, and yellowness—can be benefited simply by the daily use of sunscreen with a sun protection factor (SPF) of 15 to 25.[24]

In addition, topical tretinoin is an effective method of treatment of photoaging,[25] as are glycolic acid products and peels[26] and medium-depth chemical peeling[27] and dermabrasion.[28]

It is very helpful for the patient to understand how each of these factors is manifested in the face, how they interact with one another, and how the designed treatment program targets each of the factors to influence them individually to result in the overall improvement of this patient's particular aging face. For this reason it is best to draw out for the patient the areas that are influenced in his or her face, utilizing, for example, the model shown in Figure 1.10. A copy is given to the patient, and one is kept in her chart so that there is an understanding of what outline has been made and what suggestions have been given to the patient in terms of treatment.

Divisions of the Aging Face

Another method of evaluating the picture of the aging face is presented by Dzubow in *Cosmetic Surgery of the Skin*. It takes a slightly different approach, in that it looks at the three divisions of the face as they change with aging.

The face can be divided into equal thirds in the youthful face and, as the face ages, changes that occur within each third can be observed, and it can also be established how they interact with one another. As these changes occur, they are disproportionate and they disrupt the aesthetic perception, altering the equality between the upper, middle, and lower thirds of the face. In youth the upper third is from the hairline to the glabella, the middle third is from the glabella to the subnasal area, and the bottom third is from the subnasal area to the point of the chin.[29]

As previously mentioned, the frontalis muscle, the corrugator, and the procerus play major roles in changing the upper third of the face to produce the frowning and scowling lines in this area. In addition, if the hairline recedes, the perception of aging is going to be significantly increased, due to the picture that it presents to the observer's eye. The arched brow of the female, with its peak at a line tangential and vertical to the lateral limbus, begins to flatten, crow's feet appear from movement of the orbicularis oculi muscles, and atrophy occurs in the fat pad temporally, leading to the changes characteristic of the aged female brow.

In the middle third of the face, we are primarily concerned with the infraorbital region, the cheeks, the nose, and the eyelids. As mentioned earlier, both the upper and lower eyelids can become redundant and inelastic. Folds of redundant tissue occur, and the cheek compartment of the middle third of the face loses its volume as the buccal fat pad decreases with age. The nose enlarges both relative to the face and in actuality. There is also an enlargement of the sebaceous glands, altering the skin texture with age. The vertical height of the lower third of the face is often disproportionately decreased by bony absorption so that the middle portion of the face, with special emphasis on the nose, begins to appear both absolutely as well as relatively larger.

The most dramatic changes of the divisions occur in the lower third of the face, with height and volume loss as actual bony resorption occurs within the mandible, the maxilla, and the teeth. As the upper lip disappears and the chin begins to point downward, the nasolabial fold also forms and the face moves down

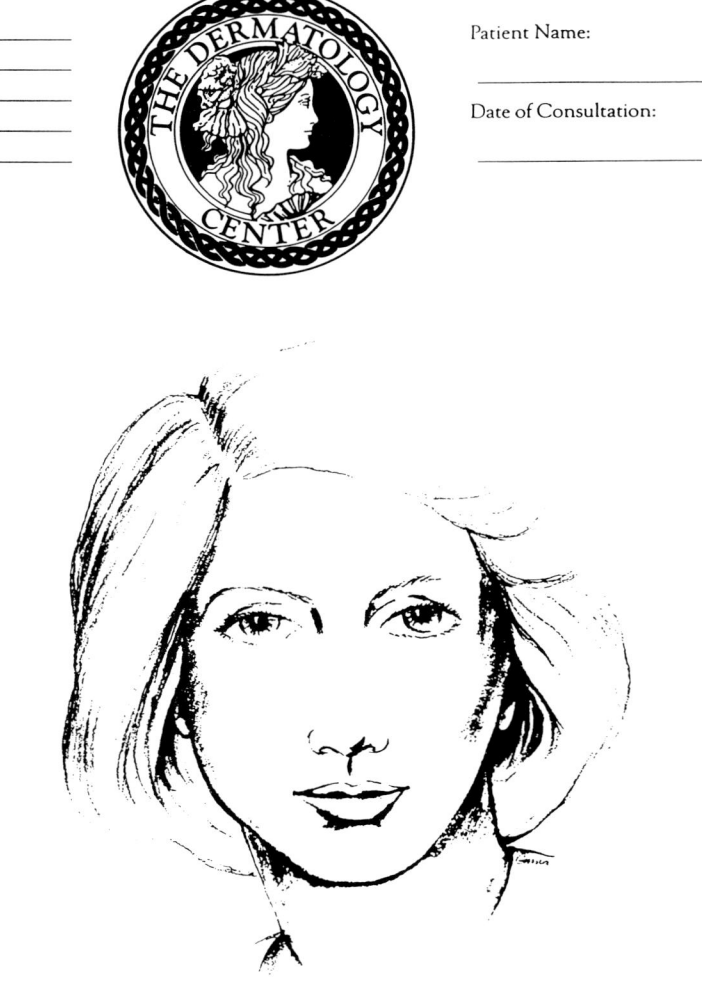

FIGURE 1.10. Worksheet for evaluation of the aging face.

toward the neck, giving a "turkey-gobbler" appearance. As aging continues the face loses height and the relative areas take on a disproportionate value, so rather than a ratio of 1.0:1.0:1.0 upper to lower, it becomes 1.3:1.1:0.6.[30]

Combining Factors and Divisions

When the five factors of the aging face as well as changes in the divisions of the face are taken into consideration, an objective method of evaluating both the patient and the effectiveness of treatment can be devised. Using a scale of 0–100, assigning value to each part of the aging face will develop a useful relative value scale.

Intrinsic aging with true loss of the submalar triangle is characteristic of the aged and, if present, must be significant; therefore, a value of 20 is assigned if there is atrophy of the submalar space.

Sleep lines play a small role in the picture of the aging face and can be quite variable, depending on many factors, such as sleep patterns and stress. Because of this they do not play a significant role in the picture. If present for part of the day, the value of 1 is assigned; presence for the whole day is a value of 2.

Assessment of the gravity factor is quite complicated and can be accomplished only by regarding both the factors and the divisions. Because of the major influence in both appearance of the aging face and available modalities for treatment, a value of 30–10 to each instead of third of the face capable of undergoing changes—is assigned.

The following factors can be present and are given corresponding value on the relative value scale:

Upper third

Greater than ⅓ of the measurement of the face	2
Flattened arch of the eyebrow	2
Lateral displacement of upper lids	3
Visual field disturbance	3

Middle third

Lower displacement of the lower lids	2
Occupying more than ⅓ of the face	1
Angle of the tip of the nose less than 90° from the face	3
Thinning of the malar eminences	2
Elongation of the ears	.5
Nasolabial fold overhangs	1.5

Lower third

Obliteration of the mandibular line	3
Chin points downward	1
Upper lip thin and flat	2
Oral commissure overhangs	2
Groove in the chin	1
Ratio less than 1.0:1.0:1.0 but less than 0.2 difference 1.0:1.0:1.0	1
Ratio less than 1.0:1.0:1.0 but greater than 0.2 difference	1

Expression lines receive an assignment in the relative value scale as follows:

Forehead lines	2
Glabellar line	1
Glabellar fold	2
Crow's feet	1
Deep crow's feet	1
Nasolabial line	2
Nasolabial fold	3
Oral commissure	3
Lip lines vertical to the lip	3
Accessory lines	4
Lower lid lines	1

Photoaging receives a relative value scale of 25:

Dry, coarse skin	4
Lentigines	4
Fine lines	3
Purpura	4
Yellowness to the skin	2
Telangiectasia	1
Enlarged pores	1
Broken vessels	2
Thin skin	4

Table 1.1—an example of three patients presenting for evaluation—reveals how useful the scale may be as an objective assessment for both the physician and the patient. See Figures 16.1, 16.2, and 16.3 for these patients.

Summary

The goal of the dermatologist and dermatologic cosmetic surgeon in treating the picture of aging is to reestablish the youthful appearance of the face, in which only the eyes and lips are visible on a clear, smooth background. Anything that detracts from emphasis on the eyes and lips—skin hanging out of the frame, unevenness to the background (sun damage), unattractive lines and folds (expression lines)—produces a picture of aging. Restoration of the face produces the illusion that only the eyes and lips are visible. Modern dermatology and dermatologic surgery can provide the physician with the necessary tools and ingredients to accomplish this goal.

TABLE 1.1. Relative value scale evaluations of three patients.

	Patient #1 (Figure 16.1)	Patient #2 (Figure 16.3)	Patient #3 (Figure 16.2)
Intrinsic aging	0	0	0
Sleep lines	2	0	2
Upper third	5	0	5
Middle third	7.5	2	6.5
Lower third	8	6	11
Expression lines	21	17	19
Photoaging	11	15	21
	54.5	40	64.5

References

1. Elson ML. Evaluation and treatment of the aging face. Cosmet Dermatol. 1990;6:11–14.
2. Dzubow L. The aging face. In: *Cosmetic Surgery of the Skin,* W Coleman, CW Hanke, T Alt, S Asken, eds. SC Daber, Inc., Philadelphia, 1991, pp. 1–10.
3. Ganske MG. Take 2 to 10 years off your face. Longevity. 1991;62–66.
4. Dubin B, Jackson IT, Hamlin A, et al. Anatomy of the buccal fat pad and its clinical significance. Plast Reconstr Surg. 1989;83:257–262.
5. Fenske NA, Lober CW. Structural and functional changes of normal aging skin. J Am Acad Dermatol. 1986;15:571–585.
6. Illouz YG. The fat cell "graft": a new technique to fill depressions. Plast Reconstr Surg. 1986;78:122.
7. Stegman SJ. Sleep creases. Am J Cosmet Surg. 1987;4:277.
8. Rees TD. Patient selection and techniques in blepharoplasty and rhytidoplasty. Surg Clin North Am. 1971; 51:22.
9. Castanares S. Correction of the baggy eyelids deformity produced by herniation of orbital fat. In: Proceedings of the 2nd International Symposium on Plastic and Reconstructive Surgery of the Eye and Adnexa, F Smith, JM Converse, eds. CV Mosley, St. Louis, 1967 (paps).
10. Johnson CM, Anderson JR. Nose-life operations. Arch Otolaryngol. 1978;104:1–3.
11. Fanous N. Aging lips. Fac Plast Surg. 1987;4:179–183.
12. Ellis DAF, Pelausa EO. Cosmetic evaluation of the lower third of the face. Fac Plast Surg. 1987;4:159–164.
13. Gonzalez-Ulloa M, Flores ES. Senility of the face—basic study to understand its causes and effects. Plast Reconstr Surg. 1965;36:239–246.
14. Elson ML. Clinical assessment of Zyplast implant: a year of experience for soft tissue contour correction. J Am Acad Dermatol. 1988; 18:707–713.
15. Elson ML. Techniques for lip augmentation discussed. Cosmet Dermatol. 1990; 3.(11):16–19.
16. Elson ML. Soft tissue augmentation of peri orbital fine lines and the orbital groove with Zyderm-I and fine-gauge needles. J Dermatol Surg Oncol. 1992; 18:779–782.
17. Yarborough JM Jr, Beeson WH. Dermabrasion. In: *Aesthetic Surgery of the Aging Face*, WH Beeson, EG McCollough, eds. CV Mosley, St. Louis, 1986, pp. 142–151.
18. Rubin LR, Mishriki Y, Lee G. Anatomy of the nasolabial fold: the keystone of the smiling mechanism. Plast Reconstr Surg. 1989;83:1–8.
19. Elson ML. Soft tissue augmentation: a review of available materials. Cosmet Dermatol. 1991; 4(1):10.
20. Kligman AM, Lavker RU. Cutaneous aging: the differences between intrinsic aging and photoaging. J Cutan Aging Cosmet Dermatol. 1988; 1:5–12.
21. Tindall JP, Palmore F. Skin conditions and lesions in the aged: a longitudinal study. In: *Normal Aging II*. Duke University Press, Durham, 1974, pp. 18–23.
22. Kligman L. Photoaging. Dermatol Clin. 1986; 4:517–528.
23. Montagna W, Carlisle K. Structural changes in aging human skin. J Inter Dermatol. 1979; 73:47–53.
24. Kligman LH, Akin FJ, Kligman AM. Suncreeens promote repair of ultraviolet radiation-induced dermal damage. J Inter Dermatol. 1983; 81:98–102.
25. Weiss J, Ellis CN, Headington JT, et al. Topical tretinoin improves photoaged skin: a double-blind vehicle controlled study. JAMA. 1988; 259:527–532.
26. Elson ML. The utilization of glycolic acid in photoaging. Cosmet Dermatol. 1992; 1:12–15.
27. Resnick SS. Chemical peeling with trichloracetic acid. J Dermatol Surg Oncol. 1984; 10: 549–550.
28. Tromovitch TE, Stegman SJ, Glogau R. *Basic Dermatologic Surgery*. Yearbook Medical Publishers, Chicago, 1984.
29. Powell N, Humphreys B. *Proportions of the Aesthetic Face*. Thieme-Stratton, New York, 1984.
30. Kaye BL. *Facial Rejuvenative Surgery*. J.B. Lippincott, Philadelphia, 1987.

2
Sunscreen: Prevention of Aging and Skin Cancer

Darrell S. Rigel

The sun provides energy for all living things on Earth. Yet along with these beneficial effects are significant negative events that may result from excessive sun exposure.

In terms of the integument, it is the ultraviolet band of the irradiance spectrum that appears to provide the greatest degree of destruction. Sun protection is therefore designed to protect the skin from the damage that occurs as a result of ultraviolet exposure.

Unprotected ultraviolet exposure leads to two significant areas of skin problems. Of primary importance is the increased risk of developing skin cancer. At current rates 1 in 6 Americans will develop a skin cancer of some sort during his or her lifetime, with more than 700,000 new cases appearing this year. The incidence of malignant melanoma, the most dangerous type of skin cancer, is increasing faster than any other cancer in the United States.[1] In 1935 the lifetime risk for an American of developing melanoma was 1 in 1,500. At current rates this risk is now 105 and is projected to increase to 1 in 75 by the year 2000. In addition, according to the World Health Organization, melanoma is increasing faster than any other malignancy worldwide.[2] Health care costs associated with the treatment of these skin cancers are more than $100 million in the United States alone. Therefore, effective mechanisms that protect the skin from skin cancer-causing UV rays are critical.

Other demographic issues have underscored the importance of effective sun protection. As the population ages, the magnitude of the problems associated with skin aging also increase. Ultraviolet rays are also associated with damage to skin texture and tone, changes that commonly are attributable to aging. Increased population aging concerns also contribute to the importance of methods that "slow" the external aging process.

History of Sun Protection

Since the majority of persons will experience at least one painful sunburn, the importance of sun protection usually has been behaviorally reinforced early in life. The importance of sun protection has also been recognized since earliest times. Ancient Egyptian art depicts persons wearing long robes and sitting in the shade of trees.

Yet it was not until the 1950s that "suntan lotions" came into usage. Their purpose was to help people tan without burning. In the early 1970s, the first true sunscreen, para-amino benzoic acid (PABA), became generally available. However, high-intensity sunscreens have been marketed only over the last decade.

Sunblocks

Sunblocks physically block the sun's ultraviolet radiation to the skin. Protective clothing, umbrellas, and trees are considered sunblocks. Sunblocks can also be in opaque forms and applied to the skin. When used in a topically

TABLE 2.1. Most commonly used sunblock agents.[3]

Zinc oxide
Talc
Titanium dioxide
Red vetenary petrolatum

applied form, these agents scatter, reflect, and primarily block ultraviolet light. They are partially effective for patients who have diseases related to light exposure, including lupus erythematous, polymorphous light eruption, xeroderma pigmentosum, and solar urticaria.[3] Sunblocks are also useful in persons spending extensive periods of time outdoors (golfers, tennis players, lifeguards, etc.) and to protect sensitive areas such as the nose, ears, and cheeks.

The most commonly used sunblock agents are listed in Table 2.1. Most topical sunblocks contain combinations of a subset of this list. The most commonly used individual agent is zinc oxide.

Certain disadvantages exist with the use of topical physical sunblocks. They tend to be messy and can stain clothing and fiberglass recreational equipment. In order to increase their cosmetic and social acceptability, newer sunblocks with "designer" coloring are now being distributed.

Sunscreens

As mentioned earlier, para-amino benzoic acid has been used in sunscreens in the United States since the early 1970s. One of the characteristics of PABA that makes it so effective as a sunscreen is its ability to bind to epidermal cells. This tends to make PABA-based sunscreens fairly water- and perspiration-resistant, but it also makes them prone to staining.[4] PABA tends to block UV radiation most effectively in the UVB zone (290–320 nm).

The PABA esters, padimate A, padimate O, and glyceryl PABA, have the absorption characteristics of PABA but the additional advantage of staining only rarely. Therefore, most current PABA-containing sunscreens use the PABA esters.

PABA, however, has a major disadvantage over other sunscreen components: There is a much higher presence of contact and photocontact allergy to PABA than to other sunscreen agents.[5,6] Among PABA-based chemicals, padimate A is often chosen for use in sunscreen compounds, due to the PABA esters' lower allergic incidence.[3] However, sunscreens with PABA esters may contain 0.2% to 4.5% PABA.[7] This may account for the many allergic reactions seen with these agents.

Benzophenones

Benzophenones are the second most commonly found component of sunscreens. Although their primary protective range is found in the UVA range (320–400 nm), a secondary protective band is noted in the UVB zone. Benzophenones were originally used alone as a PABA-free sunscreen alternative but are now combined with other sunscreen agents to provide broad spectrum coverage.

The most commonly used benzophenone agents are oxybenzone and dioxybenzone. These ingredients are much less allergenic than PABA and do not stain. However, the benzophenones are less water-resistant than PABA. Therefore, the bases that are used in benzophenone-containing sunscreens must be thicker and less cosmetically acceptable.[3]

Cinnamates

Cinnamates, a derivative of cinnamon, are also good protectors from the sun. These products are chemically related to balsam of Peru, tolu balsam, coca leaves, cinnamic aldehyde, and cinnamic oil.[8] Therefore, persons with sensitivity to these items may cross-react to sunscreens containing cinnamates.

The most commonly used cinnamates are octyl methoxycinnamate and cinnoxate. They are nonstaining but also have poor water-resistant qualities. Therefore, cinnamate products may require more frequent reapplication and/or special substantive bases.

Salicylates/Anthranilates

Salicylates are among the original sunscreen chemicals. Homomenthyl salicylate absorbs primarily in the UVB range and is typically added to other components to increase sun protection factor.[3] Octyl and triethanolamine salicylates are also used. They may cause photocontact dermatitis more frequently than homomenthyl salicylate and are therefore used less frequently.

Anthranilates, such as menthyl anthranilate, with low-level broad spectrum coverage, are also added to many sunscreens to augment protection.

Dibenzoylmethanes

Recent concerns over the effects of UVA radiation on the skin have demonstrated the need for better UVA protection in sunscreens. The newest ingredients that have been shown to have the best UVA protection are the dibenzoylmethanes.[9] Because they offer no protection from UVB rays, they must be used in combination with other ingredients.

Tert-butylmethoxydibenzoylmethane (Avobenzone, Parsol 1789) is approved for use in the United States. Its range of coverage is 310–400 nm with a peak effectiveness at 358 nm.[5] A second member of this family, isopropyldibenzoylmethane (Eusolex 8020), has been used in Europe for several years. Because of the high incidence of contact dermatitis reactions associated with its use, it has not been approved for incorporation into sunscreens in the United States.[10]

Sun Protection Factors

The effectiveness of a sunscreen is measured by the use of the sun protection factor system. SPF is the ratio of the amount of time that a person exposed to the sun takes to sunburn while wearing a sunscreen as compared to the time required to sunburn without protection.[11] Initial sunscreens, in the 1970s, had SPFs of 2 to 4. However, these sunscreens provided protection only from 50% to 75% of the UVB rays. Current high-potency sunscreens have SPFs ranging from 15 to 50, protecting from more than 95% of UVB (see Figure 2.1).

Several significant problems exist with the SPF system. First, SPFs measure only UVB protection. In natural sunlight on a summer day at noon, approximately 10% of the UV energy striking the skin is in the UVA band. In general, because UVA has so much less energy, it would take an impractical amount of time to test an SPF for UVA in a manner similar to UVB. Since 1979 the Food and Drug Administration has explored different methods for measuring the effectiveness of UVA protection that a sunscreen provides. It is hoped that there will be a resolution of this problem in the near future.[11]

Second, the SPF of a sunscreen is measured under ideal, controlled conditions. The true effectiveness of a sunscreen is a function of its usage. On average it takes approximately 1 ounce of sunscreen to cover the entire body.

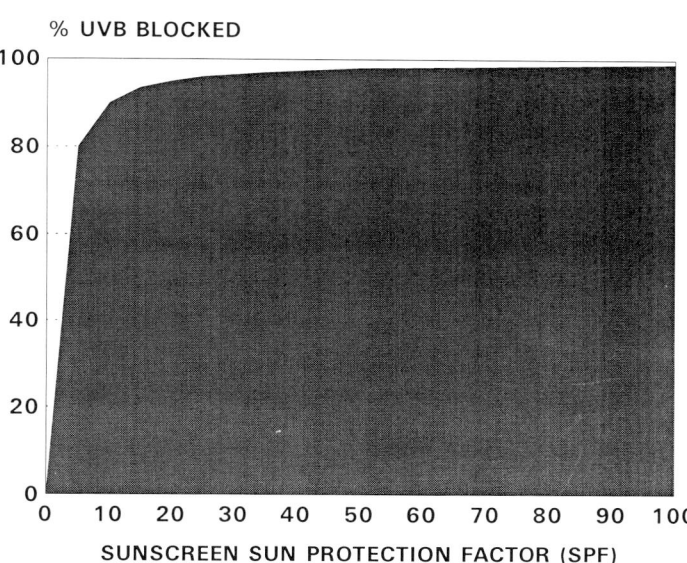

FIGURE 2.1. The percentage of UVB blocked by currently available sunscreens representing a variety of SPFs.

Using less than this amount results in lowering the true SPF.[12] Sunscreens take about 15 to 20 minutes from the time of application until they become effective. Therefore, they should be applied *prior* to the time that they are needed.

Also, depending on some sunscreen components and bases, some mixtures may be more resistant to water. The term *water-resistant* is defined as the sunscreen's having the same SPF after a person has been immersed in water for 40 minutes as it did initially. *Waterproof* is similar, except no degradation of protection is present at 80 minutes. Sunscreens with less substantivity (water resistance) may need to be reapplied more frequently to maintain their predicted SPF level of protection.[13]

A debate exists as to the value of additional protection provided by sunscreens with SPFs higher than 15. In a controlled environment, the marginal protection provided by these high SPF sunscreens is only 2% to 4%. However, since most persons underapply sunscreens, the higher-SPF sunscreens have a margin of safety, hopefully giving the user at least an SPF 15 level of protection.

Recent studies have shown that higher-SPF sunscreens may provide more effective protection than those with SPFs of 15. Cesarini et al.[14] described the first occurrence where there were fewer sunburn cells (markers for acute sun damage) in fair-skinned individuals using sunscreens with greater than 15 SPF. These sunburn cells are regarded as markers for UV radiation-induced damage to DNA. Since altered DNA is thought to be the effector of photocarcinogenesis, it was hypothesized that higher-SPF sunscreens offered better protection from skin cancer.[15] Further studies are needed to verify the clinical relevance of these findings (see Table 2.2). Nevertheless, SPF > 15 sunscreens can be recommended for persons with type I skin, with a personal or family history of skin cancer, or who will not adequately apply sunscreen. A list of commonly used sunscreens, their SPFs, and their components is presented in Table 2.3.

Vehicles

One of the most common objections to sunscreen usage is lack of cosmetic acceptability of the product.[8] The ingredients used to formulate sunscreen vehicles include mineral oil, petrolatum, isopropyl esters, lanolin, aliphatic alcohols, triglycerides, fatty acids, waxes, propylene glycol, emulsifiers, thickeners, preservatives, and fragrance.[5] A sunscreen acceptable to one person or for use in a given area of the body may not be acceptable for others. Oil-based sunscreens may be comedogenic.[16] Recently, water- and perspiration-resistant formulations with SPF 15 or greater that do not sting upon eye contact have been developed for athletes (for example, Coppertone Sport, Plough, Memphis, and TN). The development of better vehicles in the future may help to enhance sunscreen usage.

Protection from Immunologic Effects of UV Radiation

UV radiation to the skin results in various forms of local and systemic immune suppres-

TABLE 2.2. Common sunscreens and their UV protective wavelengths.

Sunscreen	Range of protection (nm)	Maximal effect of protection (nm)
PABA and PABA esters		
PABA	260–313	283
Padimate O	290–315	311
Padimate A	290–315	309
Glycerol aminobenzoate	260–313	297
Cinnamates		
Octyl methoxycinnamate	280–310	311
Cinnoxate	270–328	290
Salicylates		
Homosalicylate	290–315	306
Octyl salicylate	260–310	307
Triethanolamine salicylate	269–320	298
Octocrylene	287–323	303
Etocrylene	296–383	303
Benzophenones		
Oxybenzone	270–350	290, 325
Dioxybenzone	206–380	284, 327
Sulisobenzone	250–380	286–324
Menthylanthranilate	200–380	336
Dibenzoylmethanes		
Tert-butylmethoxy-dibenzoylmethane (Parsol)	310–400	358
4-isopropyldibenzoyl-methane (Eusolex)	310–400	345

Adapted from O'Donoghue.[3]

TABLE 2.3. Selected sunscreen formulations available in the United States.[5]

Trade name	SPF	Active ingredients
Four sunscreening ingredients		
Coppertone (Plough)	30	Padimate O, Parsol MCX, octyl salicylate, oxybenzone
Sundown (Johnson & Johnson)	30	Parsol MCX, octyl salicylate, oxybenzone, titanium dioxide
	20	Padimate O, Parsol MCX, octyl salicylate, oxybenzone
Cancer Garde (Eclipse Labs)	30	Padimate O, Parsol MCX, oxybenzone, titanium dioxide
T/I Screen (T/I Pharmaceuticals)	30+	Parsol MCX, octocrylene, octyl salicylate, oxybenzone
Block Out (Carter Products)	30	Parsol MCX, padimate O, octyl salicylate, oxybenzone
Supershade (Plough)	44	Parsol MCX, padimate O, homosalate, oxybenzone
Three sunscreening ingredients		
Solbar (Person and Covey)	50	Parsol MCX, octocrylene, oxybenzone
PreSun for Kids (Westwood)	39	Parsol MCX, octyl salicylate, oxybenzone
PreSun 29	29	Parsol MCX, octyl salicylate, oxybenzone
Bain de Soleil (Bain de Soleil)	30	Padimate O, Parsol MCX, oxybenzone
Ultrashade (Plough)	23	Padimate O, Parsol MCX, oxybenzone
Total Eclipse (Eclipse Labs)	15	Padimate O, octyl salicylate, oxybenzone
Sundown (Johnson & Johnson)	15	Padimate O, Parsol MCX, oxybenzone
Two sunscreening ingredients		
Supershade (Plough)	8, 15	Parsol MCX, oxybenzone
Coppertone (Plough)	4, 6, 8, 15	Padimate O, oxybenzone
Shade (Plough)	4, 6	Padimate O, oxybenzone
PreSun (Westwood)	8, 15	Padimate O, oxybenzone
Water Babies (Plough)		15 Parsol MCX, oxybenzone
Sundown (Johnson & Johnson)	4, 6, 8	Padimate O, oxybenzone
Block Out (Carter Products)	15	Padimate O, oxybenzone
Photoplex (Herbert Labs)	15+	Padimate O, avobenzone
One sunscreening ingredient		
Coppertone (Plough)	2	Octyl salicylate
Bain de Soleil (Bain de Soleil)	2, 4	Padimate O
Eclipse (Eclipse Labs)	5	Padimate O
Eclipse (Eclipse Labs)	10	Glyceryl PABA

sion. Release of preinflammatory cytokines (IL-1, IL-6, TNF) and prostaglandins are inhibited. Langerhans cells in the skin are depleted and inactivated. Autoimmune diseases, such as systemic lupus erythematous, can be activated. Similar activations of herpes virus eruption are noted. Allergic contact dermatitis can be suppressed. In addition, in mice, skin cancer surveillance and rejection mechanisms are suppressed.[17]

Can sunscreen prevent UV-induced immunologic damage? Clinically, sunscreens appear to reduce outbreaks of perioral herpes simplex. In 15 studies conducted from 1981 through 1992, 5 showed no protection, 17 showed partial protection, and 3 demonstrated complete protection from general immune damage. Further studies will be needed to better understand the relationship between sunscreens and immunologic response.

Sunscreen "Reactions"

Many types of sunscreen reactions have been reported. People often complain of a reaction to a specific sunscreen and subsequently will not use the product. These types of reactions include allergic contact dermatitis, photoallergic contact dermatitis, irritant dermatitis, acne, and aesthetic issues.

Because sunscreens are applied topically to the skin frequently and in relatively high concentrations (up to 26%),[5] contact sensitization can occur. Since the active agents in sunscreens absorb radiation, they also have the potential to cause photosensitization. Both types of reactions can occur not only from the sunscreen agents themselves but also from components of the vehicles. The most common offending agents in vehicles and preservatives are found in Table 2.4.

PABA is sunscreen agent that most commonly causes an allergic reaction. It has been estimated that 3% to 7% of the U.S. population are PABA-sensitive. Both contact and photoallergic reactions have been reported.[6] Benzophenone sensitization has been estimated at 1% to 2%.[18] Other sunscreen agents also can cause contact reactions.

By far the most common sunscreen reaction is due to "sensitive" skin. It is estimated that up to 1 in 3 persons using sunscreens will at some time complain about sunscreens irritating his or her skin. Complaints include subjective signs, such as stinging, burning, and itching; as well as objective findings, such as urticaria, acnegenicity and pustule formation.[5] The most effective method for alleviating these findings is to choose an alternative sunscreen from a different chemical family or with a different base.

True sunscreen reactions need to be both patch and photopatch tested to determine whether the reaction is merely allergic or if it is light-related. Use of too low a concentration of the testing materials may result in a false negative result.[5]

Future Trends

Many other substances are currently being investigated for their potential as sunscreens. Psoralen derivatives that enhance the production of melanin are being studied. Natural substances, including derivatives of coral from Australia's Great Barrier Reef, have shown some early promise. Ultimately, oral preparations with appropriate concentration delivery to the skin to make the sunscreen effective will be developed.

Summary

The usage of sunscreens has grown dramatically worldwide over the past decade. Except for total sun avoidance, sunscreens remain the best method of protection from UV-induced damage to the skin: aging and skin cancer.

References

1. Friedman RJ, Rigel DS, Kopf AW, et al. Malignant melanoma in the 1990s: the continued importance of early detection and the role of physician examination and self-examination of the skin. CA 1991, 41:201–226.
2. Koh H, et al. MMWR, CDC Atlanta, February 1991.
3. O'Donoghue MN. Sunscreen: one weapon against melanoma. Dermatol Clin. 1991; 9:789–793.
4. Willis I. Sensitization potential of para-aminobenzoic acid. Cosmet Toilet. 1976; 91:63.
5. Dromgoole SH, Maibach HI. Contact sensitization and photocontact sensitization of sunscreening agents. In: *Sunscreens: Development, Evaluation and Regulatory Aspects*, NJ Lowe, NA Shaath, eds. Marcel Derker, New York, 1991.
6. Wennerstein G, Thone P, Broathagen H, et al. The Scandinavian multicenter photopatch study: preliminary results. Contact Dermatit. 1984; 10:305–309.
7. Bruze M, Fregert S, Gruvberger B. Occurence of para-aminobenzoic acid and benzocaine as contaminants in sunscreen agents. Photodermatology. 1988; 5:162.

TABLE 2.4. Vehicles and preservatives that can cause contact or photocontact dermatitis.[5]

Avocado oil
t-butyl alcohol
Methyl parabens
Phenyldimethicone
Solvent red 1
Solvent red 3
Triethanolamine stearate
Benzyl alcohol
Cetylstearyl alcohol
Sorbitan sesquiolate
Imidazolidinyl urea (Germall 115)
Methylisothiazolin one/methylchloroisothiazolin one (Kathon CG)
Glyceryl monostearate
6-Acetoxy-2, 4-dimethyl-m-dioxane
Carbowaxes
Ethyl alcohol
Glycerol
Isopropyl alcohol
Isopropyl myristate
Petrolatum
Stearyl alcohol

8. Dromgoogle SH, Maibach HI. Sunscreening agent intolerance: contact and photocontact sensitization and contact urticaria. J Am Acad Dermatol. 1990; 22:1068–1078.
9. Gange RW, Sproker A, Matzinger E, et al. Efficacy of a sunscreen containing butyl methoxydibenzoylmethane against ultraviolet A radiation in photosensitized subjects. J Am Acad Dermatol. 1986; 15:494–499.
10. Roberts DL. Contact allergy to Eusolex 8021. Contact Dermatit. 1989; 20:74.
11. Kaidbey K, Gange, RW. Comparison of methods for assessing photoprotection against ultraviolet A in vivo. J Am Acad Dermatol. 1987; 16:346–353.
12. Taylor CR, Stern RS, Leyden JJ, et al. Photoaging/photodamage and photoprotection. J Am Acad Dermatol. 1990; 22:1–15.
13. Leroy C, Dompmartin A. Sunscreen substantivity: comparison between water and sweat resistance tests. Photodermatolrogy. 1988; 5:49–50.
14. Cesarini JP, Chardon A, Binet O, et al. High-protection sunscreen formulation prevents UVB-induced sunburn cell formulation. Photodermatology. 1989; 6:20–23.
15. Kaidbey KH. The photoprotection potential of the new superpotent sunscreens. J Am Acad Dermatol. 1990; 22:449–452.
16. Mills OH, Kligman AM. Comedogenicity of sunscreens. Arch Dermatol. 1982; 118:417–419.
17. Gurish MF, Robert LK, Kruegen GC, et al. The effects of various sunscreen agents on skin damage and their induction of tumor susceptability in mice subjected to ultraviolet radiation. J Invest Dermatol. 1981; 76:246–251.
18. Knobler E, Almeida L, Ruzkowski AM, et al. Photoallergy to benzophenone. Arch Dermatol. 1989; 125:801–804.

3
Topical Tretinoin Can Correct the Structural Abnormalities of Human Photoaged Skin

Albert M. Kligman

Retinoids have revolutionized medical practice, especially in dermatologic disorders. A multitude of publications have demonstrated that retinoids have an extraordinary diversity of biologic effects. These include regulation of epidermal differentiation,[1] increased synthesis of collagen,[2] inhibition of tumor promotion,[3] therapeutic antitumor effects on a variety of epithelial neoplasms,[4-7] membrane integrity,[7] and enhanced healing of cutaneous wounds.[8]

Basic scientists are expanding knowledge at a stunning rate, uncovering novel biologic effects in a great variety of in vivo and in vitro systems.[9] Topical and systemic retinoids have brought about dramatic therapeutic benefits in a variety of dermatologic disorders, particularly those related to abnormalities in epidermal proliferation and differentiation.[10]

The introduction of corticosteroids at midcentury marked the first great revolution in the therapy of chronic dermatoses. The introduction of topical tretinoin for the treatment of acne vulgaris more than 25 years ago inaugurated the second revolution.[11] The ability of tretinoin to prevent horny cells from sticking together to form impactions (comedones) explains its therapeutic efficacy. In addition, tretinoin has some poorly characterized antiinflammatory action. Recently, it has been demonstrated that topical tretinoin can partially reverse the skin damage induced by excessive exposure to sunlight.[12]

It has been shown beyond doubt that ultraviolet radiation is the principal cause of the appearance of premature aging, with its baleful portfolio of unattractive alterations, viz, wrinkles, blotches, excrescences, yellowing, and rough, uneven texture. The term *photoaging* refers to those changes that occur in sun-exposed skin (*extrinsic aging*).[13] The aging changes that occur in protected skin are much less drastic and are termed *intrinsic aging,* which is doubtless genetically programmed.

Features of Photoaged Skin

All the structural components of skin are damaged by chronic exposure to the sun. The clinical manifestations are numerous and varied. These include a dry, scaly surface; various irregularities in pigmentation (mottling, blotchiness); wrinkles (fine lines, deep furrows, creases); sagging, loose skin from loss of elasticity; telangiectasias; and various benign and premalignant neoplasms. Actinically damaged skin has a rough, leathery texture whose unsightliness is worsened by a yellowish, pebbly coarseness.[14]

These signs of photoaging are most likely to become manifest by early adulthood in so-called type I, Celtic persons who show the following phenotype: pale, thin-skinned, blue-eyed blondes and redheads with childhood freckles. These persons burn and blister easily and tan poorly. Although the visible signs of photoaging may not appear for many years, microscopically, there may be striking damage in the dermis by age 15. Thus, the damage is hidden, allowing the victim to continue heedless exposure and making it exceedingly difficult to educate the public regarding the hazards of sunlight exposure. In contrast to caucasians, darker-skinned persons experience photoaging at a slower rate but are certainly not immune to the harmful effects of prolonged sunlight exposure.

Even in clinically normal, smooth-skinned adolescents, biopsies show dramatic histological derangements. The dermal matrix is strongly affected. An early development is hyperplasia of elastic fibers, which become thickened, curled, and branched, resulting many years later in massive accumulations of degenerated, elastotic material.[15] Ultrastructurally, the elastic fibers show early on a moth-eaten appearance due to many electron-lucent areas.[16] Much later the elastin matrix disappears, leaving a tangled mass of microfilaments. Under low-power microscopic scanning, there is a striking increase in abnormal elastic tissue, ending in the complete disorganization known as *elastosis*. Accompanying this process is a continuous loss of collagen, the main source of the tensile strength of skin. Hence, the fibrous network disintegrates, resulting in loose, hanging skin that does not rebound after being stretched.

The third component of the dermal matrix is the ground substance, made up mainly of glycosaminoglycans (GAGs) and proteoglycans. These are hygroscopic substances that keep the matrix supple and allow fibers to slide over one another during movement. Ground substance is abundant in fetal skin, decreasing with age and remaining low throughout adulthood. However, the quantity of GAGs increases markedly in photoaged skin, resulting in huge accumulations. It is not known whether or not these are normal GAGs.

Fibroblasts, especially in the upper dermis, are also affected by chronic sun exposure. As photodamage evolves they become more numerous, larger, and apparently more metabolically active, showing hypertrophy of the endoplasmic reticulum.[17] At a later and final stage of severe elastosis, the dermis becomes relatively acellular. Macrophages, mast cells, and endothelial cells diminish greatly.

A constant factor during development of photodamage is a perivascular histiocyte-lymphocytic infiltrate containing a conspicuous admixture of mast cells, often in close proximity to fibroblasts.[17] We have termed this *chronic heliodermatitis*. The ruddy skin of farmers and sailors is a prime example of heliodermatitis. We postulated that various enzymes, especially proteases (elastase and collagenase), produced by macrophages and mast cells lead to the dissolution of the fibrous network.

Other changes in severely photodamaged skin include an irregular thickening of the stratum corneum, a flattening of the dermoepidermal junction, and a retention of melanin granules in basal keratinocytes.[18] The cells of the epidermis show a great many distinctive abnormalities, including keratinocytes, that are irregular in size, shape, and staining properties, with many shrunken, dying cells, called *atypia* by pathologists. Disarray, loss of polarity, and abnormal differentiation are termed *dysplasia*. The microvasculature is also drastically damaged by sun exposure. Deeper venules become dilated and tortuous, seen on the surface as telangiectasis. Eventually, the horizontal superficial plexus of small vessels becomes sparse and irregular. Lymphatic vessels also regress. Finally, neoplastic growths—benign, premalignant, and malignant—flourish in photoaged skin. The growths that are common in this terrain are seborrheic and actinic keratoses, solar lentigines, keratoacanthomas, basal cell epitheliomas, squamous cell carcinomas, and lentigo malignant melanoma.

By comparison intrinsic or chronological aging is in many respects the opposite of photoaging. There are few structural alterations until after about age 50. Thereafter regressive changes occur slowly, noticeable in all patients over age 70 as thin, dry, wrinkled, pale skin. Knowledge of the changes that take place in intrinsic aging derives from the histological study of protected skin, such as that of the upper inner arm, which never shows dermatoheliosis.[18] The process is essentially one of general atrophy without the extraordinary heterogeneity and disorder seen in photoaged skin. Cellular depletion properly describes the dominant change.

Efficacy of Tretinoin in Photoaged Skin

The beneficial effects of tretinoin have become evident by comparing it with the nonmedicated vehicle. Clinical and histologic studies have demonstrated the capacity of tretinoin to reverse partially photodamaged facial and dorsal forearm skin.

Our laboratory has had extensive clinical experience in treating the facial skin of more than 500 patients, covering all degrees of photoaging in men and women, middle-aged adults, and the elderly. Generally speaking, the histological improvements are more obvious than the clinical ones. The greatest effects are noted in the most severely photodamaged skin.[19] In early photodamage the amelioration is less obvious, clinically and histologically. A purely clinical study on the effect of tretinoin on wrinkles, roughness, and hyperpigmented "age spots" will underestimate the value of tretinoin in ameliorating photoaging. The best use of tretinoin is in the prophylactic mode, that is, at the earliest stage, on skin showing only a few wrinkles and pigmented spots.

Skin treated with topical tretinoin examined by light and electron microscopy showed a variety of structural improvements, including normalization of epidermal atypia, the deposition of new collagen subepidermally, and the formation of new vessels (angiogenesis).[20]

In untreated skin with severe actinic damage, the epidermis was atrophic, with abnormal cells of variable size and shape. After 3 months of once-daily treatment with 0.05% topical tretinoin, the epidermis became acanthotic, with hyperplastic keratinocytes containing prominent nuclei, evidence of hyperproliferation. The granular layer became prominent and the horny layer more compact. Polarity was restored and differentiation normalized. Computerized measurement of thickness of viable epidermis confirmed these findings. A 40% increase in thickness was observed in forearm skin treated with tretinoin, as compared to an insignificant increase of 10% with the cream vehicle.[21] Because of the thinning of the horny layer, there was also an increase in transepidermal water loss.[11] However, after a year of treatment, the stratum corneum had returned to its original thickness and quality.

The epidermal improvements may be thought of as restoration of normal epithelial differentiation. This is the process by which proliferating keratinocytes are transformed into terminal corneocytes, an action that promotes the orderly shedding of corneocytes, with a resultant decrease in skin roughness.

Of great importance was the formation of a band of new collagen just below the epidermis. Before treatment there was a thin Grenz zone of collagen, beneath which there was a massive amalgam of elastotic, degenerated dermis. After 26 months of once-daily therapy with 0.05% tretinoin, the Grenz zone expanded greatly and new, fine bundles of normal collagen were laid down, pushing down the old elastotic tissue. With the reticulin stain, which identifies newly synthesized collagen, many fine new fibers were formed in the collagen-poor mass.[11] New, fine elastic fibers had also developed. This was accompanied by the appearance of hyperactive, large fibroblasts. The entire process was one of restoration toward the normal, associated with a perceptible improvement in elasticity and firmness.

The ability of tretinoin to increase the number and metabolic activity of fibroblasts promotes collagen synthesis, especially in the upper papillary dermis. This process is responsible for the clinically observable improvement in fine wrinkles and skin turgor. It may take many months to see these results. Patients must be cautioned not to expect rapid results. Similar findings have been reported by others.[22,23] Double-blind studies compared the effects of 0.1% tretinoin with its vehicle in photoaged facial and forearm skin. Significant clinical improvement occurred in patients treated with tretinoin, while the vehicle-treated group showed practically no change. Fine wrinkling was the feature most improved. Histological changes included increases in epidermal thickness, with correction of epidermal atrophy, atypia, and dysplasia.

A prominent effect of tretinoin is the formation of new blood vessels, that is, angiogenesis.[11] After 14 months of therapy, alkaline phosphatase-stained specimens of severely photoaged skin showed an increased number of small vessels with more regular diameters in the superficial dermis. The microvessels were broad, branching, and well distributed. Correspondingly, we also noted increased bleeding upon biopsying treated skin.

Angiogenesis is undoubtedly responsible for

the rosy glow and improved color that fair-skinned patients notice after several months of tretinoin. Angiogenesis can also explain the increased reactivity to chemical stimuli observed in patients treated with tretinoin.[11] Lymphangiogenesis also occurs, though this is less well known. These findings have been confirmed by Leyden, et al.[24] A laser Doppler instrument was used to measure blood flow in photoaged forearms. After 6 months skin treated with tretinoin showed significantly higher concentrations of moving red blood cells than did placebo, a reflection of a greater number of vessels to transport erythrocytes.[25] Forearms treated with tretinoin also showed significantly greater peak blood flow in response to the vasodilatory stimulus of trafuril, a nicotinate ester. Enhancement of the microvasculature improves not only color but physiological functions as well. An additional benefit is that drugs are more rapidly cleared from the skin. Of course, transport of nutrients are be enhanced.

Finally, pigmented spots and lentigos fade and become far less noticeable. The dense clusters of melanin in the basal layer become dispersed.[26] There is a simple reason for this removal of pigment. Tretinoin markedly stimulates cell turnover so that keratinocytes move rapidly toward the surface. Melanin cannot accumulate in a rapidly proliferating epidermis; instead, it is transported to the surface and dumped in the shedding process.

Side Effects

Side effects with 0.05% tretinoin have been limited to moderate irritation, dryness, and occasional erythema. These usually occur within the first few weeks of treatment. The skin usually adjusts in a month or so and returns to near normal.[11] It is rare for patients to discontinue therapy because of discomfort, provided they are adequately counseled.

A conservative approach is to start with a low concentration of tretinoin, with upward titration as the patient's skin adjusts. The availability of 0.025% tretinoin cream is helpful in this regard. This lower concentration may take somewhat longer to show improvement, but the trade-off, in terms of enhanced patient compliance, is worth the additional wait. Well-motivated patients, under proper supervision, can be treated more aggressively, starting with the 0.1% cream.

Treatment Guidelines

We usually initiate treatment with 0.05% tretinoin cream applied to the face at night for 8 to 12 months.[19] We recommend heavy-duty moisturizers in the morning, since the treatment can be somewhat drying and most patients are in an older age group, showing varying degrees of dry skin. In fact, most white people over age 30 have photoaged skin and should use emollients on a regular basis. We recommend simple, old-fashioned moisturizers such as Eucerin Cream, Nivea Cream and Lubriderm. Petroleum jelly is excellent but too greasy for many. Creams are more effective than lotions. Complicated, pricey moisturizers with exotic ingredients are not worth the money.

During the first months of therapy, patients with fair or sensitive skin are likely to experience some irritation. For those with an undue reaction, the treatment schedule can be adjusted to an alternate-night regimen until the skin adjusts. For patients with extremely sensitive skin, application only every third night might be necessary. Tolerance develops within 4 to 6 weeks in practically all patients. Darker-skinned individuals and older persons whose skin is less able to express inflammation may be able to use twice-daily applications and higher concentrations of tretinoin to accelerate the response. The drug should be increased according to tolerance; treatment should be individualized. Extra amounts can be applied to keratotic growths such as actinic keratoses.

Because the stratum corneum thins down and the vasculature is enhanced, skin treated with tretinoin usually becomes more vulnerable to certain cosmetics and toiletries that would otherwise be well accepted. Accordingly, astringents, abrasives, and harsh soaps should be avoided.

Patients have to be made aware that their skin will become more sensitive to the sun as well as to fragrances and detergents. Accordingly, patients must protect themselves from further photodamage by using sunscreens with high sun protection factors. A product with an SPF of at least 15 should be used. Some sunscreens may cause stinging and burning. There is a wide choice, however, and all patients should be able to find a product to suit their skin type. We also counsel patients to look for broad spectrum products, especially those that absorb in the UVA range, to protect against the entire spectrum of damaging rays. A recent innovation has been the elimination of chemical UV absorbers and replacement by ultra-fine suspensions of titanium dioxide. These are truly broad spectrum sun filters and provide protection against UVB, UVA and infrared radiation. They are also water-resistant and do not cause tearing after entering the external eye.

After 3 to 5 weeks of therapy, macular, erythematous flares of subclinical actinic keratoses may appear in severely photodamaged skin. Patients should be told that this is a desirable response because it is indicative of the lighting-up of premalignant lesions, which are undergoing obliteration. Erythematous spots may persist for months and should not be viewed as a toxic side effect.

After about a year, when maximum benefits have been obtained, it is possible to reduce the therapy to a maintenance schedule of twice weekly (weekend) applications. Although treatment is usually confined to the face, the dorsal hands and forearms can also benefit from tretinoin use. The principles of treatment are the same.

With the cessation of treatment, the clinical effects may fade somewhat, especially if treatment is stopped after less than 6 months. But the antitumor effects, once obtained, remain. What is more, the full range of benefits obtained with tretinoin therapy will be sustained for as long as treatment continues.

We made histologic observations on patients treated daily for 5 to 6 years. We were impressed by the resorption of elastotic material and its replacement by new collagen, resembling the effect of a face peel. Again, the benefits were more dramatic histologically than clinically.

It is important to have realistic expectations and to communicate the limitations to patients. Clinical improvement is slow and may not be evident for months. Tretinoin is not a substitute for a facelift, dermabrasion, or collagen injections. We emphasize that topical tretinoin is a prophylactic agent to prevent or slow the progress of photoaging. Light-skinned, type I persons who tan poorly are at greatest risk for photodamage, particularly if they spend a great deal of time outdoors. These individuals might first begin topical tretinoin therapy in their twenties. In contrast, darker-skinned individuals who tan easily and deeply, such as those of Mediterranean ancestry with type IV skin, may not seek therapy until their thirties or forties.

Summary

Many studies have validated the usefulness of tretinoin in the prevention and treatment of photoaged skin.[27-29] Tretinoin is the first drug to demonstrate such effects. Tretinoin can repair many of the structural derangements found in photodamaged skin. The most dramatic clinical results occur in those persons with moderately photodamaged skin. These effects are retinoid-specific and are not the result of low-grade tissue damage or irritation, as some have maintained. We have tried to obtain similar results in humans using several nonspecific inflammogens—for example, cationic and anionic surfactants. However, repair could not be demonstrated. No evidence of reversal of epidermal dysplasia, enhanced collagen synthesis, angiogenesis, or antitumor activity could be demonstrated. In fact, chronic inflammation appears to promote elastolysis and collagenolysis. We conclude that the sum of the effects attributable to tretinoin is unique and cannot be mimicked by other weak acids designed for the treatment of photoaging.

References

1. Elias PM, Williams ML. Retinoid effects on epidermal differentiation. In: *Retinoids. New Trends in Research and Therapy,* JH Saurat, ed. S Karger, Basel, 1985, p. 138.
2. Kligman LH. Effects of all-trans retinoic acid on the dermis of hairless mice. J Am Acad Dermatol. 1986; 15:779.
3. Sporn MG, Newton DL. Chemoprevention of cancer with retinoids. Fed Proc 1979; 38:528.

4. Bollag W, Ott F. Retinoic acid topical treatment of actinic keratoses and basal cell cancers. Agents Actions. 1970; 1:172.
5. Meyskins FL. Studies of retinoids in the prevention and treatment of cancer. J Am Acad Dermatol. 1982; 6:824. 1982.
6. Levine N, Meyskins FL. Topical vitamin A therapy for cutaneous malignant melanoma. Lancet. 1980; 2:224.
7. Elias P, Fritsch PO, Lampe M. Retinoid effects on epidermal structure, differentiation and permeability. Lab Invest. 44:531. 1988
8. Lee KH, Tong TG. Mechanism of action of retinyl compounds on wound healing. J Pharm Sci. 1970; 59:1195.
9. Tsambaos O, Orfanos CE. Ultrastructural evidence suggesting an immunomodularity activity of oral retinoid. Br J Dermatol. 1981; 104:33.
10. Bradshaw, Cashen CH, Kennedy AJ. Antiinflammatory effects of retinoids. In: *Retinoid Therapy,* WJ Cunliffe, ed. MTP Press, Lancaster, p. 335. 1991
11. Kligman AM, Fulton JE, Plewig G. Topical vitamin A acid in acne vulgaris. Arch Dermatol. 1969; 99:469.
12. Kligman AM, Grove GL, Hirose R, Leyden JL. Topical tretinoin for photoaged skin. J Am Acad Dermatol. 1986; 15:836.
13. Gilchrest BA. *Skin and Aging Processes.* CRC Press, Boca Raton, 1984.
14. Kligman LH, Kligman AM. The nature of photoaging, its prevention and repair. Photodermatology. 1986; 3:215.
15. Kligman AM. Early destruction effects of sunlight in human skin. JAMA. 1969; 210:2377.
16. Braverman IM, Fonferko E. Studies in cutaneous aging: the classic fiber network. J Invest Dermatol. 1982; 78:434.
17. Lavker RM, Kligman AM. Chronic heliodermatitis. J Invest Dermatol. 1988; 90:325.
18. Lavker RM. Structural alterations in exposed and unexposed aged skin. J Invest Dermatol. 1979; 73:59.
19. Kligman AM. Guidelines for the use of topical tretinoin for photoaged skin. J Am Acad Dermatol. 1989; 21:650.
20. Weiss JS, Ellis CN, Headington JT, Hamilton TA. Treatment of photodamaged facial skin with tretinoin. JAMA. 1988; 259:527.
21. Weinstein GD, Nigra TP, Pochi PE. Topical tretinoin for treatment of photodamaged skin. Arch Dermatol. 1991; 127:659.
22. Olson EA, Katz HI, Levine N, Shupak J, Bellys MM. Tretinoin emollient cream: a new therapy for photodamaged skin. J Am Acad Dermatol. 1992; 26:215.
23. Ellis CN, Weiss JS, Voorhees JJ. Tretinoin: its use in repair of photodamage. J Cutan Aging Cosmet Dermatol. 1988; 1:33.
24. Leyden JJ, Grove GL, Thorne EG, Lufano L. Treatment of photodamaged facial with topical tretinoin. J Am Acad Dermatol. 1989; 21:635.
25. Grove GL, Zerwick CR, Leyden JJ. Determination of topical tretinoin effect on cutaneous microcirculation. J Cutan Aging Cosmet Dermatol. 1988; 1:27.
26. Zelickson AS, Mottae JH, Weiss JS. Topical tretinoin in photoaging: an ultrastructural study. J Cutan Aging Cosmet Dermatol. 1988; 1:41.
27. Lever L, Kumar P, Marks R. Topical retinoic acid in the treatment of elastotic degeneration. Br J Dermatol. 1990; 122:91.
28. Caputo R, Monti M, Motta S, Barbaresch M. The treatment of visible signs of senescence. Br J Dermatol. 1990; 122:97.
29. Voorhees JJ. Clinical effects of long-term therapy with topical tretinoin. J Inter Med Res. 1990; 18:26.

4
Treatment of the Aging Skin with Glycolic Acid

David R. Harris

Legend has it that in Old Rome, layers of acid formed in the bottoms of wine barrels. When the women of the day could get it, it was rubbed all over their faces to brighten up the skin.

Introduction

Alpha hydroxy acids (AHA) are a class of naturally occurring compounds derived from fruit and dairy products. This group consists of a large number of substances, the better known of which include lactic acid (from sour milk), glycolic acid (from sugar cane), malic acid (from apples), tartaric acid (from grapes), as well as citric, pyruvic, gluconic, mandelic, and benzylic acids. In 1974 Van Scott and Yu reported on the efficacy of lactic acid in the treatment of conditions predisposing to dry, rough skin, including ichthyosis.[1] Since then our knowledge of the therapeutic efficacy of alpha hydroxy acids has increased, and it is still unfolding.[2,3]

As a class, these compounds, when applied topically, seem to mediate specific, distinct, and unique effects on the stratum corneum, the epidermis, the papillary dermis, and the pilosebaceous units. Because of these effects, therapeutic benefits have been reported with not only dry skin conditions but also in the treatment of acne; hyperplastic epidermal lesions such as keratoses, both seborrheic and actinic, and warts; and problems related to aging, including dyschromia, dullness, and wrinkling.[3]

The compound in this series that has been used more extensively than the others in the treatment of cutaneous problems related to the aging skin is glycolic acid. The purpose of this chapter is to describe our expanding knowledge concerning the use of AHAs, especially glycolic acid, in the treatment of actinically injured and aging skin.

Chemical and Physiological Properties of Alpha Hydroxy Acids

Glycolic acid, the smallest in molecular size of the AHAs, contains two carbon atoms ($H_2C(OH)COOH$). Next in size is lactic acid, containing three carbons ($CH_3CH(OH)COOH$), which converts to pyruvic acid (a keto acid). Other AHAs have longer chains, including malic and tartaric, alpha methyl lactic (four carbons), and citric, gluconic, mandelic, and benzylic acid (six carbons).[3] All the AHAs, when applied topically in various concentrations, reduce corneocyte cohesion and stratum corneum thickening. In higher concentrations these substances, some more effectively than others, will cause detachment of keratinocytes and epidermolysis. These actions have been demonstrated clinically as well as histologically.[4]

The effect on corneocytes occurs predominantly among cells at the lower levels of the stratum corneum, with little response at the outer layers. Corneocyte cohesion is greatly influenced by hydration—in other words, by water. AHAs apparently improve hydration and decrease cohesion, in part by allowing improved imbibing as well as binding of water to the stratum corneum.[1,5] Decreased cohesion may also be due to a modification of ionic bonding. The specific biochemical process may be a prevention of cross-linking of extracellular matrix proteins, which in turn initiate those events responsible for corneocyte and keratinocyte cohesion.[4]

Another possible mode of action has been suggested by Ziboh.[6] He points out that the skin is an organ that displays a highly active metabolism of polyunsaturated fatty acids. Deficiency in dietary fatty acids (or the aging process itself) may result in scaly dermatoses and disruption of the skin barrier system. Skin possesses an enzyme system to metabolize and convert a variety of lipids. Some of these mono hydroxy fatty acids have potent antiinflammatory properties. Thus, it seems possible that an elevation of these AHAs by dietary or topical means could suppress the cutaneous inflammatory reactions elicited by excessive generations of prostaglandins and leukotrienes.

Evolving Uses

Regardless of the specific mode of action, the AHAs have penetrating and profound effects on the skin. These effects depend on the AHA, its concentration, vehicle, exposure time, and preexisting conditions of the skin. Besides thinning stratum corneum, these effects include reduced keratinocyte cohesion, complete epidermolysis, epidermal separation, and impact on the papillary dermis, particularly the dermis, leading to a new synthesis of collagen, elastin, and regeneration of protein.[7] Moreover, studies demonstrating the sparing effect of AHAs on skin thinning with topical corticosteroid treatment also reveal an increase in glycosaminoglycans in the dermis. This is a reversal of the compaction of the dermis seen with corticosteroid atrophy.[8]

That AHAs have the ability to influence abnormal keratinization is apparent in treating ichthyosiform genodermatoses, xerosis,[9-12] and acne.[13] Their effects are readily appreciated, with improvement in wrinkles, warts, abnormal pigmentation, benign and premalignant keratoses, and in enhancing and modifying the action of other topical agents applied concomitantly.[1,7,14] Van Scott noted that most lentigines are really keratoses with varying degrees of hypermelanization. This is based on work with numerous shave biopsies obtained during AHA treatment. Most brown patches on the hands and forearms are evenly divided between lentigines and keratoses. Van Scott noted that after treatment with AHAs, the brown patches faded and the skin took on a healthy glow and shine. He began the use of glycolic and pyruvic acid in higher concentrations successfully, to stimulate epidermolysis and desquamation in warts and keratoses.[15] Our own work has shown that treatment of these disorders with high concentrations of pyruvic acid is less predictable than desired. Moreover, delayed healing and depigmented scars have been noted in a few of our patients.

More useful in our hands are glycolic and lactic acids in concentrations between 15% and 20% for hyperkeratotic eczema, tinea pedis, and conditions resulting in thickened palms and soles.

The use of these compounds, especially glycolic acid, in the treatment of acne has revealed decided therapeutic benefit. The action of the acids in reducing cohesion of follicular corneocytes and subsequent desquamation of keratinous plugs is the probable cause of therapeutic benefit.[13] In fact, successful treatment of linear follicular keratoses and nevus comedonicus has been reported.[16-17]

Glycolic Acid and the Aging Skin

Over the past decade, those who have used the AHAs, first as substances for the treatment of conditions related to xerosis and hyperkeratinization and then in combination with other therapies, have noted beneficial effects on the aging skin.[18-19] For the purposes of this discussion, *aging skin* is defined as exposed skin that has suffered the ravages of photodamage, intrinsic aging, and exogenous insult. Histologically, photoaging involves epidermal atypia, thickening of the stratum corneum, melanocytic proliferation, and elastic changes in the papillary and upper reticular dermis. These changes are directly related to sun exposure.

Clinically, this skin has lost youthful luster and translucency. There is an obvious dryness and dullness to the tone. Aging skin is commonly associated with abnormal pigmentation, numerous lentigines, a muddy, irregular melasma, and telangiectasia. Moreover, there may be frank or subclinical cancers and keratoses causing erythema, pigmentation, scaling, or crusting. Finally, we see evidence of rhytids, or "wrinkle lines," either fine or deep, accentuating the natural lines of expression. All these insults associated with aging affect the quality of the skin. The remainder of the discussion will deal primarily with the use of glycolic acid in ameliorating, softening, and eliminating these histological and clinical changes in aging.

Our considerations defining the use and effects of glycolic acid on the aging skin are derived primarily from our own experience and that of others over the past half dozen years. The literature that recently has been accumulating validating the effectiveness of glycolic acid on the aging skin is necessarily sparse and evolving. We can cite only the work of several others as well as our own in outlining to the reader a successful approach to treatment with this compound.[3,7,14,18,19]

In many ways our use of glycolic acid mirrors the experience of cosmetically oriented physicians employing tretinoin (Retin A) in aging problems.[20-23] In the early years after topical retinoids were available, they were utilized almost exclusively in the treatment of acne. However, after a decade of use, it became obvious that a subset of patients was enjoying effects that reflected improved skin quality as well as amelioration of acneiform dermatitis. So it has been with the AHAs. Lactic and glycolic acids, used in the treatment of conditions other than aging, revealed to the careful observer, over time, effectiveness in improving photodamaged skin. For the most part, our patients reported that atypical pigmentation was diminished, finer rhytids were softened, and the tone of the skin took on a more lustrous and translucent quality. These reports have not been merely anecdotal; they have been found to be reproducible and have been monitored with before and after photography (see Figures 4.1A and B).

Glycolic Acid-Based Products

There is an ever-increasing number of glycolic acid-containing over-the-counter topical agents available to both the physician and the esthetician. Products currently marketed for treatment include astringents, either in an alcohol or alcohol-and-propylene glycol base, water-based creams, lotions and gels, cleansers and shampoos in a detergent base, and various strengths of peeling solutions, from 40% to 70%. Most products utilizing glycolic acid for the treatment of aging skin employ concentrations from 2% to 15%.[24] These products, in turn, will have a pH as low as 1.5 unbuffered, and as high as 4.0 when buffered.[25,26]

The products seem to be falling into two distinctive groups. Lower-strength glycolic acid-based preparations, between 1.2% and 8%, are being marketed by cosmetic firms through drug and department stores. Higher-strength modalities, between 8% and 30% in similar bases, are being distributed by smaller pharmaceutical companies through dermatology and plastic surgery practices and at salons through estheticians.[27,28] We do not know how effective preparations as low as 2% or 3% may be in improving the quality of actinically injured skin, but it is clear that products above 8% can make a difference in as little as 2 to 3 months. Some patients with severe photodamage are beginning to use preparations with concentrations between 15% and 20% with satisfying results. However, tolerance must be developed over some period of time with the use of lower-strength preparations before working up to the higher concentrations. We are even seeing 30% creams for limited application over the dorsa of the hands to enhance desquamation.

The Effect of Buffering on Glycolic Acid

Virtually all commercially available products are buffered. Is there an effect on the efficacy

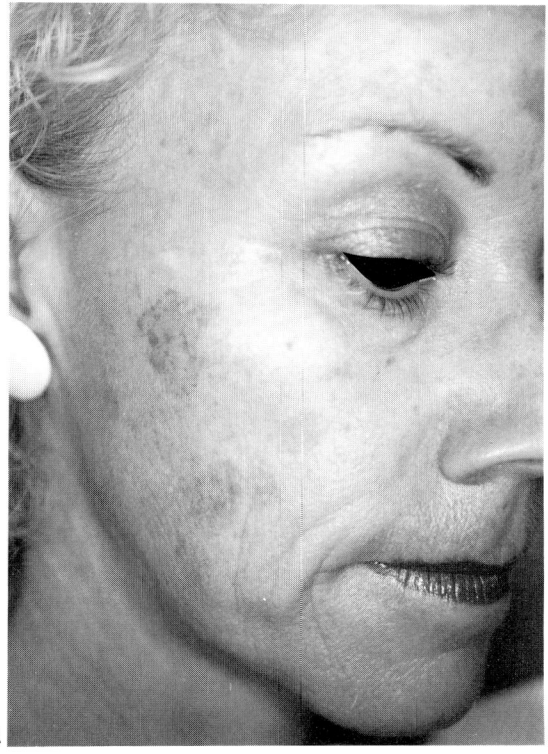 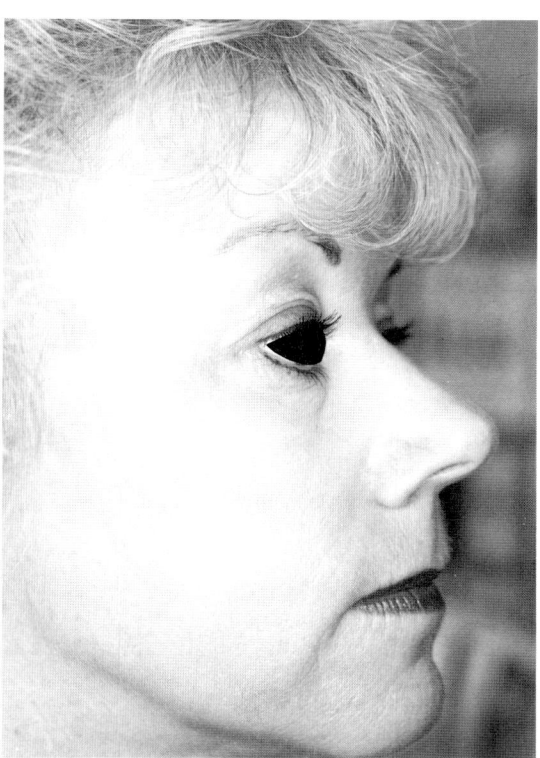

FIGURE 4.1. A. Pretreatment with basic glycolic acid topical program. B. Seven months after beginning the program. Note the brighter skin with much less dyschromia.

with buffering? Alpha and beta hydroxy acids have, at concentrations between 0.5% and 1%, a pH in the range similar to citric acid, acetic acid, and lemon juice (between 2.2 and 2.5). At 2% the pH of glycolic acid is 2.1; at 5% pH is 1.9; and at 10% it is 1.7.[25]

In the early 1970s, pharmaceutical chemists began using substantial percentages of buffer to adjust acidity of the AHAs to pH closer to 5.5.[20] Most glycolic acid products are now buffered to a pH closer to 4.5 with ammonium salts, the more bioavailable of the commonly used buffers. At pH 4.5 there is still a fair amount of the free acid, enough for a pleasing result with less irritation than an unbuffered product; however, the buffered product is somewhat slower acting.[26] Although this information has not been worked out in studies, the buffered glycolic acid products may give equivalent results to unbuffered products over months rather than weeks. Therefore, we have a trade-off when we buffer glycolic acid:

There is less irritation, but there is also slower action.

One reason why the physiological action of glycolic acid seems to continue in spite of buffering as high as pH of 4.5, is that a hydroxy group on the alpha carbon makes this acid more potent in its action on the skin than most other AHAs.[20]

Our Approach to the Use of Glycolic Acid in the Treatment of Actinically Injured and Aging Skin of the Face

Basic Strategy

In treating photoaged, not easily irritated, acne-prone, or excessively pigmented skin, our basic strategy includes the application of an 8% to

TABLE 4.1. Glycolic acid treatment of aging skin: basic strategy utilizing glycolic acid.

Basic strategy utilizing glycolic acid
1. Use soap-free cleansers only (Cetaphil Lotion, Aquanil Lotion, SFC Lotion) morning and night.
2. Apply a No. 15–25 SPF sunscreen in the morning, with or without glycolic acid product.
3. Apply 8%–12% buffered glycolic acid lotion or cream nightly.

TABLE 4.3. Glycolic acid treatment of aging skin: dry and easily irritated skin

Dry and Easily Irritated Skin
1. Use soap-free cleansers only.
2. Introduce a well-tolerated sunscreen first.
3. Cautiously add a low-strength (5% or less) glycolic acid product once daily or on alternate days (8%–12% products can be diluted with a moisturizer or by wetting the skin before application).
4. Increase use over time. Use astringents carefully, only on the acne-prone.

12% buffered lotion or cream, generally after soap-free cleansing in the morning and evening. We also advise the use of an appropriately tolerated sunscreen in the morning with a glycolic acid preparation in equal parts, if tolerated (see Table 4.1).

Acne-Prone or Excessively Oily Skin

In the acne-susceptible or oily skinned patient, the addition of oil in water-based creams and lotions may exacerbate the disease. For this group we have successfully used glycolic acid-based cleansers or mild soaps in concert with 5% to 13% glycolic acid-based astringents or toners, used twice daily, that is, morning and night. We add a glycolic acid lotion or cream as tolerated, because most patients note a measure of dryness over time with the use of alcohol- or water-based astringents and toners alone. In addition we recommend an oil-free or clear gel- or lotion-based sunscreen (refer to Table 4.2).

Dry or Easily Irritated Skin

A few patients will prove completely intolerant to any glycolic acid-based preparation. Short of this small group, there is a larger pool of patients who generally complain about intolerance to a range of substances, from soap to sunscreen. This group demands a cautious approach to treatment. We begin with soap-free cleansers and a sunscreen that we know is tolerated. Then we add diluted and buffered glycolic acid-based cream or lotion preparations once daily, or start on alternate days. Furthermore, we encourage additional use of moisturizer on an ad hoc basis. We introduce toners and astringents only at a later time, if at all, in the acne-prone (see Table 4.3).

Expected Results

Like the retinoids, notable improvement in skin quality occurs slowly over time, generally in 3 months to a year. Most of our patients begin to appreciate a brighter, less dull, and more uniform complexion during the first 3 months of treatment (see Figures 4.2A and B). Keratoses and pigmentary abnormalities as well as fine rhytids may take several more months to respond without combining treatment with additional modalities, including peeling procedures.

It is valuable to give your patient some realistic expectations when first outlining treatment; Compliance and satisfaction will certainly be improved. Never promise too much too soon.

Handling Untoward Side Effects

A degree of stinging or burning is a common side effect of glycolic acid application, especially at the beginning of treatment. Some patients also sense a moderate amount of dryness, irritation, and mild desquamation, but less than with tretinoin. *The patient must be*

TABLE 4.2. Glycolic acid treatment of aging skin: acid-prone or excessively oily skin.

Acne-Prone or Excessively Oily Skin
1. Substitute a mild soap, acne wash, or glycolic acid-containing cleanser for soap-free cleanser.
2. Utilize clear lotion or gel sunscreens or an oil-free product in the morning.
3. Provide a glycolic acid alcohol-based astringent or toner (5%–13%) instead of a lotion or cream. Use in the morning before applying sunscreen and again in the evening.

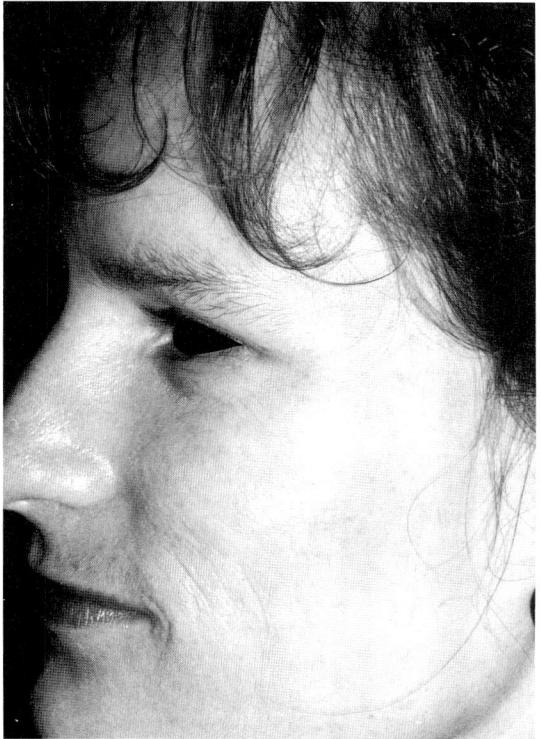 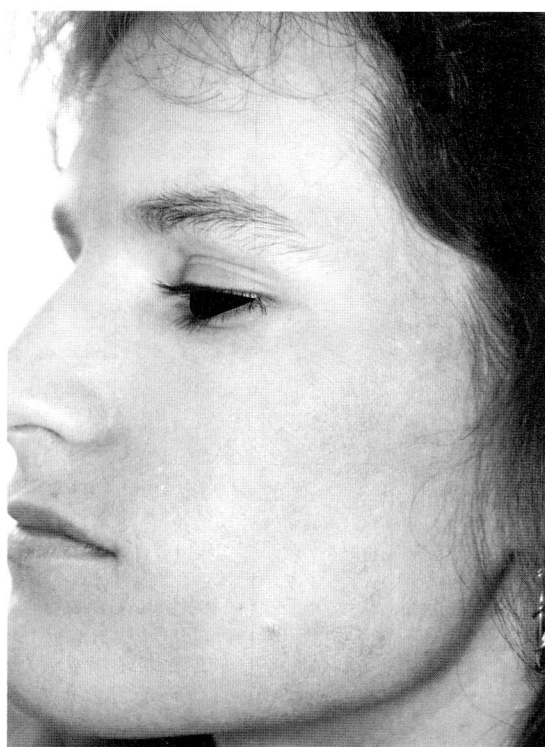

FIGURE 4.2. A. Pretreatment with glycolic acid program. B. Four months after beginning the program. Note the brighter, more uniform tone.

forewarned. We have found most patients cooperative if of these potential problems beforehand. However, many will stop applications immediately, fearing dire consequences, if untoward side effects are not understood to be harmless.

We suggest that a handout be given to each patient treated with glycolic acid. Suggestions concerning strategies for handling side effects should be included as well as an admonition to call the doctor or nurse instead of discontinuing therapy (see Table 4.4). These strategies include stopping the modality for a few days and restarting the treatment and adding a moisturizer in equal parts in order to decrease the concentration of glycolic acid until the patient is more comfortable with the treatment. Wetting the skin with water before application will also dilute glycolic acid-containing preparations. All these strategies have merit, but the urging of continued communication if problems persist is most important.

Advantages over Retinoic Acid

Glycolic acid may prove superior to retinoic acid. There is no formulation of retinoic acid that can be applied to the skin in a short interval, such as an office peeling procedure, in concert with daily use of the product. Moreover, patients tend to complain more about dryness and irritation with tretinoin than glycolic acid. In addition, there is no photosensitivity, nor are AHAs contraindicated during pregnancy. Also, telangiectasias can be an emerging problem with the use of retinoic acid. In some people there seems to be a degree of angiogenesis. Finally, glycolic acid tends to cost less than retinoic acid, which is a prescription drug.[7,13]

In spite of these deficiencies, retinoic acid has proven to be an excellent modality in treating the aging skin.[21,22] When combined with a glycolic acid program, it may have greater merit.

TABLE 4.4. Glycolic acid treatment of aging skin: sample instruction handout.

Sample instruction handout

A. Morning Care
     1. _____
     2. _____
     3. _____
     4. _____
 B. Evening Care
     1. _____
     2. _____
     3. _____
     4. _____
 C. Cosmetic Suggestions
     1. _____
     2. _____
     3. _____
     4. _____
 D. **IMPORTANT: What to expect from your personalized glycolic acid skin care program**:
     The preparations selected for you include products that may initially cause a degree of dryness, irritation, or flaking of the skin. Moreover, some medications have a tendency to tingle or burn when first applied. This is an entirely natural phenomenon, representing the nature of the active ingredients, and is in no way detrimental to the skin.
 E. **If irritation, stinging or burning occurs, we suggest that you take one or more of the following steps**:
     1. Stop using the medications for 1 or 2 days until the skin returns to normal.
     2. Wet the skin before applying the topical preparations; this dilutes everything by about 50%.
     3. Add a favorite moisturizer to the preparations prescribed, again to dilute the effect. Ask us about our special moisturizers.
 IF THERE ARE ANY QUESTIONS OR PROBLEMS CONCERNING YOUR PERSONALIZED PROGRAM, PLEASE CALL OUR OFFICE AND ASK TO SPEAK TO A NURSE—WE KNOW HOW TO HELP.

Combining Modalities for Improved Results

Glycolic acid is a superb modality for enhancing the effects of other topical medications. It has been observed that the addition of alpha hydroxy acids to corticosteroid or antifungal preparations enhance the action of these drugs, probably through the process of decreasing the keratin barrier to absorption,[2] although they may also act in another manner, as described earlier. When treating the aging skin, one can take advantage of the adjunctive effects of glycolic acid in concert with retinoids, 5-fluorouracil, and/or hydroquinone (see Table 4.5).

Combining Glycolic Acid with Retinoic Acid

Our experience is mirrored by others who have observed enhanced response to retinoic acid with less irritation when combined with glycolic acid. We combine an 8% to 12% glycolic acid-based night cream with retinoic acid, 0.025% to 0.1%, in equal parts, although we begin with one or the other before combining both. We feel that the desired goal of improved skin quality is reached more quickly when these modalities are used in concert.

TABLE 4.5. Glycolic acid treatment of aging skin: combining modalities for improved results.

Combining modalities for improved results
1. For average photodamaged skin, add *retinoic acid cream 0.025 to 0.1%* in equal parts glycolic acid cream or lotion 8%-12% nightly.
2. For severely photodamaged skin, add *fluorouracil 1%-5%* in the morning and at night twice weekly or every other week over a glycolic acid cream or lotion 8%-12%.
3. For resistant hyperpigmentation, add *hydroquinone 4%-10%* to equal parts of a 15%-25% sunscreen in the morning and/or equal parts of glycolic acid cream or lotion 8%-12% at night.
Variations
Any of the above can be applied after application of a glycolic acid astringent or toner in the acne prone.

Combining Glycolic Acid with Hydroquinone

We have found, as have others,[2] that the addition of hydroquinone 4% to 10% in equal parts of a 10% buffered glycolic acid lotion or cream enhances the effects of the lightening agent. When faced with dyschromia, lentigines, melasma, or simply a "muddy" complexion resistant to the basic strategy outlined, adding hydroquinone as part of a daily regimen enhances and accelerates the lightening effects of the treatment (see Figures 4.3A and B).

Combining Glycolic Acid and 5-Fluorouracil

For more severely actinically injured skin, when diffuse actinic keratoses and lentigines are obvious, the addition of 5-fluorouracil on a periodic basis with daily applications of glycolic acid is a useful strategy. Our current regimen for the face, arms, and hands is to apply a 10% glycolic acid-based lotion or cream once or twice daily and then add 5-fluorouracil cream, 1% to 5%, twice daily every other Monday and Tuesday. This "pulse" therapy greatly diminishes the inflammatory effects of daily applications of 5-fluorouracil and decidedly enhances improvement of actinically injured skin. The results are usually obvious to a striking degree, to both patient and observer, over a 2- to 4-month period. First the skin is softer and smoother to the touch, then keratoses and lentigines are greatly diminished. For those who are more tolerant, we sometimes increase applications of 5-fluorouracil to twice weekly rather than staying at every other week.

Combining Topical Programs with Glycolic Acid Peeling

Glycolic acid in a buffered solution for chemical peeling is increasingly becoming available through dermatological pharmaceutical houses.

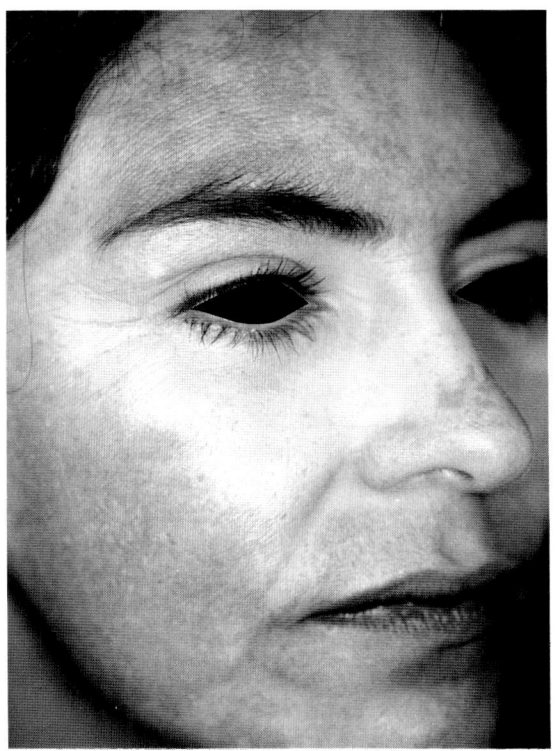
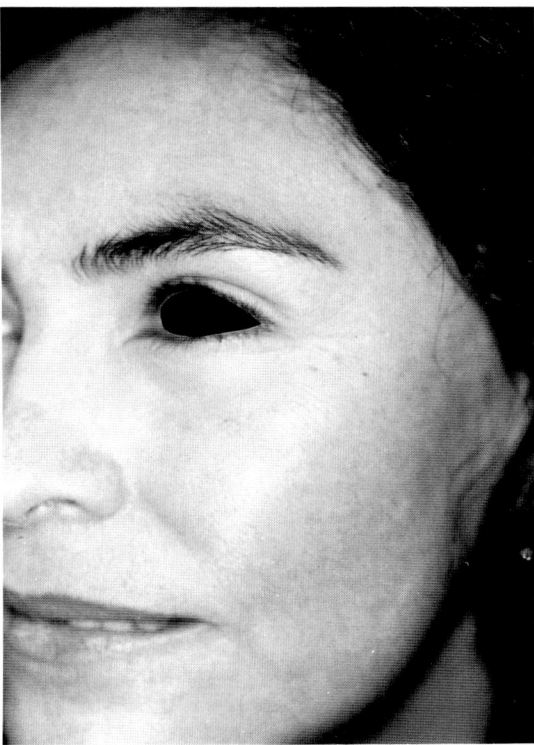

FIGURE 4.3. A. Pretreatment combining glycolic acid astringent plus 10% hydroquinone. B. Two months later. The patient received 2 67% glycolic acid peels.

Unbuffered glycolic acid 70% solution is also available from some chemical supply houses and pharmacists. Both buffered and unbuffered preparations enhance and accelerate the effects of topical programs, both for the treatment of aging skin and for acne.[29] We have found that application of 55% to 67% buffered glycolic acid solution at 2- to 3-week intervals is the best-tolerated and most efficacious approach. We also find, for most people, that between 3 and 5 peels are necessary for desired enhancement of topical care. Like others,[7,29] after cleansing and defatting with acetone or astringent, we apply the buffered glycolic acid solution evenly to the integument and wait for 3 to 10 minutes until stinging or burning is appreciated (see Figure 4.4). Following this period of application, the material is neutralized with tap water.

In contrast to peeling with trichloroacetic acid, where concentration of the material is paramount for certain depths of peeling, AHAs act, in large measure, over time. That is to say that the longer the glycolic acid-based peeling agent is in contact with the skin, the deeper the response. While for most the ideal length of application is between 3 and 10 minutes, some patients need and tolerate longer applications. This tends to vary, both with the number of repeated peels and with skin pretreated either with retinoic acid and/or glycolic acid.

There are decided differences among patients. Some are quite intolerant, needing either lower strengths, between 40% and 50%, or less application time to achieve a desired result. In any event, an appropriate end point with any application is increasing discomfort, with stinging and burning or obvious frosting. Unbuffered preparations work much faster and the results less uniform.

Results of Glycolic Acid Peeling

Buffered glycolic acid solutions tend to cause "subliminal peeling"[2,7]. That is for most patients there is little burning or irritation, virtually no obvious frosting as seen with trichloroacetic acid, and little actual peeling, especially in concentrations below 67%. The principal effect of both buffered and unbuffered glycolic acid peels, in our experience, is to improve and accelerate the effects of topical glycolic acid programs. This, we feel, glycolic acid peeling does efficiently (see Figures 4.5A and B). The peels are particularly helpful with persisting dyschromia and dullness of the integument.

In spite of the mild reaction experienced by most, some patients pretreated with glycolic acid, retinoic acid, or a combination of both topicals may have an accelerated cutaneous injury when glycolic acid peels are utilized. This may mean that these individuals have spots on the integument that "take" the glycolic acid more effectively and form a degree of crust, especially in percentages over 55% and with unbuffered material. Therefore, we like to begin a series of glycolic acid peels with 40% to 55% concentrations and observe the response before moving to 67% peels.

Maintenance peels, at monthly or alternate monthly intervals once the desired improvement is obtained, are enjoyed by an increasing number of our patients.

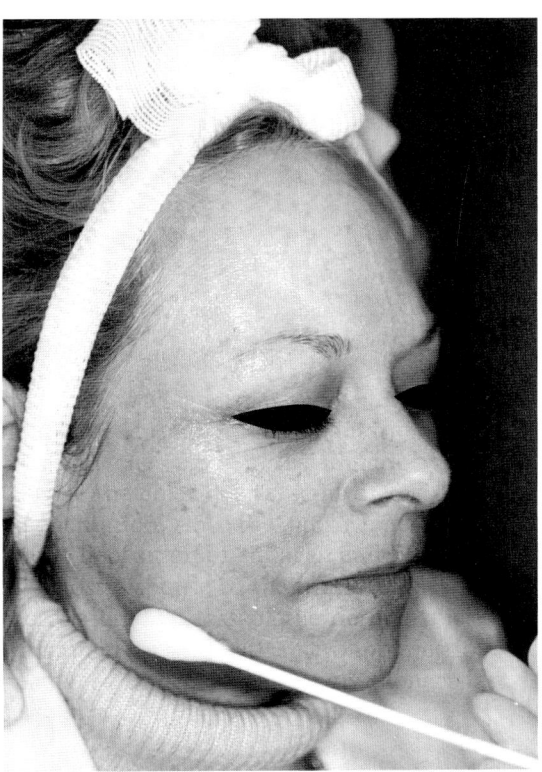

FIGURE 4.4. Glycolic acid peeling solution is applied evenly to the entire face and allowed to remain from 3 to 10 minutes as tolerated before removing.

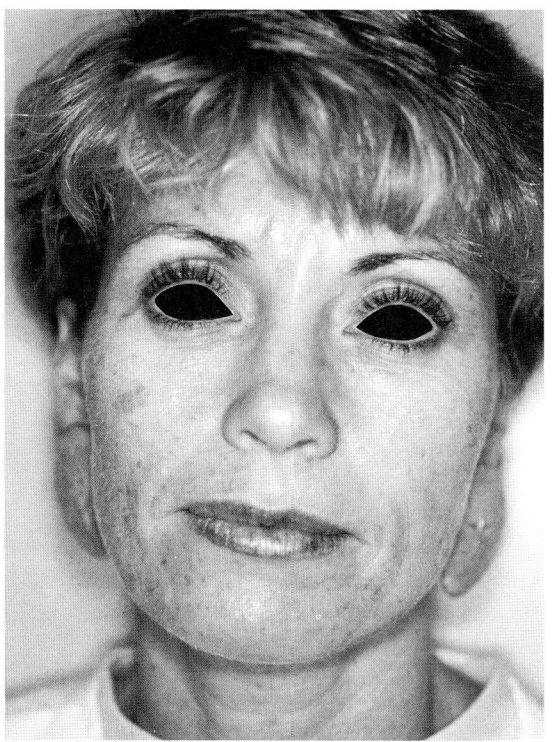 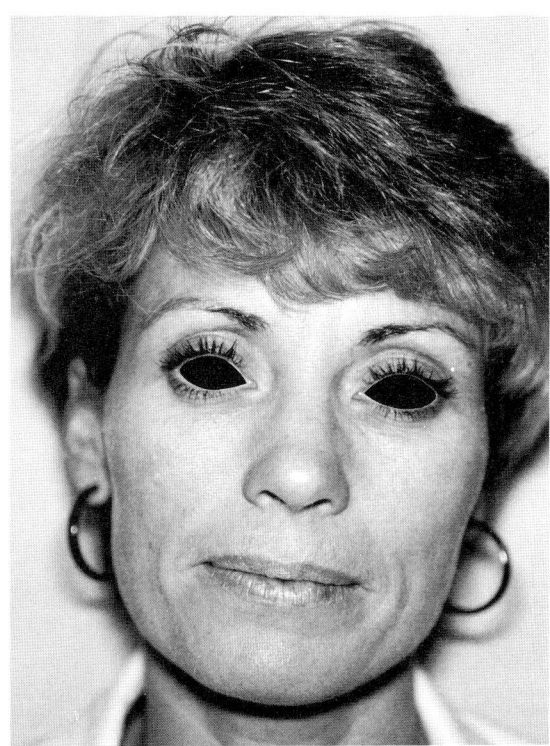

FIGURE 4.5. A. Preglycolic acid, 67% peel (unbuffered). B. Postglycolic acid, 67% peel. Improvement in general tone is noted.

Treatment of Other Photodamaged Areas

Treatment of the Forearms and Hands

One can utilize any of the discussed strategies, both topical and peeling, in a concurrent manner for treating the forearms and dorsa of the hands while improving the aging skin of the face. Many patients also find that this same approach is effective for dyschromia involving the neck and anterior chest. In fact, we encourage our patients to allow us to use the peeling solutions at the same time on the neck, anterior chest, forearms, and dorsa of the hands when we are doing a series of facial peels. Pretreating lentigines of the arms and hands with a very light application of liquid nitrogen can accelerate the effects of a topical glycolic acid program on these unwanted disfigurements. We utilize a freeze–thaw cycle of less than 1 second, so that a light frost appears only momentarily (see Figure 4.6). This is sufficient. Topical care generally consists of daily applications of glycolic acid cream or lotions between 10% and 20%.

Treatment of Actinic Cheilitis and Leukoplakia

We apply a 5% glycolic acid-based emollient to photodamaged lips several times daily. Trial-and-error has revealed the best vehicle to be petrolatum stiffened with silicone ointment and paraffin wax (this is also an excellent modality for treating brittle nails). We augment topical care with periodic applications of fluorouracil lotion or cream and/or light TCA peels.

Summary

Alpha hydroxy acids, in particular glycolic acid, as described in this communication, have profound physiological effects on photoda-

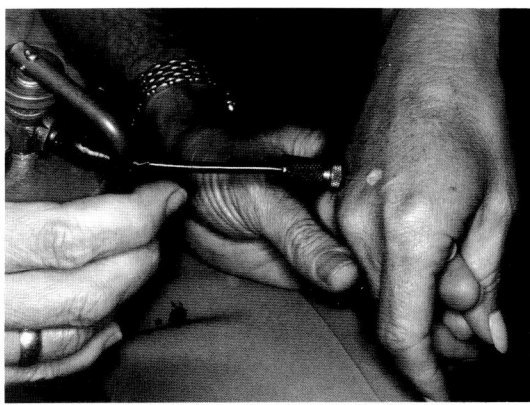

FIGURE 4.6. On the hands, lightening of lentigines with glycolic acid can be accelerated with liquid nitrogen using a freeze-thaw cycle of 1 second or less.

maged skin. These effects include decreased corneocyte cohesion, various levels of epidermal separation and thickening, and an impact on the papillary and deeper dermis. There is a synthesis of new collagen and elastin as well as an improvement in the concentration of glycosaminoglycans.

The clinical relevance of these changes is appreciated with smoother, more uniform, and more lustrous skin. A decrease in pigmented keratoses, lentigines, and melasma, and a softening in fine wrinkle lines, especially in the periorbital and oral areas, are noted over time. The approach to treatment most favored by the dermatological community includes a mixture of topical programs on a daily basis consisting of glycolic acid lotions, creams, and toners between 8% and 12%; and periodic applications of higher concentrations of glycolic acid, between 55% and 70%, at regular intervals. The application of AHAs in this manner has much to offer, including a minimal problem with irritation and photosensitivity reactions and reasonable cost.

Finally, combining glycolic acid application with specific topical agents to improve resistant problems has much to offer. The effect of retinoids, 5-fluorouracil, and hydroquinone on photodamaged and hyperpigmented skin is enhanced, probably through better percutaneous penetration, when combined with glycolic acid.

References

1. Van Scott EJ, Yu RJ. Control of keratinization with alpha hydroxy acids and related compounds: 1. topical treatment of ichthyotic disorders. Arch Dermatol. 1974;110:586–590.
2. Van Scott EJ. The unfolding therapeutic uses of alpha hydroxy acids. In: *Med Guide to Dermatol.* 3:1988;1–5.
3. Van Scott EJ, Yu RJ. Alpha hydroxy acids: therapeutic potentials. Canadian J Dermatol. 1989;1:108–112.
4. Van Scott EJ, Yu RJ. Hyperkeratinization, corneocyte cohesion, and alpha hydroxy acids. J Am Acad Dermatol. 1984;11:867–879.
5. Van Scott EJ, Yu RJ. Substances that modify the stratum corneum by modulating its formation. In: *Principles of Cosmetics for the Dermatologist,* P Frost, SN Horwitz, eds. CV Mosby Co., St. Louis, 1984, pp. 70–74.
6. Ziboh VA. Prostaglandins, leukotrienes, and hydroxy fatty acids in epidermis. Sem Derm. 1992;11 (2):114–120.
7. Moy LS. The use of glycolic acids in the treatment of various skin disorders. Communication at 17th Annual Clinical and Scientific Meeting of the American Society for Dermatologic Surgery. Reported in Canadian Medical News, July 27, 1990.
8. Lavker RM, Kaidbey K, Leyden JJ. Effects of topical ammonium lactate on cutaneous atrophy from a potent topical corticosteroid. J Am Acad Dermatol. 1992;26:535–544.
9. Dahl MV, Dahl AC. 12% lactate lotion for the treatment of xerosis. Arch Dermatol. 1983;119:27–30.
10. Buxman M, Hickman J, Ragsdale W, et al. Therapeutic activity of lactate 12% lotion in the treatment of ichthyosis. active vs. vehicle and active vs. a petroleum cream. J Am Acad Dermatol. 1986;15:1253–1258.
11. Vilaplana J. Clinical and non-invasive evaluation of 12% ammonium lactate emulsion for the treatment of dry skin in atopic and non-atopic Subjects. Acta Dermatol Venerol.1992;72:28–33.
12. Wehr FR. A controlled comparative efficacy study of 5% ammonium lactate lotion vs. an emollient control lotion in the treatment of moderate xerosis. J Am Acad Dermatol. 1991;25:849–851.
13. Murad H, Shamban AT, Moy LS, et al. Study shows that acne improves with glycolic acid regimen. Cosmet Dermatol. 1992;5:32–35.
14. Van Scott EJ, Yu RJ. Alpha hydroxy acids:

procedures for use in clinical practice. Cutis. 1989;43:122-128.
15. Griffin TD, Van Scott EJ. The use of pyruvic acid in the treatment of actinic keratoses: a clinical and histopathologic study. Cutis. 1991;47:325-329.
16. Thomas I, Shockman J, Epstein JD. Linear keratosis follicularis: a specific entity? report of a case responding to combined topical retinoid and alpha hydroxy acid therapy. J Am Acad Dermatol. 1989;20:1122-1123.
17. Milton JP, DiGiovanna JJ, Peck JL. Treatment of nevus comedonicus with ammonium lactate lotion. J Am Acad Dermatol. 1989;20:324-328.
18. Alpha hydroxy acids help protect skin; editorial. Am Pharm. 1992;32:26.
19. Burke KE. Facial wrinkles. Prevention and non-surgical correction. Post Grad Med. 1990;88:207-210.
20. Hermitte R. Aged skin, retinoids and alpha hydroxy acids. Cosmet Toilet. 1992;107:63-66.
21. Kligman AM, Grove GL, Hirose R, et al. Topical tretinoin for photoaged skin. J Am Acad Dermatol. 1986;15:836-859.
22. Weiss JR, Ellis CN, Headington JT, et al. Topical tretinoin improves photoaged skin: a double blind vehicle controlled study. JAMA. 1958;4:527-532.
23. Brodell LP, Asselin D, Brodell RT. Reversible ectropion after long term use of topical tretinoin on photodamaged skin. J Am Acad Dermatol. 1992;27:621-622.
24. Dial WF. Preparations prescribed in anti-wrinkling therapy. Cosmet Dermatol. 1990;3:6-7.
25. Merck Index. Merck and Co., Rahway, 1976, pp. 7, 300, and 583.
26. Personal Communication. Steven Hernandez, Pharmagen, Inc., 1992.
27. Asnes M, Malkin N. A skin miracle. Mirabella. 1993; January:60-61.
28. Beauty Report. The acid test for skin. Mademoiselle. 1993;March:102-106.
29. Dial WF. Uses of AHAs add new dimensions to chemical peeling. Cosmet Dermatol. 1990;3:32-34.

5
Chemical Face Peeling

Paul S. Collins

Chemical peeling of the face, also described as chemexfoliation, chemosurgery, and facial surface surgery, may be defined as the application of an irritant chemical solution onto the skin for the purpose of improving or removing facial surface defects. The peeling solution causes a facial burn that results in the partial destruction of the epidermis and dermis, followed by replacement with rejuvenated epidermal and dermal tissues. Ideally, one expects the removal, correction, or improvement of rhytides, lentigines, actinic keratoses, superficial in situ skin cancers, basophilic degeneration of collagen, superficial telangiectasia, pigmentary abnormalities, and skin diseases (acne vulgaris, acne rosacea, seborrheic dermatitis, sebaceous hyperplasia, seborrheic keratoses), with improvement in the quality as well as a tightening of the skin.

History

There has been a remarkable resurgence in interest in chemical peeling during the last several decades. With the marked increase in ultraviolet damage that the average individual has suffered, chemical peeling has offered a ray of hope in eliminating the resultant skin changes. Certainly not a new procedure, it has been practiced since ancient history, as recorded in the Ebers Papyrus, written 3,500 years ago.[1] Early records state that the Egyptians, Assyrians, and Babylonians rubbed pumice on the skin to cause exfoliation. While dermatologists have always been at the forefront of peeling, the procedure is not exclusively practiced by dermatology.

The emergence of peeling during this past century is clouded in legends and secrecy. It is apparent that physicians and nonphysicians alike were aware of not only the cutaneous effects but also the histology of peeling agents.[2] Roberts reported the results when a number of acids were applied to the skin, including trichloroacetic acid (TCA), carbolic acid, and resorcin, ". . . drugs most familiar to dermatologists. . . ." In addition, salicylic acid was also noted as a peeling agent for rosacea. In all likelihood, carbolic acid, while being utilized as an antiseptic on war victims during the 1800s and early 1900s, was noted by astute individuals as improving facial scarring. There are numerous references to lay individuals who treated the face with some unknown peeling agent, with dramatic results.

An article in 1941 discussed the skin peeling procedure for obliterating or lessening cosmetic defects.[3] Peeling was used for treatment of chloasma, marked freckling, excessive oiliness, recalcitrant acne, rosacea, and pitted scars, and to improve the tone of the skin. Eller and Wolff stated that the following chemicals were used for peeling: salicylic acid, resorcinol, phenol, betanaphthol, and solid carbon dioxide. The concern of systemic absorption was noted especially with the use of phenol, and contraindication was recommended in patients with kidney disease. Numerous pastes and lotions were listed. The authors stated that the lotions are easier to apply and that the intensity of skin reaction, along with the depth of peeling, can be controlled by varying the concentration of the solutions and the number and intervals of their applications. Two lotions causing intense inflammation are as noted:

Salicylic acid	6.0%
Phenol	30.0%
Alcohol (95%)	64.0%

The number of applications is determined by the sensitivity of the skin, with a period of observation after the first application. The number of applications should be limited to 4 and given over a period of 1 hour. The second lotion had the following formulation:

	gm or cc
Resorcinol	60.0
Salicylic acid	30.00
Lactic acid	30.0
Oil of Rose	0.195
Ethyl hydrate	240.0

Apply to the entire face with a cotton applicator every 10 minutes for 5 to 8 applications. After the third application, frosting occurs, and after the sixth, swelling. The patient should be well hydrated and should be instructed to drink 5 or 6 glasses of water during the period between applications. This lotion was an adaptation of a peeling paste described by Unna in 1882[4] (Polano) that is still, in some variation, widely used in France for peeling. The original formula is as follows:

Zinc paste	40 gm
Resorcinol	40 gm
Echthammol	10 gm
Petrolatum	10 gm

Unna applied the paste daily for 3 or 4 days until the skin became brown and shriveled. A mask of zinc gelatin (the Unna boot) was then applied and left overnight. The next day the mask and adherent dead skin were lifted off the face and a soothing emollient cream applied. Indications included treatment of wrinkled skin with irregular pigmentation and actinic keratoses.

In 1946 Urkov described his treatment of more than 2,000 patients over a period of 15 years and after considerable experimentation with various exfoliative agents and different techniques of application.[5] He eloquently described the desires and tribulations of chemical peeling: ". . . The degree of exfoliation must be controlled not only to avoid the risk of producing disfigurement more serious than the original defect, but also enable the physician to adjust the treatment in accordance with the severity of that defect. He must be able to produce superficial or deep exfoliation, over small or large areas, as the case requires. . . ." Urkov experimented with various exfoliative agents and different techniques of application before settling on the following formulas.

Superficial exfoliation was achieved with an exfoliative agent composed of:

Salicylic acid 12	gm
Resorcinol	70 gm
Lactic acid (85%)	24 cc
Ethyl alcohol (95%) qs ad	180 cc

The ingredients were allowed to stand 24 hours, then filtered, exposed to ultraviolet light (75 polarity at a distance of 12 inches) for 1 hour, and then bottled. Unused solution was discarded after 10 days. Irradiation apparently produced an effective solution, while the nonirradiated solution was ineffective. The skin was prepared by exposing it to ultraviolet light (75 polarity at 24 inches) for 2 to 3 minutes, producing a mild erythema. Five separate applications of the solution were then made with drying between applications. Twenty minutes after completion, rubberized adhesive tape was applied to increase tissue destruction. The tape was removed 24 hours later, and the skin was covered with powdered zinc stearate (USP) with additional applications for the next 5 days. There was no exposure to water or soap during this time. On the sixth day, a light liquid petrolatum was applied liberally, with complete exfoliation by the following morning. Erythema disappeared in only 4 to 5 days. This regimen is similar to that utilized decades later with the Baker-Litton phenol formula peels.

A deeper exfoliation for deep lines and wrinkles utilized phenol along with electrocautery of the deeper lines and crevices. A mixture of liquefied (88%) phenol and alcohol (30 drops of each) was brushed over the face, followed by electrocautery. Adhesive plaster was applied and removed on the third day. The rest of the procedure was the same as followed with the superficial exfoliation.

Additional documentation of chemical peeling performed by dermatologists since the turn of the century is noted in the literature with the publication in 1952 of a paper by MacKee and Karp.[6] The article described their procedure in utilizing phenol liquefactum U.S.P. to obtain improvement in acne scarring. Histological results were described, reporting the epidermis as flattened, with obliteration of the rete ridges, and the collagen bundles denser and more compact. Urine and blood chemistries revealed only a slight increase in conjugated phenols, "... of low toxicity...." MacKee noted that he had utilized phenol peels since 1903. It is not known from whom he learned this procedure.

Marmelzat expanded on the history behind this publication.[7] He noted that Karp, born in Russia, trained in Switzerland, and who practiced in both Russia and France, was a Parisian emigrant who arrived in the United States in 1936. Under MacKee's chairmanship, Karp established a phenol peeling clinic at the New York Skin and Cancer Hospital in the 1940s. Marmelzat, who trained at the hospital, recorded in his notes several phenol preparations utilized by Karp, including the following:

Phenol crystals	80 parts
Glycerine	10 parts
Water	10 parts

A much stronger preparation was used only on deep scarring, not for the entire face:

Acetic acid	
Boracic acid	
Salicylic acid	
Glycerine	aa 15.00
Citric acid	1.625
Phenol 88% liquefied	q.s. 480.00

A careful history was always obtained to determine if the patient had atopy, kidney, liver, or heart disease. While only patients with scarring were treated, it was noted that the peeling procedure improved fine rhytides, freckles, and various benign keratotic lesions. Marmelzat also outlined the details of the procedure. Karp later developed another formula, which became her treatment of choice and was named the "Phoenix Formula":

	gm or cc
Acetic acid	0.3
Sodium salicylate	1.0
Glycerine	2.0
Water	1.0
Phenol crystals	30.0

It was during the end of the 1950s that interest in chemical peeling rapidly gained popularity for treatment of wrinkles, pigmentation, and scarring. Two lines of peeling agents gained popularity during this time. Phenol gained its popularity due to the dramatic results it could obtain with the aged face; while trichloroacetic acid, not as dramatic an agent, offered simplicity and minimal pain for adequate results and improvement of actinic changes. It was not until the 1980s that we encountered the widespread use of additional peeling agents as well as the simultaneous use of multiple peeling agents to achieve more dramatic results with less pain and fewer complications.

LaGasse, a lay operator, practiced facial phenol peeling in the Los Angeles area during the 1930s and 1940s. She used a formula that she had brought from Europe.[8] LaGasse's father was a French physician who, during World War I, treated powder burns on the faces of soldiers with phenol solutions. Apparently, this was a common treatment at the time. Scars, blemishes, and other cutaneous disfigurements, when treated with the phenol solution and covered with an adhesive tape, healed with cosmetic improvement. The elder LaGasse refined the formula and technique in his private practice after the war. The younger LaGasse worked as a nurse in his office and brought the formula and technique with her when she immigrated to the United States. Gross and Maschek modified her technique and reported peeling approximately 3,000 patients.[8] They described multiple phenol formulas and stated that all were adequate for peeling.

In 1960 Brown, Kaplan, and Brown published their experience on peeling with a phenol solution.[9] They recorded the death of a surgeon's wife who underwent a phenol peel by a lay operator and that of another individual at the hands of yet another lay operator, as reported by the local newspaper. The deaths were attributed to the application of phenol to large skin areas. By varying phenol concentration and surface tension, the penetrating power and toxicity of the solution could be controlled (in general, the lower the phenol concentration and surface tension, the greater the penetration). Surface tension could be controlled by adding soap or bentonite or minute amounts of oil. They described the quintessential use of the phenol peel, the ablation of fine rhytides, which was not amenable to facelifting. Microscopic exam postpeel revealed the collagenous fibers to have become stratified, or laminated, and compacted.

The typical formula utilized was:

Phenol	60% to 95%
Saponate solution of cresol	0.3%
Olive oil or sesame oil	0.25%
Distilled water, q.s.	100%

These proportions are by volume. If the test area behind the ear developed ulceration, the solution was buffered with the addition of oil, added in increments of 0.5%, but not more than a total of 10%. Potency was increased with the increment addition of either phenol or saponated cresol. Once the appropriate solution was chosen, the patient was sedated and the face divided into 5 treatment zones. After each zone was coated, it was taped with a rubber or plastic adhesive tape that was impermeable. Application required 2 days, with an interval of at least 2 hours between zones. The tape was removed no sooner than 48 hours and the skin dusted with antiseptic powder. The dead epithelium took 1 week to peel off.

Combes, Sperber, and Reisch in 1960 declared that their "buffered" phenol formula had less irritating qualities, offering their patented formula for purchase.[10] This formula was not revealed until 1964:

Sodium salicylate	0.3 gm
Powdered citric acid	0.3 gm
Glycerine	4.0 cc
Water	1.0 cc
Anhydrous (99.5%) phenol crystals	30.0 gm

The success of this formula was overwhelmed by the acceptance of the phenol formula that Baker published in 1961:[11]

Phenol	5 cc
Distilled water	4 cc
Croton oil	3 drops
Septisol	5 drops

It was modified in 1961 to the following most popular phenol peel formula:[12]

Phenol	3 cc
Distilled water	2 cc
Croton oil	2 drops
Septisol	8 drops

Baker states that it was the considerable attention given to the chemical peels performed in secret by nonprofessional people during the 1950s that brought them to his attention.

During the same time, Litton was utilizing a similar phenol formula for peeling.[13] The formula was presented at the meeting of the American Society of Plastic and Reconstructive Surgeons in New Orleans in September 1961.

Liquefy one pound of phenol crystals by heating in warm water until melted, and adding 8 cc of distilled water and 8 cc of glycerin. Stir well. Take 4 oz. of liquefied phenol and 1 cc of croton oil. Stir well.

Into an 8 oz. bottle, place 4 oz. of distilled water, and then add the phenol and croton oil mixture. Shake well before applying.

Over the ensuing years, Baker's and Litton's formulas became the most popular of the phenol peeling formulas utilized. This is probably attributed to their willingness to share their formulas and their experiences with peeling.

Ayres described his use of trichloroacetic acid for treatment of actinically damaged skin utilizing concentrations of 25% to 50% and occasionally, with greater caution, even 75% to full-strength concentrations.[14,15] He obtained good results with the treatment of fine, delicate wrinkles with 1 or 2 treatment sessions. Patients with relatively deep rhytides of the upper lip or below the eyes were treated with 2 or more sessions, at intervals of 1 to several months, for optimal improvement. There was no set scheme of concentration used because of the wide variation in individuals' skin, area treated, and age. Ayres warned that 50% TCA can produce scarring on the face. The utilization of superficial chemosurgery and local dermabrasion for deeper lesions achieved more significant results.[15] The addition of superficial chemosurgery produced a blending of areas that were difficult to abrade, such as along the hairline, nose, and lips.

A formula used by Ayres with less risk than 50% TCA was a combination of two major peeling agents:

Phenol	⅓
Trichloroacetic acid	⅓
Alcohol	⅓

This resulted in a moderate peel, not a deep peel, as was expected with Baker's or Litton's formula. Many other variations of phenol peeling agents have been described. Arohnson gave us his formulation in 1971 to be used for lighter peels and without taping:[16]

Phenol 88%	15.0 cc
Anhydrous glycerine	1.25 cc
Ethanol	0.5 cc

In the 1980s the concept of light-, medium-, and deep-depth peels emerged, along with the use of enhancers to obtain deeper peels, but without the dangers of utilizing more potent peeling agents or solutions. Collins, in 1985[17] and 1987,[18] emphasized the importance of repetitive peeling to obtain deeper inflammation with less risk, and thus the fact that TCA could be utilized to produce a superficial and a deeper peel. He noted that these peeling depths were to be differentiated from the still deeper penetration obtained by the Baker and Litton phenol formulas. Brody and Hailey expanded this concept with the introduction of combining two peeling agents (solid carbon dioxide and trichloroacetic acid) to obtain a medium-depth chemical peel.[19] They were able to obtain a peeling depth comparable to a much stronger acid (60% TCA) but without the inherent dangers of the stronger acid. Monheit reported on his experience with the combined use of Jessner's solution and TCA.[20] The Jessner's solution is used as an "absorbing agent" to enhance the effectiveness of a less concentrated solution of TCA. Jessner's formula is as follows:

Resorcinol	14 gm
Salicylic acid	14 gm
Lactic acid (85%)	14 cc
Ethyl Alcohol (95%) qs ad	100 cc

Recently, Coleman reported the use of glycolic acid as another enhancing agent for TCA peels.[21] Many physicians advocate the use of retinoic acid for several weeks prior to peeling, to enhance the depth of penetration and to allow an even depth of peeling. The reasoning for the use of retinoic acid is based on the fact that it will strip the stratum corneum of loose cells and debris, increase blood flow, and stimulate new collagen formation.

The use of *enhancers* or *absorbers*, which may be defined as substances added to, or used prior to, a peeling agent to increase its effectiveness, has been studied extensively by Fulton.[22] He tested a variety of substances added to TCA, including croton oil, phenol, saponin, salicylic acid, and alpha hydroxy acids, on the rabbit ear to determine their degree of TCA potential. The following formula was deemed ideal:

Trichloroacetic acid	30 gm
Distilled water (mix until dissolved)	64 gm
Polysorbate 20 (mix)	1 gm
Methyl salicylate (mix well before using)	5 gm

Although not without some complications—herpes simplex flares, postinflammatory hyperpigmentation, skin infection—no scarring was reported.

Alpha hydroxy acids, as a facial peeling agent, gained popularity during the late 1980s, although initially use was limited for other conditions during the previous decade.[23] Their utilization, specifically that of glycolic acid, has proliferated due to ease of application, relative lack of both complications and morbidity, and the improvement seen with the treatment of facial skin diseases such as acne. The use of glycolic acid in self-applied creams and lotions attests to its relative lack of complications.[24] It has also become a cornerstone in combination treatments for the aging face.[25]

The future development of chemical peeling in all likelihood will not produce a single agent that will be a panacea for all facial skin-aging changes. It is also doubtful that any one single peeling solution or procedure will dominate the field. The utilization of enhancers or accelerators to maximize peeling depth while minimizing complications of scarring will proliferate. Repetitive peeling will remain a viable method for obtaining satisfactory results with minimal morbidity and risk. The combined utilization of different peeling-depth solutions remains an alternative for areas that are relatively resistant to improvement.

Peeling Agents and Methods

The Chemistry of Peeling Ingredients

Phenol

Phenol exists as a crystal in its pure state. Phenol (C_6H_5OH) OH

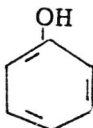

or carbolic acid (hydroxybenzene, oxybenzene, phenic acid, and phenylic acid are other names for the same substance) is an aromatic organic hydrocarbon derived from benzene and obtained from the distillation of coal tar. The addition of 10% water converts it into a clear liquid. Liquefied phenol (phenol liquefactum) USP is an aqueous solution of phenol containing not less than 89% by weight of phenol. Since the formula does not contain the carboxyl (COOH) group, it is at variance with the structural characteristics of organic acids. This hydroxyl group indicates that it is closer to being an organic base or alcohol rather than an acid.

Liquefied phenol USP is a protein precipitant and keratocoagulant, causing extremely rapid denaturation and coagulation of the surface keratin. Phenol denatures the surface keratin proteins, loosely combining with them to form larger molecules with different physical and chemical properties. This coagulum becomes a protective barrier to further phenol penetration into the dermis. At concentrations over 80%, phenol is a keratocoagulant, precipitating the surface protein and thus preventing an extension of the peel solution into the deeper layers of the skin.[26] Thus, increasing the concentration enhances the keratocoagulation and hinders dermal penetration. Conversely, when phenol is diluted, deeper penetration and greater systemic absorption occurs, increasing the danger of adverse reactions. This is because at a 50% dilution, phenol becomes keratolytic, disrupting sulfur bridges in the keratin layer and causing greater dermal destruction. Therefore, dilution of phenol with water makes the resultant mixture stronger and more toxic systemically, not weaker. It is the keratolytic ability of phenol that allows it to penetrate for greater effectiveness without an unacceptable incidence of scarring.

Phenol is an extremely stable compound. Litton[13] and Wexler and others[27] noted that after phenol is absorbed into the bloodstream, it is rapidly conjugated with gluceronic acid or sulfuric acid and excreted as such by the kidneys, or it is detoxified by oxidation to hydroquinone or pyrocatechin. It can also remain as free phenol in the bloodstream and be excreted by the kidneys. Phenol toxicity symptoms include central depression, fallen blood pressure, headache, and/or nausea. There can be a direct effect on the blood vessels of the myocardium, which usually causes the fallen blood pressure. Pure phenol is a protoplasmic poison particularly affecting the central nervous system. It is readily absorbed from all mucous membranes, wounds, and intact skin.[28]

Trichloroacetic Acid

Trichloroacetic acid is a chemical cauterant that coagulates the proteins of the skin. As the concentration of the acid increases, the depth of dermal damage increases, as evidenced by edema, cellular infiltration, and necrosis. It is concentration-dependent, with greater concentrations resulting in greater tissue damage. The acid is eventually neutralized, and the barrier produced from the protein coagulant prevents further destruction, even if the acid is not diluted or neutralized (see Figures 5.1A and B). Concentrations of TCA above 50% can result in extensive necrosis and the inability for normal tissue regeneration to occur. The ability of different regions of facial tissue to regenerate after a TCA cutaneous burn varies, as evidenced by eyelid tissue recovery after treatment of xanthelasma with 80% TCA.

Trichloroacetic acid has no systemic absorption and, therefore, no systemic toxicity. It is less melanotoxic than phenol and thus unlikely

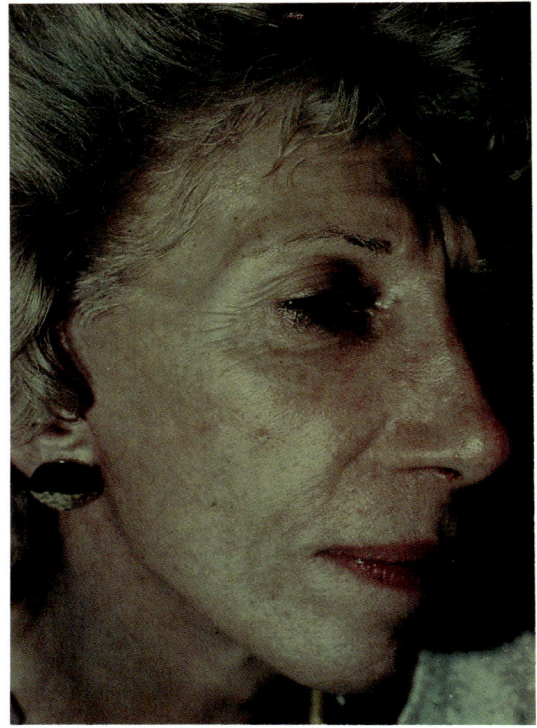

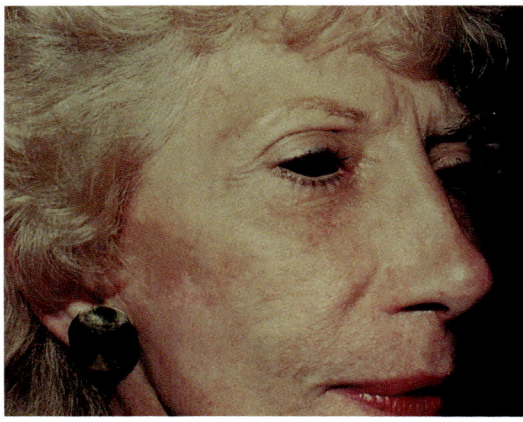

FIGURE 5.1. A. Trichloroacetic acid 35% peel. Preoperative photograph demonstrating fine wrinkling of the periorbital region, scattered actinic lentigines, and actinic pallor of the facial skin. B Postoperative after a single 35%. There are diminution of fine rhytides, elimination of lentigines, and a brightening of the facial skin.

to produce a permanent bleaching of the skin. TCA is stable in glass- or acid-resistant plastic containers for at least 2 years. The correct TCA formula is based on a weight in volume method:

$$\frac{\text{TCA USP(crystals) 35g}}{\text{Distilled water qs a.d. 100 ml}}$$

This is a true 35% (W/V) and the formulation one should utilize for TCA peeling solutions.

Alpha Hydroxy Acids

The alpha hydroxy acids include glycolic and lactic acids as well as malic, tartaric, gluconic, and citric acids. Pyruvic acid, which is a keto acid, is the most potent, followed by glycolic acid and then lactic acid. All will reduce corneocyte cohesion and thus facilitate desquamation. Glycolic and pyruvic acids can be formulated at higher strengths, which will reduce keratinocyte cohesion to a degree that results in epidermolysis. Both glycolic and pyruvic acids seem to penetrate readily through the stratum corneum (see Figures 5.2A and B). Alpha hydroxy acids block hyperkeratosis, maintain a smoother skin surface, keep follicular canals from being occluded, and restrain the development of various types of dermatoses. The tissue reaction to AHA is said to be time-dependent rather than concentration-dependent; therefore, in general, the greater the time exposure, the greater the effects. Glycolic acid can be diluted with water or ethanol, whereas pyruvic acid must be diluted with 100% ethanol.

Resorcin

Resorcin, resorcinol or *m* dihyroxybenzene, is a phenol derivative having keratolytic properties and precipitates cutaneous proteins. It reputedly has 1/40th the strength of phenolic acid. Resorcin separates the stratum corneum and the most superficial layers of the epidermis from the deeper ones. The split occurs in the stratum granulosum.[29] Histologically, there are superficial epidermal separation, increased mitoses of the stratum germinativum, and increased glycosamines in the intercellular spaces, all resulting in a thicker epidermis. Dermal changes include prolonged vasodilatation and proliferation of fibroblasts, with increased fibrillar collagen producing a thickening of the papillary dermis.

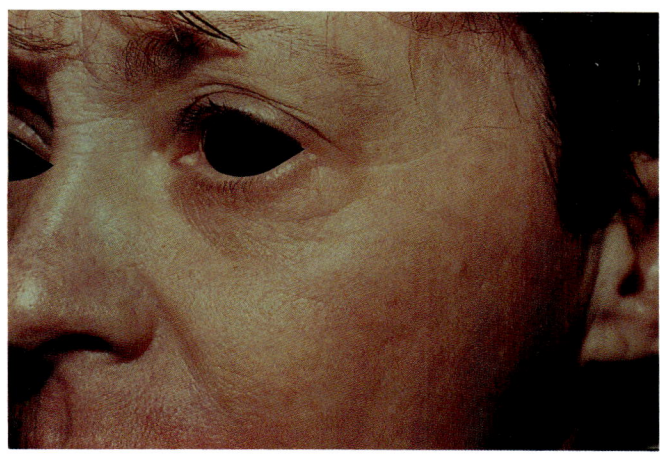

FIGURE 5.2. A. Combination trichloroacetic acid and glycolic acid peels. Periorbital fine rhytides with actinic pallor of the facial skin. B. Repetitive light peels with 70% glycolic acid and 20% TCA with minimal frosting of the skin. The peels were repeated every 2 to 4 weeks over a period of 6 months.

Baker's and Litton's Phenol Formulas

Baker's and Litton's formulas contain four substances: phenol, croton oil, water, and an emulsifier—either glycerol (in Litton's) or septisol (in Baker's). The liquefied phenol is diluted to approximately a 50% concentration by the addition of distilled water. This converts the phenolic reaction from keratocoagulation to keratolytic. Croton oil is a commercially prepared extract of the seed from the plant *Croton tiglium*. It is a viscous liquid capable of causing significant skin injury, including inflammation, desiccation, and collagen destruction.[13] It irritates the skin and causes additional maceration. This allows consistent penetration of the phenol through the epidermis. Septisol, a liquid soap, reduces surface tension and aids penetration of the phenol and croton oil into the skin. Glycerol is miscible with water, dilutes the phenol, and keeps the formula in solution.

Jessner's Solution

The formulation of resorcinol, salicylic acid, and lactic acid was created to lower the concentration of each agent (and the incidence of toxicity) and to intensify the effects as a keratolytic, exfoliant, and protein coagulant. Jessner's solution is thought to break the intercellular bridges between keratinocytes and thus destroy the barrier function of the epidermis. By itself Jessner's solution will produce a partial epidermal exfoliation that heals within 3 days. When used as an absorber, these actions remove the epidermis as a barrier for the penetration of TCA. A 35% TCA concentration can thus penetrate deeper into the papillary dermis. Its destructive burn induces new collagen formation, which accounts for whatever degree of lessening of wrinkles or improved texture is seen after a peel.[20]

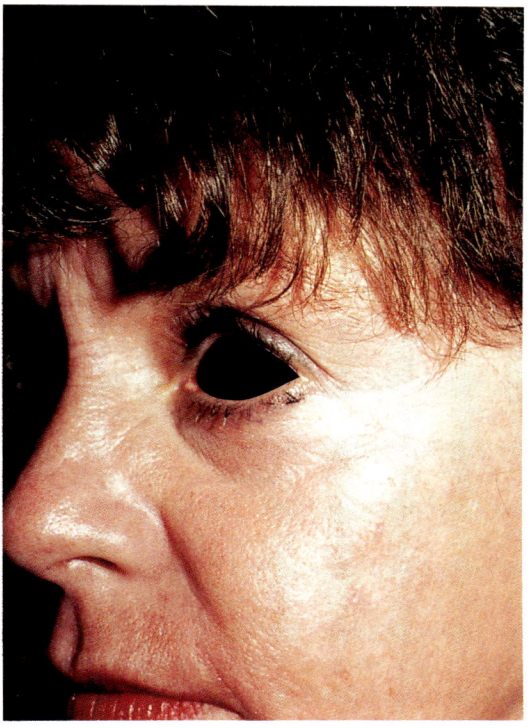

Histology

While there are several excellent histological studies demonstrating the depth of destruction or burn obtained by a peeling agent, none address the full spectrum of variability seen in skin thickness, adnexal density, aging, actinic changes, and other factors. To be fair, none probably ever will, due to the multiple factors that must be accounted for. Therefore, an examination of the findings produced must be correlated with the quality of skin to be peeled in the particular patient. Peeling is not an all-or-nothing accomplishment but is laced with nuances that can add or subtract from the ultimate result. The importance lies with the reality that some individuals will respond with a deeper burn than that expected for the peeling agent utilized. What results in an excellent peel in one patient may produce disastrous results in another. Therefore, know what the peeling agent is capable of producing and adjust according to the skin to be treated.

The histologic findings after treatment with phenol have been documented by numerous authors.[14,30-32] Immediately after application there is necrosis of tissue with homogenization replete with ghost cells. This is followed by massive edema and neutrophilic invasion. The intensity of the inflammatory response varies, with the taped phenol resulting in the greatest response. A thin crust of keratin, necrotic epidermis, and a proteinaceous precipitate interspersed with a cellular exudate forms at the surface. Dermal thickening secondary to the inflammatory response and intercellular edema then is replaced by a fibroblastic proliferation and finally deposition of collagen. The deposition of collagen is in a wide band, and within the collagen bundles, numerous, fine, new elastin fibers develop.

Stegman reported his findings comparing the effects of several peeling agents and dermabrasion on normal and sun-damaged skin, with the 1980 study performed on guinea pigs and the 1982 study based on the results from the neck of a 55-year-old male.[33,34] Significantly, his studies showed that phenol is dose-dependent and does not produce an all-or-nothing reaction; and, in guinea pig skin, the effects on normal and sun damaged skin are similar. Overall the wound was deeper in sun-damaged skin.

Baker's phenol formula, occluded and non-occluded, resulted in necrotic but intact epidermis and massive edema of the entire dermis (see Figures 5.3A, B, and C). Phenol, under occlusion, resulted in necrosis to a deeper level, with cellular infiltration and edema extending deeper into the reticular dermis with a slower recovery. The addition of croton oil resulted in a deeper injury. Trichloroacetic acid, 40% and 60%, did not produce complete necrosis of the epidermis but did induce edema, cellular infiltrate, and changes in the staining of collagen. These more shallow wounds crusted more quickly and formed a lighter crust than the deeper wound produced by phenol. The greater the damage, the more likely abnormal elastin in the papillary dermis was removed and damaged collagen was replaced by new collagen, with glycosaminoglycans completely removed.[35] This was most evident with phenol. Therefore, the main difference noted among the various peeling solutions was the depth of inflammation produced, with the most effective solutions creating inflammation into the deep reticular dermis.

It was believed that the use of phenol resulted in the destruction of melanocytes. In a long-term histological study by Kligman and his associates, melanocytes were found to be present and even spottily increased.[36] Melanin was still being synthesized and passed to the surrounding epithelial cells. Phenol causes hypopigmentation and not depigmentation. This is obvious as some phenol-peeled patients can still develop lentigines and splotchy pigmentation when overexposed to the sun. The skin alterations of a new, wide band of dermis with horizontally arranged compact collagen bundles, regenerated elastin fibers, a normalization of the epidermis with basal layer of columnar cells without cellular irregularities, and a PAS basement membrane of uniform thickness and staining seen soon after the peel, remain for decades when compared to nonpeeled skin in the same patient. They noted that within this reconstruction zone the small vessels appeared to be normal and telangiectatic vessels were confined to the deep dermis, not removed by the peel. Significantly, the benefits of peeling were found to be more than cosmetic. There was a marked decrease in the rate of appearance of new neoplasms in peeled versus non

5. Chemical Face Peeling

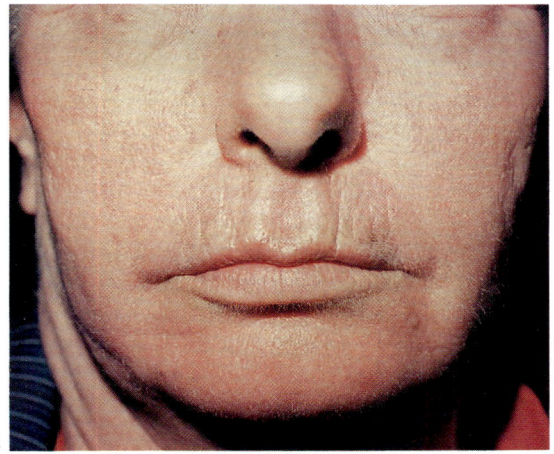

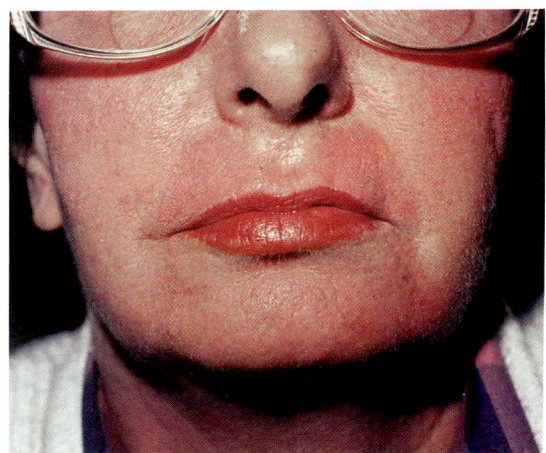

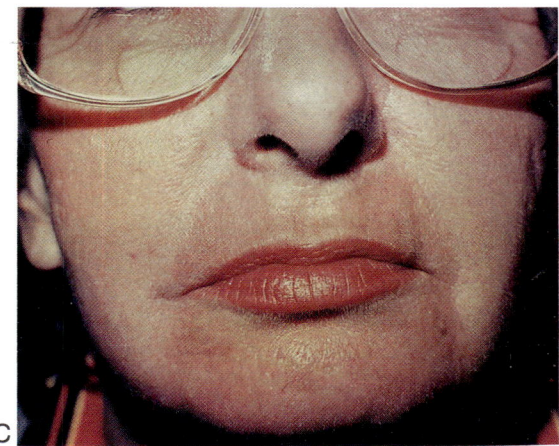

FIGURE 5.3. A. Phenol formula peel (Baker's) of the upper lip. Multiple deep rhytides with basophilic degeneration of collagen. B. Good improvement with postinflammatory erythema commonly seen with phenol peels. C. At 3 months the erythema is fading. Now the difference in skin quality between the lip and cheek is obvious. Peeling the face with 25% or 35% trichloroacetic acid will lessen the difference in skin quality.

peeled skin. The effects of this last observation have been reported by several authors.[14,28]

The effects of alpha hydroxy acids in low concentrations are limited to diminishing corneocyte adhesion and the subsequent prevention of stratum corneum thickening.[37] This effect predominantly occurs among the cells at the lower levels of the stratum corneum, with no effect on the cells of the outer layers. Applied to the skin in higher concentrations, AHAs cause detachment of the keratinocytes, epidermolysis with epidermal separation and edema, and inflammatory response of the papillary and upper reticular dermis. Glycolic acid promotion of new collagen and cellular DNA is not dependent on a marked dermal inflammatory response.[38]

Griffin and Van Scott reported pyruvic acid 60% produced a thinner epidermis with efface-ment of the rete ridges, consistent with a reepithelialized epidermis.[39] At 2 weeks there was a mild lymphohistiocytic infiltrate in the papillary dermis and the formation of edematous cellular new collagen. Between the third and eighth week a thin band of denser, more eosinophilic collagen was present. This thin band of new collagen in the papillary dermis represents healing in response to injury.

Peeling Techniques

There have been and are countless protocols for peeling the face. Each peeling nuance is done in the belief that it must be the correct and optimal approach to accomplish the goal desired. Selection of a peeling solution and technique of application should be based on the patient, the patient's schedule, the quality and color of the facial skin, the pathology, and the skin preparation. Each patient should be viewed as unique and a treatment regimen planned. This does not mean that a routine cannot be followed with most patients, only that the physician must recognize patient variation requiring an individualized plan of attack. The greater the number of techniques and peeling solutions the physician is familiar with, the wider the spectrum of patient selection and treatment plans that can be utilized for satisfactory results.

Preparation of the skin is, and remains, important. Unless superficial debris, oils, cosmetics, and moisturizers are removed, one cannot expect a uniform effect from the peeling agent. Traditionally, preparation was just prior to the peel and involved vigorous debridement of the skin with a degreasing agent such as acetone or ether. The skin was literally abraded during the cleansing. Recently, the tendency has shifted from a less vigorous attempt at physical cleansing to the use of preoperative adjuncts, accelerators, or enhancers. These include the use of retinoic acid, Jessner's solution, glycolic acid, solid carbon dioxide, topical ascorbic acid, Accutane, and other agents. Some of these are used for several weeks prior to the peel, while others are applied to the skin immediately prior to the peeling solution. The purpose remains the same: preparation of the skin to enable a uniform peel while utilizing a less potent peeling agent to obtain substantial results without the additional risk of scarring. Some of the reputed differences or effectiveness of the prepeel preparation may be anecdotal. It was reported in a double-blind study that tretinoin, applied for 2 weeks prior to peeling, accelerated recovery after a TCA peel.[40] While this led to greater patient satisfaction, the authors could not find any difference between pretreated and nontreated skin.

There are other factors, besides the cleansing of skin and preoperative preparation, that are essential in peeling. The different qualities of skin—including thinness, atrophy, degree of actinic damage, types and location of rhytides (fine or deep, periorbital, perioral, glabellar, forehead, nasal, cheek), sebaceousness and skin tone—must be evaluated. The method of application of the peeling solution and the addition of peeling enhancers can result in widely divergent results. Application of the solution can vary with the utilization of Q-tips or gauze sponge. The total number of wipes or rubs the solution is applied, the total number of reapplications of the solution, the time duration of application, the degree of frosting (light, medium, or heavy), the time span allowed until dilution or neutralization, the agent utilized for dilution or neutralization, and the immediate postoperative treatments are all additional important factors in determining peel results. Repetitive peels, done at intervals of several weeks to months, result in continued inflammation of the dermis, which can lead to dermal restoration because of new collagen formation. All these factors should be noted and recorded, enabling the physician to determine and follow a set, reproducible course for the same specific type of skin.

The art of application is also important, specifically to avoid potential complications. The peeling solution should always be brought around, never over or across the face, to the region treated. The patient's eyes should be closed to prevent accidental or careless spillage onto the cornea. A readily available eye irrigating solution is indispensable for these hopefully rare accidents. Tearing is quickly mopped with a dry, unused sponge, which is then discarded (during sponging, acid may be absorbed and, if the sponge is reused, possibly applied directly to the eyelids; since the upper eyelids are exposed when shut, excess acid can produce a significant burn). Tearing can also allow retrograde flow of the peeling solution into the conjunctiva and onto the cornea. A small fan will alleviate some of the discomfort of the burn. It will also provide air circulation when phenol is utilized and minimize patient, as well as medical personnel, inhalation of the vapors.

A special note should be made for the perioral region, a common area requested for improvement. The patient desires all the rhytides to be removed from the region while puckering to emphasize their presence. Unfortunately, some women suffer not only from rhytides but also from significant subcutaneous atrophy of the surrounding perioral tissues. It is reputed that perioral rhytides are more prominent and common in females because of the male–female difference in pronunciation of sounds (women pucker more readily while speaking as well as during eating), and the lack of density of upper lip hair in females results in the lack of subcutaneous support with aging. When subcutaneous atrophy is prominent, there are not only numerous rhytides, but also the entire perioral region is sunken. This creates a formidable problem that is not easily corrected by a chemical peel, even if a phenol formula is utilized. The sunken, depressed subcutaneous tissues naturally accordion the surface, aggravating the depth and number of rhytides present. Unless the subcutaneous tissue atrophy is corrected, improvement will be short of the desired effect. Restoration of the previous subcutaneous bulk is required prior to the chemical peel for optimal results.

It is important to realize that a chemical peel is a surgical procedure and as such should be treated with similar protocol. The patient should be given material (preferably written) outlining the procedure; its potential abilities, inadequacies, and pitfalls; and common complications, recovery time, and postoperative care. A consent form should be read, any questions answered, and the form signed and witnessed. In addition, photographs should be obtained for deeper peels and, if warranted, medium or even light peels. Pigmentary problems, scars and notable skin changes should also be photographed and documented for possible future use. Many patients soon forget the severity of the original problem and may question the effectiveness of their treatment. This is a greater problem with dermabrasion than with chemical peeling, but in any case, photo documentation often awakens forgotten memories to the physician's advantage. Patients undergoing a phenol peel may require a medical clearance for surgery as well as blood chemistries (specifically for renal and hepatic function) and an electrocardiogram. Finally, note your findings, the patient's desires, probable results and failures, and the plan of action in the chart. It becomes a valuable reference point for future treatment and care. Specifically, record the procedure, including preoperative care, preoperative medications, type of peel, details of region variation in the peel, and the routine for postoperative care. All telephone calls can be easily documented by answering only if the chart is present. Your personnel should know that they must first have the patient's chart available before the physician will answer a call. Note all missed appointments or failures of the patient to follow the instructions or care recommended. This is especially important when it involves postoperative ultraviolet light exposure, the most common cause of postpeel pigmentation. This entire routine, while affording the physician protection, is to regimen the peel procedure and to minimize omissions in patient treatment and care.

As alluded to previously, there are numerous solutions and pastes that are effective peeling agents. The ensuing discussion will focus on three peeling agents: phenol, trichloroacetic acid, and alpha hydroxy acids, specifically glycolic acid. One should realize that although only a limited number of peeling agents are discussed, the general principles and complications can be extrapolated to any peeling agent.

Phenol Peels

This author has little doubt that a phenol formula peel, specifically one employing either Baker's or Litton's formula, produces the most dramatic results of any single procedure for the aging face. Remarkable denouements can be observed in individuals exhibiting decades of facial actinic radiation abuse supplemented by the effects of smoking. Not only are rhytides, both superficial and deep, amendable, but there is also a tightening and condensing of the skin, which is drawn back, at times snugly, over the bony facial frame. Skin tightening is to be expected, but there is a limit. It is not a therapy or substitute for surgical procedures designed for treatment of sagging skin and skin folds. It will also dissolve severe actinic dermatitis and associated lentigines, basophilic degeneration of collagen, actinic lentigines, actinic keratoses, superficial epitheliomas, and squamous cell carcinomas in situ.[36]

Unfortunately, many individuals are not ideal candidates and the procedure carries some inherent problems and risks. It can be a very painful procedure that, for some individuals, requires heavy sedation when the full face is peeled. Phenol is also cardiotoxic. The use of intravenous sedation and application of a cardiotoxin often dictates cardiac and respiratory monitoring and the assistance of an anesthesiologist or anesthetist. Some physicians maintain the patient in an overnight facility where pain and sedative medication can be administered under supervision. Certainly, phenol peels are being performed without the above paraphernalia, as they have been for several decades. Regional peels do not require sophisticated monitoring and are not usually associated with extraordinary pain and discomfort. Phenol will eventually produce a porcelainlike appearance to the skin. This may not eventuate until many months later. Cosmetics are usually needed to add color to the skin. It is imperative that the patient avoid excessive solar exposure to prevent further actinic damage to skin that now has a reduced capacity to tolerate solar radiation.

The ideal patient is a fair-skinned woman, with actinic changes compounded by the effects of smoking, resulting in a face that is etched with multiple fine rhytides, lentigines, and associated actinic dermatitis. She should use or be willing to use cosmetic makeup, as she will need to do so after the peel. Darkly tanned individuals may be unsuitable, due to the pigment color differential that will be produced at the neck and the necessity to avoid excessive solar exposure postpeel. Unless the lifestyle is changed, the eventual porcelain color can be a harsh contrast that will be impossible for the patient to deal with. Men can also obtain good results, but with reservations. Male skin is thicker due to the presence of beard. It also tends to be significantly more sebaceous than a woman's. The sebaceousness can hinder penetration, and the final depth of penetration obtained with the phenol solution may not be adequate when the dermis is so thick. A thick neck beard can, however, be helpful with blending, if the physician zig-zags the solution onto the neck to minimize a line of demarcation. Skin color is especially important in male patients because of the reluctance to utilize makeup. If the patient exhibits significant sebaceous hyperplasia, treat this condition first with electrodesiccation at a separate date prior to the peel.

The consultation for a phenol peel differs from that of other peel consultations in several aspects. It is imperative that the patient and any supporting personnel fully comprehend the expected course. They must realize that pain is to be expected for the first 8 to 24 hours and that medications often will not completely alleviate the pain. Grotesque edema of the entire face, at times so intense that the swelling closes the eyes shut, is common after the first 24 to 48 hours and will remain for several days. The appearance of the facial skin will mimic a severe burn but will heal without scarring. Uninformed individuals may construe the resultant state as requiring medical intervention and seek inappropriate care and advice. Most medical personnel are not familiar with the progression of a phenol peel and may panic unduly.

Patients must be evaluated and screened for myocardial, hepatic, and renal disease because of the systemic absorption and toxicity of phenol and the utilization of anesthetics and narcotics during and subsequent to the procedure. Evaluation may necessitate a medical clearance as well as blood chemistries and an electrocardiogram. Systemic absorption of phenol can occur either through the skin or respiratory tract, resulting in toxicity, the most immediate danger being cardiac arrhythmias. Once absorbed, 25% of phenol is metabolized to carbon dioxide and water and excreted through the lungs. The bulk (75%) of phenol, however, is excreted by the kidneys either unchanged or conjugated with glycuronic or sulfuric acid.[41] Liver detoxification also occurs with the conversion of phenol to hydroquinone and pyrocatechol. Phenol is a myocardial toxin that can produce arrhythmias even in patients with normal electrocardiograms.[42,43] Renal, myocardial, or hepatic disease patients can be unsuitable candidates for a full face phenol peel if their ability to detoxify and excrete phenol is seriously compromised or if the myocardium is unduly sensitive to toxins. This still provides the physician the option of regional peels with minimal exposure to phenol.

Renal excretion is vital to detoxification, and an adequately hydrated patient with normal renal function reduces toxicity. Intravenous hydration with 500 ml of Ringer's lactate prior to peeling, with an additional 500 to 1000 ml during and after, enhances phenol excretion. If during cardiac monitoring an arrhythmia is noted, continued application of phenol should be stopped, intravenous hydration be increased, and the arrhythmia be appropriately treated. Transient arrhythmias need no treatment other than observation and prolongation or possibly discontinuation of the peel process.

Full face phenol peels have been performed utilizing an assortment of anesthesia, ranging from simple oral pain relievers to general anesthesia. Pain will occur, and the duration and intensity are widely variable. Some patients will have pain for only a few hours, while others can be uncomfortable for several days. The intensity may be severe, uncontrollable by oral or intramuscular narcotics. Certainly, patients who experience intolerable pain will not easily forget the experience and are apt to relate the unpleasant experience to others, thus discouraging potential candidates. Amnestic anesthesia, such as with midazolam, while not eliminating the resultant pain, will eliminate the unpleasant memories. With utilization of more potent anesthesia, monitoring of respiratory and cardiac function takes on a greater priority. The assistance of an anesthetist or anesthesiologist can facilitate the procedure and increase patient comfort.

Controversy exists as to whether the phenol formula should be freshly mixed prior to each peel or whether a previously solution, properly stored in an amber bottle and out of direct sunlight, can be used. The simplicity of the Baker's solution facilitates rapid formulation prior to peeling. The formulation results in a solution volume of approximately 6 cc, the remainder of which after a peel is scarcely worth storing. In contrast, Litton's peel formulation will produce a substantial volume that can be stored. The author has used the same store Litton's phenol formula for several years without obvious variation in results.

The most common indication for a phenol peel is widespread, deep rhytides, especially those in the perioral region, and the physician accordingly should avail his or her efforts to obtain the maximal potential benefits. Skin preparation still requires meticulous cleansing of the skin and the depths of all rhytides. The rhytides are stretched out and vigorously scrubbed of all debris, oils, and cosmetics utilizing acetone or a similar degreasing agent. The solution is either mixed or, if stored, first shaken thoroughly and then poured into a wide-mouthed beaker. The phenol formula in the beaker must be carefully mixed prior to each application because the solution does not stay in suspension but quickly separates. Cotton-tipped applicators are stirred into the solution, rolled along the beaker to eliminate excess and the possibility of dripping, and then brought to the area to be peeled. The applicators should never cross over the patient's face, thus eliminating the possibility of accidental spillage on the skin or periorbital region. The solution is carefully rubbed into the region, with the skin stretched, for uniform application, especially into the depths of all rhytides. A uniform frosting of the skin will eventuate. This frosting need not occur immediately, even with an adequate application. The physician must not be hasty and reapply too much solution.

The face is always divided into peeling units, with each additional unit peeled only after an appropriate time interval. This lengthens the total time of the surgical procedure, maximizing the time between applications while minimizing the blood concentration of phenol. The face may be divided into forehead, right cheek, left cheek, perioral and chin, and nasal and periorbital regions, with the entire procedure approximately 60 minutes in duration. The physician must blend the peel into adjacent areas. The initial frosting eventuates into a rubber, dusky red in color, accompanied with edema and vesiculation. Swelling soon follows.

The solution should be rubbed into the hairline and brows; it will not affect hair growth or color. The peel is continued onto the mucosa of the lips and the nasal columella and alar rims. The earlobes are also peeled, as is the skin immediately behind the lower ear. The solution is applied to the upper neck (above a line perpendicular to the thyroid cartilage, but with light strokes, in a zig-zag pattern and incompletely, preventing excess burning of the neck while minimizing the development of a demarcation line along the mandible). Some physicians may feel more comfortable utilizing trichloroacetic acid, 25% or 35%, in peeling the upper neck.

Improvements of the perioral rhytides is an important aspect of phenol peels. It is imperative that the physician meticulously apply the solution to each rhytid and the border of the mucosal lip. The border of the mucosal lip often had advanced changes, with basophilic degeneration of collagen as well as deep rhytides that actually extend not only onto the lip vermilion but also onto the mucosal lip. The solution must be applied to these areas too if results are expected.

Care is mandatory when peeling the periorbital region. Phenol will cloud the cornea. Retrograde flow into the conjunctival sac can occur during tearing. All tears should be wiped immediately with a cotton sponge, which should then be discarded. Additional tears should be wiped with a new, fresh sponge. While the upper lids should be peeled, it is not necessary to peel on the tarsus. Indeed, it is unwise to apply phenol on any surface that is intertriginous, where the phenol can pool and produce a deeper burn than expected. The lower eyelid is peeled within 2 to 4 mm of the ciliary border.

Initially, all physicians taped the skin after a phenol peel. The application of tape is thought to enhance the depth and thus the effect of the peel (see Figures 5.4A, B, C, and D). The tape is removed at 48 hours.

Less discomfort is expected if a serious exudate is allowed to form under the tape mask, literally lifting it off the underlying facial tissue. This usually takes 48 hours to form, thus the author's preference in tape removal at that time. Once the tape is removed, either a dry or wet technique may be followed. Thymol iodide powder is applied to hasten drying; it decreases exudative oozing and is bacteriostatic. Once a dry crust has formed, the patient can then moisturize the skin, inducing the final sloughing of debris and peeled tissue. Patients may report discomfort because drying results in uncomfortable stiffness of the facial skin. As a result most physicians who still tape the face will use an emollient after tape removal.

Beeson and McCollough reported the use of an emollient immediately postpeel avoiding any taping.[44] By keeping the burn moistened, wound healing was hastened, and they observed no difference in peel effectiveness (see Figures 5.5A and B). This also avoided the unpleasant, often painful experience of tape removal. The popularity of postpeel emollient use has magnified. However, it is still believed by most physicians that application of tape produces a more effective peel in the treatment of multiple, deep rhytides. Taping also hastens the removal of the sloughing skin during removal. Application of a moisturizer may result in a thick layer on the face that requires scrubbing for removal. Occasionally, patients are too timid in facial cleansing and do not remove the moisturized debris effectively. Tape or no tape, the utilization of moisturizers for postoperative care is becoming typical. It eliminates the uncomfortable state of crusting while hastening wound healing. It does add to the problem of development of occlusive acne, however, a condition more likely to be seen in younger patients.

Trichloroacetic Acid Peels

Trichloroacetic acid peels do not require the magnitude of patient consultation and preparation necessary for a phenol peel. There is no systemic absorption nor systemic toxicity; consultation is thus limited to discussion, selection, and treatment regimen for the appropriate skin. Pain is less severe and of shorter duration than phenol; and anesthesia, either intramuscular, intravenous, or general, is optional even with medium-depth TCA peels. Understandably, the use of anesthesia demands a more comprehensive patient evaluation.

Depending upon the concentration utilized and the addition of preoperative enhancers, TCA can produce light, medium, or deep peels. Since use of a 50% or greater concentration of TCA is associated with the possibility of scarring, most peels produced with a TCA of 45% or less are either light or medium in depth. Light peels with TCA are accomplished with concentrations of 10% to 30% and often are repeated at intervals of 2 weeks to several months. The more vigorous the method of application, the greater the penetration of

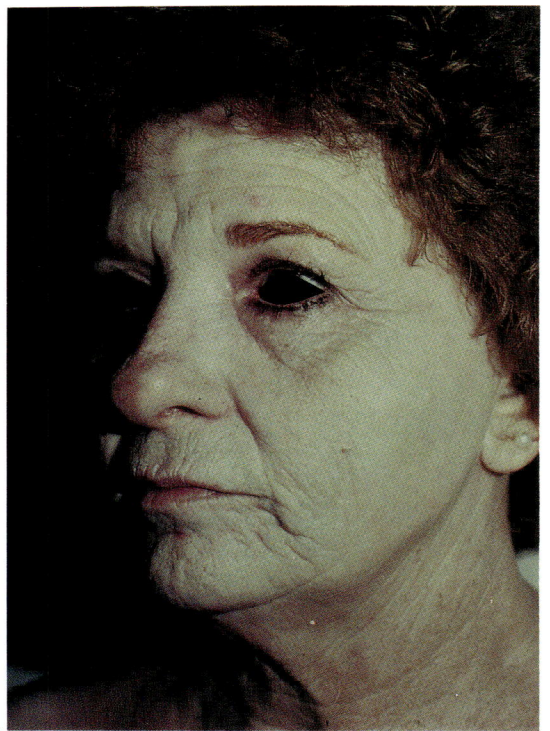
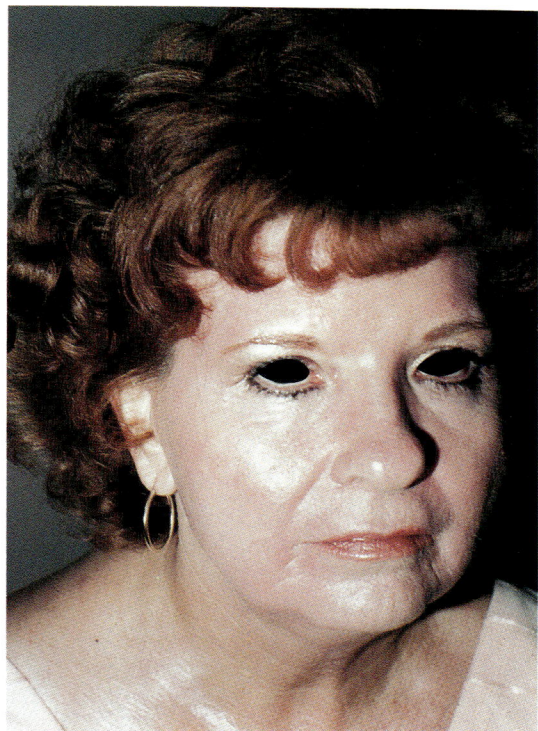
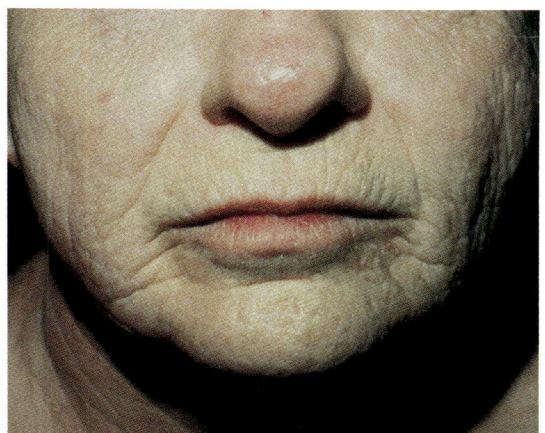
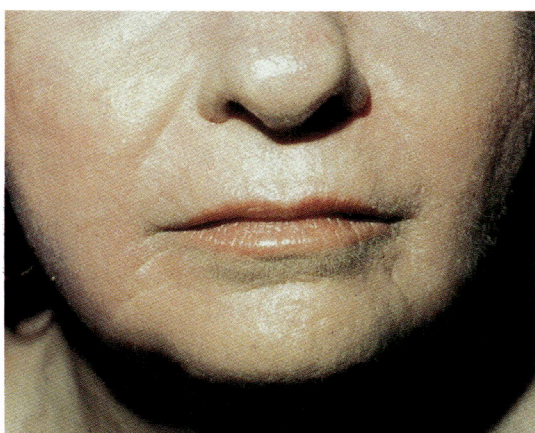

FIGURE 5.4. A. Full face phenol formula peel taped. Preoperative multiple deep rhytides of the perioral and periorbital regions as well as the cheeks. The pallor of the facial skin is from actinic damage and years of smoking. B. Spectacular results with removal of rhytides, tightening of facial skin, as evidenced by retraction of the periorbital skin, and improvement of the skin quality and tone, resulting in a more youthful appearance. C. Preoperative closeup of the perioral region. D. Postoperative closeup demonstrating improvement in the rhytides and skin tone and quality.

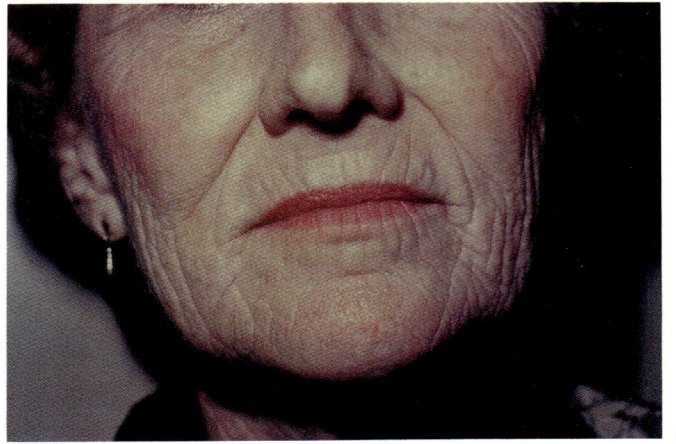

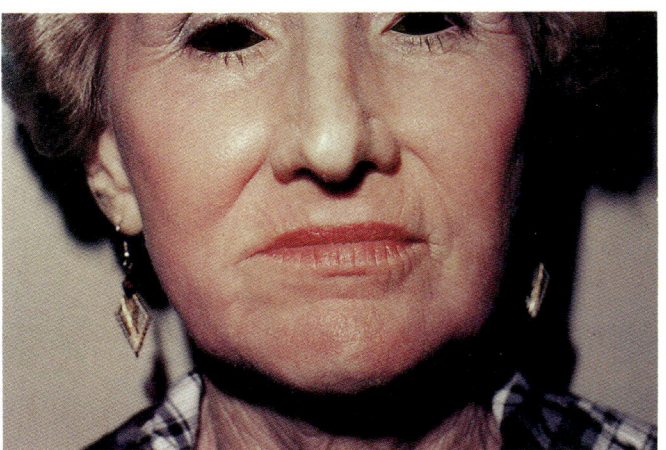

FIGURE 5.5. A. Full face phenol formula peel nontaped. Checkerboard rhytides with tissue atrophy of the perioral region. B. Satisfactory improvement of the rhytides as well as skin quality and tone. There are still residual rhytides in the perioral region due to the accordion effect of tissue atrophy. Further correction can be obtained with the utilization of dermal fillers.

TCA, thus potentially changing a light peel to one of medium depth despite no change in the concentration of TCA. Usually the degree of frosting becomes the endpoint, heavy frosting being associated with the maximal burn for that concentration of TCA.

Light peels, performed with a 10% to 30% concentration of TCA, are applied to the endpoint of either light (frosting is visible, but not complete, and faint in color) or medium (frosting is more widespread and involves the entire peeled area, but is of a faint white color). Obviously, a 30% concentration, if rubbed vigorously into the skin and allowed to develop a heavy frost, will produce a medium peel. Only by applying a delicate skin coating with a light frosting will a light peel be accomplished with a 30% concentration. The author believes that dilution with alcohol controls the degree of frosting and aids in epithelial desiccation after the initial tissue injury by the acid. It is important to realize that some individuals do not exhibit immediate frosting. There is a delay in onset of frosting, and during this time the skin may develop a deeper burn than desired. Typically, the burning sensation of the acid will be noticeable to the patient. If a light peel is expected and if there is indecision on the depth of burn achieved, dilute immediately and reevaluate. Additional applications of TCA can always be done if the desired effect has not been reached.

Typically, the patient will experience the onset of skin flaking 3 to 5 days after the peel. Some areas, specifically those with a deeper burn, may turn a brownish color prior to peeling. Glycolic acid may be better suited for lighter peels because it will cause epidermal flaking without the appearance of brown skin or sheets of separating skin typical of TCA.

Trichloroacetic acid is a good peeling agent for medium-depth peels and can be used with a variety of agents that enhances its effects. Medium-depth TCA requires vigorous application of the acid with development of a heavy (the entire area should be completely white) frost. The face is washed prior to application and lightly cleansed with acetone. An enhancer, such as 70% glycolic acid or Jessner's solution, is used to obtain a uniform peel. It is applied with cotton-tipped applicators and typically left on for 2 minutes before the face is again washed and dried. TCA 25% or 35% is applied with a gauze sponge and rubbed into the skin. The application can be recorded by either time or the number of strokes per area. Certain areas, such as the forehead and central cheeks, may be treated in appropriate candidates with 45% TCA. The entire face is allowed to develop a uniform heavy frost before dilution with alcohol. The patient is then requested to rinse the face with water to prevent any chance that undiluted acid may still be present. It is possible that the acid may be spent, and application of the alcohol or water has no diluting effect.

Brody and Hailey utilized another method[19] to obtain peels of an intermediate depth between superficial TCA peels and those with Baker's phenol. They combined solid CO_2 treatment with the application of 35% to 50% TCA. The ice is dipped in a 3:1 solution of acetone and alcohol to prevent it from sticking to the skin. By varying the pressure applied, microepidermal vesiculo-bullous lesions are created. Pressure designations of CO_2 mild, moderate, or hard are recorded. TCA is then applied liberally with cotton applicators. After 5 minutes a soothing emollient is applied, such as bacitracin or a live yeast cell ointment. Considerable edema occurs during the first few days, but discomfort is generally mild. Erythematous areas become brownish as crusts form, with separation beginning between the fourth and eight day and complete within 14 days, depending upon CO_2 pressure and TCA strength. Histological examination of the resultant tissue reaction documents the depth of the peel.

Postoperative care can vary from dry to wet. Some physicians prefer that the patient apply no moisturizers until the skin turns a brown color and begins to crack, flake, and peel. Application of water, either by soaks or spray bottle, enhances separation of the skin. Once drying is complete, usually within 2 to 3 days, moisturizers are then applied. Other physicians prefer use of moisturizers immediately after the peel. When there is considerable serous exudate, eczematization and pruritus, topical or even oral or intramuscular corticosteriods are warranted. Hydroquinone is useful as a post-peel prophylactic to minimize hyperpigmentation, which can plague trichloroacetic acid peels.

Alpha Hydroxy Acids

Whether desquamation or epidermolysis occurs is dependent upon the concentration of the acid, the type of formulation, frequency of application, the condition of the influencing delivery, and the absolute amount of acid delivered to the particular skin compartment over a given period of time.[45] The alpha hydroxy acid, glycolic, and the alpha keto acid, pyruvic, are currently the most utilized. Glycolic acid produces a light peel, without the obvious frosting seen with trichloroacetic acid. It is important that the physician or aide time and record the duration of application and then exposure before neutralization or dilution. Because a light peel is produced, glycolic acid is administered in a series of treatments, ideally at 2-week intervals. The acid is applied to the face over a 2-minute interval, rubbing it into all crevices with either a cotton Q-tip, a cotton ball, or gauze. The initial treatment is then left on for an additional 1 to 2 minutes, with subsequent peels of longer duration (increasing by 30 to 60 seconds) if tolerated.

The time for application and penetration must be carefully recorded, as glycolic acid does not normally produce frosting of the skin. Between treatments glycolic acid can be applied to enhance results in selected patients. It is important to realize that skin treated with retinoic acid will peel deeper and may vesiculate and crust. For this reason the physician may request that no retinoic acid be applied the night before the peel to assure that the skin has not suffered an unapparent retinoic burn. The physician should wear protective gloves during application to avoid peeling of the fingers. The effects are not immediately noted, and these precautions are wise.

Complications

Chemical peeling, even in the best of hands, can be a trying experience, fraught with unexpected results. There is no peeling agent that will produce ideal results in all individuals. And there is no peeling agent that will not produce complications. It is only the incidence and severity of complications that differentiate peeling agents. Any claims to the contrary are made either in ignorance or with duplicity.

The physician must determine what the skin can tolerate while producing the desired peel. Expertise only reduces the incidence of unexpected results to a tolerable level and prepares the physician for the seemingly impossible task of reversing the untoward sequelae of chemical peeling. Due to the countless variables that influence the depth of acid penetration,[17] it is important to be cognizant of the various potential complications associated with peels and the steps that can be taken to reduce complications.[46] The ideal patient—one with fair skin, no pigmentary abnormalities, and moderate actinic damage—seldom experiences a problem unless treated with too aggressive a peel. Unfortunately, many patients who can benefit from chemical peeling do not have the ideal skin complexion. This group is susceptible to a myriad of untoward effects, especially pigmentary anomalies. One must therefore expect some individuals to experience complications. The object is to minimize or avoid those complications that are nonreversible and disfiguring while providing optimal effects.

The extent of untoward results encountered is dependent upon the ability of the peeling agent to produce not only cutaneous effects (melanocytic function toxicity and a cutaneous burn) but also its systemic symptoms. The most widely used agents for facial peeling solutions are various formulas of either phenolic acid, trichloroacetic acid, or the alpha hydroxy acids. Phenolic acid has the ability to produce toxic effects on melanocytic function and produce systemic symptoms when absorbed in sufficient quantities. In contrast, TCA and AHA have no systemic absorption[47] and do not have a direct toxic effect on melanocytes. Complications of TCA and AHA are limited to the skin. Preoperative blood evaluation is not necessary because there is no systemic absorption and the body does not have to detoxify these peeling agents. They can be used in patients with myocardial, hepatic, or renal disease without cardiac monitoring, provided the patient does not have incapacitating systemic disease and can tolerate the discomfort of acid application. Remember, pain can induce a cardiac arrhythmia.

It is mandatory that the physician inform the patient of the more common and serious untoward sequelae. This information should always include the possibility of cutaneous pigmentary anomalies, scarring, and any systemic effects from absorption of the peeling chemical, as with phenol or salicylic acid. While there are other problems, these are the most common and disastrous complications that can require extended postoperative care and recovery. They are also the typical problems that culminate in litigation. It is wise to provide the patient with a handout prior to the consult. It should explain the procedure, the expected postoperative course, and the common problems and complications. The patient then has time to read, digest, and, hopefully, comprehend the procedure, its possible benefits, and its undesirable side effects. While verbal informed consent is acceptable, an instructional handout documents the discussion and can be retained as a reference. It is better that the patient realize that such problems can occur and decide not to undergo the procedure than to proceed with reckless abandon. It is advisable to follow the recovery of the patient with scheduled visits or phone contact to assure that healing is proceeding normally. After all, a normal recovery denotes an absence of complications.

The remaining portion of this chapter is divided into the following sections: cutaneous complications common to all peeling agents,

5. Chemical Face Peeling

avoidance and treatment of complications, complications specific to phenol, and specific effects of miscellaneous peeling agents.

Cutaneous Complications Common to All Peeling Agents

Peeling complications can be classified as either major or minor. *Minor complications* are defined as those that are relatively common, that are usually responsive to therapy, that dissipate quickly with treatment, and that leave no or insignificant sequelae. While responsive to therapy, a minor complication cannot be ignored because of its potential to progress to a major complication such as the development of scarring and/or pigmentary abnormalities. A *major complication* can be unpredictable in occurrence, is difficult to treat, has an unpredictable response to therapy, and responds slowly, if at all, to therapy.

Major Complications

Pigmentation Anomalies

Of all the possible complications that can occur from chemical peels, abnormal pigmentation is the most common. It can be unpredictable and unexpected. The pigmentary changes may be generalized or restricted to an area. The pigmentary problems encountered may be hyperpigmentation, hypopigmentation, mottled, blotched, streaked, whorled, or variegated pigmentation, and poikilodermalike changes. Poikiloderma changes produce irregular and uneven hyperpigmentation over a background of erythema and telangiectasia. The most common cause of pigmentation anomalies is the patient's inherent tendency to respond nonuniformly to the peeling agent. However, whorled or streaked pigmentation and uneven skin texture may be due to faulty technique, improper cleansing of the skin, inadequate mixing of the solution, suspension, nonuniform application of the chemical solution, ocular tearing with acid dilution, and nonuniform occlusion of the tape mask. The result is differences in the depth of peel with variations in the skin texture and color.

The frequency of pigmentary abnormalities is especially high in patients who either have a familial tendency for, or have brown, yellow, or red skin. It is paramount to remember that not all individuals with Asian, Latin, Indian, Mexican, or Mediterranean heritage exhibit brown skin. Unfortunately, they still can retain the ability to develop postinflammatory pigmentation anomalies. The pigmentary problems encountered in this group can be persistent and inconsistently responsive to all treatments. It is important to realize that treatment may actually exacerbate an already difficult pigmentary complication.

Abnormal pigmentation can occur at any area of the face and neck. Pigmentation is most likely to develop over the malar and lateral periorbital areas. Pigmentation can be preceded by the inflammatory erythema of the peel that was slow to resolve. It is aggravated by, but not necessarily caused by, excessive exposure to ultraviolet radiation. Poikiloderma normally can be seen along the lower lateral cheek and upper lateral neck. Peeling of poikilodermal skin is inconsistent and best approached with light peels rather than a deep peel. A deep peel can not only exacerbate the condition by markedly accentuating pigmentary differences but also induce or uncover prominent telangiectasia. Occasionally, the emergence of a dark nevus or multiple nevi can be seen after a peel. This is thought to be due to the irritant factor of peeling. It represents a postinflammatory hyperpigmentation reaction to preexisting flesh-colored nevi.

Darkly pigmented individuals can respond to a deeper peel with a uniform hyperpigmentation. This fades with time, usually within several months, but can be alarming and disconcerting to the uninformed patient. Hyperpigmentation can occur in patients with fair skin but tends to be less intense and of shorter duration. The pigmentation also responds well to treatment.

Hypopigmentation is of greater concern. If widespread, it produces a pale, ghostly appearance. This is more common with phenol and unusual with TCA and AHA. Patchy hypopigmentation can also be the result of cutaneous scarring. It presents difficulty because it is not easily camouflaged by cosmetics. Loss of pigmentation can thus be permanent and disabling in darker individuals. It does not present such a serious problem if the individual is pale-complexioned, as the color differential will be minimal.

Scarring

Scarring is related to the depth of dermal injury produced by the chemexfoliation process. Fortunately, scarring is not so common as pigmentary problems. Unlike pigmentary problems, which may correct themselves and actually disappear over time, scarring is permanent. Early intervention will limit its extent and prominence. The most common cause is application of a peeling agent too strong for the skin treated, with a resultant deep cutaneous burn. Scarring can also occur as the result of a minor complication that has been neglected. Herpes simplex, bacterial skin infection, pruritus complicated by excoriation, and eruptive cystic acne can all result in scarring or pigmentary abnormalities if left unattended.

Scarring can present itself in several forms: hypertrophic, contracture, and atrophic. Atrophic scarring appears as an area of white pigmentation or hypopigmentation that can havea lacy appearance. It is seen on the lower face, especially on the cheeks and the chin. Contracture scarring occurs at the lower eyelids with development of ectropion and at the perioral region with lip contracture. It can be seen along the nasolabial fold, due to pooling of the acid. Thin or atrophic skin will be more susceptible to hypertrophic scars. The preauricular cheek and the skin along the mandible are common areas of involvement, due to the thinner skin found here. Isotretinoin[48] treated skin can develop bizarre hypertrophic scarring that typically occurs in the mid-cheek region. This skin, because of its thickness and adnexal gland density, is normally resistant to scarring.

Certain areas are prone to scarring. They are either contiguous to a region that normally exhibits significant actinic changes and rhytides and/or the area does not have the inherent capability of normal recovery after a deeper peel. The mandible is one such area, due to the thinness of the overlying skin and the torsion produced as the edematous facial skin is stretched over the underlying bone.

The perioral region is an area of significant aging changes in women and is thus one of the more important, if not the most important, area requiring improvement from chemical peeling. The upper lip may be disproportionately aged, with basophilic degeneration, cobblestoning, and rhytides when compared with the rest of the face. This scenario is common in smokers. Unfortunately, the upper lip is also an area that is resistant to significant improvement by many modalities, thus the tendency to treat with a deeper peel. Herpes simplex is a frequent upper lip infection. While herpes simplex infection usually does not cause scarring, the combination of a peel and herpetic infection can.

The lower eyelid develops laxity with age. Scar contracture along the lower eyelid can eventuate in an ectropion. Retinoic acid and other modalities are often used in the periorbital region for treatment of fine rhytides. Application of a peeling agent may result in a deeper burn than expected if the physician is unaware of the use of these medications. The lower eyelid along the zygoma is also prone to development of bright erythema. The persistence of the erythema can be alarming to the patient and physician. Inappropriate therapy to the erythema can result in scarring by aggravating what once was a superficial burn into a deep one.

An area of persistent erythema or the late development of an area of erythema, especially along the mandible or cheek, should alert the physician to the possible development of scarring. Scratching, picking, and excoriation can traumatize healing skin and produce injury. Intercurrent infection may add to tissue injury and enhance scarring. When there is abnormal tissue sloughing, it is advisable to treat for a secondary infection with topical and, if preferable, oral antibiotics.

A word of caution: All peeling agents can induce scarring. Actinic, atrophic skin and skin severely irritated and thinned by topical antiaging creams and lotions are prime candidates. The addition of a minor complication aggravates the problem. Mild peeling acids, when used inappropriately or without caution or forethought, can scar facial tissue.

Minor Complications

Recrudescence of Herpes Simplex Infection

Recrudescence of a herpes simplex infection is common after a chemical peel. Typically, it is manifested by the appearance of superficial, exquisitely tender ulcerations. Characteristic vesicles are not seen, because the epidermis that forms the roof of the vesicle has been stripped away by the chemical peel. The appearance of superficial ulcerations can mimic the results of a deep peel, but the presence of pain and location should clue the physician as to etiology. Involvement can be widespread, covering the entire upper lip and portions of the cheeks. Scarring, while not common, can occur. Pigmentary changes can also be a sequelae of the infection. The discomfort and pain of a herpetic infection responds rapidly to acyclovir. Herpes can appear as late as a week after a peel, and delayed healing is to be expected.

It is important to differentiate the viral infection from bacterial infections. A *Staphylococcus* or *Streptococcus* impetigo will produce a similar superficial ulceration. In contrast, bacterial skin infections are not initially accompanied by pain. Infection can cause scarring if unrecognized or left untreated, and associated pruritus and scratching can exacerbate the situation.

Bacterial Infection

Two factors minimize the incidence of cutaneous infections of the face after peels. Acids are germicidal, and the facial skin is richly vascularized. However, accumulation of tissue debris aggravated by occlusion with ointments such as vegetable fat, Vaseline, or similar nonantibacterial moisturizers can promote the growth of bacteria and development of impetigo or folliculitis by *Staphylococcus*, *Streptococcus*, or *Pseudomonas*. The accumulation of molting skin and debris lends to bacterial overgrowth. Contact should be avoided with any individual with streptococcal pharyngitis or skin infections. The peeled, denuded facial skin is susceptible to infection by a streptococcal impetigo. The use of topical antibiotic ointments as moisturizing agents minimizes this complication but may produce a contact dermatitis. Acne and acneiform dermatitis are also common because of the above factors. Fortunately, scarring usually does not result from a skin infection. A neglected or unrecognized or traumatized infection can produce scars and pigmentary changes. Pruritus may accompany the cutaneous infection, and excoriation can promote scarring. LoVerme et al, report two cases of toxic shock syndrome from a toxin-producing *Staphylococcus aureus* after a Baker's formula phenol peel.[49] Symptoms appeared on the third and fourth postoperative day, respectively. Both patients had taped peels, and thymol iodide powder was applied after removal.

Erythema and Demarcation Lines

Generalized erythema may be marked and persistent for weeks, occasionally months. While most common with phenol, it can occur with TCA or any other deep peel. Regional erythema can also occur when the perioral or periorbital region is treated. Erythema will fade with time, and treatment is not indicated. However, any area of persistent erythema (lasting more than 1 week) must be carefully observed, as it may be the first sign of hypertrophic scarring. This needs to be treated aggressively, as noted previously. Sun exposure and application of photosensitizing agents, including cosmetics, can also be responsible for prolonged erythema. Repetitive peels performed at too close a time interval produce the problem, due to inflammation. A common region of involvement is the periorbital cheek on and above the medial zygoma.

Erythema is to be expected after phenol application; it usually takes 6 to 8 weeks to fade. Persistent erythema occurs occasionally, with redness lasting for months before slowly resolving. A special problem area is the perioral region. Phenol formula peels (Baker's or Litton's) are very effective in removing perioral rhytides. However, the expected erythema may be marked and persistent for many months. When the upper lip is the only area peeled, the intense redness is difficult to mask with cosmetics. The generalized erythema seen after TCA is less severe. Unlike the erythema associated with phenol, it can be followed by pigmentary changes. Localized erythema that is slow to resolve should be suspect for development of pigmentation or hypertrophic scarring.

An obvious line of demarcation can also form between peeled and nonpeeled areas. This is most commonly seen along the mandible and the periorbital region. The demarcation line may be the result of pigmentation at the border of the peeled area or due to a quality difference between peeled and nonpeeled skin. Patients with marked actinic and pigmentary abnormalities are likely to exhibit these changes. The phenol demarcation line is due to loss of pigmentation, which may not be initially noticeable; with time the hypopigmentation from the phenol manifests itself. The importance of this depigmented demarcation line is with the future performance of facial surgery. The sagging cheek and neck skin is lifted during a facelift, and in the process of doing so, the demarcation line can be raised onto the lower cheek and into a visually obvious zone.

Dermographism and Pruritus

Erythema may be accompanied by dermographism and pruritus. They can also occur separately from erythema. Dermographism associated with intense pruritus may cause the patient, especially during sleep, to excoriate the healing tissue, eventuating in scarring and pigmentary changes. Itching and burning are usual complaints and typically start in the first 2 weeks posttreatment.

Facial Swelling

All peeling agents can cause some degree of facial swelling. Deeper peels of the entire face or a regional peel of the forehead can produce upper eyelid edema. The edema occurs 24 to 72 hours after the peel. It is worse in the morning but improves with ambulating. The swelling can be severe enough to close the eyelids, thus inhibiting normal vision for work or driving. It is certainly frightening if unexpected, and thus the patient should be warned of this possible complication. The eyelid edema usually takes several days to resolve.

The patient and any individual who administers postoperative care should be warned of the subsequent appearance. Chemical peeling agents, especially phenol, can induce extreme facial swelling, with the face ballooning to hideous proportions. The addition of the chemical burn, with blistering and discoloration, can produce a terrifying effect. But while the appearance may look painful, it typically is not. The uninitiated may construe the appearance as a threatening complication and seek emergency medical care elsewhere. Here the real danger is when an uneducated physician misinterprets the patient's condition and initiates grossly inappropriate treatment.

Milia

Development of small facial inclusion cysts is common. They result from the use of occlusive thick ointments. They do not appear until several weeks after the peel and can persist for months. Located on the cheeks and forehead, their number can vary from a few to a hundred or more.

Telangiectasia

Telangiectasia are relatively common and can be caused by actinic radiation, acne rosacea, and estrogens. They may be prominent on the central cheeks, nose, and lateral neck. Superficial telangiectasia can disappear after a deep peel. Those telangiectasia located deeper within the skin are not destroyed by peeling agents and may become more prominent postoperatively. The chemical peel strips the overlying aged skin of keratoses, lentigines, basophilic degenerative changes, and actinic dermatitis. This removes the overlying tissue camouflaging these deeper, underlying telangiectasia. They are now closer to the surface and have greater visual prominence.

Avoidance and Treatment of Complications

General Considerations for Avoidance of Complications

Succinctly stated, choosing a suitable candidate, carefully evaluating the quality of the skin, utilizing the appropriate peeling regimen, and providing meticulous postoperative care eliminate or mitigate complications. Unfortunately, many patients who can benefit from chemical peeling do not have an ideal skin complexion or skin quality. This group is susceptible; one must, therefore, expect some of these individuals to experience complications from peeling. The extent of untoward results encountered is dependent upon the ability of the physician to be consistent with patient care and chemical peel selection. The physician must minimize and avoid those complications that are nonreversible and disfiguring and still provide satisfactory results.

There are a multitude of variables that affect the penetration of acid into and through the epidermis and the subsequent cutaneous burn produced. Among the significant variables that may affect the depth of an acid peel include the following: the concentration and type of peeling agent utilized; the technique of acid application; prior and continued utilization of retinoic acid or skin exfoliants; the effectiveness of prepeel skin preparation and degreasing; sebaceous gland density and activity; the thinness of the epidermis and dermis from atrophic actinic changes; ingestion of any agent that causes epidermal sloughing and thinning such as vitamin A, beta-carotene, and Accutane; and the application of prepeel keratolytic agents and solutions.[17]

Chemical peeling is not necessarily an all-or-nothing phenomenon.[33] The depth of penetration and tissue destruction can vary even if given the same concentration of acid and similarly prepared skin. For instance, several applications of an acid (the total quantity of acid applied) increases the cutaneous burn and enhances penetration. Vigorous, repetitive rubbing of the acid onto the skin increases penetration by progressively stripping the epithelium that is being loosened and blistered by the acid. The importance of a clean cutaneous surface without any elements that may hinder penetration is implicit. Scrubbing can cause localized abrasions and enhanced acid penetration at these sites. Vigorous rubbing of the acid into the skin increases penetration by removing the superficial debris that can block penetration.

This is more important when weaker acids are used because penetration will be greater than expected with possible complications. This technique of enhanced penetration can be desirable when treating deep rhytides or skin with hyperkeratosis. Conversely, these techniques may increase the incidence of complications, especially scarring and pigmentary anomalies. The physician must individualize the application of acid to the area treated to obtain optimal results and minimal complications. Some regions of the face can tolerate a deeper burn than others without complications. Facial areas with a higher incidence of complications include the perioral, mandibular, and lower eyelid regions.

The necessity of thoroughly cleansing the skin has always been emphasized. A vigorous scrubbing of the skin with acetone or ether was advocated for removal of all cosmetics, debris, and heavy oils, which inhibit penetration. During this vigorous attempt at cleansing the skin, superficial epithelial abrasions are produced, thus enhancing penetration of the acid solution. It can be difficult to scrub the entire face equally, and variation in acid penetration is to be expected. For this very reason, several authors have advocated the use of a prepeel accelerator to prepare the skin for the definitive peeling solution. Among the popular accelerators are frozen CO_2, Jessner's solution,[20] and glycolic acid.[50] By applying the accelerator, the epidermis is cleansed of its superficial layers along with any oils, cosmetic, and seborrhea present, thus eliminating the need to scrub the skin and, in theory, providing an evenly prepared skin surface for the subsequent peeling agent to penetrate.

Manipulation of any variable may produce inconsistent, unexpected, and disparate peel results. Although the application of a peeling regimen is simplistic, the controlling factors that determine acid penetration are not. They should be standardized in order to obtain a consistent chemical peel. The common denominator behind any complication with a chemical peel is the assumption that all skin reacts equally. Chemical peeling is not a cookbook recipe. Each individual patient must be evaluated before choosing the appropriate peeling regimen. Thick, sebaceous male facial skin will tolerate a TCA solution concentration of 50%, whereas scarring can result if the same solution is applied to the thin, fine, atrophic facial skin of an elderly woman. Furthermore, any substance that reduces the thickness of the horny layer enhances the depth of penetration and chemical burn by the acid. Consequently, a seemingly weak peeling agent produces a cutaneous burn deeper than expected, with unexpected disastrous results.

The patient should be instructed not to apply cosmetics or moisturizers on the day of the peel and preferably for several days prior to the peel. Thick layers of cosmetics may plug the skin creases and pores. These must be thoroughly cleansed or be dissolved by a prepeel accelerator of all scales, sebum, moisturizers, dirt, cosmetics, and other debris. This can be difficult to achieve. The physician should take this into account when applying the peeling agent. Deep rhytides need to be stretched apart and flattened, cleansed, and peeled evenly without pooling to prevent inadequate peeling and complications. The peeling solution must not be allowed to pool into creases and wrinkles nor to run freely on the skin to dependent regions.

Inadequate shaking of the bottle and mixing of the solution, prior to application, can result in crystals of TCA that precipitated along the rim of the jar being applied with the solution. An inconsistent and higher than expected concentration of TCA is thus applied to the skin. Phenol solution (Baker's or Litton's) does not stay in solution but must be mixed prior to each application. Failure to apply a thoroughly mixed solution results in variation in the strength of the formula and the depth of the peel. Simply swirling mixture into solution prior to dipping the Q-tip prevents this problem.

A consistent uniform peel is the essence of good results. Uniformity enables the physician to avoid problems because he or she now understands what the peel is capable of accomplishing. A recordable peeling regimen promulgates consistency. Recording the following parameters can be helpful in developing consistency: patient use of skin irritants (retinoic acid, glycolic acid creams, etc.), skin color (brown, fair, etc.), skin quality (sebaceous, actinic, atrophic, melasma, etc.), prepeel accelerator and duration of skin contact, chemical peeling agent and concentration, time to dilution, degree of frosting if appropriate, postpeel care regimen, dates of repetitive peels, and so on. It is very helpful when determining what peeling agent, concentration, and preparation to utilize with repetitive peels.

Abnormal Pigmentation

Abnormal pigmentation can be a normal physiological response to cutaneous irritation, whether caused by a skin disease or injury such as a chemical peel. It is aggravated by, but not necessarily caused by, excessive exposure to ultraviolet radiation. Hyperpigmentation is common in patients who are or have a family background of brown skin. It can occur in patients with fair skin but tends to be less intense and of shorter duration. A simple history can determine a majority of, but not all, individuals prone to hyperpigmentation. Some individuals may not know their family background or be unaware of its significance. Examination of the non-sun-exposed forearm can be helpful in determining the presence of brown color.

A test spot peel is reasonable in patients who are anxious or are prone to develop hyperpigmentation. A negative test result is encouraging but does not ensure that hyperpigmentation will not develop. Development of hyperpigmentation in the presence of a negative test result may cause the patient to question the physician's peeling procedure. Conversely, the physician may suspect that the patient has been exposed to an exacerbating factor, such as excessive solar exposure. For these reasons the author believes that the best utilization of skin testing is for discouraging a chemical peel in susceptible or anxious patients. The absence of hyperpigmentation is interpreted as an inconclusive test, and not as an assurance of a good result, in these individuals. Do not bend to the wishes of an unrealistic patient, especially in the presence of adverse factors. Light peels, with minimal expected improvement but minimal risk, may be an alternative in patients who are insistent.

The tendency for pigmentary anomalies can be magnified by medications such as estrogens, progesterones, birth control pills, phenothiazine, pituitary melanocyte-stimulating hormones, adrenocorticotropic hormones, thyroid hormones, and other photosensitizing medicines and chemicals. Some sunscreens and perfumes may actually contain photosensitizing chemicals that result in not only hyperpigmentation but also poikilodermal changes. Pigmentation can occur months after the peel, during which interval the melanocyte remains hypersensitive. It is advisable to avoid and, if possible, to eliminate any provoker of pigmentation, both prior to and after a peel. Furthermore, these medications or other exacerbating factors may need to be stopped before the pigmentation resolves or can respond to therapy such as a topical depigmentary agent or a second peel.

Improper skin cleansing of cosmetics, moisturizers, dirt, and oils prevents uniform penetration of the peeling agent. Poor, inconsistent, or uneven skin cleansing results in incomplete penetration. As previously noted, to combat the problem of inadequate and irregular penetration, some physicians utilize an enhancer or accelerator to assure uniform penetration. The use of Jessner's solution, glycolic acid, or another accelerator prior to application of the peeling solution assists in achieving an even penetration. Some authors believe that this will also enhance the effects of the peeling solution. Thus, similar results may be produced from a weaker agent without the undue risks of an alternative stronger peeling agent.

It is mandatory to emphasize the importance of minimizing exposure to the sun after a peel. Use of a wide spectrum sunscreen for both the UVA and UVB range is necessary, as both UV spectra can induce pigmentation. The newer sunscreens now provide protection over a wider UV spectrum, extending into the UVA spectrum. Although cosmetic makeup does offer protection, the author advises use of a sunscreen under the makeup. Fluorescent lighting can also be a source of ultraviolet rays. Ultraviolet radiation avoidance must be accompanied by the use of sunscreens. Most individuals have significantly greater ultraviolet exposure than they realize.

Pigmentary problems can occur despite reasonable avoidance of solar radiation. Pigmentation is a normal physiological response to cutaneous irritation, and in some situations, it is due to melanocytic sensitivity caused by the irritating effect of the peel. This melanocytic hypersensitivity can last for months, during which time pigmentation can be induced. Irritation, leading to pigmentation, may first start as erythema. The use of a topical mild steroid ointment, applied 3 or 4 times daily, will reverse the irritation. If there is a delay before treatment is initiated, a stronger fluorinated steroid may be used.

In susceptible individuals treatment for possible hyperpigmentation can be considered prior to its appearance. In any case, prompt, early treatment will often mollify the extent and duration of the pigmentation. All patients should be instructed to inform the physician's office immediately if they believe that pigmentation is developing. The limiting factor is the time interval between the appearance of pigmentation and the initiation of treatment. One of several fading formulas available is:

Hydroquinone 3% solution	30 ml
Retin-A solution	7.5 cc
Hydrocortisone	400 mg

Apply this solution at least twice daily. This solution can be irritating, causing an erythematous, flaking dermatitis. While undesirable, this reaction will often quickly remove any hyperpigmentation present. If the patient dislikes the dermatitis or if the physician wishes to avoid it, the addition of 7.5 cc of fluocinolone acetonid 0.01% solution to the bottle in substitution for the hydrocortisone.

A less irritating depigmentary formula in a cream is as follows:

Eldopaque forte 4%	15 gm
Aristocort A cream 0.1%	15 gm
Retin-A cream 0.1%	15 or 20 gm
Ascorbic acid	250 mg
Water	1 ml

Apply this cream twice a day. The Eldopaque forte contains a sunscreen. Any cosmetic makeup or sunscreens should be applied over the fading formulas.

Postinflammatory hyperpigmentation may respond to treatment only if the exacerbating factor is eliminated. It is advisable to avoid or eliminate any inducer of pigmentation, both prior to and after a peel. This is of greater importance with deeper, more inflammatory peels than with light peels. Abnormal pigmentation can be persistent and inconsistently responsive to any type of treatment. Treatment may actually exacerbate an already difficult pigmentary complication in some individuals. The pigmentation can correct itself with time and without treatment, a course that is conservative but does no additional harm.

Hypertrophic and Contracture Scars

There is no single standard peeling agent. Nor is chemical peeling an all-or-nothing phenomenon. Each individual patient must be evaluated before choosing the appropriate agent and concentration. A common denominator behind any complication with chemical peeling is the assumption that all skin reacts equally. The eyelids can tolerate a powerful peeling agent while the mandibular skin may not. In general, the greater the cutaneous burn, the greater the risk for scarring. This is certainly true for trichloroacetic acid. Application of a 50% TCA solution will produce more spectacular results than a 35% solution. The risk of scarring, however, is significantly greater with 50%, while with 35% it is unusual. In contrast, a phenol formula peel (Baker's or Litton's) produces a deep penetration and burn but is less prone to scarring than a similar burn from TCA. Scarring can be due to a mild variant of Ehlers-Danlos syndrome, mitis for, which may be present in as much as 9% of the population. A good exam and history should detect any joint hypermobility, increased skin elasticity, abnormal scarring, or easy bruising.

Facial areas with the highest incidence of scarring are the perioral, mandibular, and lower eyelid regions. The mandible is prone to scarring, due to the thinness of the overlying skin and the torsion produced as the edematous facial skin is stretched across the bone. Acid should be applied here carefully and not as vigorously. White atrophic scarring of the mandible and chin regions is usually seen in individuals with thin, atrophic skin treated with higher concentrations or stronger solutions of acid. Once this scarring occurs, there is little that can be done. Fortunately, cosmetic makeup can camouflage the scarring. Since these regions do not usually manifest significant rhytides and actinic changes as compared to the upper lips, cheeks, and forehead, they usually do not require as deep a peel.

The perioral region, an area of significant aging changes, is relatively resistant to significant improvement by many modalities. Heroic treatment attempts must be tempered to avoid scarring and other complications. Correction is very difficult if deep rhytides are associated with atrophy of the underlying tissues, producing an accordion effect. Only by increasing the bulk of the underlying tissue will one expect significant improvement of the deep rhytides. Taping of a perioral area can induce scarring, and therefore many physicians avoid it or tape 0.5 cm above the vermilion lip. Zealous treatment complicated by a labial herpes simplex infection may also produce scarring. A combination of modalities such as soft tissue augmentation, repetitive milder peels (remember, phenol and phenol formula peels may be applied very superficially), and superficial dermabrasion can produce good and possibly excellent results with less hazard.

The integrity of the lower eyelid must be carefully evaluated. Tissue tightening or scar contracture along the lower eyelid can eventuate in ectropion. Laxity of the lower eyelid, as evidenced by abnormal horizontal lid excursion and lid lag, an incipient ectropion, and a history of previous blepharoplasty should alert the physician. Minimal application or even avoidance of the peeling solution on the susceptible eyelids should be done and duly recorded in the operative note. If an ectropion develops, massage of the eyelid and taping up of the lateral lid at bedtime may resolve the problem. The addition of topical steroids or diluted doses of intralesional steroids can be used.

Patients treated with isotretinoin have been reported to develop bizarre hypertrophic scarring.[48] The scarring can occur in patients who have undergone a chemical peel or dermabrasion. Exposure to isotretinoin, either before, during, or after the surgery, can predispose the patient to scarring. The atypical scarring has surfaced months after treatment with isotretinoin. The germinal calls in the adnexal structures are an integral component in normal cutaneous recovery and healing after injury. Isotretinoin has a known effect of shrinking adnexal structures and inhibiting the expression of collagenase and procollagen production. The resultant reduction in epithelial cell growth leads to delayed wound healing and appears to be the mechanism that can cause scarring. Any individual who has received or who will receive isotretinoin for treatment of acne, or any oral retinoid, must be carefully evaluated and warned of this possible complication. The performance of surface surgery (specifically, dermabrasion and deep chemical peels) and the use of isotretinoin within a 12-month period are unadvisable. Even this time duration may be too short, as scarring has been reported when this time span has been over 36 months.

The importance of recognizing the genesis of scarring and initiating treatment is paramount to the effectiveness of therapy. The impact from scarring can be reduced if the early signs are aggressively treated. An area of persistent duration, edema, or the appearance of an area of erythema should alert the physician to the possible development of scarring. Early application of a topical fluorinated steroid is very effective in reducing or preventing hypertrophic scars. Steroids, administered either p.o. or intramuscular, are effective when scar formation or tissue contracture has started to form. The author's preference is Celestone Soluspan, 1.0 to 1.5 cc IM, given every 1 to 2 weeks, for a total of 3 doses. Intralesional steroids are also effective, but one must be aware of possible steroid atrophy at the injection site. Scratching and excoriation can traumatize healing skin and produce scarring. A cutaneous infection may add to tissue injury and enhance scarring. Any cutaneous infection must be closely observed for a complicating scar. When there is abnormal tissue sloughing, it is advisable to treat for secondary infection with topical and, if necessary, oral antibiotics.

Formulating a treatment plan based on the skin quality and pathology to be treated is important. Repetitive application (on a bimonthly or monthly schedule) of a weaker peeling solution enhances penetration and improvement. Although there is the inconvenience of undergoing several peels, the safety factor is significant. Complementing a weaker peel with fading or peeling agents can also produce adequate results and minimize pigmentary and scar complications. Several formulas have been previously described. The following is a peeling solution that a pharmacist can formulate:

Hydroquinone 3% solution	30 ml
Retin-A 0.05%	7.5 cc
Hydrocortisone	400 mg
Glycolic acid 70%	5 ml

This can be applied twice a day and will enhance the results of the peel. It can be started 1 or 2 weeks after the peels or used between repetitive peels to enhance results. If it is too irritating, 7.5 cc of fluocinolone acetonid 0.01% can be substituted for the hydrocortisone or just added to the above.

Herpes Simplex and Bacterial Infections

Herpes can appear a week or later after a peel and may delay healing for several weeks (see Figure 5.6). It is important to differentiate the viral infection from impetigo, caused by *Staphylococcus* or *Streptococcus* or a *Pseudomonas folliculitis*. Bacterial infections may also produce superficial ulceration but, in contrast, are not accompanied by painful ulcerations initially. The location of the outbreak is also

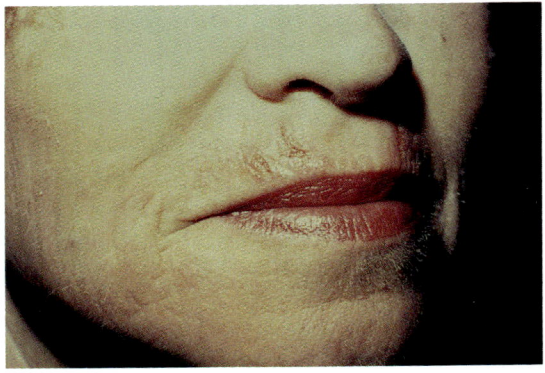

FIGURE 5.6. Postpeel herpes simplex eruption. A very common occurrence with phenol. Prophylaxis with acyclovir is reasonable in all patients undergoing phenol peels. Herpes simplex may disseminate and involve the entire area peeled, mimicking a bacterial infection. Disseminated herpes simplex infection is painful while bacterial infections typically are not.

helpful in differentiating bacterial and viral infections. Herpetic infection occurs typically in the perioral region, while a bacterial infection commonly involves the cheeks. Acyclovir may prevent an outbreak of herpes simplex in a patient with a history of recurrent herpetic infections. A prophylactic dose of acyclovir (400 mg bid, or, if preferable, 200 mg tid) starting several days prior and continuing for 5 to 7 days after the surgery can prevent the outbreak. All herpetic infections should be treated immediately with acyclovir (400 mg qid) to minimize the incidence of scarring. The discomfort and pain respond rapidly to the therapy. Should the diagnosis and treatment be delayed and there is evidence of nascent scarring and pigmentation, a potent topical steroid can mollify the cutaneous response.

Acneiform dermatitis with cystic, comedonal, and pustular acne lesions are common with excessive and prolonged use of occlusive ointments. The patient should be instructed to cleanse the face to prevent accumulation of molting skin and debris, which lends itself to bacterial overgrowth. Frequent facial rinsing with plain water or washing with a gentle soap such as Basis or Purpose will remove debris and minimize bacterial growth. It is not unreasonable to start acne antibiotic therapy to prevent a flare of cystic acne prior to its development. *Pseudomonas folliculitis* involves occluded, improperly washed skin and mimics acne. It is resistant to the typical antibiotics used in acne.

Pyogenic infections are unusual because of the inherent resistance of the facial skin to infection. Impetigo can occur because the skin is denuded and has no resistant barriers. It can mimic herpes simplex, but there is no associated pain. Impetigo can be caused by both *Streptococcus* and *Staphylococcus*.

Toxic shock syndrome has been reported following a Baker's phenol peel.[51] It is a rare but potentially fatal complication. The patient developed a fever, hypotension, vomiting, and diarrhea 2 to 3 days after the peel, accompanied in 2 to 6 days postpeel by scarlatiniform rash with subsequent desquamation. Toxic shock syndrome can produce myalgias, mucosal hyperemia, and hepatorenal, hematologic, or central nervous system involvement. Treatment with a β-lactamase-resistant antibiotic for *Staphylococcus aureus* and large volumes of parenteral fluid are necessary to prevent vascular collapse.

Demarcation Lines and Blending

Differential penetration of areas of the face may be desirable for blending and to prevent lines of demarcation, due to the difference in cutaneous surface quality. By gently stroking a peeling solution-moist Q-tip in a zig-zag motion on the neck, a lessening of the demarcation line can be created. This is the same principle applied with the use of a W-plasty instead of a straight-line excision for scar formation camouflage. In men the line of demarcation is easily hidden in the bearded skin. The same problem of blending is also important when treating perioral rhytides. The peeling solution must be placed onto the mucosal vermilion of the lip to avoid an unsightly border surrounding the lips, and the solution is applied to the nasolabial fold. When peeling only the lower lip, the acid is applied to the mentolabial sulcus rather than treating the entire chin. This results in a smooth blending and does not violate the more porous, sebaceous tissue of the lower chin.

Milia

Milia occur from use of occlusive facial creams and ointments. A reduction in the duration of use of occlusives can markedly reduce their occurrence. The use of retinoic acid prior to and after peeling can also reduce the number of milia. Retinoic acid can produce a cutaneous burn, induce hyperpigmentation, and interfere with cutaneous wound healing if initiated too soon after a peel.[52] The author generally resumes use of retinoic acid 1 to several weeks after a peel, depending on the depth of the peel. A large eruption of milia can be cosmetically unacceptable to the patient. It is wise to carefully extract these lesions with a small finger lancet. Milia are resistant to "picking" by the patient, this should be discouraged.

Erythema

The severity of the erythema should determine the treatment. If the patient is unconcerned and is willing to await resolution, no treatment is necessary. Early use of a topical steroid will help reduce the duration of the erythema in patients who are anxious or in physicians who are leery of possible evolution in scarring. The use of a mild topical steroid cream is usually sufficient. More potent topical steroids are indicated if there is a fear of scarring. Prolonged use of fluorinated topical steroids can be associated with aggravation or the appearance of telangiectasia and acne. Celestone soluspan, 1.0 to 1.5 cc intramuscular, is effective and avoids use of topical steroids. It is usually reserved for generalized erythema, while topical steroids are utilized for localized erythema. Diphenhydramine (50 mg qhs or upon the development of symptoms) is given in conjunction with celestone to minimize or prevent the hyperactivity, tremulousness, and nervousness that occasionally occur with the use of intramuscular celestone soluspan.

Erythema, accompanied by dermographism and pruritus, often responds to hydroxyzine, 25 to 75 mg nightly (given at night to minimize the sedative effect). Diphenhydramine, 25 to 50 mg, can be added if the dermographism and its associated pruritus are controlled by the hydroxyzine. It should be continued for 7 days to prevent a relapse of symptoms.

Facial Edema

Facial edema implies a good peel, as it indicates significant dermal inflammation. Unfortunately, upper eyelid edema can impair vision. Its occurrence is unpredictable, and the mainstay of treatment is time. It is an inconvenience to an individual who planned to remain active despite the facial appearance. The patient's schedule for the first week may need to be modified to take into account this sequelae of peels. Consumption of salty foods probably exacerbates the condition. Firm pressure with cool compresses may hasten resolution. It is worse in the morning and improves during the day, especially if the patient is up and about. Sleeping with the head propped up is recommended to reduce the extent of the edema.

Telangiectasia

Appropriate patients should be warned prior to surgery that the presence of facial telangiectasia may become more noticeable and widespread. By eliminating some of the signs of aging skin, an uncovering of telangiectasia can occur.

However, unless there is an extensive network of telangiectasia present, it is doubtful that this will become a significant problem. It is important to examine the face carefully without cosmetics and determine if a significant number of telangiectasia is present. The patient may need to make a decision weighing the benefits of the peel versus the appearance of telangiectasia. Prominent telangiectasia are difficult to camouflage with makeup.

Peels Combined with Surgery

Never insult the skin by peeling and undermining the same area simultaneously. It is not advisable to peel an area recovering from a compromised blood supply, such a flap created during surgery on the forehead, face, neck, or eyelids. The ensuing edema may produce pressure necrosis and vascular compromise. Tissue, already injured, may not tolerate the subsequent peel and develop scar tissue. Litton recommended a 6-month elapse before peeling after blepharoplasty to prevent ectropion and possible scarring.[53] This is probably too conservative, as it is often recommended during seminars to wait 3 months. The same applies for a face-neck lift.

Complications Specific to Phenolic Acid

Phenol Cardiotoxicity

Potentially the most serious complication of phenolic acid is its immediate cardiotoxic effect. This has been documented by Truppman and Ellenby[42] and later Gross.[43] They described in patients undergoing a full face phenol peel a variety of arrhythmias, including premature ventricular contractions, ventricular bigeminy, ventricular tachycardia, and premature atrial tachycardia. Significantly, the arrhythmias occurred even in the presence of a normal preoperative electrocardiogram. No parameter could be used to predetermine patient susceptibility. There was no apparent relationship to sex, age, phenol serum levels, administration of oxygen, or use of either a saponified (Baker's formula) or nonsaponified (Litton's formula) phenol peeling formula.

The toxic oral dose of phenol is 8 to 15 gr,

with fatality usual within 24 hours. Since only 1 to 1.5 cc of phenol are applied to the face when utilizing Baker's formula, it is obvious that the margin of safety is very adequate. The systemic toxic manifestations of phenol are evident after a few minutes and include muscular weakness, faintness, weak and irregular pulse, constricted pupils, coma, and possibly even death.[28]

During a peel phenol is absorbed into the bloodstream through both the skin and respiratory tract. Phenol is metabolized in the liver and excreted by the kidneys. It is a potential hepatorenal toxin. Phenol is also excreted by the lungs. Absorption through the skin and thus toxicity are directly related to the quantity applied to the skin, the total surface area treated, the duration of time for the phenol to be applied to the skin, and the rate of excretion.[27] Restricting application to a single facial region, such as the forehead or the right cheek, and then waiting 15 minutes before treatment of the next region limits absorption. This will prevent cardiotoxicity in an adequately hydrated patient without renal, hepatic, or significant cardiac disease. Avoid preoperative dehydration with the administration of intravenous hydration during and after the procedure. This accelerates the excretion of phenol, decreasing the incidence and severity of systemic toxicity.

Cardiac and blood pressure monitoring with adequate hydration is recommended for a full face phenol formula peel. Administration of intravenous fluids (Ringer's lactate), 500 ml preoperatively and 500 to 1000 ml during and after the peel, ensures adequate hydration and rapid diuresis of the absorbed phenol molecule. The appearance of an arrhythmia should immediately suspend further application of phenol. Assuming that the arrhythmia resolves immediately, a timely delay before additional application is advisable. Cessation of the procedure and administration of lidocaine may be required for recurrent or persistent arrhythmias.

The respiratory tract can also be a source of phenol absorption. The physician should not idly hold the phenol-soaked applicator in front of the patient's nose. The room should be well ventilated, for both the patient's and the physician's safety. A small fan in the room aids in the flow of room air. Klein and Little had 3 patients develop laryngeal edema, respiratory stridor, hoarseness, and tachypnea with 24 hours after a phenol peel.[54] Symptoms resolved within 24 hours to 48 hours on warm-mist therapy. Recovery was complete, without evidence of permanent laryngeal injury. All the patients were 1- to 2-pack-a-day cigarette smokers.

If phenol is inadvertently applied to an area of the skin where it is not desired, it can be removed effectively with 50% alcohol or even water, if done immediately.[28] Brown et al. tested a number of treatments for cutaneous decontamination of phenol.[55] The most effective treatment was with a mixture of polyethylene glycols (PEG-300)/industrial methylated spirit, 2:1 by volume). It not only prevented death in the test animals but also effectively reduced the burn capabilities of phenol with only a 20-second swab. This mixture is also nontoxic to the eye. The authors reported that a 60- to 120-second swabbing with water was nearly as effective.

Pain

Application of any peeling agent can cause pain. The pain of phenol is unique. It is described as similar to the burn produced from hot cooking grease. In general, the larger the area treated, the greater the pain. In all cases there is an extreme burning sensation noted within seconds after application. At times the burning sensation reaches its peak immediately and remains for several hours before disappearing completely. Other patients may have an immediate burning sensation that dissipates after several minutes. However, within 30 to 60 minutes, the discomfort returns and remains for approximately another 8 to 12 hours. An occasional patient may experience discomfort for several days.

The pain intensity experienced varies from moderate to the "most intense pain I have ever experienced." The pain is not controlled by oral or intramuscular narcotics. Patients should be warned of this intense discomfort. Midazolam's ability to produce amnesia is helpful. The patient may complain of pain, but its discomfort, as an unpleasant aspect of the surgery, will not be remembered. The author has noted that if

TCA (25% or 35% medium to heavy frost) is applied to the entire face before applying a phenol formula peel to the upper lip, the patient does not seem to experience the usual intense pain. Instead, the pain is typically mild and of short duration in most patients.

Removal of the Facial Tape

Normally, the tape is removed 24 to 48 hours after the phenol peel. If a significant serous exudate has developed, the tape is literally lifted off the face; removal is easy because the tape is not adherent to the facial skin and there is minimal pain with removal. Unfortunately, not all patients produce a copious exudate. The tape remains adherent to the skin, producing pain as it pulls the peeling but incompletely separated skin off the face. Administration of narcotics may be necessary prior to attempting removal. Soaking the tape and face facilitates removal and minimizes trauma to the deeper layers of the newly exposed skin. The physician should apply the tape carefully and avoid taping hair. Taping after a phenol peel is losing its popularity. Application of a moisturizing agent such as Vaseline, vegetable fat, or aquaphor is now more commonly practiced.

Skin Bleaching

The bleaching effect of phenol is to be expected, although it may not manifest itself until many months later. Initially, as the erythema fades, the skin takes on a refreshed, healthy tint. This phase persists for months before fading into a porcelainlike hypopigmentation. The facial skin tone then appears lifeless and ghostly. Proper patient selection can avoid most problems associated with loss of pigmentation. Sunbathers, or individuals not accustomed to applying cosmetic makeup, do not appreciate the new color tone. In contrast, a fair-complexioned individual who shuns sun exposure and skin tanning and who is accustomed to utilizing makeup will find this pigmentary change perfectly acceptable, except for the expected line of demarcation.

The porcelain color is the result of hypopigmentation and depigmentation.[36] Melanocytes are not actually decreased, and there may even be an increase in the number of melanocytes. The melanocytes can still synthesize melanin and distribute the melanin granules to epidermal cells. This explains the mild freckling and uneven pigmentation of the skin that occurs after prolonged sun exposure in some individuals. Hyperpigmentation is not to be expected after a phenol peel, but it can occur. Pigmentation is due to melanocytic stimulation by medications such as estrogen, progesterone, and phenothiazine, which are known to produce hyperpigmentation in susceptible individuals.[46]

Demarcation Lines

Phenol peels are very likely to produce an obvious line of demarcation between peeled and nonpeeled areas. The most common area is along the mandible after a full face phenol peel, but it can also be seen around the lips and hairline. Should the patient undergo a facelift, the line of demarcation formerly hidden just below the mandible is now raised onto the cheeks. Obviously, the greater the extent of solar dermatitis, with its associated pigmentary changes, the greater the contrast that is created. A demarcation line can be produced around the lips if the physician fails to apply the phenol solution onto the lip vermilion. An unsightly, thin border of aged skin outlining the lips would be the result.

Specific Effects of Miscellaneous Peeling Agents: Rare and Unusual Complications

Resorcinism

Resorcinol can cause chronic poisoning, resulting in paralysis, methemoglobinemia, and myxedema[56] along with damage to the capillaries, kidneys, heart, and nervous system. Resorcinol, like phenol, is a hydrocarbon with germicidal properties. Applied extensively, resorcinol can produce systemic toxicity and symptoms similar to phenol poisoning. Resorcinol, however, is only one-third as potent as phenol and requires widespread and protracted skin-surface contact to produce any degree of toxicity. Excess absorption can occur when several large areas are peeled, such as the face and back, or if the paste remains in contact with the skin for a long time.

Salicylic Acid

Salicylism is the toxic effect of an excessive dosage of salicylic acid or its salts, usually marked by tinnitus, nausea, and vomiting. Salicylic acid is utilized as one of several ingredients in several types of peeling pastes and lotions, including Jessner's and Comb's formulae. The combination of oral ingestion of aspirin and widespread application of a paste containing salicylic acid can produce symptoms.

Summary

Over the last decade, a myriad of facial chemical peel solutions and techniques have been developed and improved. The search for a perfect peeling agent, however, a formula that will evaporate wrinkles, can be applied to any skin type, and is relatively free of complications, is still fruitless and exasperating. In general, the more dramatic the results that a peeling agent can produce, the more likely it is that one will also experience major complications. But chemical peeling has become more sophisticated. Repetitive peels, spaced to increase effectiveness while minimizing complications; use of adjuvants to enhance the depth of the peel; and pre- and postpeel regimens have been developed and improved, resulting in safer peels. While improvements have been made, no revolutionary new peeling agent has been discovered.

Essentially, two cutaneous complications cause the majority of disabling, untoward effects of chemical peeling. They are pigmentary alterations and scarring. While there are other complications, these are the most common and disastrous and may require extended postoperative care and recovery. Proper patient skin selection with the appropriate peeling agent, concentration and procedure can avoid most, but not necessarily all, these difficulties. Many of the other peeling complications can usually be easily treated with minimal disability. It is imperative that the physician inform the patient of the more common and serious untoward sequelae.

References

1. Sperber PA. Chemexfoliation for aging skin and acne scarring. Arch Otolaryngol. 1965; 81:278-283.
2. Roberts HL. The chloracetic acids: a biochemical study. Br J Dermatol Syph. 1926; August/September:382.
3. Eller JJ, Wolff S. Skin peeling and scarification. JAMA. 1941;116:934.
4. Polano. J. Am. Acad. Dermatol. 1988;18:1149.
5. Urkov JC. Surface defects of skin: treatment by controlled exfoliation. Ill Med J. 1946; 75.
6. MacKee GM, Karp FL. The treatment of post-acne scars with phenol. Br J Dermatol. 1952;64:456.
7. Marmelzat WL. Bits of history, bits of mystery—a historical review of chemical rejuvenation of the face. In *Chemical Rejuvenation of the Face,* R. Kotler. Mosby-Year Book, St. Louis, 1992.
8. Gross BG, Maschek F. Phenol chemosurgery for removal of deep facial wrinkles. Int J Dermatol. 1980;19:159.
9. Brown AM, Kaplan LM, Brown ME. Phenol-induced histological skin changes: hazards, technique, and uses. Br J Plast Surg. 1960;13:158.
10. Combes FC, Sperber PA, Reisch M. Dermal defects: treatment by a chemical agent. NY Phys Am Med 1960; 56:
11. Baker TJ. The ablation of rhytides by chemical means. J Fla Med Assoc. 1961;48:451.
12. Baker TJ. Chemical face peeling and rhytidectomy. Plast Reconstr Surg. 1962;29:199.
13. Litton C. Chemical face lifting. Plast Reconstr Surg. 1962;29(4):371-380.
14. Ayres S III. Dermal changes following application of chemical cauterants to aging skin (superficial chemosurgery). Arch Dermatol. 1960;82:578.
15. Ayres S III. Superficial chemosurgery in treating aging skin. Arch Dermatol. 1962;85:385.
16. Arohnson RB. Facial Chemosurgery. Eye Ear Nose Throat Monthly 50:20, 1971.
17. Collins PS. Trichloroacetic acid peels revisited. J Dermatol Surg Oncol. 1989;15:933-940.
18. Collins PS. The spectrum of chemical peeling. American Academy of Dermatology Annual Meeting, Las Vegas, December 1985.
19. Brody HJ, Hailey CW. Medium-depth chemical peeling of the skin. J Dermatol Surg Oncol. 1986;12(12):1268-1275.
20. Monheit GD. The Jessner's + TCA peel: a medium-depth chemical peel. J Dermatol Surg Oncol. 1989;15(9):949-950.
21. Coleman WP III. Chemical peel seminar. Amer-

ican Academy of Dermatology Annual Meeting. San Francisco, December 1992.
22. Fulton JE Jr. Step-by-step skin rejuvenation. Am J Cosmet Surg. 1990;7:199.
23 Van Scott EJ, Yu RJ. Control of keratinization with alpha hydroxy acids and related compounds: 1. topical treatment of ichthyotic disorders. Arch Dermatol 1974;110:586.
24. Van Scott EJ. The unfolding therapeutic uses of the alpha-hydroxy acids. Mediguide to Dermatology, AR, ed. Shalita ed. 1988;3(4):1.
25. Elson ML. The utilization of glycolic acid in photoaging. Cosmet Dermatol. 1992;5:12.
26. Matarasso SL, Glogau RC. Chemical face peels. Dermatol Clin. 1991;9:1.
27. Wexler MR, Halon DA, Teitelbaum A, et al. The prevention of cardiac arrhythmias produced in an animal model by the topical application of a phenol preparation in common use for face peeling. Plast Reconstr Surg. 1984;73:595–598.
28. Mosienko P, Baker TJ. Chemical peel. Clin Plast. Surg. 1978;5(1):79–96.
29. Letessier SM. Chemical peel with resorcin. In: *Dermatologic Surgery: Principals and Practice*, RR Roenig and HH ed. Roenig, Marcel Dekker, New York, 1988.
30. Spira M, et al. Chemosurgery—a histological study. Plast Reconstr Surg. 1970;45:247.
31. Baker TJ, et al. Long-term histological study of skin after chemical face peeling. Plast Reconstr Surg. 1974;53:522.
32. Behin F, Feuerstein SS, and Marovitz WF. Comparative histological study of mini pig skin after chemical peel and dermabrasion. Arch Otolaryngol. 1977;103:271.
33. Stegman SJ. A study of dermabrasion and chemical peels in an animal model. J dermatol Surg Oncol. 1980;6:490–497.
34. Stegman SJ. A comparative histological study of the effects of three peeling agents and dermabrasion on normal and sundamaged Skin. Aesthet Plast Surg. 1982;6:123.
35. Hannon DP. American Academy of Dermatology, Dallas, December 1991.
36. Kligman AM, Baker TJ, Gordon HL. Long-term histologic followup of phenol face peels. Plast Reconstr Surg. 1985;75:652–659.
37. Van Scott EJ, Yu RJ. Alpha hydroxyacids: therapeutic potentials. Canadian J Dermatol. 1989;1:108.
38. Moy LS. A comparison of the histologic depth of wounds created by several peeling agents vs. alpha hydroxy acids. update on skin peeling. MG, Rubin Course Director, La Jolla, May 1992.
39. Griffin TD, Van Scott EJ. Use of pyruvic acid in the treatment of actinic keratoses: a clinical and histopathologic study. Cutis. 1991;47:325.
40. Hevia O, Nemeth AJ and Taylor JR. Tretinoin Accelerates Healing After Trichloroacetic Acid Chemical Peel, Arch Dermatol. 1991;27: 678.
41. Koopmann CF Jr. Phenol toxicity during face peels. Otolaryngol Head Neck Surg. 1982;90: 383.
42. Truppman ES, Ellenby JD. Major electrocardiographic changes during chemical face peeling. Plast Reconstr Surg. 1978;63:44–48.
43. Gross BG. Cardiac arrhythmias during phenol face peeling. Plast Reconstr Surg. 1983;73: 590–594.
44. Beeson WH McCollough EG. Chemical face peeling without taping. J Dermatol Surg Oncol. 1985;11:985.
45. Van Scott EJ. The unfolding therapeutic uses of the alpha-hydroxy acids. in Mediguide to Dermatology, AR, Shalita ed., 3:1, 1989.
46. Collins PS. The chemical peel. Dermatol Clin. 1987;5:57–74.
47. Stagnone GJ, Orgel MG, Stagnone JJ. Cardiovascular effects of topical 50% trichloroacetic acid and Baker's phenol solution. J Dermatol Surg Oncol. 1987;13:999–1002.
48. Pinski K. Does isotretinoin cause scarring with chemical peels? Dermatol Times. 1992 (September); 13:6.
49. LoVerme WE, et al. Toxic shock syndrome after chemical face peel. Plast Reconstr Surg. 1987;80:115.
50. Coleman WP III. Chemical peel seminar. American Academy of Dermatology Annual Meeting, San Francisco, December 1992.
51. Brody HJ. Complications of chemical peeling. J Dermatol Surg Oncol. 1989 (September); 15(9):1010–1019.
52. Hung VC, Lee JY, Zitelli JA, Hebda PA. Topical tretinoin and epithelial wound healing. Arch Dermatol. 1989;125;1:65–69.
53. Litton C, Szachowicz EH, Trinidad GP. Present day status of the chemical face peel, Aesthet Plast Surg. 1986;10(1):1–6.
54. Klein DR, Little JH. Laryngeal edema as a complication of chemical peel. Plast Reconstr Surg. 1983;71:419.
55. Brown VKH, Box VL, Simpton BJ. Decontamination procedures for skin exposed to phenolic substances. Arch Environ Health. 1975; 30:1.
56. Thomas AE, Gisburn MA. Exogenous onchronosis and myxedema from resorinol. Br J Dermatol. 1961;73:378–81.

6
Dermabrasion

Bruce E. Katz

History

The earliest efforts to improve surface irregularities of the human skin date back to antiquity. In the Egyptian Papyrus Ebers, which was published circa 1500 B.C., descriptions of abrasive pastes of pumice and alabaster particles in honey and milk used to smooth skin defects are found. These formulations endured in a host of variations over many centuries. In fact, the great European dermatologist Unna, in the late nineteenth century, applied compounds of pumice to facial skin to improve its cosmetic appearance.

Kromayer, in 1905, described rudimentary motor-powered dermabrasion instrumentation which he used to plane down facial scars and defects.[1] Considered the father of modern dermabrasion (see Table 6.1), he first applied cylindrical knives and then dental burrs and rasps to treat a variety of conditions, including freckles, pigmentation, nevi, tattoos, warts, and scars. His innovations also included freezing with carbon dioxide snow and ether spray to provide the rigidity and anesthesia that are suitable for dermabrasion. Kromayer's book *Cosmetic Treatment of Skin Complaints* detailed the evolution of his technique and its applications.[2] There was little interest, however, in this new area of surgery until the 1930s.

In 1935 Janson reported the use of a stiff-bristled brush to remove a tattoo, with good cosmetic results.[3] Twelve years later Iverson drew more attention to skin abrasion by successfully removing traumatic tattoos with common carpenters' sandpaper.[4] McEvitt applied sandpaper abrasion to the treatment of acne pits with a satisfactory outcome.[5] However, this method of abrasion had several significant limitations: General anesthesia was usually necessary; selective abrasion of anatomical sites was obscured by the bloody field; and the development of foreign-body silica granulomas was a frequent complication.

In the early 1950s, Abner Kurtin refined much of Kromayer's original work and reawakened the interest of dermatologists in this field.[6] His contributions included developing motor-driven wire brushes and using ethyl chloride as a skin refrigerant. This permitted controlled abrasion in a relatively bloodless field. Kurtin's technique was applied successfully to such conditions as fine wrinkles, freckles, keratoses, acne pits, traumatic scars, and tattoos.

Indications

Dermatoheliosis refers to the clinical changes seen in the skin as a result of photoaging (chronic exposure to solar radiation). These include yellowed and mottled pigmentation; rhytides; leathery and rough surface; telangiectasias; skin laxity; and neoplastic proliferations, including actinic keratoses, lentigos, seborrheic keratoses, and, eventually, basal cell and squamous cell carcinomas.

Dermabrasion is an extremely versatile mo-

TABLE 6.1. Early pioneers of dermabrasion.

Kromayer	1905
Janson	1935
Iverson	1947
McEvitt	1948
Kurtin	1953

dality. It has been applied to more than 50 skin conditions[7] for therapeutic as well as cosmetic purposes.

The indications for dermabrasion in dermatoheliosis or photoaging can be considered in terms of its therapeutic effects (i.e., treatment of actinic damage) and cosmetic effects (i.e., treatment of rhytides, solar lentigines, and altered pigmentation). The efficacy of dermabrasion in the prevention and treatment of actinic keratoses and in prophylaxis against development of skin carcinomas has been well documented.[7-12] In a recent study, further confirmation of the beneficial therapeutic effects of dermabrasion was found.[13] Benedetto et al. reviewed predermabrasion skin biopsies in 10 patients and compared them to postdermabrasion biopsies as long as 8 years later. All predermabrasion specimens showed epidermal thinning, focal effacement of rete pattern, dyskeratosis, and abnormal keratinocyte polarity. There was thinning of the Grenz zone of the papillary dermis, decreased density of collagen fibers, and absence of elastic fibers. Predermabrasion, all patients showed clinical signs of photoaging, including rhytides, yellow and mottled pigmentation, telangiectasias, a leathery and pebbly surface, and tissue laxity. Normalization of the histologic signs of photoaging persisted for more than 2 years postdermabrasion. Clinically, the dermabraded skin was found to be soft and smooth, with the absence of signs of dermatoheliosis. In some cases these changes persisted for up to 8 years. While the nonabraded skin of the trunk and extremities of these patients continued to develop actinic keratoses and basal cell and squamous cell carcinomas, the abraded facial skin did not.

Patients with severe photoaging resulting in multiple actinic keratoses of the face are often treated with liquid nitrogen, curettage, or other destructive techniques. Such therapy is usually prolonged and requires many visits. The patchy hypopigmentation resulting from this intermittent treatment is often cosmetically displeasing. Though topical 5-fluorouracil therapy is effective in ablating both active and latent actinic keratoses, the 6 to 8 weeks of discomfort and physical disfigurement resulting from this treatment is often a deterrent to its use. This compares to the 7 to 10 days required for wound healing after dermabrasion with subsequent uniform facial pigmentation (see Figures 6.1A and B).

Dermabrasive treatment of cosmetic lesions, such as wrinkles, solar lentigines, seborrheic keratoses, and mottled pigmentation, is effective and long-lasting (refer to Figures 6.2A and B and Figures 6.3A and B). This assumes continued use of photoprotection postoperatively. Full face dermabrasion is preferred to segmental dermabrasion, as the latter treatment may lead to differences in pigmentation between abraded and nonabraded skin.

When compared to deep phenol peels in the treatment of photoaged skin, dermabrasion may have advantages in selected cases.[14] This is particularly true when the control of depth of treatment is critical. In more darkly pigmented individuals, dermabrasion produces less of a bleaching effect than phenol and therefore less color contrast between treated and untreated skin.

Patient Selection

The initial consultation is often critical in determining the patient's ultimate satisfaction with the outcome of the dermabrasion procedure. As in any assessment for a cosmetic procedure, the psychosocial as well as medical characteristics of an individual must be considered. Careful attention should be given to developing good rapport with the patient. He or she should feel able to discuss any questions or problems openly with the physician, in an unhurried fashion. The patient should have realistic expectations of the anticipated surgery and how the cosmetic outcome will affect his or her

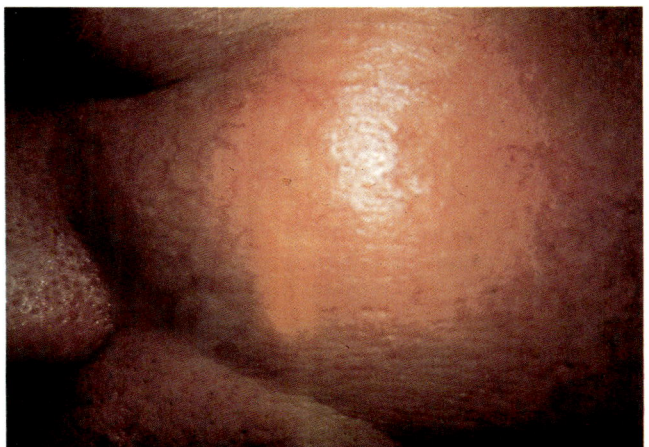

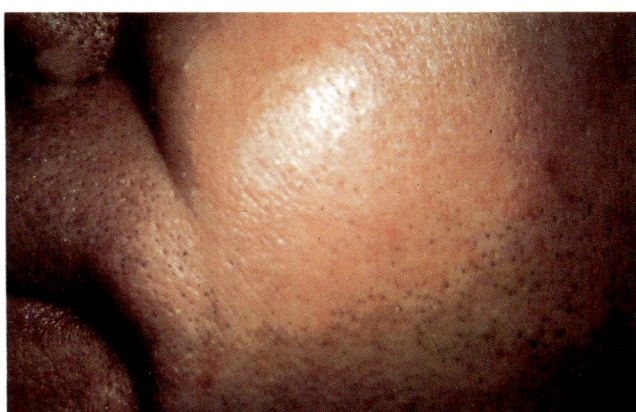

FIGURE 6.1. A. Severe photoaging of the face before dermabrasion. B. Two months after dermabrasion, with clearing of actinic keratoses, lentigines, and telangiectasias.

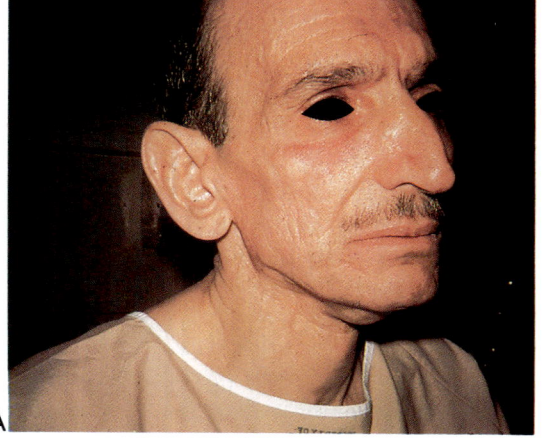
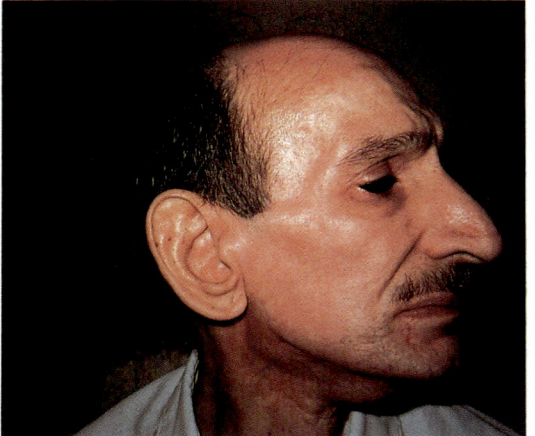

FIGURE 6.2A. Multiple rhytides and telangiectasias before dermabrasion. B. Significant improvement 6 months after dermabrasion.

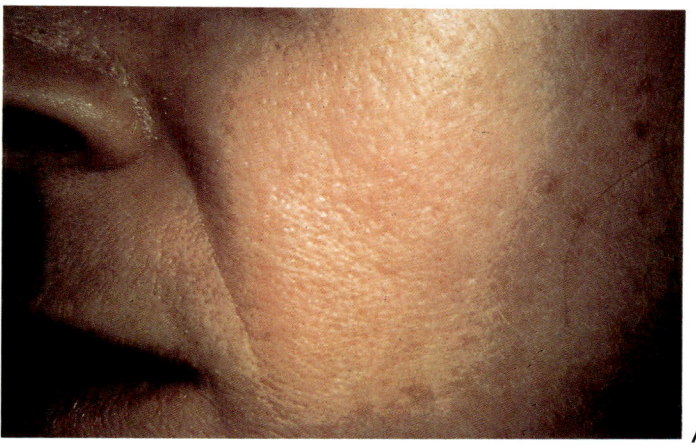

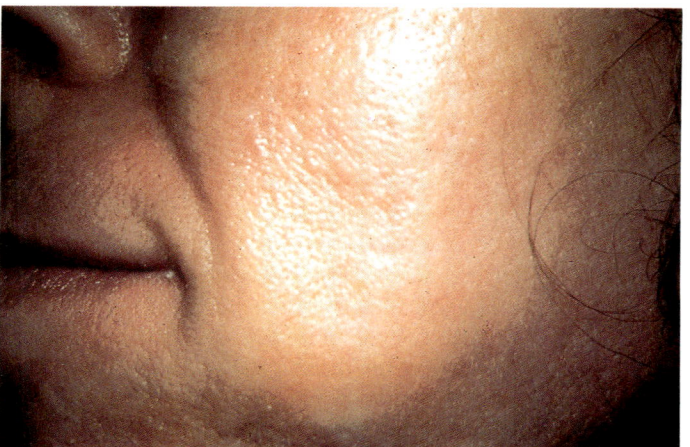

FIGURE 6.3. A. Fine rhytides and lentigines in a 38-year-old female before dermabrasion. B. Clearing of rhytides and lentigines 6 months after dermabrasion.

life. The individual who believes that the removal of wrinkles and dark spots from one's face will significantly improve one's love life or job status is a poor candidate for dermabrasion. One who is greatly disturbed by a slight imperfection will never be completely satisfied by the benefits afforded by this technique.

Adequate time should be spent outlining all aspects of the surgery, from preoperative preparation to postoperative care. The risks as well as benefits of the procedure should be described and alternative therapy reviewed. Adjunctive techniques such as microlipoinjection or collagen injections that can enhance the outcome may be discussed.

It is helpful to have an assistant show before and after photographs of patients who have undergone dermabrasion for a similar problem. However, the identity of the patients shown in these photos should be protected, as there have been instances in which such individuals have been recognized. Well-produced videotapes (for public viewing) describing all aspects of the procedure have been found to be an excellent vehicle for informing the patient. Written information can be provided to the patient to reinforce details of the interview that may have been forgotten.

Pigmentary alteration as a result of dermabrasion is a concern that should be addressed from the outset. The lightest and darkest skin colors are least likely to exhibit pigmentary change. Persons of intermediate color (e.g., light-colored Hispanic or Asian) often develop hyperpigmentation after dermabrasion, which is temporary if treated early. Topical hydroquinone applied twice daily usually resolves this problem within several weeks of onset. The physician should also evaluate scars and pigmentary changes in other areas of the body to assess how the individual's skin responds to trauma in general. If there is evidence of major pigmentary changes from just the slightest trauma, dermabrasion may provoke similar responses and should probably be deferred. Evidence of significant numbers of keloids and hypertrophic scars also makes the patient a poor candidate for dermabrasion.

Complete chart documentation of all aspects of the patient interview, examination, and the audiovisuals shown is a necessity. All patients must be told that adequate sunscreen use is mandatory for at least 6 months after surgery and preferably longer-term in order to prevent the recurrence of dermatoheliosis.

Isotretinoin (Accutane) and Scarring

Atypical scarring may develop in patients undergoing dermabrasion after having recently completed a course of isotretinoin (Accutane).[15-17] Such scarring has been called *atypical* because it occurs in areas of the face (e.g., the hollows of cheeks) usually not considered at high risk for dermabrasion scarring. The author has recently reported a case where atypical scarring of the cheek developed in a patient who took a course of isotretinoin a short time after having had a full face dermabrasion.[17]

Although opinions differ as to the exact time interval that should elapse between the use of isotretinoin and undergoing dermabrasion, at least 6 to 24 months is considered the range of time between each treatment. It is therefore prudent to elicit any history of isotretinoin use and to weigh carefully its possible impact on the outcome of dermabrasion.

Contraindications

Patients with a history of chronic radiodermatitis or extensive burn scars are considered contraindications to dermabrasion. Due to a reduction in the number of adnexal structures, these patients usually heal poorly. Xeroderma pigmentosum is a contraindication as well as cryoglobulinemia or cryofibrinogenemia, particularly when topical refrigerants are used. In cases of active discoid lupus erythematosus and scleroderma, dermabrasion should be deferred. Dermabrasion is not advised for patients with psychoses or severe neuroses—in addition to having unrealistic expectations, these patients may compromise the results by following directions poorly and not keeping the required follow-up appointments.

Active verruca plana, pyoderma, and HIV are also considered contraindications to dermabrasion. The risk of spread of these infections through contact and aerosols poses a serious problem for the surgeon and staff. In the case of HIV, the immunocompromised state may lead to a suboptimal cosmetic outcome due to poor healing.

Herpes simplex has been considered a relative contraindication to dermabrasion. It has been suggested that patients in whom there is a history of herpes simplex involving a localized area of the face (e.g., herpes labialis) should take prophylactic acyclovir (Zovirax) orally before and during dermabrasion.[18] It has been the author's experience, however, that even patients who have not reported a history of cutaneous herpes may develop an episode postdermabrasion. Such cases can be extensive and cause scarring. Whether it occurs in an area of previous subclinical infection or as a result of primary infection is not clear.

Since acyclovir is relatively safe, with few side effects, it is now given routinely at a dose of 200 mg, 3 times a day, to all patients having a full face dermabrasion, beginning 3 days before surgery and continuing for 10 days. There have been no cases of herpes simplex postdermabrasion since this regimen was begun and no side effects from the medication.

Preoperative Preparation

Preoperative laboratory studies include CBC, platelet count, SMA-20, prothrombin time, partial thromboplastin time, syphilis serology, hepatitis B surface antigen, and HIV serology.

At the time that these tests are ordered, pre- and postoperative care instructions are given to the patient. He or she then has time to review this material and can call if there are any questions. The patient is also reminded to have someone accompany him or her home after the procedure. Topical retinoic acid applied nightly, beginning at least 2 weeks before dermabrasion, may reduce the incidence of milia postoperatively.

Prescriptions are also given at this time so that the patient will have the required postoperative medications before the day of surgery. These include acetaminophen with codeine (30 mg q4-6h prn) for pain, mupirocin ointment (bid), and acyclovir (200 mg tid) beginning 3 days before surgery and continuing for 10 days. Prednisone (40 mg per day) is given in a tapering dose over 7 days to reduce postoperative edema.

Standard and close-up photographs with adequate lighting should be taken preoperatively for documentation as well as medicolegal purposes.

Anesthesia

A number of different approaches can be taken with predermabrasion anesthesia in order to relax the patient and reduce pain. Intramuscular meperidine (50 to 100 mg), midazolam (HCL 2.5 to 5.0 mg) and hydroxyzine (25 mg) is one popular combination of premedications. Prechilling of the skin with ice packs potentiates the effects of cryoanesthesia. The surgeon or assistant sprays either Frigiderm or Fluro Ethyl topical refrigerants on the area to be abraded in a circular fashion for 10 to 20 seconds. This produces a rigid, frozen surface on which to perform dermabrasion. With this regimen, however, patients may complain of discomfort from the freezing produced by the cryogens or burning from the actual dermabrasion. The use of facial regional nerve blocks with 0.5% Xylocaine obviates this problem to a great extent.

There are some individuals who refuse to have regional blocks due to the number of needle sticks employed. Others are very nervous or restless during the actual dermabrasion and, by constantly moving, make the procedure more difficult to perform. For these and other patients, intravenous sedation with agents such as fentanyl citrate and midazolam HCL can be very efficacious. An anesthesiologist works with the surgeon and oversees the use of all intravenous medications. This approach allows for a less stressful and more facile dermabrasion, as the patient is comfortable and at rest. It is more expeditious and less time consuming, as regional blocks are not employed and intramuscular agents need not be readministered midway through the procedure. As the responsibility for supervising the administration of medication is the anesthesiologist's, the surgeon can concentrate exclusively on performing the best possible dermabrasion.

Equipment

It is optimal to have one well-ventilated air-conditioned operating room set aside in which to perform dermabrasion. The room temperature should be maintained at between 60°F to 65°F to allow for adequate use of skin refrigerants. An adjustable operating table, sufficient lighting, and emergency equipment should be standard apparatus.

Fluid-impervious surgical gowns, boots, caps, gloves, eye goggles, and face shields should be worn by the operator and assistant. Recent work has raised concern about the possible inhalation of particulate matter produced by dermabrasion through standard surgical masks.[19] Of concern also is the persistence of this material in the ambient room air for hours after the procedure. Although the actual risk of infection from these aerosols is unknown, it seems prudent to use high-filtration surgical respirators instead of regular surgical masks. The latter were designed to prevent exhaled particles from escaping the mask and not for reducing the risk of the operator for contracting a disease. Respirators were designed to protect against specific respiratory hazards and offer a better fit than traditional masks (see Figure 6.4). An efficient ventilation system in the operating room is desirable. All counters and furnishings in the room should be cleaned

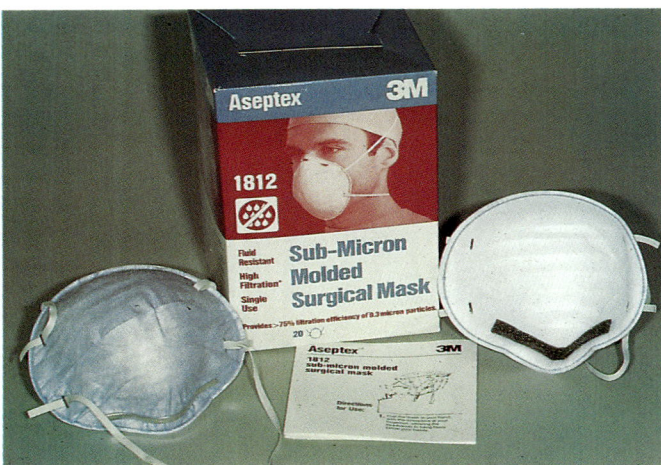

FIGURE 6.4. Example of a high-filtration surgical respirator.

with appropriate germicidal agents on a regular basis.

Dermabrading machines used in the past included the cable-driven Robbins type and compressed nitrogen gas units. Currently, the most popular are small, hand-held electric engines, such as the Bell and Osada models.

The abrading tools or end pieces for dermabrasion are either the wire brush, the diamond fraise, or the serrated wheel (see Figures 6.5 and 6.6). The wire brush consists of a stainless steel wheel with wires projecting at an angle. Diamond fraises are stainless steel cones, cylinders, or wheels of various sizes to which diamond chips are bonded. Serrated wheels combine features of the wire brush and the diamond fraise but are rarely used. Proponents of either the wire brush or diamond fraise claim superior results with one or the other tool. However, the skill and experience of the operator are probably the greatest determinants of cosmetic outcome.

Fluro Ethyl and Frigiderm are the most popular skin refrigerants used today. Fluro Ethyl is a mixture of Freon 114 and ethyl chloride, and Frigiderm is pure Freon 114.

Technique

The patient lies in the supine position so that the face can be moved from side to side. Some operators prechill the skin with ice packs for 15 to 20 minutes, but this is not required. Skin markers or gentian violet is used to outline the areas to be abraded. Lines are usually drawn just below the jawline, at the infraorbital rims, and to highlight any areas that may need deeper abrasion. This is done in the sitting position to account for any effects of gravity.

Dermabrasion is usually performed in segments. Surgical towels or sterilized baby diapers are used by the assistant to delineate the area to be abraded and to protect the eyes, nose, and mouth from the refrigerant spray. The use of gauze is to be avoided, as it easily becomes tangled in the spinning handpiece.

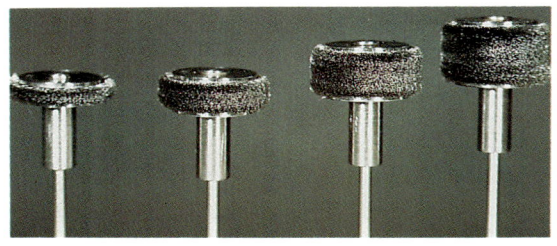

FIGURE 6.5. Wire brushes in various sizes.

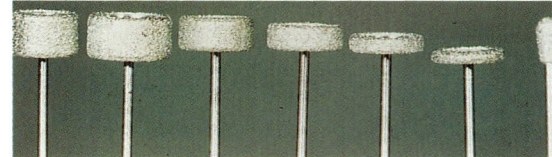

FIGURE 6.6. Diamond fraises in different sizes and shapes.

Skin refrigerants such as Frigiderm or Fluor Ethyl are sprayed over each segment for 10 to 20 seconds to produce a solid surface on which to abrade. It is important that the skin be frozen in the natural, nondistended position so that rhytides and other lesions can be abraded to the proper depth. If the skin is stretched before freezing, margins of the rhytides may be distorted or missed and not blended with the surrounding skin.

Dermabrasion is performed on the dependent areas of the face first, followed by the central and upper areas. If this order is reversed, blood running over areas to be abraded obscures the surgical field. The handpiece is moved with slow, steady strokes, with attention given to blending the interfaces of the various segments of the face. Moving the fraise or wire brush in different directions will result in a uniform abrasion and avoid the appearance of "brush strokes." Care should be taken when abrading in the periorbital areas. Some recommend covering the eyelids with Vaseline, lead shields, or goggles, but careful use of towels to protect the eyes usually suffices.

Areas such as the mandible, malar eminence, zygomatic arch, and bosses of the forehead and chin are considered "danger zones" and should be approached with care. Excessive freezing or abrading too deeply may result in scarring.

Dermabrasion should be carried onto the vermilion of the lip in order to remove as much of the perioral rhytides as possible. Failure to do so will result in short, fine wrinkles radiating out from the lips. Abrasion should also be carried into the hairline and eyebrows so that a border of unabraded, "weathered" skin is not apparent.

Dermabrasion of the entire face results in the best cosmetic outcome; however, certain patients may wish that only segmental dermabrasion be performed. The abrasion should then be confined to an entire cosmetic unit. For example, a patient may wish to have only the "lip lines" treated. However, the entire chin, upper lip, and skin extending to the nasolabial folds should be abraded so that pigment or texture changes are less evident (see Figures 6.7A and B). Even when the entire cosmetic unit is dermabraded, the patient should be advised in advance that slight differences in appearance may be detectable between the treated and adjacent untreated skin. Any differences in pigment can usually be camouflaged by makeup.

Postoperative Management

There are a number of approaches to postoperative care after full face dermabrasion. The traditional method has been to apply an antibiotic ointment to the face, over which a petro-

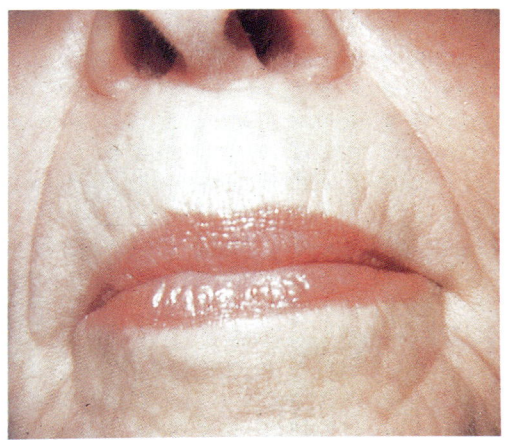
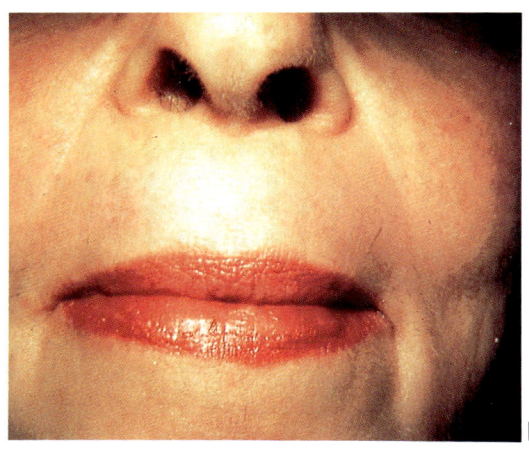

FIGURE 6.7. A. Upper and lower lip rhytides before segmental dermabrasion. B. One year after dermabrasion of the entire cosmetic unit, including the lips, chin, and nasolabial folds.

latum-impregnated gauze is kept in place with a cloth face mask tied behind the back of the head. Acetaminophen and codeine usually suffice for pain management. Sleeping with the head on two pillows on the night of the procedure reduces the amount of facial edema and is more comfortable. The patient comes to the office the next morning to have the bandage removed. Warm tap-water compresses are done 2 or 3 times a day, followed by the application of antibiotic ointment. Lubricating the wound with ointment keeps the crust soft, allows for faster healing, and is more comfortable for the patient. After several days the face can be washed with mild soap and water, followed by ointment applications.

More recently, biologic dressings such as Vigilon, Tegaderm, Bioclusive, Biobrane, Omniderm, and others have become available. Reepithelialization proceeds more quickly with the use of these materials.[20] Vigilon is the most popular dressing, as it absorbs a substantial amount of exudate and has a soothing effect. After one side of the polyethylene film is removed, it is applied directly to the abraded skin, with or without antibiotic ointment. Gauze and tape or a face mask is used to hold it in place. The dressing is changed daily. Three to 4 days postoperative, when the amount of exudate is minimal, Vigilon can be discontinued and only antibiotic ointment applied.

A short course of systemic corticosteroids may help to reduce facial edema. Avoidance of sun exposure must be stressed and the patient instructed in the use of adequate sunscreens once they can be tolerated. The freshly abraded skin will be sensitive to sun exposure for at least 3 to 6 months. The pruritus that occurs as healing proceeds can be managed with noncomedogenic emollients. Strenuous exercise should be avoided for several weeks postoperative.

Patients are usually seen at 1, 3, 6, and 12 weeks postdermabrasion, and more frequently if warranted. After the crusts have cleared, the face may be erythematous for several weeks. Instructing the patient in the use of paramedical cosmetics to camouflage the abraded areas allows the return to normal activities more quickly. Patients are often very appreciative of the surgeon's attention to this "social" aspect of their recovery in addition to the medical considerations.

Side Effects and Complications

The most common side effects and complications of dermabrasion include hypopigmentation, hyperpigmentation, persistent erythema, keloids, milia, herpes simplex, and telangiectasias.

Hypopigmentation and hyperpigmentation are frequent side effects and are usually transitory. Excessive prolonged hypopigmentation may be related to overuse of skin refrigerants with destructive effects on melanocytes. Hyperpigmentation is seen more often in darkly complected individuals, usually at the borders of the dermabrasion. It may, however, be diffuse and/or patchy. Postinflammatory hyperpigmentation usually clears in several months but may persist longer (refers to Figures 6.8A and B). Topical hydroquinone may speed its resolution. Erythema is a natural sequela of dermabrasion appearing once crusts have come off. It usually lasts for several weeks but in certain cases may continue for longer. Twice-daily applications of hydrocortisone 2½% ointment (Hytone-Dermik) help these areas to fade more quickly.

Once generalized erythema of the face has subsided, one should be attentive to persistent areas of localized erythema, particularly over the jawline. This may indicate early development of persistent erythema or hypertrophic scarring. Application of Cordran tape or short courses of superpotent corticosteroid creams can help these areas fade. If localized skin induration begins to develop, indicating early hypertrophic scar or keloid formation, intralesional corticosteroid injections may be administered.

Recent work with silicone gel sheeting has shown it to be effective in preventing the development of hypertrophic scarring.[21-23] A piece of gel sheeting is taped over the involved area, with the shiny side facing the skin. It should be kept in place for 12 to 24 hours a day. The gel sheet is washed once a day with a soap and water solution and replaced with a fresh piece every 7 to 10 days (when it begins to crumble).

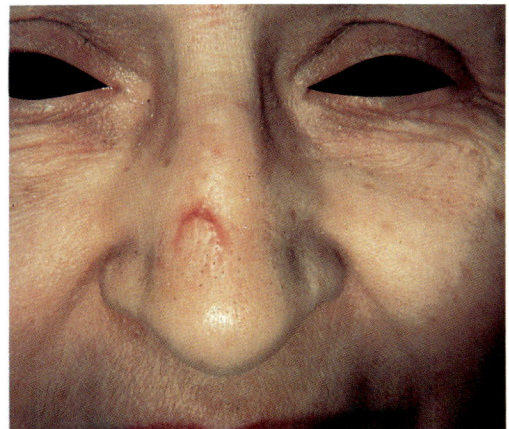 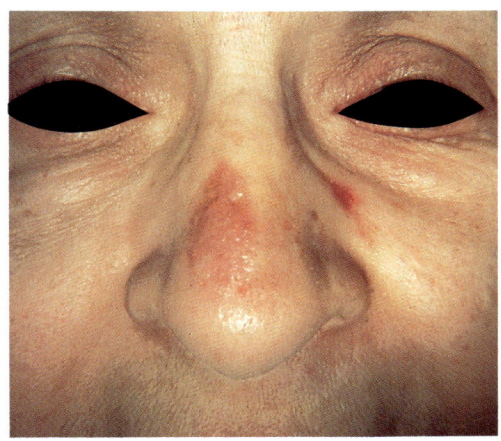

FIGURE 6.8. A. Before dermabrasion of nasal scar. B. Postinflammatory hyperpigmentation after dermabrasion of nasal scar.

It is worn until the area of erythema or hypertrophy returns to normal.

Milia formation is a common side effect of dermabrasion and usually clears spontaneously after several months (see Figure 6.9). The incidence of milia may be reduced by the use of topical tretinoin before dermabrasion. If milia are present in large numbers or are cosmetically displeasing to the patient, they may be treated with light electrodessication or incision with a #11 blade.

Herpes simplex infection after dermabrasion is a complication that can usually be avoided by the prophylactic use of oral acyclovir. Although some have advocated its use only inpatients in whom there is a prior history of herpes infection, cases of generalized herpes with subsequent scarring after dermabrasion have been seen in patients with no personal history of the infection. This may represent previous subclinical infection or primary infection from exposure to another individual with the condition. Since the risks of a short course of oral acyclovir are minimal, its use in the prevention of herpes infection and potential scarring after dermabrasion appear to be justified. If severe, disseminated herpes simplex occurs, hospitalization and intravenous acyclovir are indicated.

Telangiectasia, or petechiae, are a rare complication. They may be due to skin torsion or overly aggressive treatment of hypertrophic scars with intralesional corticosteroids. These lesions usually resolve over time.

Gouging or grooving of the skin is usually due to poor technique. Careful attention at all

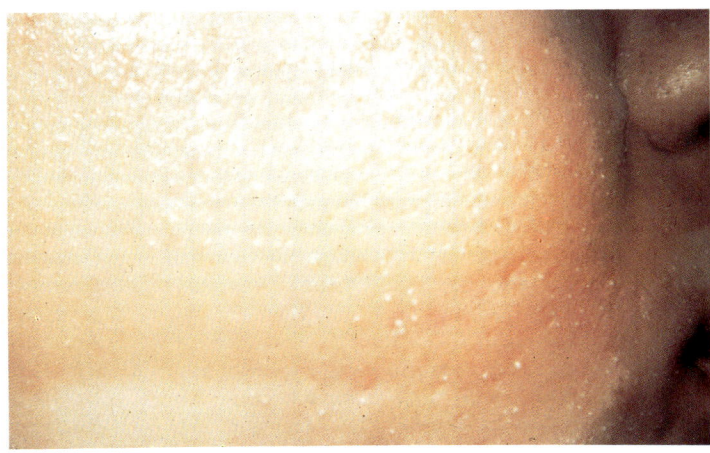

FIGURE 6.9. Milia formation after full face dermabrasion.

times to the direction of rotation of the fraise or wire brush reduces the possibility of gouging or tearing of skin. Grooving can be avoided by moving the handpiece in short strokes and abrading each area from different directions. Regular inspection and maintenance of the hand engine and endpieces will prevent injuries to both patient and staff from equipment failure.

References

1. Kromayer E. Rotationsinstrumente: ein neues technisches Verfahren in der dermatologischen Kleinchirurgie. Dermatol Z. 1905; 12:26.
2. Kromayer E. *Cosmetic Treatment of Skin Complaints.* English translation of the second German ed (1929). Oxford University Press, New York, 1930.
3. Janson P. Eine einfache methode der entfernung. Dermatol Wochenschr. 1935;101:894-895.
4. Iverson PC. Surgical treatment of skin lesions by abrasion. Plast Reconstr Surg. 1953;12:27-31.
5. McEvitt WG. Acne pits. J Mich Med Soc. 1948;47:1234-1244.
6. Kurtin A. Corrective surgical planing of the skin. Arch Dermatol. 1953;68(supplement):389-397.
7. Alt TH, Coleman WP, Hanke CW, et al. Dermabrasion. In: *Cosmetic Surgery of the Skin,* WP Coleman, CW Hanke, TH Alt, et al., eds. BC Decker, Philadelphia, 1991, pp. 147-195.
8. Field L. Dermabrasion versus 5 fluorouracil in the management of actinic keratoses. In: *Controversies in Dermatology,* I Epstein, ed. WB Saunders, Philadelphia, 1984, pp. 62-102.
9. Epstein E. Dermabrasion for therapeutic purposes. In: *Skin Surgery.* E Epstein, E Epstein Jr, eds. WB Saunders, Philadelphia, 1987: pp. 344-347.
10. Burks J, Marascalco J, Clark W. Half-face planing of precancerous skin after five years. Arch Dermatol. 1963;88:572-582.
11. Burks J, Brewer J, Chernosky ME. Surgical planing for the prevention of cancer of the skin. South Med J. 1960;53:86-91.
12. Epstein E. Planing for precancerous skin—a ten-year evaluation. Calif Med. 1966;105:26-27.
13. Benedetto AV, Griffin TD, Benedetto EA, et al. Dermabrasion: therapy and prophylaxis of the photoaged face. J Am Acad Dermatol. 1992;27:439-447.
14. Stuzin JM, Baker TJ, Gordon HL. Treatment of photoaging: facial chemical peeling (phenol and trichloroacetic acid) and dermabrasion. In: *Clinics in Plastic Surgery,* MH McGrath, ML Turner, eds. 1993, 20:9-25.
15. Rubenstein R, Roenigk HH, Stegman SJ, et al. Atypical keloids after dermabrasion of patients taking isotretinoin. J Am Acad Dermatol. 1986;15:280-285.
16. Zachariae H. Delayed wound healing and keloid formation following argon laser treatment or dermabrasion during isotretinoin treatment. Br J Dermatol. 1988;118:703-706.
17. Katz BE, MacFarlane DF. Atypical facial scarring after isotretinoin therapy in a patient with previous dermabrasion. J Am Acad Dermatol. 1994;30:852-53.
18. Silverman AK, Laing KF, Swanson NA, et al. Activation of herpes simplex following dermabrasion. J Am Acad Dermatol. 1985;13:103-107.
19. Wentzell MJ, Robinson JK. Physical properties of aerosols produced by dermabrasion. Arch Dermatol. 1989;125:1637.
20. Pinski JB. Dressings for dermabrasion: new aspects. J Dermatol Surg Oncol. 1987;13:673-677.
21. Katz BE. Silastic gel sheeting is found to be effective in scar therapy. Cosmet Dermatol. 1992;5:32-34.
22. Ahn ST, Monafo WW, Mustoe TA. Topical silicone gel for the prevention and treatment of hypertrophic scar. Arch Surg. 1991;126:499-504.
23. Katz BE. Dermabrasion for scar revision. In: *Surgical Dermatology: Advances in Current Practice,* RK Roenigk, HH Roenigk, Jr, eds. Martin Dunitz, London, 1993, pp. 391-392.
24. Roenigk HH. Dermabrasion. *Dermatologic Surgery: Principles and Practice,* In: RK Roenigk, HH Roenigk, Jr, eds. Marcel Dekker, New York, 1989, pp. 959-978.
25. Stegman SJ, Tromovitch TA. *Cosmetic Dermatologic Surgery.* Year Book Medical Publishers, Chicago, 1984, pp. 47-76.
26. Burks JW. *Dermabrasion and Chemical Peeling in the Treatment of Certain Cosmetic Defects and Diseases of the Skin.* Charles C. Thomas, Springfield, 1979, pp. 45-138.
27. Yarborough JM. Preoperative evaluation of the patient for dermabrasion. J Dermatol Surg Oncol. 1987;13:652-653.
28. Alt TH. Facial dermabrasion: advantages of the diamond fraise technique. J Dermatol Surg Oncol. 1987;13:618-624.
29. Yarborough JM. Dermabrasion by wire brush. J Dermatol Surg Oncol. 1987;13:610-615.
30. Dzubow LM. Survey of refrigeration and surgical technics used for facial dermabrasion. J Am Acad Dermatol. 1985;13:287-292.
31. Alt TH. Technical aids for dermabrasion. J Dermatol Surg Oncol. 1987;13:638-648.
32. Roenigk HH Jr. Dermabrasion: state of the art. J Dermatol Surg Oncol. 1985;11:306-314.

7
Soft Tissue Augmentation

Melvin L. Elson

Soft tissue augmentation — the ability to soften and build up the tissue of the face by means other than surgical — has actually been attempted for centuries. Substances used in the past such as beeswax and paraffin were not only not particularly effective but often caused devastating complications, even death.[1] In the modern era, various substances have been used to augment and soften the features of the face, but no perfect material yet exists.

The perfect material for soft tissue augmentation would have certain characteristics: It would be readily available; be easily administered; be forgiving for the physician; induce no allergy, infection, or disease; be noncarcinogenic; feel and look like natural tissue; require little time off work or social activities on the part of the patient; be inexpensive; and, over time, be replaced by host tissue.[2] Obviously, there is no material that meets all these criteria.

Of the substances recently used (such as silicone), the substances currently in use (such as bovine injectable collagen, Fibrel, Koken Atelocollagen, Bioplastique, autologous fat, autologous collagen, autocol, and Gore-Tex), and certain substances under investigation (such as hyaluronic acid and human collagen), bovine products set the standard to which others must be compared with regard to both safety and efficacy. Zyderm and Zyplast collagen have now received approval in 31 countries and have been injected in more than 1,000,000 patients worldwide.

Bovine Collagen

The use of bovine collagen in surgery and medicine is certainly not new — suture material, hemostatic sponges and other devices have utilized this technology for decades (see Table 7.1). In July 1981 the U.S Food and Drug Administration (FDA) approved Zyderm-I as the first device for cosmetic use in soft tissue augmentation.[3] It consists of 95% Type I and 5% Type III bovine collagen prepared from cow hide to produce a final product, a sterile suspension in a concentration of 35 mg per cc buffered with physiologic saline containing 0.3% lidocaine. In 1982 Zyderm-II was approved, which is 65 mg per cc concentration. Zyplast was approved in 1985.[4] Like Zyderm-I, Zyplast is 35 mg per cc concentration, but during processing it is cross-linked with glutaraldehyde across lysine residues to produce a lattice that maintains its integrity with less syneresis upon injection. This acts as a more robust filler and can be used to augment tissue as well as as a filling material for scars, lines, and wrinkles, especially when used in conjunction with Zyderm-I or Zyderm-II.

More recently, Zyderm-I with fine-gauge needle has become available. It is identical to Zyderm-I with the fibrils now uniform and giving it the ability to flow through finer gauge needles (*i.e.*, 32- or 33-gauge needles). This completes the current family of products of bovine collagen available from Collagen Corporation.

TABLE 7.1. Collagen as a biomaterial currently marketed medical devices.

Currently marketed medical device	Use	Collagen source	Years of use
Suture	Closure of surgical incisions	Bovine or ovine tissue	100
Suture	Closure of surgical incisions	Bovine tendon	30
Hemostat	Antibleeding agent	Bovine and porcine skin	30
Dermal implant	Correction of scars, wrinkles, and contour deformities	Bovine skin	10
Synthetic blood vessel	Vascular prosthesis	Bovine artery	10
Wound dressing	To aid in wound-healing process	Bovine skin	5
Corneal shield	Temporary covering for damaged cornea	Bovine tendon	5
Catheter cuff	Anchors catheter into skin	Bovine	3
Alveolar onlay	Jawbone augmentation for improved denture fit	Bovine skin	3

The materials are prepared by pepsin digestion and purification, and the telopeptide regions of the molecule are hydrolyzed to decrease the antigenicity. Although this does decrease the antigenicity, the potential for allergy remains in this xenogeneic material, necessitating skin testing in the forearm prior to injection in the face. Although no significant problems were evident in the use of bovine collagen materials in the past in other medical uses, it was thought prudent to institute skin testing in the cosmetic use of these products.

Skin Testing

Three percent of the population are allergic to the material, probably through dietary exposure, and cannot undergo augmentation. It is the purpose of skin testing to select out this population. The current package insert directs the physician to skin test the patient by injecting 0.1 cc Zyderm-I into the dermis of the volar surface of the forearm. This test is to be read in 48 to 72 hours and again at 4 weeks. A *positive test* is defined as: "erythema of any degree, induration, tenderness, or swelling at the test site, with or without pruritus, which persists for more than six hours or appears more than 24 hours following implantation."[5]

This method of skin testing will detect most patients allergic to the material, but not all of them. This incomplete detection allows for adverse reactions to bovine collagen to occur. *Adverse reactions* are defined as sensitization reactions of an immunologic nature that occur at the treatment site after the patient has demonstrated clinically negative skin test results.[6] The incidence of these reactions is reported to be 1% to 6% but probably occurs in fewer than 3% of the patients undergoing augmentation. The vast majority (89.6%) occur with the first treatment; this has eventuated in all physicians at the forefront of soft tissue augmentation recommending double skin testing. The initial study by Elson in the *Journal of Dermatologic Surgery and Oncology* compared 200 patients with a single skin test and 200 patients with double skin tests in the following manner. The groups were comparable as to sex, age range, and diagnoses. The first group underwent skin testing according to the package insert, as previously outlined. Five (2.5%) had a positive skin test and did not undergo augmentation. Of the 195 who did, 6 developed allergic reactions.

Two hundred patients underwent double testing as follows: the first test was administered in the right volar forearm, read at 48 to 72 hours, and the patient returned in 2 weeks for another test in the left volar forearm, which was administered in the same manner. Both tests were then read at a total of 4 weeks from the first test (2 weeks from the second test). The first test in the right volar forearm was positive in 5 patients (2.5%, see Figure 7.1). Of the 195 who received the second test in the other arm, 7 (3%) developed a positive reaction while the first test remained negative (see Figure 7.2). One hundred seventy-one patients who had two negative skin test results and decided to undergo augmentation were then treated with injectable collagen, and none had adverse reactions.[7]

This has led to a number of other studies and confirmation that double skin testing does decrease the incidence of adverse reactions to

7. Soft Tissue Augmentation

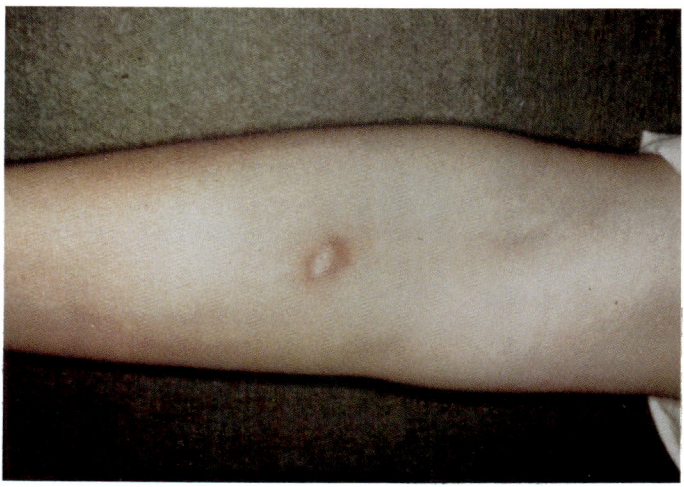

FIGURE 7.1. Positive skin test to bovine collagen.

collagen injectable material.[8] Although adverse reactions still may occur, the incidence is certainly decreased and the severity of the reactions appears to be less, probably because the patients who are more allergic and would have more severe reactions are screened out through this process.

Technique

Once the patient undergoes skin testing, the augmentation can proceed, utilizing the materials previously described. Although many monographs are available on technique and the use of collagen injectable materials, a few important items can be pointed out at this juncture.

Zyplast is injected into the mid-dermis with the needle parallel to the defect and is dependent more on the feel for augmentation than on sight. Zyderm is generally injected perpendicular to the defect in a serial puncture technique overlying the Zyplast and is dependent upon sight rather than feel for correction. Overcorrection with Zyderm is necessary in all areas to a degree of 150% to 200% to afford correction, with the exception of the area around the eyes, which should not be overcorrected.

The technique with Zyderm and fine-gauge needles is to be very gentle around the area of the eyes, injecting parallel to the crow's feet and

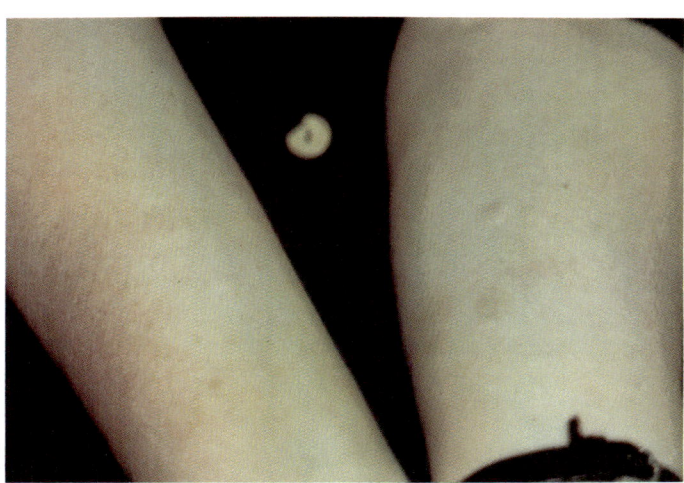

FIGURE 7.2. Right arm: negative first test. Left arm: positive second test.

with no overcorrection, as well as under the eyes with no overcorrection. Hiding of the orbital groove can also be accomplished by injecting Zyderm into the area and allowing it to flow to the caruncle to augment the area with no overcorrection[9] (see Figures 7.3 and 7.4).

Adequate softening of the features and correction can be obtained utilizing Zyplast and Zyderm collagen, as can be seen in the photographs in Figures 7.5 through 7.12.

Side Effects

Side effects that can occur and have been reported with injectable bovine collagen material range in severity from mild to rather significant. Probably one of the most common side effects is disappointment stemming from unrealistic expectations on the part of the patient. It is necessary for the physician to educate the patient as to exactly where collagen injectable material fits into the treatment of the aging face so that the patient can understand what can and cannot be accomplished.[10]

Discomfort is minimized with the 0.3% lidocaine that is included in all the collagen material around the world (recently having been approved in France). Icing the area to be injected not only helps in relieving some of the discomfort but also affords better correction, since this keeps the material cold until it starts to warm up to body temperature, causing the fibers to increase.

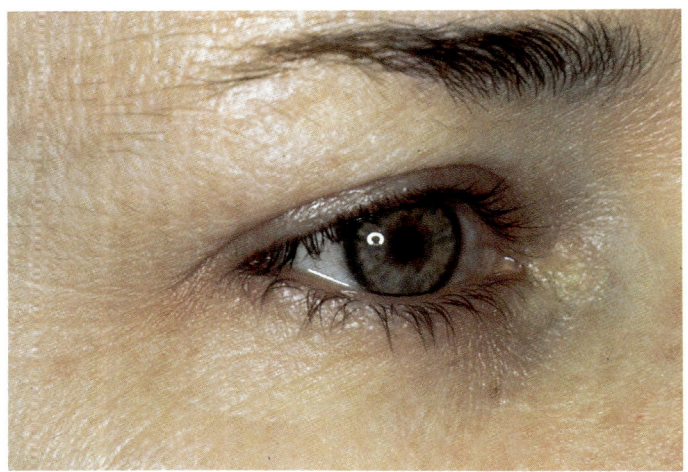

FIGURE 7.3. Before augmentation.

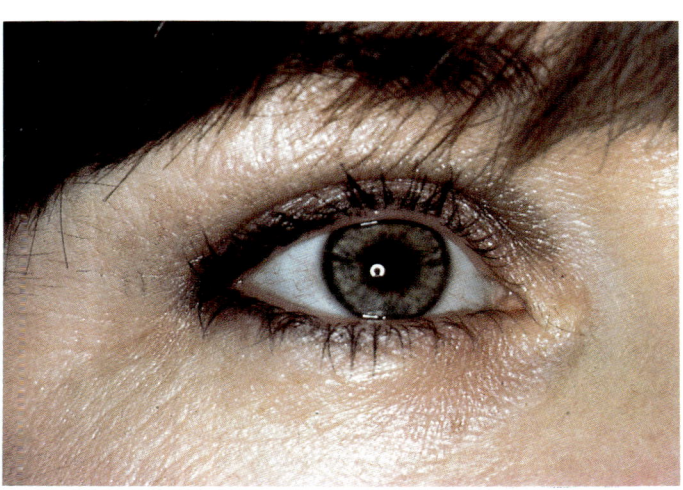

FIGURE 7.4. After augmentation.

FIGURE 7.5. Nasolabial folds prior to injection.

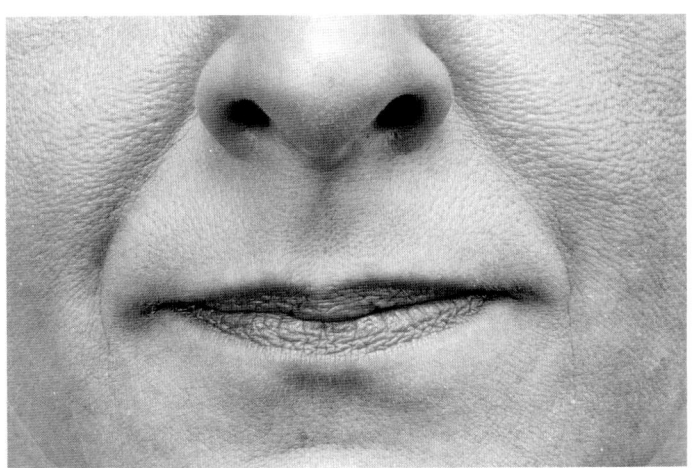

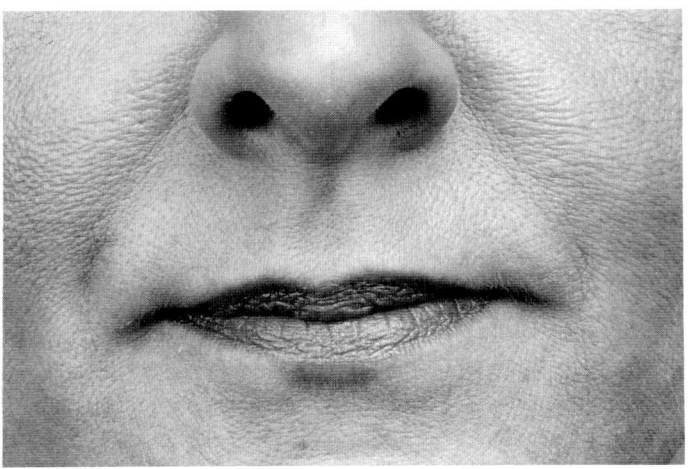

FIGURE 7.6. Following injection with 1.0 cc Zyplast.

Some physicians have found Hurricaine Jelly and eutectic mixtures such as EMLA to be of benefit in certain areas, especially around the mouth,[11] and nerve block certainly can benefit the patient undergoing augmentation of the lips. Needle marks may occur but are very short-lived and with the use of the finer-gauge needles virtually do not occur. Bruising may occur and will last a few days and disappear. Beading after the injection is a frequent complaint of patients and can be eliminated to a certain degree by obtaining expertise in the use of the material so that it is possible to have the material flow in the dermis rather than having skip areas after the injection.

Transient erythema occurs in a few patients (usually fewer than 10%) and is of no consequence, disappearing within hours. Fewer than 1% of the patients experience episodes of erythema and occasionally edema upon exposure to alcohol, exercise, sun exposure, hay fever, emotional upset, and other vasodilatory episodes. They are self-limited, and the patients do not have anti-Zyderm antibodies, will not experience adverse reactions, and may continue to undergo augmentation.[12]

One episode of partial blindness in one eye has been reported,[13] occurring during injection of the glabellar area. This is a side effect of injection of this particular area rather than a true side effect of collagen injectable material.

Infection is extremely rare and is not an inherent side effect of the injection of this sterile material; but since this is not a sterile procedure, the possibility of transcutaneous transmission of bacteria always exists. The

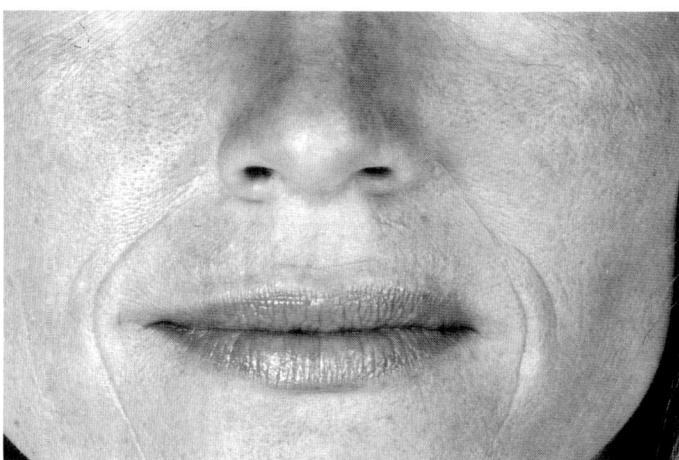

FIGURE 7.7. Nasolabial folds before injection.

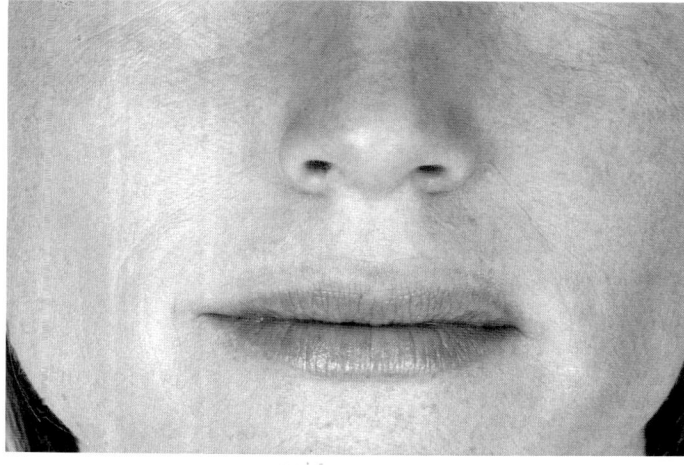

FIGURE 7.8. Nasolabial folds after injection of 1.0 cc Zyplast, 1.0 cc Zyderm-I.

practice of recapping syringes by the physician for the same patient to be used at a later injection session is discouraged since sterility cannot be guaranteed once the syringe has been opened.

Systemic complaints are very infrequent and have been reported to the manufacturer by fewer than 0.01% of patients. They have consisted of nausea, rash, arthralgia, myalgia, and headache. Although these complaints are reported to the manufacturer and are associated with the collagen injected, there is no documentation of the relationship of these systemic complaints and the injection of this material. A single anaphylactoid response has been reported that included an episode of hypotension and difficulty in breathing.[14]

Obviously, as more and more patients are injected, side effects that are not particularly common will manifest themselves due to the sheer numbers. Two of these are abscess formation and local necrosis. Local necrosis, based upon reports from physicians to Collagen Biomedical, has an incidence rate of 0.09%. Although this is quite low, there appears to be an increase in the rate of this side effect since the introduction of Zyplast in November 1985. Local necrosis following the injection of the material results from the interruption of the vascular supply of the area that is injected and is not really dependent upon the material itself. The material may compress or injure a blood vessel in the area of injection, compromising the oxygen flow and leading to the slough.

The first manifestation is discomfort in the area and a blanching of the area during injec-

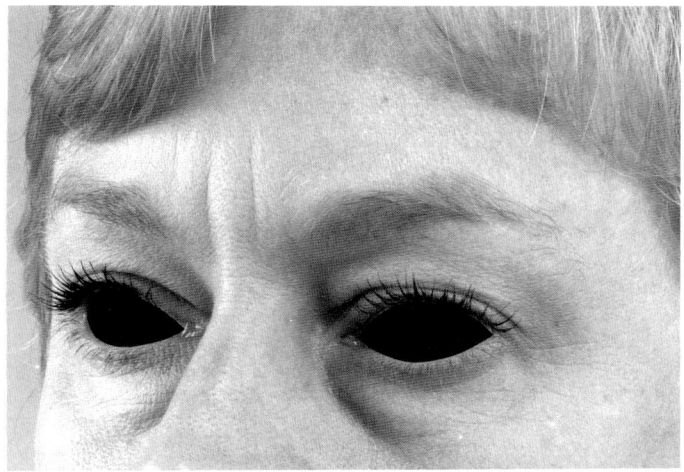

FIGURE 7.9. Before injection in the glabella area.

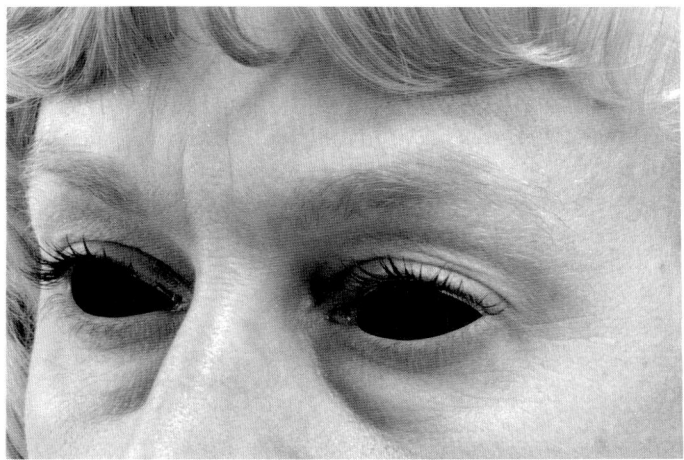

FIGURE 7.10. After injection of 0.5 cc Zyderm-I.

tion, followed by duskiness, which then gives way to bruising and necrosis over the next couple of days. It may take months to heal and may eventuate in scarring.

According to the manufacturer, 56% of all reported instances of this side effect have occurred in the glabella and with Zyplast. Hanke et al. reported that when the skin of the forehead is examined in the cadaver, the bilateral supratrochlear and supraorbital arteries, which are branches of the ophthalmic, lie in superficial fascia and ascend the forehead in company of the supratrochlear and supraorbital branch of the ophthalmic nerve.[15]

They stated that the bilateral symmetry of the superficial neurovascular bundles is carried over into the deeper hypodermis of the glabella.

Sections taken from the glabella revealed large-caliber vessels on either side of a median fat pad. The absence of large vessels in the mid-line dermis and the hypodermis suggests that the perfusion of mid-line tissues is dependent on smaller branches of these larger lateral vessels and may account for the higher incidence of this side effect in this area. Since Zyplast is injected deeper into the dermis and undergoes less syneresis, vascular compromise would be more likely to occur with this material; it is, therefore, recommended that Zyplast not be used in the glabella to achieve correction. Zyderm-I or -II can be substituted instead.[16]

Once it is apparent that vascular compromise has occurred, it is prudent to discontinue the injections at the site immediately. Some physi-

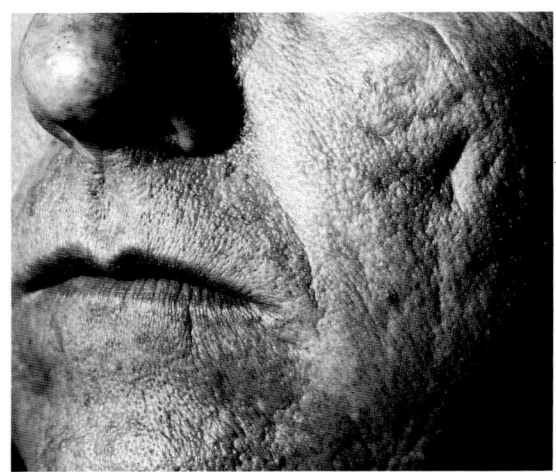

FIGURE 7.11. Oral commissure and nasolabial folds, as well as the accessory lines prior to injection.

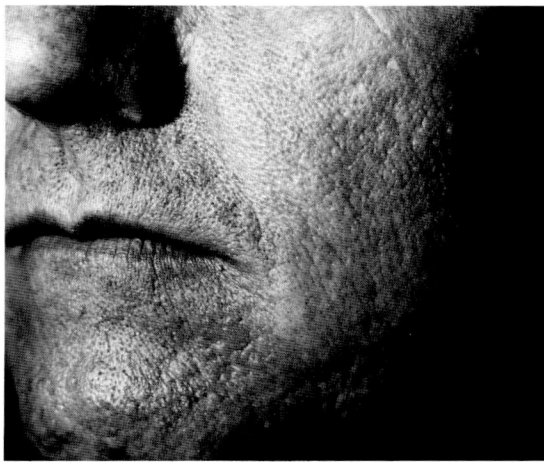

FIGURE 7.12. After injection with 1.0 cc Zyplast, 1.0 cc Zyderm-I.

cians advocate the use of ice, some heat, and some nitroglycerin paste. Application of 50% DMSO at the immediate time of compression of the vessel appears to provide some benefit; studies are ongoing to determine the efficacy of this modality.

Abscess formation is the most serious complication of injectable collagen. The incidence is placed at 0.04% and has remained at a steady level of reporting since 1981, with the introduction of the first injectable collagen (Zyderm-I). It can occur upon the first exposure to collagen but may also occur upon any subsequent exposure. The onset is delayed; the delay may be as short as 7 days or as long as 22 months after the injection. There is also a great deal of variability reported in the clinical description of the event, from a small draining lesion at the site to severe fluctuant lesions surrounded by a great deal of induration and erythema. These reactions differ from routine hypersensitivity reactions to collagen implants in that, although the adverse reaction may be indurated and erythematous, they are not fluctuant.

Hanke et al. reported that in many patients, some injection sites react and others do not. This is also characteristic of allergic reaction to collagen materials in general. There may be long periods of remission followed by exacerbation, and the severity of the reaction tends to decrease over a period of time. All available evidence at this point indicates that this reaction is dependent upon some degree of hypersensitivity, as 86% of the patients in the original study had elevated titers against bovine collagen as determined by ELISA.

Treatment consists of drainage of the lesion, which affords considerable relief when the pressure is released. Intralesional steroids may be used, and one should wait 6 months following resolution before attempting to revise the resultant scar. Scar revision may be performed using any of the modalities available to the dermatologic cosmetic surgeon with the exception of injectable collagen.

Although there is no basis for allegations linking collagen injectable materials with autoimmune disease, it is necessary to discuss this due to the media reports and litigation in the United States. As discussed previously, adverse events may occur with the use of injectable collagen, and it is these adverse events that have led to the false linking of autoimmune disease, especially dermatomyositis/polymyositis, to the injection of bovine collagen.[17]

Antibodies to bovine collagen do occur in the general population, probably through dietary exposure, and these antibodies remain species-specific. Adverse events are directed at the site of the bovine implant, do not produce any type of cross-reaction with the host tissue, and the patients who demonstrate antibovine collagen antibodies do not demonstrate antibodies against human collagen.

There is a vast literature relating to the safety of bovine collagen products both before and after the institution of the cosmetic use of the products. A review by DeLustro et al. in 1990 presented the pertinent facts from the presence of the antibodies in the general population to the immunohistology demonstrating host antibody in the infiltrating plasma cells and bound to bovine dermal collagen implant but not the surrounding host dermis.[18] Another study with another implant material (Koken atelocollagen) concluded that in an extensive study and follow-up of 705 patients, there was some cross-reactivity to bovine collagen type II as well as I and III, but that reactivity remained species-specific.[19] The conclusion in the DeLustro article is that an immune response to xenogeneic collagen has been demonstrated in both animals and humans and that the data clearly demonstrate immunity per se not to be associated with any adverse sequelae in vivo (see Figure 7.13).

The outdated term *collagen vascular disease* is unfortunate and creates an aura of confusion in this situation. Its original use in the medical literature denoted the organ systems of major involvement in these disease processes. The implication that collagen and the vasculature are somehow involved in the etiology of rheumatologic disease is false. We now know that these disorders involve an altered state in the immune system, with the production of autoantibodies dependent upon a variety of interacting factors.

When one looks at the data related to the reporting of problems to the company, one would expect to see an increase in the reporting of a particular side effect if that side effect were dependent upon increased usage of the material. Such is the case for cyst/abscess reaction, a known side effect of collagen injectable material. The more collagen is used, the more the side effect is reported, even though it is an uncommon event. On the other hand, the incidence of polymyositis/dermatomyositis (PM/DM) has remained the same over time, indicating no relationship (see Figure 7.14).

Looking at the epidemiologic data for this particular disease, in 1989 Lyon et al. reported the largest series of patients with DM/PM in an attempt to determine cause and incidence.[20] The overall incidence was put at between 5.0 million and 9.6 million per year. As far as etiology was concerned, no correlation was found with any type of allergic phenomena. The only apparent significant factors in the etiology of the disease were emotional factors and severe and muscular exertion. None of the patients had received injectable bovine collagen.

By May 1992, 107 patients had been reported

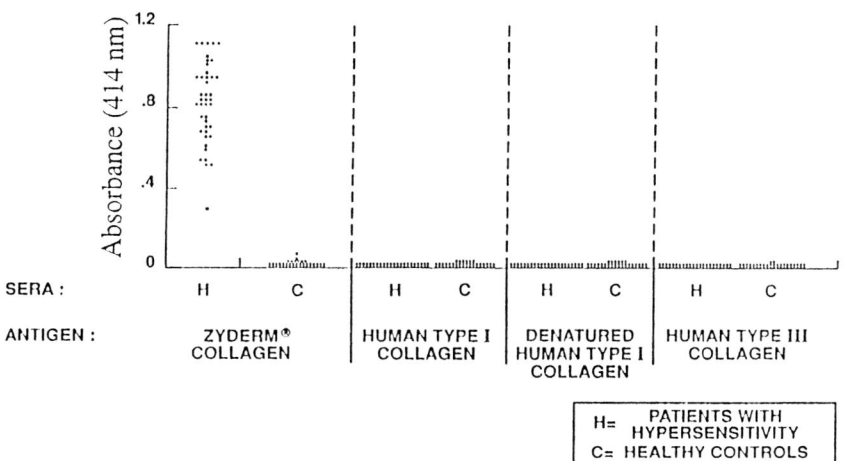

FIGURE 7.13. Antibodies against bovine collagen in patients with hypersensitivity to Zyderm collagen: ELISA results.

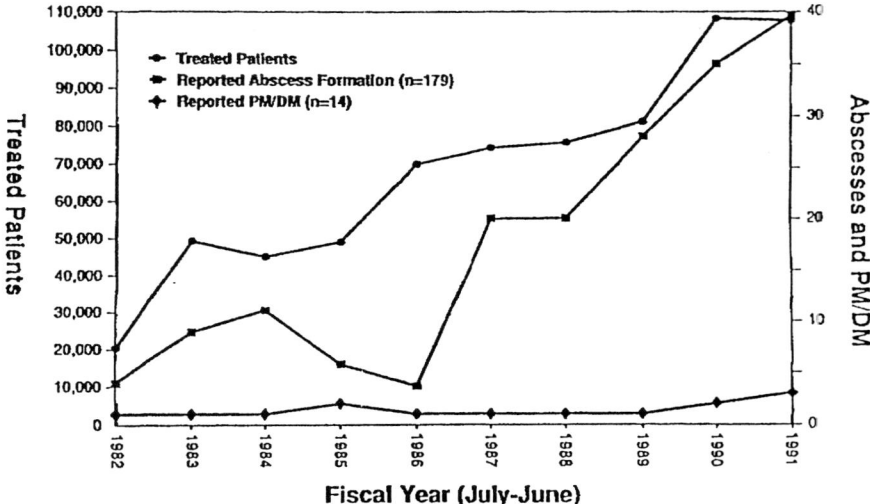

FIGURE 7.14. Comparison of reports to the Collagen Corporation of PM/DM and cyst/abscess reaction in patients undergoing augmentation with Zyden/ZP.

to Collagen Corporation by physicians with rheumatoid disease of some sort and 9 with alleged dermatomyositis. This is well below the expected numbers for a population of 650,000.[21] A statement issued by the American College of Rheumatology in 1991 stated that 100 cases of autoimmune disease had been alleged in the United States and Canada in the more than 500,000 people receiving injections in those countries. Of these, 11 cases were alleged to be PM/DM. The latest epidemiologic studies have indicated that between 12 and 23 cases of PM/DM would be expected by chance alone among these 500,000 patients and according to the American College of Rheumatology "the alleged cases of PM/DM are less than would be expected for the population."[22]

Finally, expert review panels convened by the FDA on two occasions—1989[23] and 1992[24]—reviewed all the data and concluded on both occasions that there are no data to suggest that immunity to xenogeneic dermal collagen can precipitate autoimmune disease. They also concluded that "there are considerable data that are inconsistent with the hypothesis of a relationship between injectable collagen and autoimmune disease."

In addition to the data from both the scientific and epidemiologic fronts indicating no link between injectable collagen and autoimmune disease, the courts have also ruled in favor of Collagen Corporation in every suit and on every appeal. Also, the courts recently ruled that since the FDA, an agency of the U.S. government, had approved and continues to monitor Zyderm and Zyplast as medical devices, the lawsuits should not even have been allowed to be filed in the first place.[25,26] Thus, on all fronts no link can be substantiated between the injection of bovine collagen and autoimmune disease.

Fibrel

Although Zyderm and Zyplast collagen remain the standard for filling materials, there are other substances and modalities available for soft tissue augmentation. The only other material approved by the United States' FDA for soft tissue augmentation at this time is Fibrel. It was approved for use in depressed scars in 1985 and wrinkles in 1990. The initial multicenter study was reported by Millikan et al. after studying 300 patients for 12 months and 111 of these for another year's follow-up. They reported that successful correction was maintained in 58.9% to 78.90% after 2 years.[27] Longevity after 5 years was also reported as satisfactory in a majority of patients.[28]

This substance is a sterile implant composed of a gelatin powder of porcine origin with epsilon amino caproic acid, which is mixed with 0.5 cc of the patient's serum and 0.5 cc normal saline. The theory is that upon injection, Fibrel will provide the necessary ingredients to recreate wound healing under scars and wrinkles—the absorbable gelatin powder to elevate the depression and provide a matrix, the plasma providing the necessary ingredients for collagen synthesis and epsilon aminocaproic acid to inhibit the production of fibrinolysis, allowing excessive collagen to be produced within the clot, elevating the depression and producing clinical correction.[29]

Skin testing is required with this xenogeneic material, proceeding in the manner similar to that for bovine collagen and waiting 1 month from testing to injection. Long-term, objective data with regard to efficacy in the treatment of wrinkles are not yet available, and one must be careful extrapolating data related to nonmobile scars to movable wrinkles.

According to the package insert, 1.8% of patients react to the skin test and cannot undergo augmentation. Adverse reactions that are listed in the package insert include transient swelling, redness, and discomfort usually resolving within 24 hours.[30] Of the initial clinical trials, 0.7% experienced nodules, erythema, and skin discoloration that lasted up to 4 weeks. One percent experienced treatment site discoloration, nodules, and pruritus that lasted longer than 4 weeks. As to whether or not these are hypersensitivity phenomena associated with antiporcine antibodies, no data have yet been provided. The package insert does provide antibody formation data with regards to collagen type I and III, but this is apparently antibovine data rather than antiporcine. It seems difficult to determine the true safety of the product without data relevant to the porcine implant.

Work is currently being carried out in a number of centers to decrease the pain associated with the injection of Fibrel as well as to develop methods of preparation that do not require phlebotomy and so much time by the physician and staff.

Silicone

The use of injectable medical-grade silicone, though in use in some countries around the world, has been declared illegal in the United States by the commissioner of the FDA.[31] It was used rather extensively as a filling material from the early 1950s until 1992; and, although its use has been significantly curtailed, it is a filler that is virtually permanent and has been injected into thousands of patients. Discussion of this substance and its possible side effects must therefore remain in the medical literature.

The injection of large amounts of adulterated silicone into breasts, lips, and other tissue must be condemned on all counts and plays no role in the discussion of the microdroplet technique previously advocated by Orentreich and others.[32] Certainly, there are many patients over the years who have benefited from the use of this material, though side effects do occur. Granuloma formation may occur and may be delayed for many years. This may necessitate surgical removal of the reaction and the material. Drifting has been reported, but apparently not with the proper technique of injecting tiny amounts of the material into the lowest part of the dermis and allowing the body to produce collagen in response to the deposition of the silicone, much as a pearl forms around a grain of sand in an oyster.

Although drifting may be a problem and foreign-body reaction can occur, the major concern at this time is the possibility of human adjuvant disease. Silicone gel-filled breast implants have been removed from the general market in the United States due to a number of problems.[33] Contracture with its ensuing scarring, disfigurement, and pain is a problem as well as obscuring breast tissue during mammography. The greatest concern, however, is the leakage of the silicone from the implant, with the possible induction of autoimmune disease with silicone acting as an adjuvant. If this is valid, there could be an increase in the incidence of diseases such as scleroderma and other rheumatoid diseases from the injection of liquid silicone, for it is not known whether the type of silicone is important, or the amount or the location of the material in the human body.

Patients who have been injected with liquid silicone should be monitored throughout their lives for possible side effects.

Other Materials

Although in the United States soft tissue augmentation has been primarily focused on the use of Zyderm/Zyplast collagen and silicone with some limited use of Fibrel, other substances are available around the world, and there are other materials under investigation.

Koken atelocollagen is approved for use in Japan, Australia, Canada, and some countries in the European Community. It is a clear solution in concentrations of 2% or 3.5% supplied in cartridges to fit into dental carriers for injection fitted with a 30-gauge needle. The 3.5% solution is comparable to Zyderm I, which is a suspension rather than a solution. The implant itself is prepared from young calf hide—calf rather than mature cows, because the collagen is said to be more soluble from calves. It must be refrigerated in order to prevent fibrillation. The solution contains only the helical body of the collagen molecule without the telopeptides.[34] Skin testing is indicated, as with other xenogeneic materials.[35] Studies by Dierickx and others indicate satisfactory correction with this material, even with the 2% concentration.[36] The solution is made of short fibrils uniform in the solution that form a new collagen matrix upon injection, which imprisons more glycosamino-glycans and water to produce the desired correction. In addition to the material being quite painful to inject, side effects include rare instances of persistent erythema and edema, local flare-ups after alcohol or sun exposure, and occasional hyperpigmentation.

With the increased emphasis in recent years on liposuction, fat transplantation (microlipo injection) has enjoyed a resurgence. Basically, fat is extracted from one area of the body either during liposuction or for the purpose of transplantation with either a closed cannula system or large-gauge needles and injected into other areas with 14-gauge needles or a cannula system. Over the last few years, experience has led surgeons to recommend the use of this material only for large defects with or without combination with true fillers such as Zyderm/Zyplast. The material cannot be injected into fine lines and does not persist unless fat is being utilized to replace fat rather than dermal tissue.

Although not yet perfected, one interesting development from microlipo injection has been the innovative use of the collagen portion of the removed tissue by Newman and others. A special device has been developed by Newman to be used in conjunction with the liposuction apparatus that removes the collagen portion and spins it into a substance for reinjection.[37]

Allergy is certainly not a possibility with the material obtained from the patient's own tissue, but it has not yet been possible to produce material that can be injected into fine lines or even medium ones. Longevity of correction, efficacy, and safety remain to be determined.

Another method of obtaining the patient's own material for injection has been instituted by Autogenesis Technologies, Inc., known as Autologen. This process utilizes skin from the patient, which is removed by the physician during surgery or specifically for this purpose, frozen and shipped to the company in Massachusetts, where it is processed into an injectable form of collagen and returned to the physician for injection in the same patient. It is not yet a popular method of soft tissue augmentation, due to the amount of tissue required for processing and other problems that may arise from the shipping and processing of such materials. It remains, however, an interesting beginning for the possibility of processing the patient's own skin for reinjection.

Bioplastique was recently undergoing clinical trials with a number of plastic surgeons in the United States.[38] It is a system of placement by cannula during surgery under sterile conditions of silicone gel droplets. Although it is used in some countries, clinical trials have been discontinued in the United States. Most likely this will never come to market, due to its use of silicone.

Gore-tex threads are becoming popular in some centers in Europe.[39] The placement of the fiber into the skin allowing reaction to occur and then removing the thread leaving the correction in place relies upon the ability of the tissue to react to a foreign body, much as the reaction to silicone developed. No long-term studies are yet available for the use of this fiber in soft tissue augmentation.

Hyaluronic acid is undergoing clinical trials in the United States as a filler.[40] The use of the material is based not upon its presence in the tissue, as a component of the ground substance, but as a true filling material occupying space in the dermis to eventuate in correction. There is apparently very little, if any, reaction to the material, and clinical results appear to be acceptable. Long-term data are awaited, as is approval by the FDA.

All the materials discussed so far are dependent upon the body reacting to the material to produce correction or to fill space, producing the correction. Another way of achieving the desired result of soft tissue augmentation is to treat the underlying cause of the defect—the muscular pull upon the collagen fibers. This is the basis of the use of Botulinum A exotoxin to eliminate the frown line at the glabella.[41] In the method proposed by Carruthers and Carruthers of Vancouver, one takes advantage of the ability of this substance to paralyze muscles by injecting it directly into the procerus, to prohibit the action of frowning. This is a natural sequel to the use of injectable botulinum in the treatment of ophthalmic/ophthalmologic conditions, such as blepharospasms. The results are temporary and must be repeated every few months but may have a role in patients who desire correction of the glabellar frown line and are either allergic to injectable collagen or do not desire injectable collagen. This also demonstrates that there may be a future for other treatments based upon alleviating the etiology of the expression lines rather than filling materials.

The future of soft tissue augmentation is very bright, with a number of innovative substances undergoing trials or experimentation. GAX 65 is a more concentrated form of gluteraldehyde cross-linked material that shows promise as to greater longevity in animal models. Bovine collagen linked with polyethylene glycol may be able to attach to dermal tissue, affording longer correction. In addition, the ultimate material for soft tissue augmentation, human collagen from pooled placenta, should begin clinical trials in 1994. Certainly, other materials will also come to the fore as the search for the perfect material for soft tissue augmentation continues.

References

1. Barton JL, Cunliff WJ. The subcutaneous fat: oil granuloma. In: *Textbook of Dermatology,* AS Rook, DS Wilkinson, FJ Eberling, RH Champion, JL Burton, eds. Blackwell Press, Oxford, 1986, p. 1870.
2. Elson ML. Clinical assessment of Zyplast implant: a year of experience for soft tissue contour correction. J Am Acad Dermatol. 1988;18:707.
3. FDA approval letter to Collagen Corporation, July 22, 1981.
4. FDA approval letter to Collagen Corporation, June 24, 1985.
5. Zyderm skin test package insert. Collagen Corporation, Palo Alto, California, 1991.
6. Elson ML. Soft tissue augmentation: a review of available materials. Cosmet Dermatol. 1991;4[1]:10.
7. Elson ML. The role of skin testing in the use of collagen injectable materials. J Dermatol Surg Oncol. 1989;15:301.
8. Klein AW. In favor of double testing. J Dermatol Surg Oncol. 1989;15:263.
9. Elson ML. Soft tissue augmentation of periorbital fine lines and the orbital groove with Zyderm I and fine-gauge needles. J Dermatol Surg Oncol. 1992; 18:779.
10. Elson ML. Communication is imperative regarding side effects of soft tissue augmentation. Cosmet Dermatol. 1991;4[3]:8.
11. Elson ML. Techniques for lip augmentation discussed. Cosmet Dermatol. 1990;3[11]:16.
12. Elson ML. Collagen Implantation. In: *Complications of Dermatologic Surgery,* H Harahap, ed. Springer-Verlag, Heidelberg, 1993, pp. 91–100.
13. Cucin RL, Barek D. Complications of injectable collagen implants. Plast Reconstr Surg. 1983; 71:731.
14. Zyderm/Zyplast physician package insert. Collagen Corporation, Palo Alto, California, 1991.
15. Hanke DW, Stegman SJ, et al. Abscess formation and local necrosis following treatment with Zyderm and Zyplast collagen implant. J Am Acad Dermatol. 1991;25:319.
16. Letter from Collagen Corporation to Physicians, April 16, 1990.
17. Elson ML. Dermal filler materials. Dermatologic Clin. 1993;11:361–367.

18. Elson ML. Injectable collagen and autoimmune disease [editorial]. J Dermatol Surg Oncol. 1993;19:165–168.
19. Ishikawa T, Ogura T, et al. Clinical study of injectable atelocollagen from bovine calk skin. Nishinihon Hifuka. 1985; 47(7).
20. Lyon MC, Block DA, et al. Predisposing factors in polymyositis/dermatomyositis: results of a nationwide survey. J Rheumatol. 1989;16:1218.
21. Personal communication. Dr. Dan Jolivette, Collagen Corporation, Palo Alto, California, May 1992.
22. News release from American College of Rheumatology, 1991.
23. 1989 Advisory Panel to the FDA
24. 1991 Advisory Panel to the FDA
25. Ramey vs. Collagen Corporation, case number 85-57338, District Court of Harris County, Texas, 270 Judicial District.
26. Ruling by Texas Appellant Court August 28, 1991
27. Millikan L, Rosen T, et al. Treatment of depressed cutaneous scars with gelatin matrix implant: a multicenter study. J Am Acad Dermatol. 1987;16:1155.
28. Millikan L, Banks K, et al. A 5-year safety and efficacy evaluation with Fibrel in the correction of cutaneous scars following one or two treatments. J Dermatol Surg Oncol. 1991;17:223.
29. Monheit GD. Fibrel injection techniques in cutaneous scars for soft-tissue augmentation and wrinkles. Cosmet Dermatol. 1991;5[4]:10.
30. Fibrel package insert. Mentor, Goleta, California.
31. June 11, 1991, testimony of FDA commissioner Dr. David Kessler before the House of Representatives Human Resources and Intergovernmental Relations Subcommittee re: promoting drugs for unapproved uses.
32. Selmanowitz VJ, Orentreich N. Medical-grade fluid silicone: a monographic review. J Dermatol Surg Oncol. 1977;3:597.
33. Kessler before Congress re: breast implants, February 1992.
34. Ishikawa T, Ogura T, et al. Clinical study of injectable Atelocollagen from bovine calf skin. Nishinihon Hifuka. 1985;47(7).
35. Koken Atelocollagen Implant package insert, Koken Bioscience Institute, Tokyo, Japan.
36. Dierickx P, Dermueaux L. Comparative study of the clinical efficiency of a 2% collagen solution and a 3.5% collagen dispersion on 60 patients. Presented at the 5th International Society for Dermatologic Surgery, Jerusalem, Israel, October 28–31, 1984.
37. Personal communication. Dr. A Julius Newmann, Philadelphia, Pennsylvania, May 1992.
38. Ersek RA, Geisang AA III. Bioplastique soft tissue augmentation. Plast Reconstr Surg. 1990; *693*. Vol. 85. # 6
39. Walter CC. The use of Gore-Tex for facial augmentation. Presented at the 12th International Society for Dermatologic Surgery, Munich, Germany, October 4–7, 1991.
40. Piacquadio, D. Hyalin gel: a new substance for soft tissue augmentation. Am Acad Dermat 51st Annual meeting, San Francisco, California, Dec 5–10, 1992.
41. Carruthers JD, Carruthers JA. Treatment of glabellar frown lines with Botulinum A exotoxin. J Dermatol Surg Oncol. 1992; 18:17.

8
Liposuction Surgery of the Face and Neck

Rhoda S. Narins

Since 1982, when liposuction surgery was first introduced into the United States, this procedure has been used in many ways to enhance the appearance of the face and neck. Cervical liposuction has been proven to be a safe and efficacious surgical procedure.[1] The neck is probably the easiest area on which to perform this surgery; skin retraction is excellent here.[2] Fatty deposits range from submental accumulations to a tremendous "double chin" that involves most of the neck from ear to ear. The superficial fat in the neck lies between the skin and the platysma-SMAS and can easily be removed with liposuction. A clean, sharp angle at the jawline gives a youthful appearance.

In the younger patient with taut skin, liposuction alone is the procedure of choice (refer to Figures 8.1 and 8.2). If the fat is limited to the submental region alone, this procedure can be undertaken through 1 tiny 3 mm incision in the submental crease. If the deposit of adipose tissue is large, then 2 additional incisions behind each ear are necessary.

In the realistic older patient, liposuction alone may give the patient the desired result for the morbidity of the procedure performed. Some patients do not want to undergo a neck lift. In those patients with extremely loose skin who do not want a neck lift, liposuction with a submental excision can be done easily (see Figure 8.3). This procedure is discussed later in this chapter.

Liposuction of the face and neck is a widely performed procedure both alone and in combination with a rhytidectomy. When used alone it is a simple, quick procedure that is relatively pain-free, with very little morbidity. It is not a panacea for all patients, but in those patients in whom it is indicated, it has proven to be a wonderful technique.

Liposuction of the Neck

As previously mentioned, the neck is an ideal area on which to perform liposuction surgery. This procedure can lead to dramatic changes in appearance. The immediate results are gratifying and the end results excellent. The incisions can barely be seen immediately postoperatively. The use of local anesthesia[3] using the tumescent technique[4] makes the procedure very easy for the patient.

There are some precautions to take when recommending this procedure. Liposuction alone will not take care of platysmal bands. In addition, while obliteration of the anterior cervico-mandibular angle may be due to fat, it is sometimes due to muscle or a high insertion of the Hyoid bone. This is a familial trait and limits the success of liposuction; this should be explained to the patient.[5] But for most people, liposuction alone through a single incision is all that is necessary to remove the fat from this area, doing so can take 10 years off the way they look (see Figure 8.2).

Consultation

During the consultation the patient is examined to see if he or she is a good candidate for the

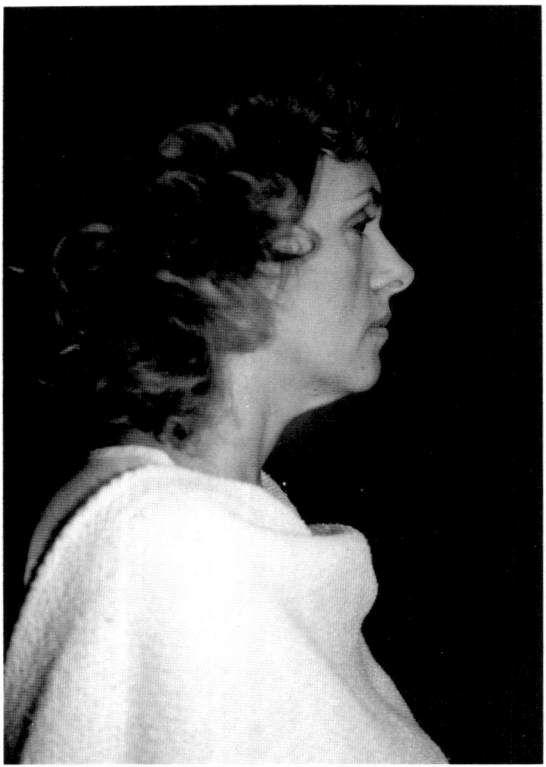

FIGURE 8.1. Preoperative cervical liposuction (patient 1).

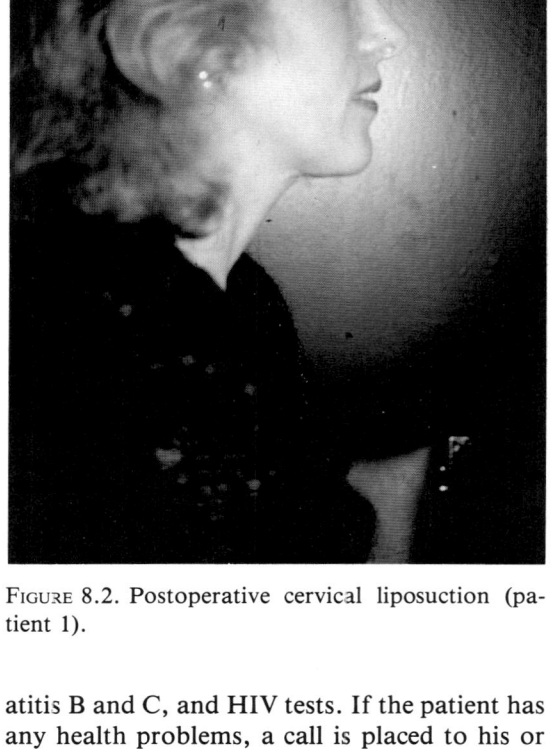

FIGURE 8.2. Postoperative cervical liposuction (patient 1).

procedure. Then the procedure is described in detail to the patient, including the number of incisions that will be required. Depending on the patients' age and skin turgor, the experienced surgeon can discuss the probable result as well as any possible complications. For those patients who are older and who have looser skin, it is important to determine if they are realistic about the results that can be achieved. It is useful at this point to show patients preoperative and postoperative photos of other patients who have similar skin turgor and fat deposits. In addition, preoperative and postoperative instructions are gone over with the patient, and the postoperative course is discussed.

Again, it is most important that the patient understand what result can realistically be achieved.

At this first consultation visit, or at the second consultation visit if the patient needs some time to think it over, blood tests are drawn, including CBC, PT, PTT, SMAC, hepatitis B and C, and HIV tests. If the patient has any health problems, a call is placed to his or her general medical doctor. At this time a Polaroid picture is taken so that the procedure can be planned preoperatively. The patient is also given antibiotics to be taken prior to surgery and is warned to stop all aspirin, aspirin-containing compounds, and nonsteroidal anti-inflammatory drugs 2 weeks prior to surgery.

Patients who are anxious should be told that they will be given Valium preoperatively and therefore should have someone come with them to take them home. Because the surgery in this area is almost painless and because most patients are not anxious and do not need preoperative medication, most can get home by themselves postoperatively.

Preoperative Procedure

1. Photography: On the morning of surgery, go over the procedure again with the patient

8. Liposuction Surgery of the Face and Neck

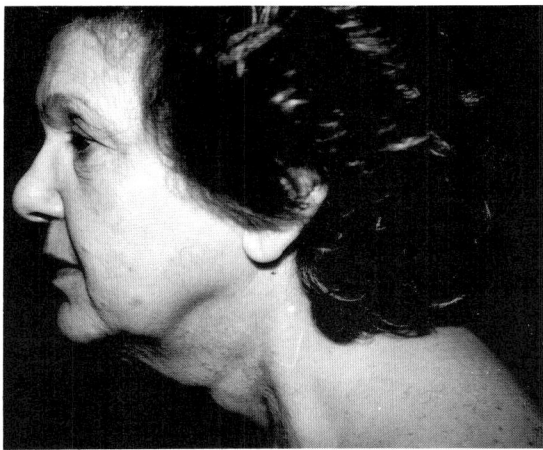

FIGURE 8.3. A preoperative patient who needs excision of excess skin along with liposuction.

and then take a series of photographs with a Polaroid camera and a 35 mm camera. Three views are taken: 90° right side, 90° left side, and frontal from the shoulders to the top of the head with the patient looking straight ahead. A matte-colored background is helpful.
2. Marking: With the patient sitting or standing, the submental crease is first outlined and 2 little marks put on either side of the intended submental incision. With the patient bending the chin downward, a line is drawn from the submental crease around the bulk of the fat and around jowls, if these are present.
3. Consent: The consent form is signed prior to any sedation or anesthesia.
4. Weighing: The patient is weighed at this time.
5. Sedation: If the patient is anxious, a small amount of Valium is given preoperatively to allay his or her fears. If the patient is not anxious, no medication is given at this point.

Liposuction Procedure

1. Preoperative preparation: After being taken to the operatory, the patient is placed onto the operating table in sterile fashion. The area is prepped with Betadine and the patient is readied for surgery with the usual sterile precautions and set-up.
2. Anesthesia: Local anesthesia with the tumescent technique is all that is necessary to perform cervical liposuction. The incision area or areas are injected first, using a 3 cc syringe filled with 2 ½ cc of 1% Xylocaine and 1:100,000 epinephrine and ½ cc sodium bicarbonate. The tumescent anesthetic is then injected through a 30-gauge spinal needle attached to a 10 cc syringe that is filled with the 1% lidocaine tumescent solution (refer to Table 8.1). This tumescent solution is injected radially into the neck fat through the incisions areas. If incisions are made behind the earlobe, then anesthetic is injected radially through these as well.
3. Surgical technique: After anesthesia is injected, wait an additional 10 to 15 minutes before starting surgery, during which time the patient is reprepped with Betadine. A ¼ inch stab incision is made with a number 11 blade. Depending upon the amount of fat present, we will use several different types of cannulas: sizes 2 and 3 for necks with small amounts of adipose tissue; and sizes 2, 3 and 4 for larger deposits. Our workhorse cannula is a 3-holed 3 mm cannula with a blunt tip that really curettes the tissue. This is one area where the cannula can be turned over so that the opening is face upward to get out as much fat as possible. Care also has to be taken so that the fat right around the incision site is also removed. Small cannulas should be used gently in the jowl area so that there is no injury to the marginal mandibular branch of the facial nerve. In general, one does not usually extract more than 10 to 50 cc in this area. The fat is collected in a disposable canister similar to but smaller than that used for liposuction of the body. This canister can then be disposed of in

TABLE 8.1. Anesthesia; tumescent technique, small volume.

90 cc 0.9% NaCl
10 cc 1% lidocaine + 1:100,000 epinephrine
 2 cc 8.4% sodium bicarbonate
Total = 10 mg lidocaine/100 cc NaCl
      = 1. 0.1% lidocaine
           2. 1:1,000,000 epinephrine

accordance with OSHA guidelines. When all the fat is removed, the incision is closed with a subcutaneous vicryl suture. Blood loss is virtually nil.

Postoperative Care

4. Immediately postoperative: An ice pack is placed on the area and is changed every 10 minutes for ½ hour. After that the Betadine is washed off and the area is scrubbed with acetone or alcohol. A dressing is applied with tape, which will stay on for 2 to 3 days. In order to avoid vertical wrinkling, which is temporary but can be upsetting, the initial piece of tape is split in half and the halves of tape applied 1 inch apart in the center and to either side (see Figure 8.4). Then longer tape strips are placed over the entire area. This method of taping serves to spread the central skin and redrape it.
5. Postoperative home care: The patient is allowed to leave after approximately 1 hour in the office. Speak to the patient that evening to make sure that there are no problems. Two to 3 days later, the dressing is removed, and the patient is seen in the office for a quick check. The patient is advised to wear a chin support at night thereafter for 2 to 4 weeks, depending on the turgor of the skin and the amount of fat that has been removed.

Complications

It is rare with this procedure to see even ecchymosis occur. In the multiple patients we have done, we have had no complications except for 2 patients with vertical creases, which were temporary. In this area we have not seen any skin pigmentation, hematomas, syromas, infections, scars, irregularities, or necrosis. We have had a few patients with dysesthesia, which was temporary, and 1 patient with temporary paralysis, probably due to trauma to the marginal mandibular branch of the facial nerve. Many patients have this temporarily during the procedure due to the anesthesia itself, but there have been no reports of permanent motor nerve injury in this area from liposuction.

Results

The patient looks better immediately and then continues to improve for 6 months. We generally take postoperative 35 mm and Polaroid photographs immediately and at the 3- and 6-month postoperative visits. The patient can immediately compare results using the Polaroid photos that are kept in the chart.

Summary

Cervical liposuction is a popular and safe procedure for the removal of cervical fat. Won-

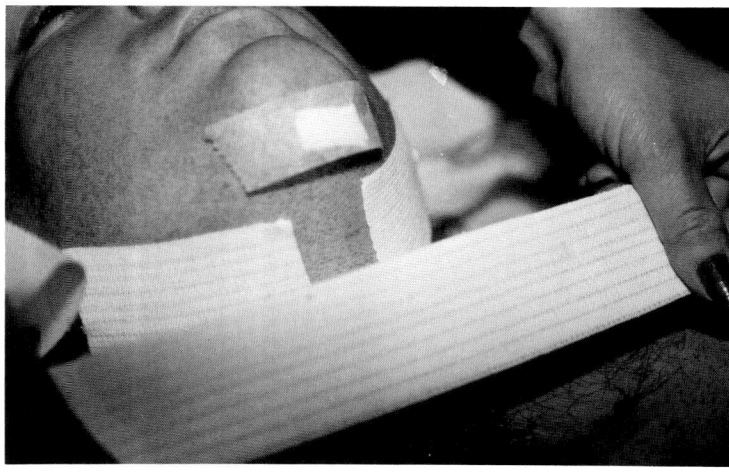

FIGURE 8.4. Postoperative taping.

8. Liposuction Surgery of the Face and Neck

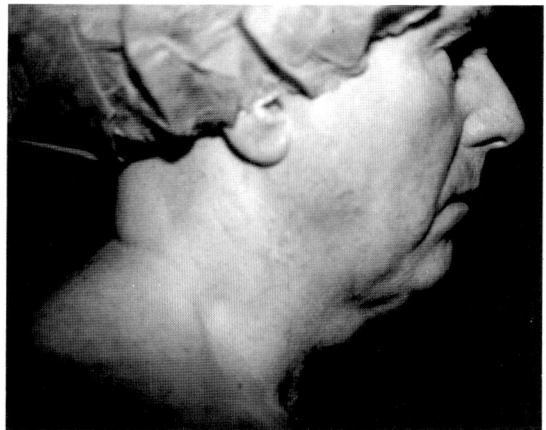

FIGURE 8.5. Preoperative: submental liposuction with excision of excess skin.

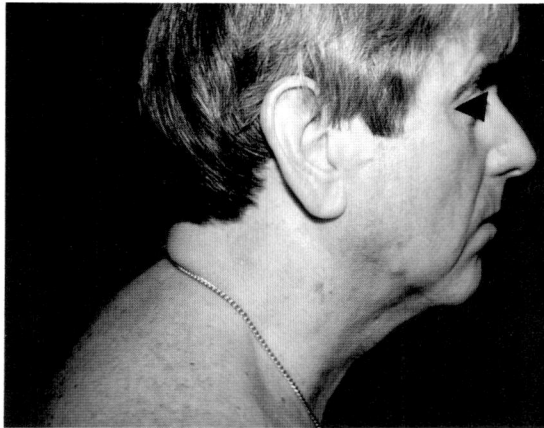

FIGURE 8.6. Postoperative: submental liposuction with excision of excess skin.

derful results can be achieved with a minimal procedure. Bleeding and infection have not proven to be problems. The procedure is almost pain-free and the postoperative recovery uneventful.

Cervical Liposuction with Excision of Excess Skin

As explained previously, cervical liposuction is an easy procedure that can be performed in the dermatologic surgeon's office through a tiny incision using local anesthesia.

Occasionally, however, one needs to take out some excess skin at the same time (refer to Figures 8.5 and 8.6). This generally occurs in the older patient with lax skin who does not want a neck lift. The excision is performed after the liposuction. This makes it very easy to remove the excess skin, as the undermining is already done. The scar from the incision is placed in the submental crease and is an extension of the incision used for liposuction. The entire procedure for liposuction is performed as described in the previous section, with certain additions.

1. Preoperative marking (see Figure 8.7):
   A. Incision sites for liposuction and borders around fat deposits.
   B. The upper excision line in the submental crease.
   C. Several lower excision lines.
2. Liposuction: Refer to the description provided in the previous section (see Figure 8.8).
3. Excise excess skin (see Figures 8.9 and 8.10):
   A. Excise through the upper excision line.
   B. Excise the central vertical line to first lower line.
   C. Pull up.
   D. Extend to the second excision line of skin.

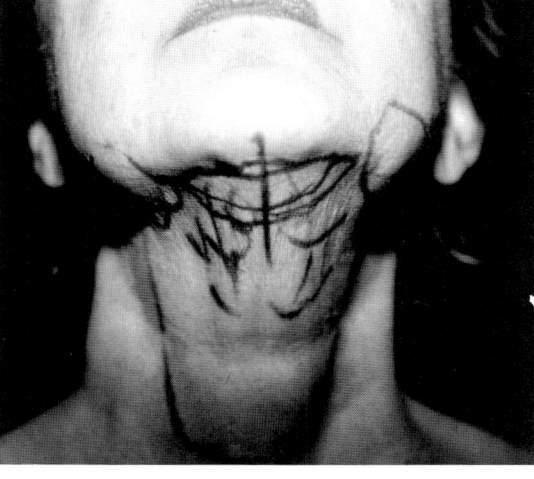

FIGURE 8.7. Preoperative marking for liposuction and excision of excess skin.

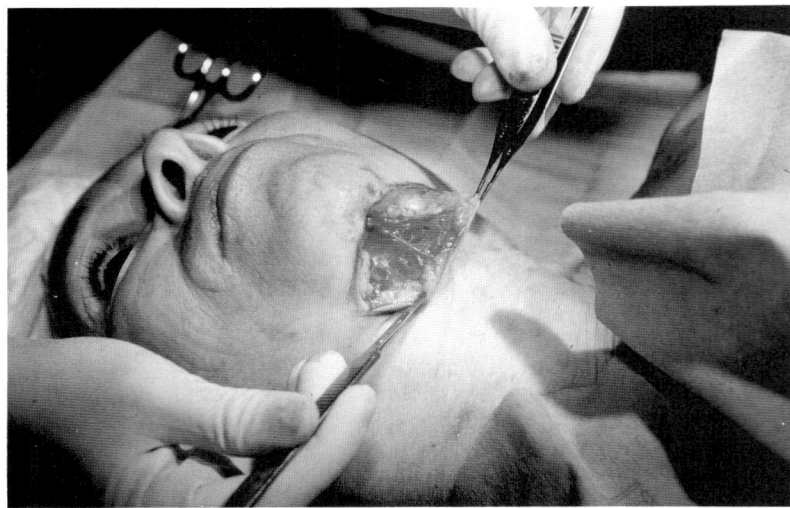

FIGURE 8.8. Intraoperative: after liposuction.

E. Keep extending until you reach the line where there is no loose skin, no skin tension.
F. Pull up, holding suture placed.
G. Excise along that lower line to meet the upper line.
H. Remove excess skin.
I. Suture the area closed.
J. Repair any dog ears.
K. Ice the area as described in the previous section.

4. Apply dressing:
Apply a dressing with telfa over antibiotic ointment over the incision area, followed by tape to compress the upper neck area, as described in the previous section. Remove the tape after 2 days. After that the incision is cared for and kept covered with Telfa and antibiotic ointment for 5 to 7 days. The sutures are removed in 5 days, and steri-strips are applied over the area with Mastisol and left on for several days.

Summary

Very few patients get any ecchymosis at all, and healing takes place rapidly, so that the line of the excision can barely be seen after a few months (see Figure 8.11).

Other Procedures

In some patients prominent platysmal bands must be ligated. A necklift is the only procedure that will give the desired result to those patients with lax skin who want a perfect result.

Liposuction of the Face

Liposuction of the face should be done with great care to avoid any surface irregularities. The layer of fat is very thin here, and the patient should be undercorrected.[6] In addition, facial liposuction, sometimes called *liposculpture*, can cause scarring and facial flattening.[7] Use small cannulas and very little suction, or use a syringe to perform the procedure by hand.

Liposuction of the face is referred to by some as *microliposuction* because very little fat may be removed and it is performed with finer instruments.[5] There is also a greater potential for significant damage to vessels and nerves in the face, so the procedure should be attempted only by trained individuals.[5]

8. Liposuction Surgery of the Face and Neck

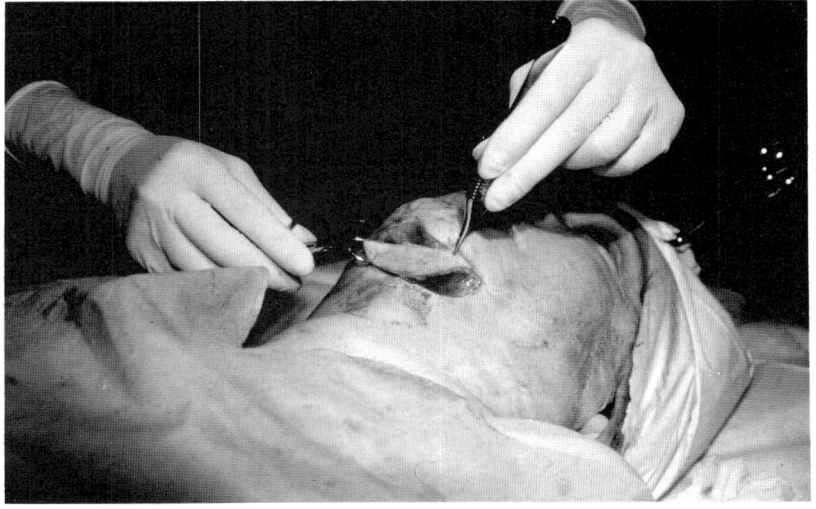

FIGURE 8.9. Intraoperative: removal of excess skin.

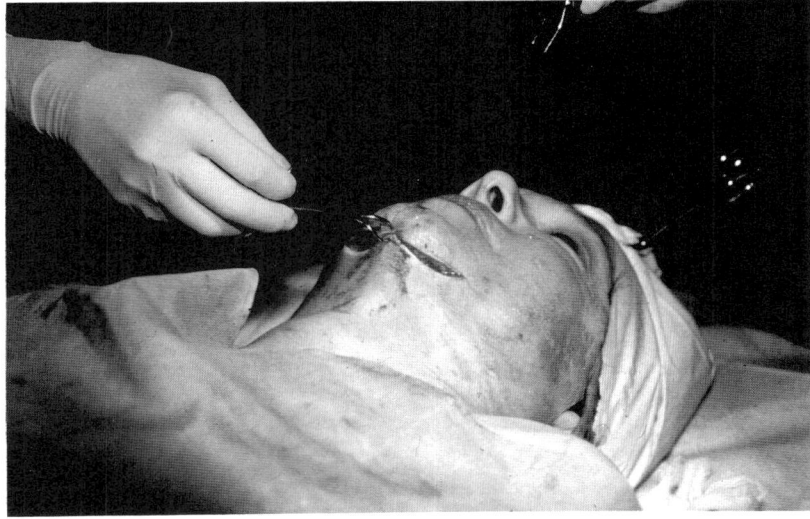

FIGURE 8.10. Intraoperative: excision line pulled together prior to suturing.

Sagging Jowls

Sagging jowls can be improved only somewhat with liposuction. This procedure can be done through a tiny submental incision along with cervical liposuction. Care must be taken not to injure the branch of the facial nerve in this area.

Nasolabial Fold

Some authors feel that unless there is a gross deposition of fat, it is difficult to get a good result in this area.[8] The entry through the pyriform aperture just inside the nostril with 2 and 3 mm short cannulas can be used. Contouring here should be conservative and cau-

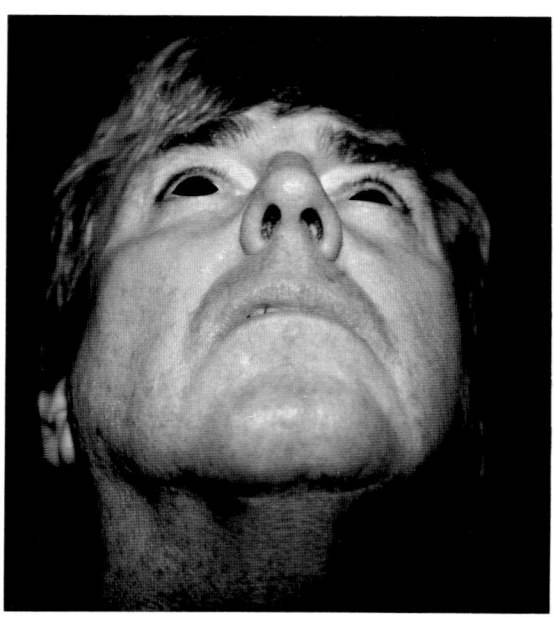

FIGURE 8.11. Posterative: suture line after excision excess of skin.

tious. Suction can be helpful in subtle contouring of young people who have full faces, but it cannot be used as the sole treatment for patients with prominent nasolabial folds, since it will not remove excess skin.[6]

Adjunct to Rhytidectomy

Submental liposuction has become a part of the vast majority of rhytidectomies. Open and closed liposuction techniques have been developed to use in conjunction with a facelift to improve definition of the facial mandibular and cervical contours. Liposuction has made the facelift procedure easier and safer.[9] Liposuction speeds the facelift procedure, lessening operator fatigue while shortening surgical and anesthesia time for the patient. Excellent results are achieved without resorting to the various complex and sometimes dangerous platysma—splitting and SMAS—undermining procedures advocated in the past decade.[9]

Liposuction of Buccal Fat Pads

Some operators use excision with liposuction, with the excision made inside the cheek,[10] and some excise buccal fat pads.[11] Most operators feel that liposuction of the cheeks is not a satisfactory procedure, because the superficial fat layer is very thin, leading to irregularities of the cheek. In addition, there is the likelihood of nerve and vessel injury in this area.

References

1. Bernstein G, Hanke CW. Safety of liposuction: a review of 947 cases performed by dermatologists. J Dermatol Surg Oncol. 1988;14:1112–1114.
2. Goddio AS. Skin retraction following suction lipectomy by treatment cite: a study of 500 procedures in 458 selected subjects. Plast Reconstr Surg. 1991;87(1):66–75.
3. Narins RS. Liposuction and anesthesia. Dermatol Clin. 1990;8(3):421–424.
4. Klein JA. The tumescent technique. Am J Cosmet Surg. 1987;4:263–267.
5. Asken S. *Liposuction Surgery and Autologous Fat Transplantation*. Appleton & Lange, Norwalk, 1988.
6. Lambros B. Fat contouring in the face and neck. Clin Plast Surg. 1992;19(2):401–14.
7. Toledo LS. Syringe liposuction: a two-year experience. Aesthet Plast Surg. 1991;15(4):321–326.
8. Asken S. Microliposuction and autologous fat transplantation for aesthetic enhancement of the aging face. J.D.S. & O. 1990;16(10):965–972.
9. Chrisman BB. Liposuction with facelift surgery. Dermatol Clin. 1990;8(3):501–522.
10. Pitman GH. Suction lipectomy of the face and body: precision and refinement instructional courses. Plast Surg Ed Found. 1988;I:71.
11. Matarasso A. Buccal fat pad excision: aesthetic improvement of the midface. An Plast Surg. 1991;26:413–418.

9
Lipotransfer

William P. Coleman III

Although autologous tissue from numerous organs has been transplanted throughout the body successfully, none of these is more appealing than fat. Theoretically, fat should provide a nearly unlimited source of host tissue for subcutaneous and dermal augmentation. It is soft and has a natural consistency, is easy to obtain access to, and is readily regenerated after harvesting.

Since at least the nineteenth century, physicians have tried to take advantage of this plentiful source of autologous tissue. Early attempts relied primarily on en bloc excision and transfer into a pouch at the host site.[1] This resulted in scars at both the donor and recipient sites. These early experiments portended future frustration with fat as a tissue source because the survival of this transplanted tissue was erratic. In the early 1950s, Peer demonstrated that transplanted fat does survive and that living adipocytes exist indefinitely after transfer.[2,3] He reported that the cells lost approximately 50% of their weight in volume 1 year after transplantation.

During the 1940s surgeons began to employ dermal fat grafts as a replacement for en bloc autologous fat, in the hope of increasing the survival of the graft. The popularity of this technique led many surgeons to abandon autologous fat. The advent of various artificial soft tissue fillers, such as silicone, further replaced fat grafting.

In the early 1980s, Illouz and Fournier, the Parisian liposuction pioneers, began to experiment with reinjecting fat that had just been removed by suction.[4,5] This new technique was termed *microlipoinjection*. A whole new era in lipotransfer had arrived. Suddenly, fat could be removed using a syringe attached to a small cannula and then immediately reinjected where needed. This could be done without the scars that resulted from en bloc fat grafts. Early experience indicated that at least some of the reinjected fat survived.[6,7]

In the initial excitement following the emergence of microlipoinjection, many dermatologists and plastic surgeons began suctioning and reinjecting fat. A period of disillusionment soon followed, because in many cases the results were not long-lasting. Many surgeons tried a few cases and then totally abandoned the procedure. Meanwhile a small number of surgeons continued to refine the technique of microlipoinjection. Fournier evolved an approach of processing the extracted fat with distilled water and then breaking the cells down with centrifugation to obtain the fibrous cell walls for dermal augmentation. He named this approach *autologous collagen*.[8] Zocchi continued this work in Italy.[9] Simplification of technique made microlipoinjection more attractive.

Now fat augmentation is reemerging as a viable and practical approach to both subcutaneous and dermal augmentation. Like all procedures, there is variation in results. The evolution of techniques to maximize the benefits of this procedure continues. However, it is clear that lipotransfer will continue to be used more and more by dermatologists in the future.

Histology of Lipotransfer

Although a number of credible studies examined the histologic behavior of en bloc transplanted autologous fat during the twentieth century, there have been only a few reports on the histology of fat grafts after microlipoinjection. These, however, have confirmed that a portion of transplanted fat does survive. Campbell et al. studied the mechanical effects on lipocytes forced through a needle.[10] Glucose oxidation determinations showed viable fat cells after suction and reinjection. They also demonstrated that the cell viability decreased with smaller-diameter needles.

Skouge et al. studied fat suctioned from the perivesical fat pad and injected into the bladder wall of New Zealand white rabbits.[11] They described an initial inflammatory reaction surrounding the grafts followed by regeneration of the lipocytes and microcyst formation. Nine months after transplantation, viable adipocytes could be seen quite clearly.

Studies of autologous collagen extracted from fat demonstrated an initial inflammatory response followed by deposition of connective tissue and complete obliteration of adipocytes when this material was injected into the dermis. This resulted in a nearly threefold thickening of the dermis as the fibrotic reaction replaced the injected lipocytic material.[12]

Patient Selection

Subcutaneous augmentation with autologous fat is primarily indicated for atrophy or defects in the subcutis. Fat seems to survive best when injected into spaces formerly occupied by fat. Injecting fat into defects that primarily contain scar tissue is usually unsuccessful. Similarly, defects that result from muscular or bony atrophy with a normal overlying subcutaneous layer cannot be effectively recontoured by lipotransfer.

One of the most reliable scenarios for using fat augmentation is to improve defects resulting from liposuction. When lipoplasty results in focal subcutaneous atrophy, correction can usually be obtained by suctioning a small amount of the fat surrounding the depression and injecting this into the defect. The survival of the fat after this technique is usually quite good. In some cases, years after liposuction, weight gain in the tissue surrounding the liposuction site may produce an obvious step-off between treated and untreated skin. Conservative liposuction around the periphery of the original liposuction site can be used to feather the edges of the defect. The fat obtained can then be injected directly into the periphery of the previously suctioned areas to achieve a more even contour (see Figures 9.1A and B).

Lipodystrophy may be congenital or result from trauma or disease or may be idiopathic.[13] Localized areas of fat loss can be corrected quite successfully using lipotransfer.[14] When due to trauma or disease, it is best to wait until the tissues have fully recovered before attempting to replace the lost fat. In extensive cases, multiple procedures may be necessary to reestablish the proper contours (see Figures 9.2A and B).

The most popular use of lipotransfer is to restore subcutaneous atrophy resulting from aging. In the chin and nasolabial areas, the tissue loss results in deep depressions, frequently with adjacent overlying loose skin. Extensive augmentation is often required to soften these defects. Obviously, traditional fillers such as Zyderm are not suitable for these patients, because so much material is required and the cost becomes prohibitive. However, fat becomes an excellent alternative when it is injected subcutaneously to fill depressions. In addition, the autologous collagen or lipocytic dermal augmentation technique can be used to correct dermal depressions overlying the subcutaneous defects[12] (refer to Figures 9.3A and B). In this application, the fat cells are ruptured by adding distilled water and then using ultrasound and centrifugation to produce a less viscous material that can be injected through a 25-gauge needle (Vide Supra).

Aging of the face is the result of changes that occur in the epidermis and dermis as well as in the subcutaneous tissue, muscle, and bone. Lipotransfer often becomes a supplemental procedure to facelift, hard tissue implants, chemical peel, and dermabrasion. Judicious combinations of these various procedures can give the patient the best rejuvenating result.

There has been great interest by physicians and patients alike in augmenting breasts with lipotransfer. Obviously, this fatty organ is an

9. Lipotransfer

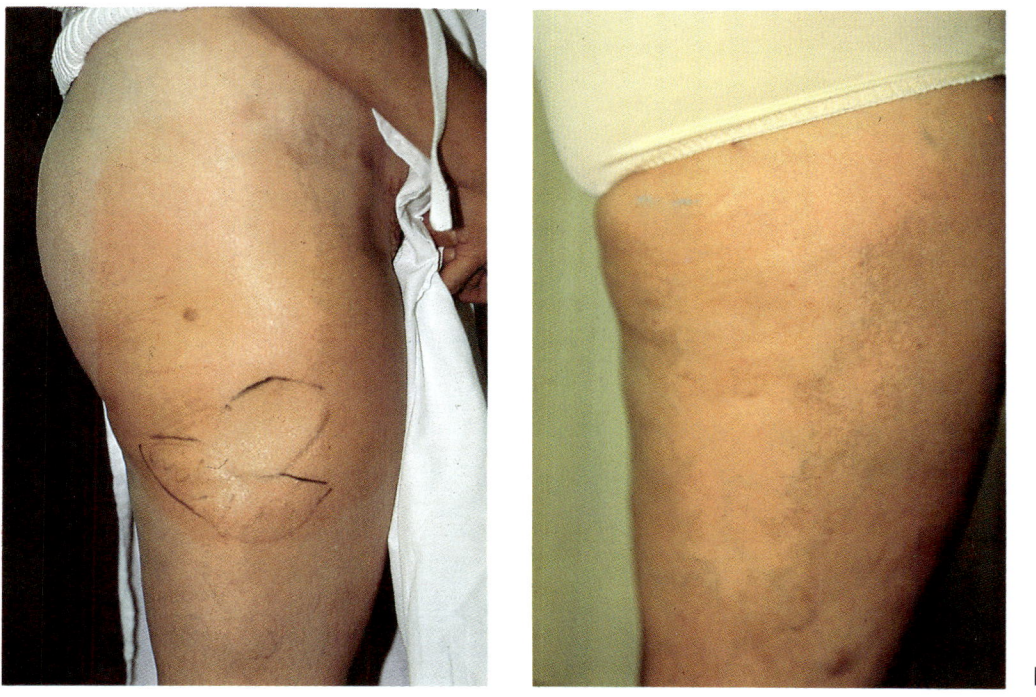

FIGURE 9.1. A. Depressed area of the thigh resulting from liposuction. B. Correction is obvious after circumferential liposuction with injection of the suctioned fat into the defect.

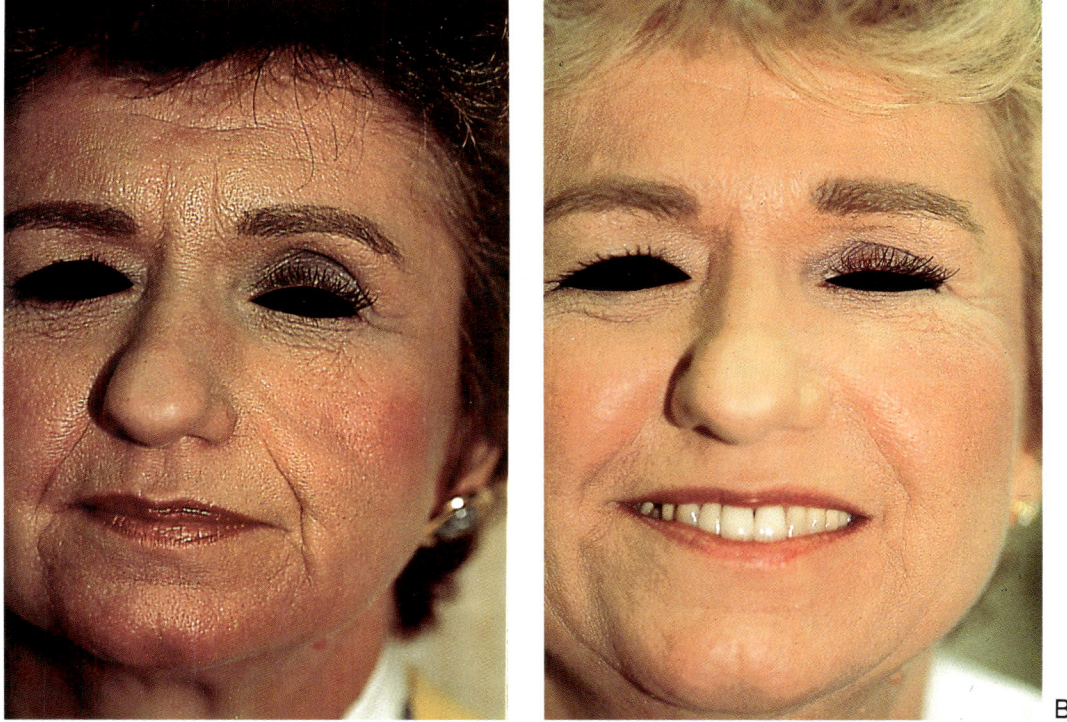

FIGURE 9.2. A. Idiopathic lipodystrophy of the left cheek. B. Excellent correction is apparent after 2 lipotransfer procedures.

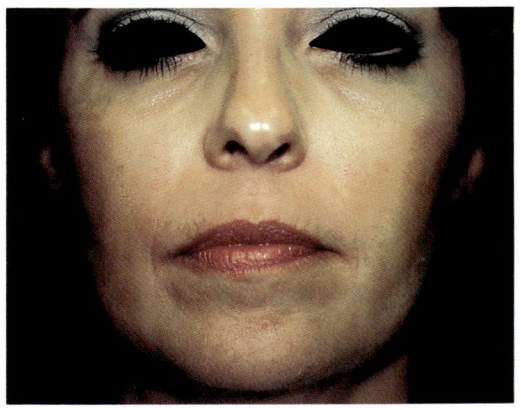
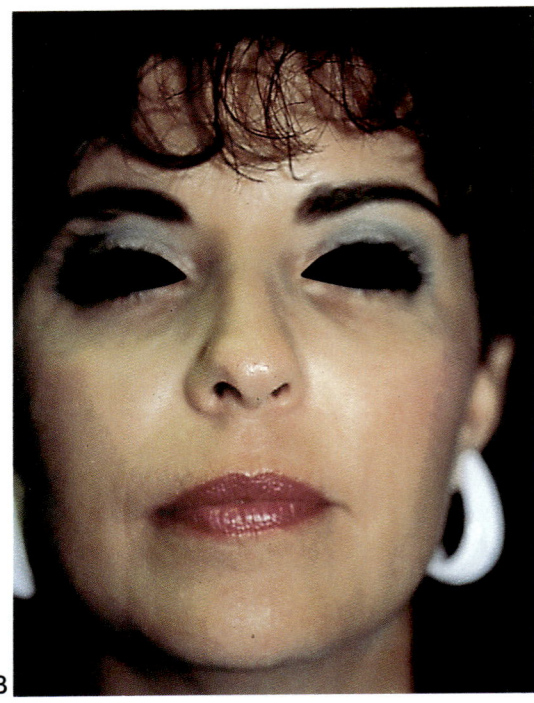

FIGURE 9.3. A. Preoperative lipotransfer with overlying lipocytic dermal augmentation. B. Improvement is maintained 7 months postoperative, 2 procedures.

appealing site for autologous fat transplantation. Unfortunately, however results to date have not been good. Large amounts of fat must be transplanted to create even a modest result. When these large amounts of fat are injected, benign calcifications often occur.[15] These may appear during mammography and make tumor surveillance confusing. The recent hysteria over the dangers of breast implants has rekindled interest in this procedure.

Lipotransfer can be beneficial in improving the appearance of the aging hand.[16] A thin atrophic dermis reveals the underlying veins and tendons and is an obvious sign of aging. This is worse in those individuals who have severe actinic damage. Fat transfer to the dorsum of the hand through a small injection site on the wrist camouflages the underlying structures and gives the appearance of much more youthful hands (see Figure 9.4).

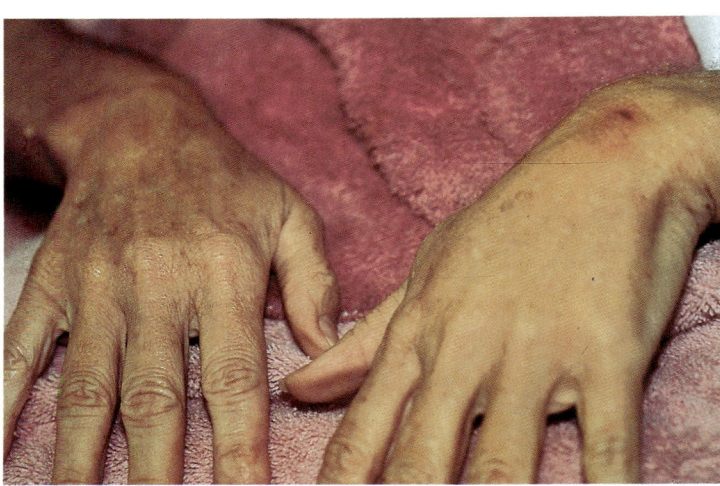

FIGURE 9.4. The left hand has been augmented with fat, whereas the right remains in its preoperative state.

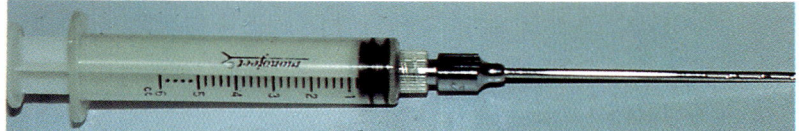

FIGURE 9.5. A 10 cc syringe attached to a minicannula ready for harvesting fat.

Lipotransfer Technique

Excess fat can be found in most patients, especially in the abdominal, thigh, and hip areas. The patients themselves should be asked where they most would like to rid themselves of some excess fat. Donor sites should be chosen and marked with patients standing.

After patients are supine, a small wheal is raised on the edge of the donor site using 1% lidocaine with epinephrine. Through this wheal, a 0.1% tumescent anesthetic solution is injected until the donor area becomes quite firm. The tumescent solution can be prepared by adding 5 cc of 2% plain lidocaine, 1 cc (1 meq) of sodium bicarbonate, and 0.1 cc of epinephrine (1:1,000) to each 100 cc of normal saline. Obvious vasoconstriction on the surface of the skin indicates adequate tumescent anesthesia.

A small stab incision can then be made with a number 11 blade, providing access to the subcutis. A 14-gauge minicannula or blunt needle can then be advanced into the engorged fat. A 10 cc syringe is then attached to the cannula and the plunger raised to exert negative pressure (refer to Figure 9.5). Holding the plunger out with four fingers of the dominant hand, a gentle to-and-fro motion through the subcutaneous tissue suctions fat into the syringe (see Figure 9.6). Once 7 or 8 cc of fat are obtained in this manner, the mechanical suction advantage is lost and a fresh syringe must be attached to the cannula. Additional syringes are filled until a sufficient amount of fat is obtained.

Once the syringes are filled, they are capped and allowed to stand, plunger up, on a testtube rack. After 5 minutes a clear or slightly red infranate appears at the bottom of the syringe and can be expelled. The remaining solid fraction is yellow fat (see Figure 9.7). With the tumescent anesthetic technique, there is usually very little bleeding, so additional washing of the fat is not required.

The harvested fat can then be injected immediately into the appropriate recipient sites. A small wheal of 1% lidocaine with epinephrine can be used as the injection site. The fat will typically pass smoothly through an 18-gauge needle. If a sharp needle is employed, then it is very important to draw back on the syringe before injecting to be certain that the needle has not penetrated a blood vessel. The fat is best injected in individual ribbons rather than as a large bolus (see Figure 9.8). Several layers of these ribbons may be required, depending upon the depth of the subcutaneous defect. With immediate manual manipulation, the fat can be molded into the proper contours.

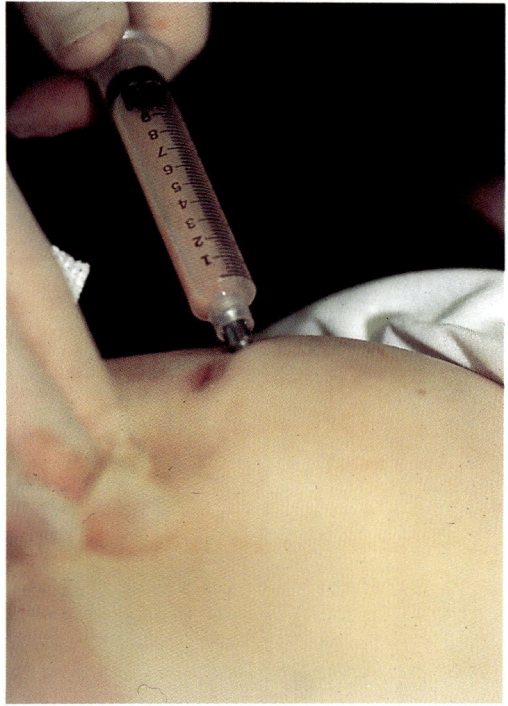

FIGURE 9.6. With the plunger raised, fat can be suctioned into the syringe.

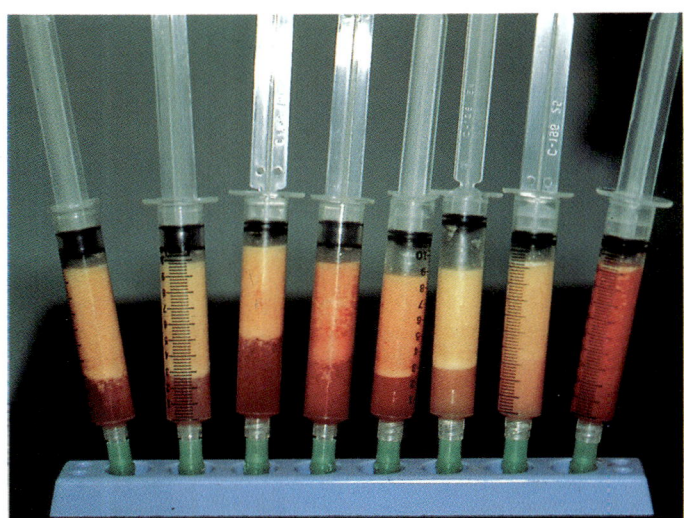

FIGURE 9.7. Syringes are allowed to stand upright until the fat separates from the blood-tinged infranate.

Postoperatively, the donor site should be compressed with elastic adhesive tape for 24 hours. After this time period, mild compression with an elastic garment is recommended for several days to minimize swelling and bruising. The recipient area should initially be covered with a light gauze dressing. No recipient-site dressing is usually required after 24 hours. Eating chewy foods or excessive talking is interdicted on the first postoperative day, in order to avoid shifting of the transplanted fat. Patients are encouraged to use icepacks to minimize swelling. Intramuscular or oral steroids can also be given to minimize swelling and bruising.

Lipocytic Dermal Augmentation

Since Fournier's and Zocchi's studies on autologous collagen in the late 1980s, there has been interest in extracting fibrous materials from fat that might be used for intradermal injection. With the FDA's banning of silicone and questions about the immunicity of Zyderm, there is interest in developing alternative substances for augmentation of dermal defects. Although fat does not contain as much collagen as other tissues, such as dermis or cartilage, there is a small amount of collagen and other connective tissue in the cell walls surrounding adipocytes.

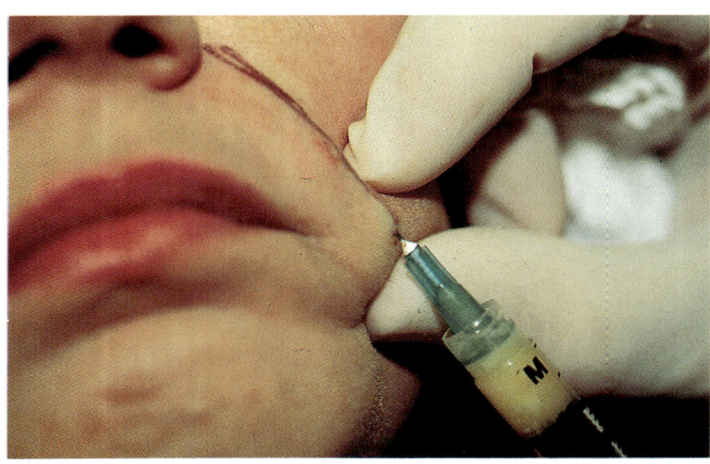

FIGURE 9.8. The fat is injected in individual ribbons rather than as a large bolus.

9. Lipotransfer

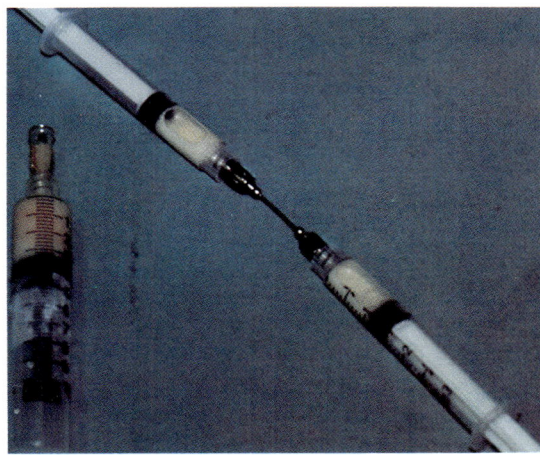

FIGURE 9.9. A bi-lurelock connector enables the surgeon to break up the adipocytes.

Recurrent emphasis has centered around breaking down the extracted fat by mechanical manipulation to render it in a nonviscous form so that it may be injected through a small-gauge needle.[8,9]

One reliable approach to processing fat for intradermal augmentation relies on rupturing the fat cells by adding sterile distilled water. After extraction of the fat, using the same method described for microlipoinjection, 1 cc of sterile water is added to 6 cc of fat. This material is then transferred to 3 cc syringes, each about half full. These are capped and then centrifuged at 1,000 revolutions per minute for 60 seconds. An oily infranate composed of triglycerides can then be expelled. Further separation of the cell walls and lipocyte contents can be achieved using ultrasound, with a common jewelry-cleaning device. The remaining solid fraction can then be further broken down by passing it back and forth between two syringes attached to a biluerlock connector of diminishing diameters (see Figure 9.9). This can be achieved by using connectors of different diameters or a biluerlock device with a screw attachment. Once the material can pass through a 23- or 25-gauge needle, it can be injected intradermally in a similar fashion to Fibrel. A small wheal verifies the intradermal location of the needle (see Figure 9.10). Slight overcorrection is usually necessary to obtain proper results.

Studies of this approach using lipocytic material for dermal augmentation have indicated that the processed fat contains about 3% collagen.[12] The material can be frozen and reused, though histology demonstrates some fragmenting of the collagen fibers when this is done. Biopsies of augmented sites indicate that at 3 months, the dermal thickness had increased by nearly threefold.[12] Evidence of new collagen formation indicates that the benefits come not only from a volume increase due to the injected material but also from the inflammatory response of the recipient tissue.

Lipocytic dermal augmentation is particularly efficient in patients who require more than 1 cc of dermal augmentation. The use of multiple syringes of Zyderm or Fibrel is cost-prohibitive. Moreover, many patients with aging changes around the mouth have evidence

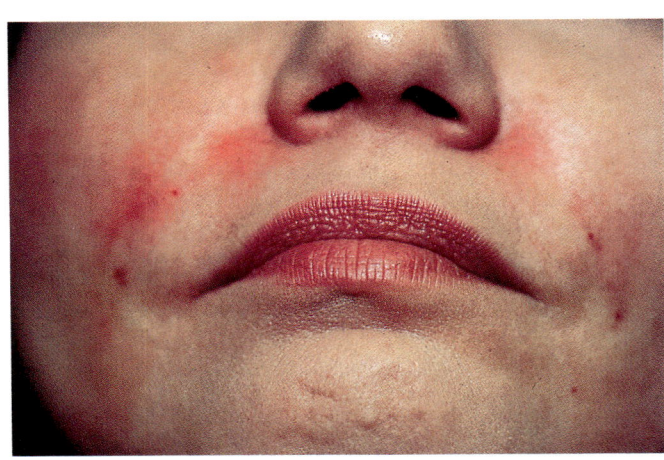

FIGURE 9.10. Small wheals indicate the intradermal location of the injected material.

of subcutaneous as well as dermal loss. Microlipoinjection can be used in these cases to build up the subcutis and lipocytic dermal augmentation to smooth out dermal depressions and wrinkles. These patients show excellent results with longevity of their improvement comparable to Zyderm or Fibrel, especially if a touch-up treatment is done 3 or 4 weeks after the initial one.

How Long Does It Last?

Although researchers continue to attempt to quantify the success rate of lipotransfer, whether used subcutaneously or intradermally, there is a great deal of individual variation.[17] At this time there appears to be no scientific evidence that the donor site choice has any effect on the longevity of the survival of the transplanted fat. The vascularity of the recipient site may affect survival.[1] Other transplanted tissues depend on the integrity of the vascular bed at the recipient site. However, further unknown factors obviously affect the longevity of transplanted fat. When lipotransfer is employed in areas of the face where there is constant movement, such as around the mouth, there is diminished survival as compared to less mobile areas. Very active locations such as the dorsal hands have poor long-term results after lipotransfer. Certainly a percentage of the injected cells survive each treatment session. Theoretically, multiple retreatments can eventually result in long-term survival.[18]

With lipocytic dermal augmentation, success does not depend on transplantation of viable lipocytes; the degree of inflammatory response may be the chief determinant of the degree of augmentation, since the improvement is largely due to deposition of collagen and fibrous tissue as a host response to the transplant. However, there is gradual loss of the dermal thickening with time. Just as with microlipoinjection, repeated treatments seem to give longer-lasting results.

Complications

Lipotransfer has proved to be a very safe technique. Although infection is rare, it is wise to use aseptic technique when performing this procedure. Overcorrection is a possible complication; but due to the incomplete take of the transplant, this usually resolves spontaneously. It is highly appropriate to overcorrect after warning the patient that this is being done in an attempt to achieve a better final result. It is important to mold the contours of the injected fat immediately after transplantation to achieve a symmetrical result. Dimples and small scars at the sites of both harvesting and transplantation are possibilities but certainly minor sequelae rather than complications.

Although there is the possibility of injecting fat intravascularly, this has not been reported widely. However, there are known cases of blindness resulting after fat transplantation in the glabella.[19] This appears to be similar to cases of sudden blindness following injection of other particulate matter in this area. Certainly great care must be taken to be certain that the needle is not placed in a blood vessel.

There is increasing consensus that repeated lipotransfer is required to achieve a lasting result. Clinically, patients often lose much of the initial augmentation within a few months. Those who have a touch-up treatment as soon as the benefits begin to fade usually have a much more lasting result after the second transplant. Similarly, the survival after a third lipotransfer is usually even longer lasting than after the second, and so on. Probably some of the transferred fat survives each treatment, so repeated transplantation results in cumulative survival.

References

1. Skouge JW. Autologous fat transplantation in facial surgery. In: *Cosmetic Surgery of the Skin.* WP Coleman, CW Hanke, S Asken, TH Alt., eds. B.C. Decker Inc., Philadelphia, 1991, pp. 239–249.
2. Peer LA. Loss of weight and volume in human fat grafts. Plast Reconstr Surg. 1950;5:217.
3. Peer LA. The neglected "fat free graft," its behavior and clinical use. Am J Surg. 1956;92:40.
4. Illouz Y. The fat cell "graft," a new technique to fill depressions. Plast Reconstr Surg. 1986; 78:122–123.

5. Fournier PF. Facial recontouring with fat grafting. Dermatol Clin. 1990;8:523–537.
6. Billings E, May JW. Historical review and present status of free fat graft autografts in plastic and reconstructive surgery. Plast Reconstr Surg. 1989;83:368–381.
7. Chajchin A, Benzaques I. Fat grafting injection for soft tissue augmentation. Plast Reconstr Surg. 1989;84:921–934.
8. Fournier PF. *Collagen Autologue: Liposculpture Ma Technique.* Arnette, Paris, 1989, pp. 277–279.
9. Zocchi M. Methode de production de collagene autologue par traitement du tissu graisseaux. J Med Esthet Chirur Dermatol. 1990;XVII,66:105–114.
10. Campbell GL, Laudslager N, Newman J. The effect of mechanical stress on adipocyte morphology and metabolism. Am J Cosmet Surg. 1987;4:89–94.
11. Skouge JW, Canning DA, Jefs RD. Long term survival of perivesical fat hervested and injection by microlipoinjection techniques in a rabbit model. Presented at the 16th Annual American Society for Dermatologic Surgery Meeting, Fort Lauderdale, Florida, March 1989.
12. Coleman WP, Lawrence N, Sherman RN, Reed RJ, Pinski KS. Autologous collagen? lipocytic dermal augmentation: a histopathologic study. J Dermatol Surg Oncol. 1993;19:1032–1040.
13. Afifi, AK, et al. Partial (localized) lipodystrophy. J Am Acad Dermatol. 1985;12:199.
14. Moscona R, Ullman Y, Har-Shai Y, Hirshowitz B. Fat free injections for the correction of hemifacial atrophy. Plast Reconstr Surg. 1989;84:501–507.
16. Lauber JS, Abrams H, Coleman WP III. Application of the tumescent technique to hand augmentation. J Dermatol Surg Oncol. 1990;16:369–373.
17. Glogau RG. Microlipoinjection. Arch Dermatol. 1988;124:1340–1343.
18. Pinski KS, Roenigk HH. Autologous fat transplantation: long term follow-up. J Dermatol Surg Oncol. 1992;18:179–184.
19. Telmourian B. Blindness following fat injections [letter to the editor]. Plast Reconstr Surg. 1988;82(2):361.

10
Facelift Surgery

Thomas H. Alt

Facelift surgery is one of the most satisfying surgeries performed. Although rhinoplasty and liposuction are more common, the facelift is considered by the layman as the most complex and, therefore, most important procedure. This is probably because the results are apparent and gratifying and, as one ages, provide benefit to all potential candidates. Although rhinoplasty and liposuction also can produce dramatic results, not all individuals will ultimately need or benefit from these procedures.

After World War I, attention was placed less on the political and economic needs of the day and individuals began to seek self-improvement, an option that had not been plausible at the turn of the century. As a result cosmetic procedures began to be developed, with the first comprehensive treatise being published by Madame Noel, a Parisian dermatologist, in 1926 and expanded in 1928.[1,2] These early attempts were quite limited by current standards.

However, Passot, a student of Noel's, was the first to publish a paper on facelift in 1919, in which he commented on her technique.[3] Joseph, in a paper published in 1921, stated that he had performed a facelift operation in 1912.[4] Then, in 1931, Lexer published a paper stating that he had performed the procedure in 1906.[5] Surgeons from across the world began to report on the early benefits of facelift procedures, including Bames of Los Angeles,[6] Bettman of Portland,[7] Booth of Seattle,[8] Bourguet[9] and Lagarde[10] of Paris, Hunt of New York,[11] Miller of Chicago,[12] and Stein of Vienna.[13] Since these beginnings hundreds of surgeons have written on the technique, effects, and complications of facelift surgery.

Definition of Purpose

Although the procedure is referred to by the layman as *facelift,* this is, indeed, a misnomer. A significant number of patients believe that the facelift will improve the entire face, including the melolabial folds, the periorbital region, and the descent of the forehead structures seen with normal aging. Within the medical community, the term *cervicofacial rhytidectomy* denotes procedures that improve the lower one-third of the face and the anterior cervical region. The procedure is designed to reinforce the underlying muscular and fascial structures and to remove excess skin. The removal of rhytides or wrinkles is not the goal of this procedure and, therefore, the patient will be disappointed if this is not clarified. The purpose of the facelift is many-faceted, with the following as major considerations:

1. Improvement of the jowling along the mandibular ramus resulting from excess fat and/or a descent of the skin secondary to loss of elasticity.
2. Removal of excess skin and fat of the neck.
3. Improved definition of the cervicomental angle.
4. Improvement of existing platysmal banding.
5. Redraping of the angles of the mouth to diminish or delete the marionette appearance.

All photographs reproduced with permission of Thomas H. Alt, M.D. © 1995 Thomas H. Alt, M.D.

It may be most appropriate for the physician to begin the evaluation at the initial consultation by asking, "What do you want a facelift to do for you?" or, a slightly different approach, "What do you think a facelift will do for you?" Patients are then asked to use a mirror to articulate their personal needs to the surgeon. It is not the surgeon's responsibility to tell patients what their needs are, but it is the surgeon's responsibility to outline the reasonable results that patients can expect when discussing their individual cases. It is, therefore, important for the surgeon to clarify the limited nature of the cervicofacial rhytidectomy, in that it has little effect upon the upper half of the melolabial folds, will have no effect on the perioral and periorbital rhytides, and will not, independently, have any effect upon the brow or the eyelids. Patients with moderate elastotic changes who have prominent bony structures and well-defined cervicomental angles are excellent candidates. Those with severe loss of elasticity or extensive actinic changes and those with an ill-defined anterior neck as the result of a low hyoid bone cannot expect to have as dramatic a result. Platysmal banding, when excessive, may be difficult or impossible to eliminate and will probably be the first defect to return as the aging process continues postoperatively.

Ancillary procedures such as chin or malar implants, facial liposuction or lipotransfer, facial chemical peel, upper and lower lid blepharoplasty, elevation of the eyebrow using procedures such as the direct browlift, coronal lift, mid-forehead lift, or a pretricheal lift are best introduced at the initial consultation so that the patient recognizes that multiple procedures are available for the type of rejuvenation necessary. With a thorough discussion of the advantages and disadvantages of each procedure, the physician becomes a responsible consultant, allowing patients to understand and evaluate their own needs in an educated sense. It is usually at this point that the surgeon will be able to evaluate the realistic or unrealistic expectations of the particular patient.

Health, both physically and psychologically, is an important factor in the acceptance of a candidate for facelift surgery. Individuals in American Society of Anesthesiologists (ASA) Class I or Class II are usually appropriate candidates for the surgery. ASA Class I are patients in excellent health; ASA Class II are patients in good health with minor systemic disease under good control, such as hypertension. Most of this information can be obtained by a history form completed by the patient prior to the consultation. Further questioning and evaluation by the patient's regular physician will assist in the acceptance or rejection of a candidate. Rarely, patients will withhold important information because they either misunderstand the history form or are so desirous of cosmetic improvement that they fear denial if their present health status is exposed. This possibility is usually eliminated if the patient's regular physician performs the preoperative history and physical examination necessary for the procedure. The psychological status of patients should also be carefully evaluated, with specific questions as to the patient's present and past well-being included on the preoperative history form. Wright has written extensively on evaluation of cosmetic surgery patients, and every surgeon performing cosmetic surgery should be familiar with identifying patients with special psychological needs.[14]

Age is not a critical factor in the acceptance of patients. The surgeon will be consulted by patients who are in their mid- to late thirties who will definitely benefit from a rhytidectomy, although the changes that will result from the surgery will be subtle. Studies have shown that younger patients will appreciate their surgery more than older patients.[15] Patients should not be denied the surgery solely on the basis of age, although benefits from the procedure diminish with advancing age. Individuals in their seventies and eighties can successfully undergo this surgery if their health warrants.

Explanation of the Procedure

In today's litigious society, it is best to clearly define the procedure or procedures to be performed along with the alternatives or options available. With the aid of a mirror, patients are shown the proposed incision lines and the options used by some other surgeons. Since most patients are unaware of these options and their disadvantages, it will be helpful to discuss the disadvantages of options that result in the

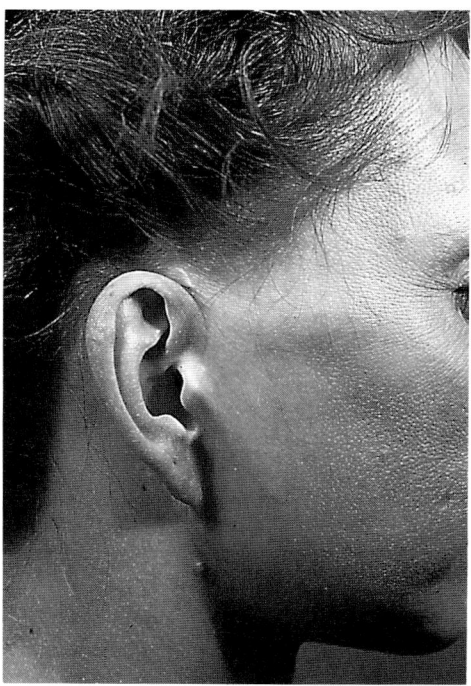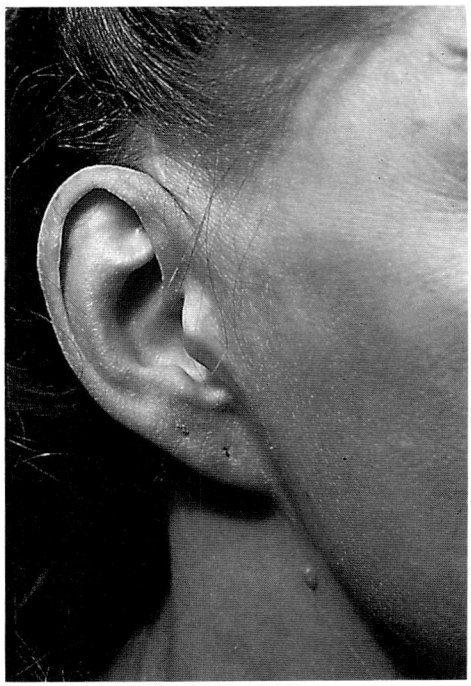

FIGURE 10.1. This patient has several abnormalities resulting from poor planning. The vertical incision in the temporal area eliminated the entire sideburn. The patient has an anterior and inferior displacement of her lobule resulting from improper positioning and disregard of the scar contracture that occurs postoperatively. A third defect is an obvious ridge present from the crest of the tragus anteriorly at a 45° angle. This is the result of excessive tension being placed on the flap.

FIGURE 10.2. This is an oblique view of the same patient shown in Figure 10.1. There is a deformed lobule resulting in an elf ear, absence of the sideburn, and a raised scar between the crest of the tragus and the lower cheek.

diminution or elimination of the preauricular tuft of hair (Figures 10.1, 10.2, and 10.3), a vertical incision anterior to the external ear (Figure 10.2), incisions that result in the formation of an elf ear with downward displacement of the lobule (Figures 10.2 and 10.3), and postauricular incisions that are inferior to the hairline (Figures 10.4, 10.5 and 10.6).

A decision on a pretragal or posttragal incision line is best made at this time, after discussion of the advantages and disadvantages. A notation should be placed in the chart so that the surgeon will clearly recall this decision. Although lifting of the skin with the fingers by the surgeon does not definitively predict the end result, the approximate tension is usually considerably less than that which is applied by patients when they attempt to visualize their concept of the results of this procedure. Excessive preauricular pressure applied by patients will usually eliminate most of the melolabial fold but will also cause gross distortion of the inferolateral aspect of the periorbital tissues. This should be pointed out to patients. It is at this point where reemphasis of the facelift's limited improvement of the melolabial folds is important.

Platysmal banding and cervical and submental fat should be evaluated and cervical liposuction should be considered, if indicated. Ancillary and alternative procedures are appropriate to discuss at this point. The surgical goals and expected results of the facelift and any other ancillary treatment should be summarized.

Prior to making a decision, it is important that patients understand the usual course following surgery. The need and extent of postoperative dressings and restrictions and the side effects and complications that might occur must be discussed. Postoperative instructions are given to patients so that they may carefully review them prior to making a final decision. An

10. Facelift Surgery

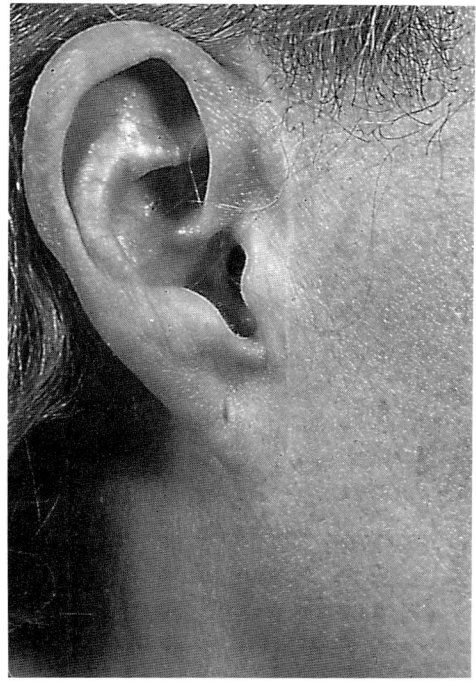

FIGURE 10.3. This patient has an obvious vertical preauricular incision that did not follow the curvature of the preauricular area. There is also absence of the sideburn resulting from the flap being advanced superiorly and posteriorly without regard to preservation of the temporal tuft of hair. This is an extreme example of the inferior displacement of the lobule resulting in an elf ear.

informed patient is usually a compliant patient, since no surprises will be forthcoming if the surgeon is thorough in this important preoperative discussion. Most patients will understand that it will require a minimum of several weeks before the edema and ecchymosis resolve sufficiently for them to return to gainful employment. Although most patients could return to work at the end of two weeks, it is our advice that patients should remain off work for 3 weeks if they wish to be covert about their surgery. Postoperative facelift instructions are detailed in Table 10.1.

Preoperative Physical and Laboratory Evaluation

Since most patients prefer to be unaware of the events during the surgery, intravenous sedation and general anesthesia are the most common methods of performing this surgery. Both of these methods of anesthesia require evaluation of the patient's physical health and a laboratory evaluation. Patients are asked to obtain a physical examination performed by their regular physicians, comparable to that which would be used for same-day surgery. A letter outlining the requirements of this physical should be provided to the patients so that the examining physicians can provide the necessary services.

Any special areas found on the preoperative history should be addressed. Laboratory evaluation will vary among surgeons. Table 10.2 shows preoperative instructions to be given to patients. Table 10.3 lists the laboratory tests and Table 10.4 lists the history and physical examination that we routinely request.

The laboratory tests and physical exam should be performed between 7 and 14 days prior to surgery and be present in the surgeon's office within sufficient time to evaluate the results, to order additional laboratory evaluation, and/or to delay or decline surgery on individuals with abnormal physical or laboratory findings.

Preoperative Medication

Attitudes vary among surgeons concerning preoperative medications. Most surgeons use systemic antibiotic therapy employing erythromycin or cephalexin 24 hours preoperatively and 48 to 72 hours postoperatively. These oral doses are supplemented by an intravenous push during surgery. Vitamin K therapy in the form of Mephyton is also favored by some, as is vitamin C (ascorbic acid) for improved wound healing. There is no definitive rule concerning the necessity of these preoperative medications.

Preoperative Photography

Preoperative photographs are advisable not only for medicolegal purposes but also for pre- and postoperative evaluation. Virtually all patients want to review their improvement, usually by the fourth postoperative week. Adequate preoperative photos will allow this. It is advisable to obtain a series of preoperative photographs 2 weeks prior to surgery if the film is being forwarded to a distant laboratory such as Kodalux when using Kodak film. If the pictures are inadequate upon return or if the

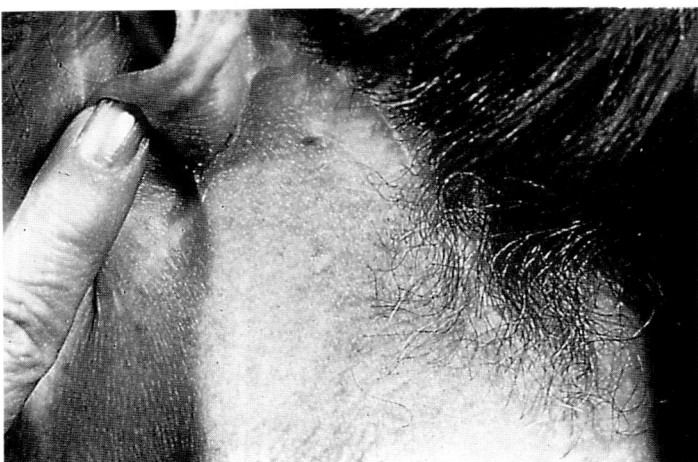

FIGURE 10.4. This patient has an obvious postauricular scar, which was placed inferior to the occipital hairline. Because of this placement, the patient must style her hair down around her shoulders.

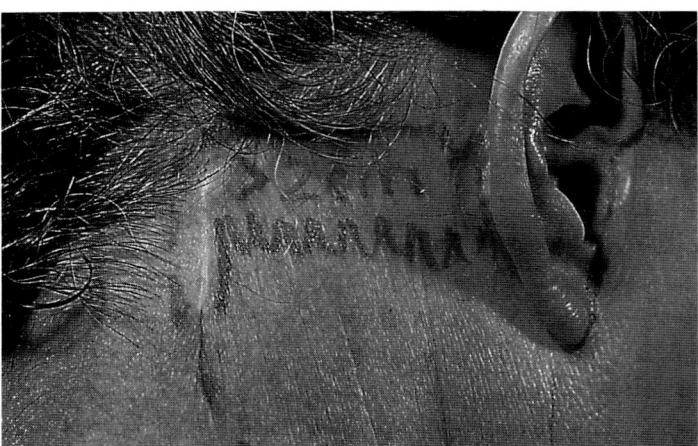

FIGURE 10.5. This patient had a very low deep horizontal retroauricular scar with its posterior limb angling 90° in the vertical position. Adequate support was not provided resulting in her sutures coming untied on the first postoperative day. Marking shows the extent of the postauricular scar which was greater than 2-cm. wide.

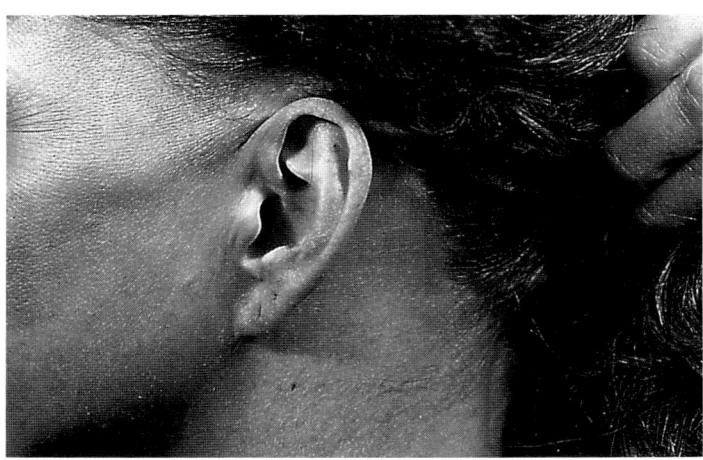

FIGURE 10.6. The same patient as shown in Figures 10.1 and 10.3 also shows poor planning with the presence of an obvious postauricular scar, which has been placed at the inferior border of the occipital hairline. The elf ear deformity is less than that shown in Figures 10.1 and 10.3, but there is a large and conspicuous band of elevated skin from the superior border of the auricle extending down to the zygomatic arch. As on the opposite side, the temporal hair has been elevated superiorly and posteriorly with the complete elimination of the sideburn.

TABLE 10.1. Postoperative facelift instructions.

Follow these instructions during your postoperative facelift recovery period:
1. Patients should be at bedrest for the remainder of the day of surgery. When up to the bathroom you should have assistance. This is because when you stand up, dizziness and fainting spells may occur. The chance of this greatly diminishes after 24 hours. Sometimes dizziness and weakness may occur following surgery; this will subside in a few days.
2. To reduce swelling, elevate the head on 2 to 3 pillows for approximately 2 weeks following surgery.
3. The turban applied at the time of your surgery should not be adjusted. Talking and visitors are discouraged the first 48 hours. We suggest using a notepad and pencil to communicate the first 2 days.
4. A chin strap will replace the turban dressing on the third day. It is to be worn continuously, except to wash, shower or shampoo, until the 14th day. Beginning the third week wear the chinstrap all hours when at home, awake, or asleep, through the third month.
5. You will experience a tight or heavy feeling of the face. Very little discomfort will accompany this surgery. *Do not take aspirin, aspirin products or ibuprofen.* To alleviate your discomfort, either Double Strength Tylenol or the pain medication prescribed for you may be taken.
6. To avoid bleeding and excess swelling, limit motion of the face. Do not bend the head forward, backward or sideways. Avoid gum and foods that are hard to chew for 2 weeks.
7. Avoid anything that could result in hitting or bumping your face. Do not hold or lift children. We advise sleeping on your back for 30 nights. *Do not roll over on your face.* A recliner at a 45° angle may be used.
8. Do not turn your head or stretch your neck for 2 weeks. Move your head and shoulders as one section. This is to avoid stretching the healing incisions.
9. No alcohol should be consumed for 1 week prior to and 1 week following surgery to avoid bleeding.
10. Do not wear clothing that must be pulled over your head.
11. There will be swelling following your surgery. This is normal. Discoloration is normal and usually subsides within 2 or 3 weeks.
12. You may experience some numbness or tingling in the area. This is usually temporary.
13. Should bleeding occur, go to bed, elevate the head, and apply pressure to that area. Call the physician immediately.
14. If you feel warm, take your temperature. A temperature of 100° or less is normal. Any persistent fever over 100° should be reported.
15. You may shower and shampoo any time after the large dressing has been removed, usually the third day.
16. You may wear your eyeglasses after the bandages have been removed. Contact lenses may be worn the day after surgery. If you have had eyelid surgery, do not wear contact lenses for 7 days.
17. Once your bandages have been removed, use full strength hydrogen peroxide on a Q-tip to clean over your suture lines 2 to 3 times daily. A generous amount of Polysporin should be applied to the suture line in front and back of the ear after each peroxide treatment while the sutures are in. Apply a small strip of Saran Wrap to each suture line on top of the Polysporin.
18. Do not bend or lift for 2 weeks to avoid bleeding.
19. Do not tweeze eyebrows for 1 week. Do not visit a hair salon for 2 weeks and do not have a permanent for 3 weeks following surgery.
20. Do not wash your face for the first week following surgery to avoid bleeding. When showering and shampooing let the soap and water stream from your scalp over your face for cleansing. Pat the face dry; do not rub it dry. *After the first week* wash your face twice a day with your fingertips and a mild soap, using an upward motion.
21. Your sutures and clips will be removed beginning 5 to 7 days after your surgery. All clips will be removed by 14 days.
22. Do not smoke for 2 weeks prior to and 2 weeks after your surgery. Some studies claim that smoking can increase serious complications *12* times. One cigarette can significantly decrease blood flow up to 20 hours. Do not use a nicotine patch or nicorette gum.
23. Do not drive for 2 weeks. It is necessary to make arrangements ahead of time for someone to drive you to the office for your postoperative visits. These visits usually include the first 3 days after surgery and usually 2 days the next week depending on your progress.
24. The average patient returns to work in 2 or 3 weeks. This will vary with your job.
25. Athletic activities and exercise should be delayed for 4 weeks. Slow walks may be taken after 4 days.
26. Restoril 15 mg will be prescribed to be taken at bedtime for sleep, if needed.
27. A laxative may be used to avoid straining.
28. Your scars will appear a deep pink following suture and/or clip removal and will diminish with the passage of time. In most cases this process takes months.
29. It is normal to have some depression. Divert your attention by reading a good book, watching television or a nice ride in the car.
30. All postoperative appointments should be scheduled in advance with the office.

(Continued)

TABLE 10.1. (*Continued*)

Office private line: 936-0922; Thomas H. Alt, M.D.: 926-1097; Dr. Alt's Pager # is: 643-5351. Call this number, then enter your number and the # sign.
Surgical Fellow: _____
Home Phone #: _____
Pager #: _____

Copyright. All rights reserved. No reproduction or use of any part allowed without prior written permission. 12/93

TABLE 10.2. Preoperative instructions for facelift.

Name: _____
Date: _____
Your facelift has been scheduled for _____ .
Please arrive at the office at _____ .
The fee for this procedure is $ _____ : $ _____ for surgery and $ _____ for anesthesia. Full payment is to be made 2 weeks prior to the surgery. Because we must preplan our nurses and operating room schedule, your surgical fee must be received by that time. We hope you understand that if this payment is not received we will have to remove your name from our schedule. If, during the 2-week period prior to your surgery, you should decide to cancel your surgery, a prorata amount of your prepaid surgical fee will be refunded, based on our ability to fill the time with another surgery and materials fee.

Please note the instructions below to be followed prior to your surgery:
1. Do not wear clothing that must be pulled over the head.
2. Shampoo your scalp with Phisoderm for 10 minutes on the evening prior to and the morning of your surgery. Following the use of Phisoderm, you may use a hair conditioner.
3. Cleanse your face for 5 minutes twice daily with Phisoderm for at least 3 days prior to your surgery.
4. Have a good night's rest. NOTHING BY MOUTH AFTER MIDNIGHT.
5. For out-of-town patients, make arrangements to stay in town for a period of 7 days.
6. If preoperative pictures have not been taken, please call our office immediately for an appointment to have them taken.

Avoid the following:
1. Aspirin, aspirin-containing products and ibuprofen—do not take for 7 days before surgery.
2. Vitamin E—do not take for 14 days before surgery.
3. Alcohol, mood-altering drugs or substances—do not use for 7 days before surgery. Prescription drugs administered under the care of your physician and reported on the history form you completed at the time of consultation may be taken unless you were instructed otherwise.
4. A prescription for Mephyton is enclosed. This medication controls bleeding during surgery. Take 1 tablet 4 times daily for 5 days, taking the last tablet the evening before surgery. If you prefer a vitamin K injection at no charge, in place of Mephyton, please make arrangements with our office to have it administered 1 to 3 days prior to your surgery.
5. Cephalexin, the antibiotic prescribed for you, should be started 1 full day before surgery and continued for a total of 5 days. Take 1 capsule 3 times a day. Omit the morning of surgery. A prescription is enclosed.

The following items should be purchased prior to surgery:
1. Phisoderm—for scalp and facial washings prior to surgery.
2. Saran Wrap—to cover suture lines following surgery.
3. 2 tubes of Polysporin ointment—to be used on suture lines.
4. Q-tips—to cleanse and apply Polysporin ointment to suture lines.
5. Hydrogen peroxide—to cleanse suture lines.
6. Cotton balls—to wash your face following surgery.
7. Neutrogena soap—to cleanse face following surgery.

Following your surgery:
1. You must have a RESPONSIBLE ADULT, friend or relative, 21 years or older, drive you home following surgery and remain with you for the first 24 hours postoperatively. We will not allow you to ride home in a taxi following surgery.
2. Arrange for a driver to transport you to the office for your postoperative visits, as you WILL NOT be allowed to drive for 2 weeks. Your first visits will be at 24 hours and 48 hours following surgery.

Copyright. All rights reserved. No reproduction or use of any part allowed without prior written permission. 1/94

TABLE 10.3. Laboratory tests given prior to surgery.

You must fast for 8 hours prior to having these tests performed:
1. Complete blood count with differential
2. Platelet count
3. Prothrombin time
4. Partial thromboplastin time
5. SMA 12 — to include sodium and potassium
6. HIV
7. Hepatitis B surface antigen
8. Urinalysis
9. Urine pregnancy test (even for those using contraceptive techniques)

If over 40 years of age, provide the following, done within the past 24 months:
10. Chest xray
11. EKG

developed film does not return, the surgeon should be aware of this prior to surgery and must repeat these essential photographs. We use 17 views to document photographically the preoperative status. These views are described and shown in Figures 10.7 through 10.23.

TABLE 10.4. History and physical examination routinely requested.

Please have a history and physical done by your physician. The physician should then send it and the blood test results to our office at least 2 weeks prior to your surgery date.

Past and present history

Physical exam:
  Head and neck:
  Breasts:
  Chest and lungs:
  Heart:
  Abdomen:
  Extremities:
  Other:
  Summary of positive findings:

Please note any changes in health that may contraindicate the safe use of anesthesia, i.e., present medications, bleeding, upper respiratory infection, allergies, fever, et cetera and notify our office immediately. Thank you.

To make the photographs, the patient is placed in a neutral position, avoiding extension or flexion of the neck. Earrings and jewelry should be removed. Photoflood lights are highly recommended over a camera-attached flash, since the former will show the subtle contouring and wrinkling of the face which is the reason the patient seeks improvement. In contrast to the oblique light produced by a photoflood lamp, a camera with an attached photoflash will produce flat light, which may completely eliminate all the shadows created by the subtle contours and wrinkling that are the result of aging.

Occasionally, a patient will be unable to have photographs completed until the day of surgery. In this case it is wise to obtain two series of preoperative photographs using two different cameras on two different rolls of film. It is recommended that these films be sent for processing at different times so that if the film is destroyed or lost, the surgeon will have a second available source. If any asymmetry or anatomical peculiarity is noted during the initial consultation or the photographic session, this should be discussed with the patient and carefully documented photographically.

Operative Preparation and Marking

The patient is advised to wash the face and shampoo the hair the night prior to surgery, as outlined in the preoperative instructions (Table 10.2). Preoperative oral medications are used as instructed per prescription. Makeup, particularly eyeliner, should be thoroughly removed by the patient on the evening prior to surgery. The patient should arrive at the surgical facility without jewelry and in appropriate clothing such as a blouse or shirt that buttons so that clothing need not be put on or taken off over the large, bulky head dressing. Jewelry, money, and articles of value should be left at home and the patient should take no tranquilizers or mood-altering substances prior to reading and completing the preoperative consent form. An interim history is completed to assure that there

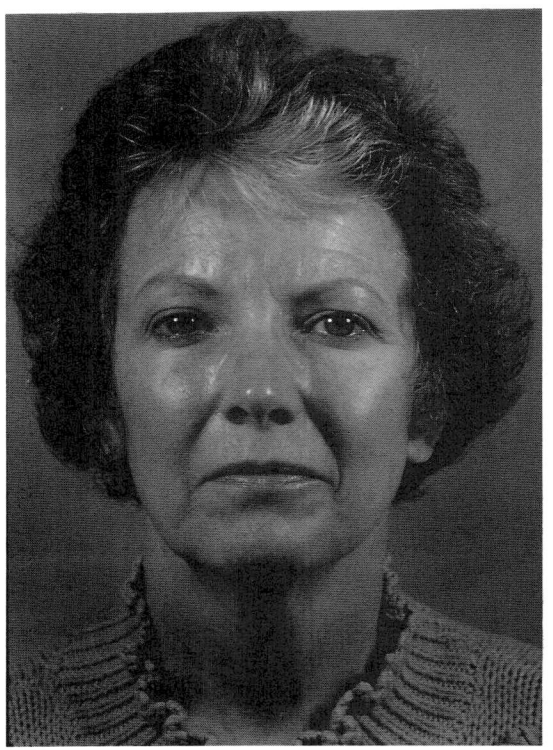

FIGURE 10.7. The preoperative photographs are taken with the patient in a neutral position, eyes in forward gaze with two photo floods using 250-watt Tungsten bulbs of 3200 Kelvin temperature on movable stands. A 100-mm macro lens is used on a 35-mm camera. This view is taken at four-foot, frontal view, vertical position of the camera body.

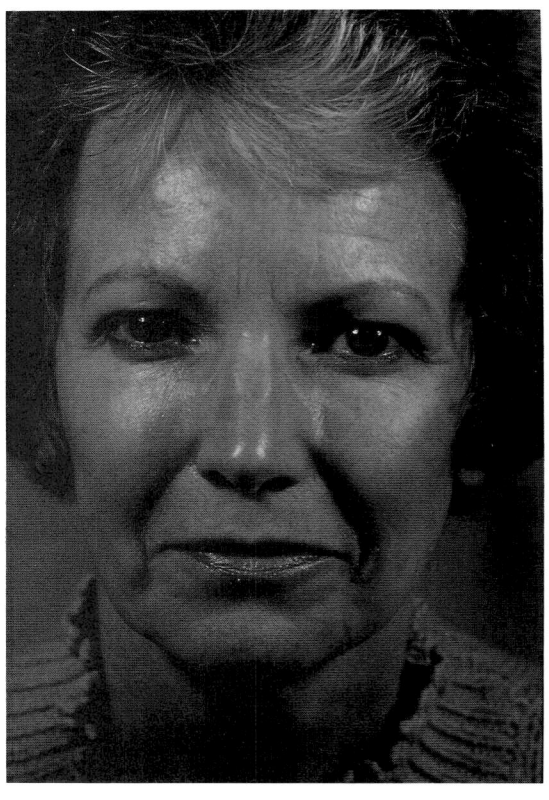

FIGURE 10.8. Three-foot, frontal view, vertical position.

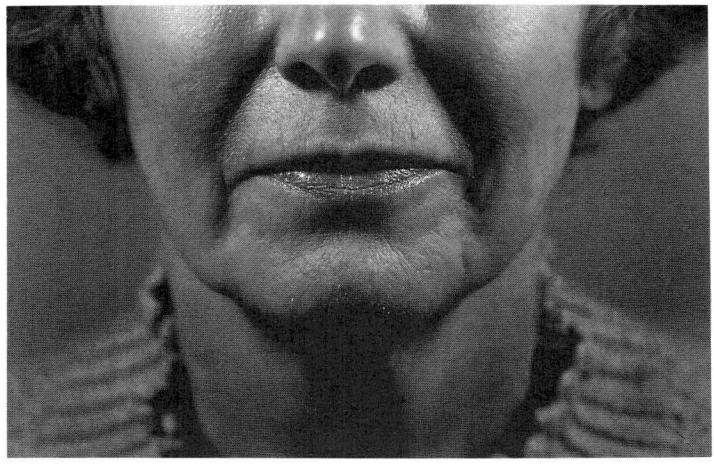

FIGURE 10.9. Two-and-a-half foot, frontal view, horizontal position. From tip of nose including the chin and neck.

10. Facelift Surgery

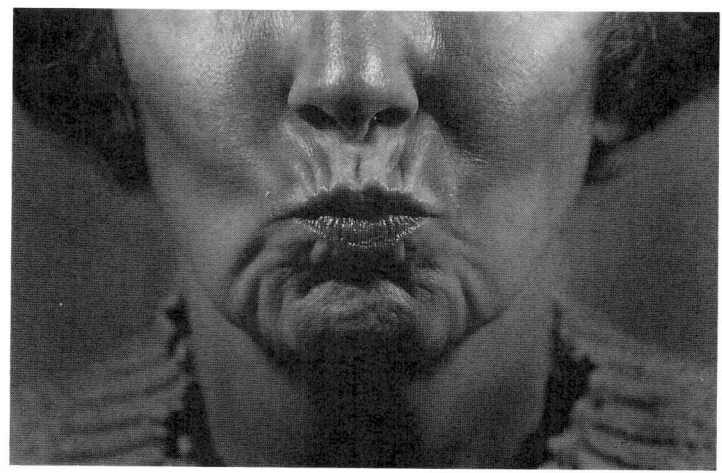

FIGURE 10.10. Two-and-a-half foot, frontal view, horizontal position with lips pursed.

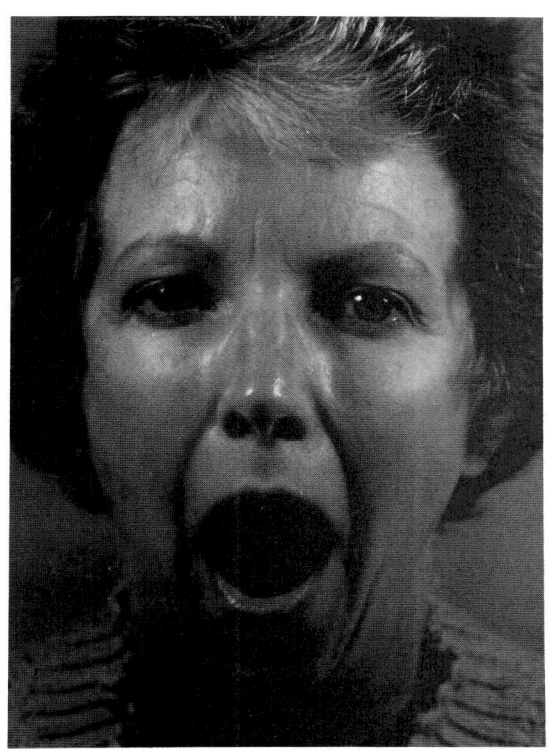

FIGURE 10.11. Four-foot, frontal view, vertical position, mouth open.

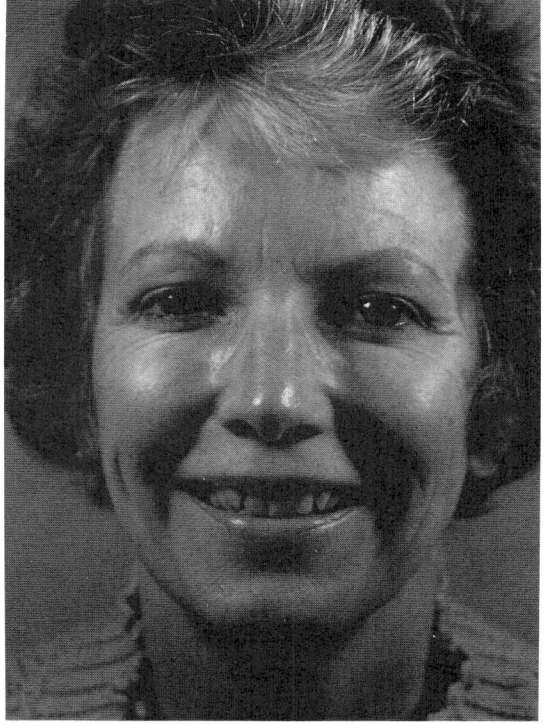

FIGURE 10.12. Four-foot, frontal view, vertical position, patient smiling.

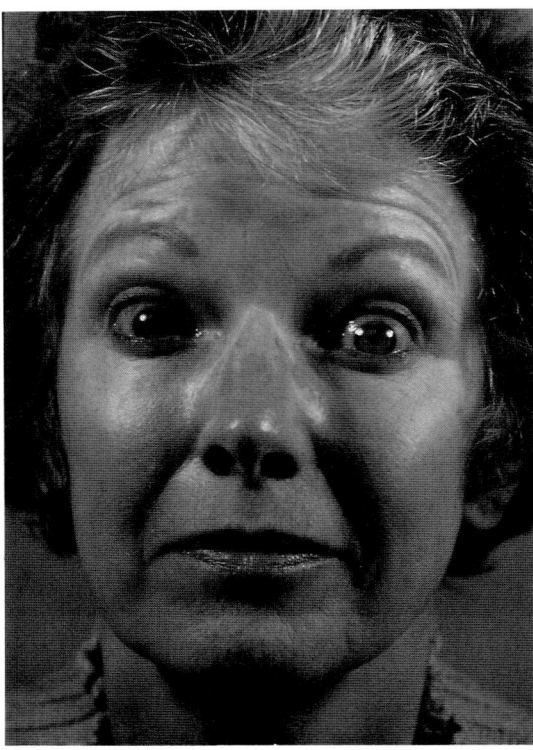

FIGURE 10.13. Four-foot, frontal view, vertical position, frontalis muscle contracted with eyebrows elevated.

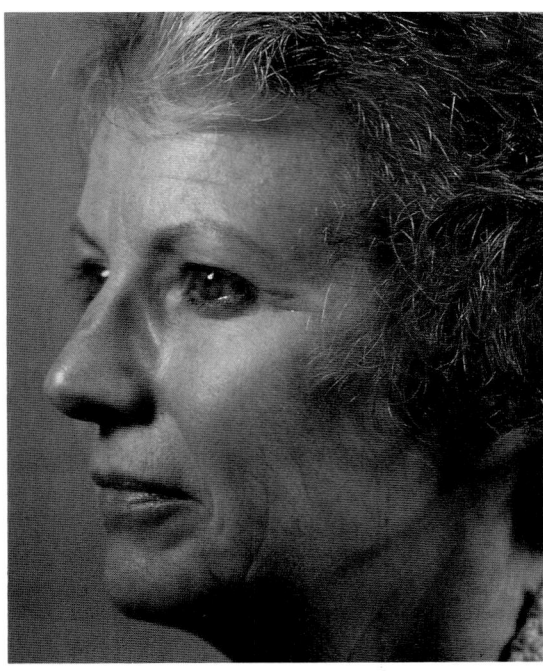

FIGURE 10.15. Three-foot, left oblique view, vertical position.

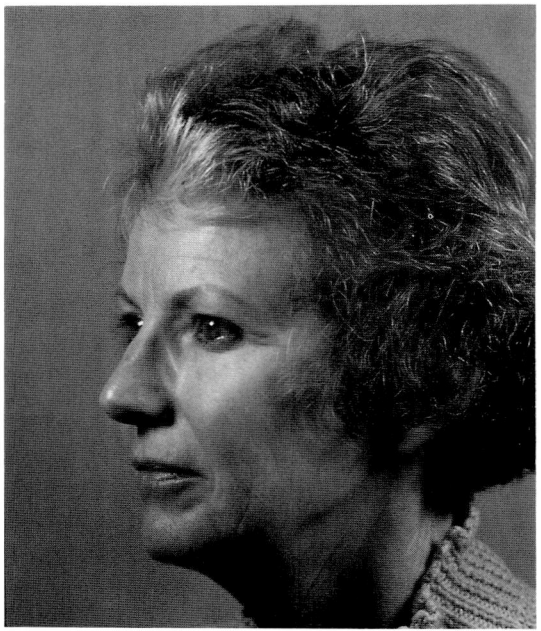

FIGURE 10.14. Four-foot, left oblique view, vertical position.

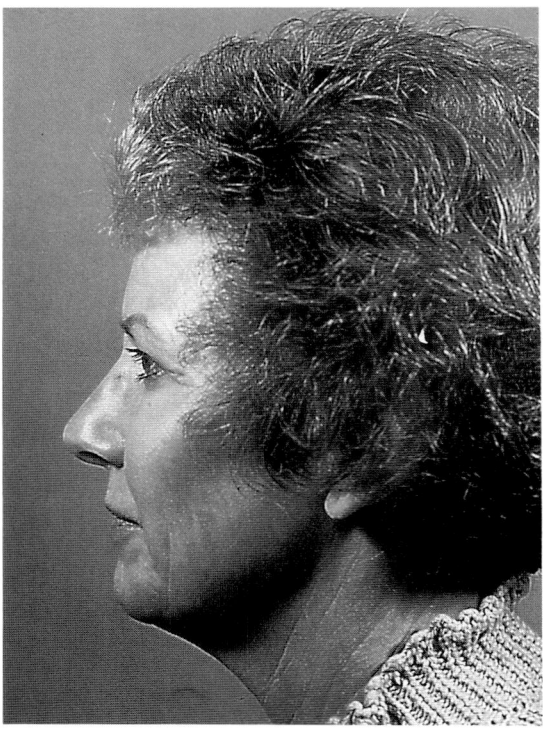

FIGURE 10.16. Four-foot, left lateral view, horizontal position.

10. Facelift Surgery

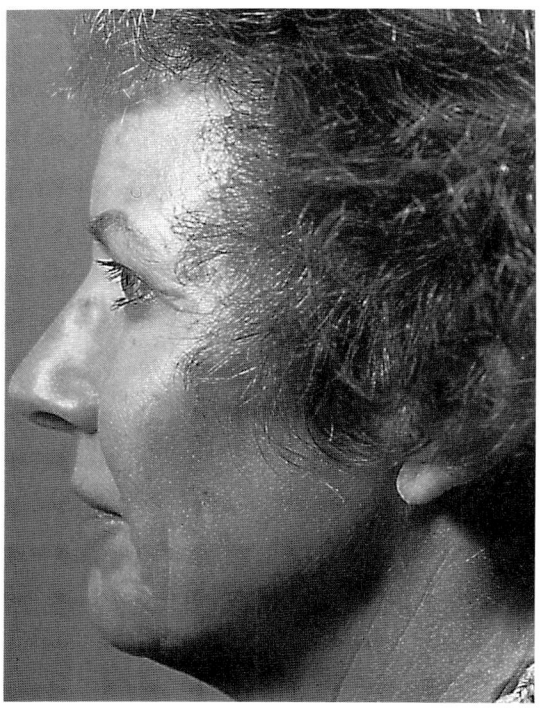

FIGURE 10.17. Three-foot, left lateral view, vertical position.

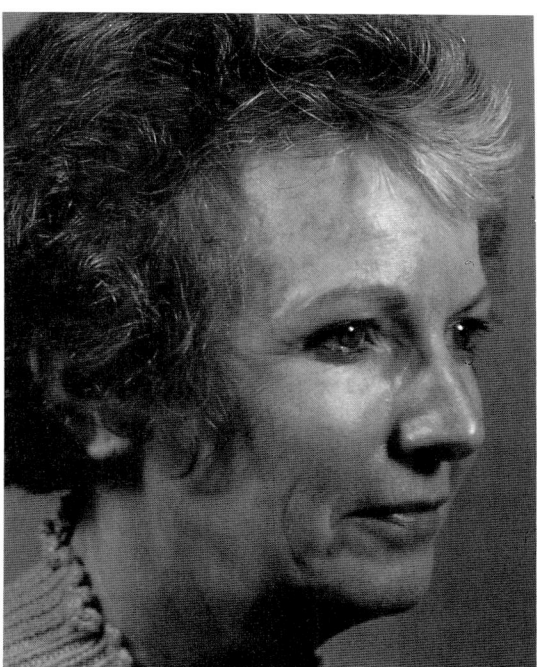

FIGURE 10.19. Four-foot, right lateral oblique view, vertical position.

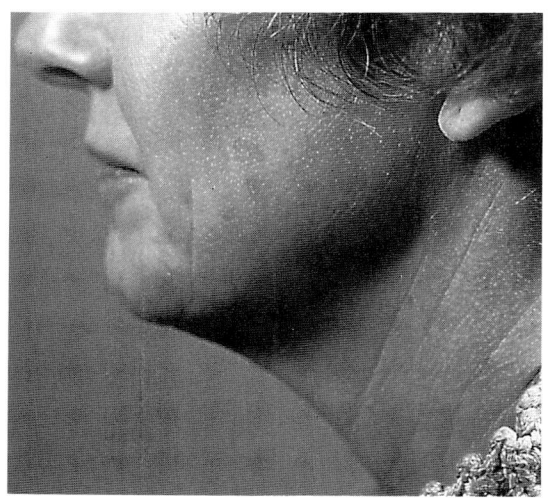

FIGURE 10.18. Two-and-a-half foot, left lateral view, horizontal position from tip of nose including chin and neck.

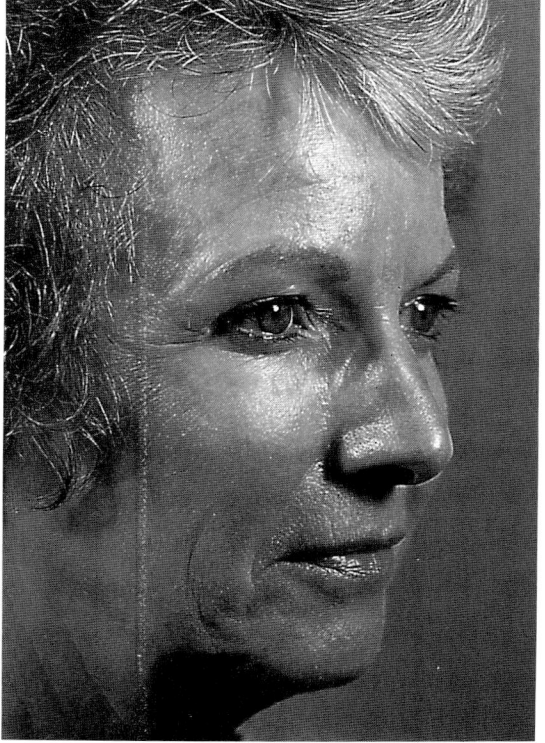

FIGURE 10.20. Three-foot, right oblique view, vertical position.

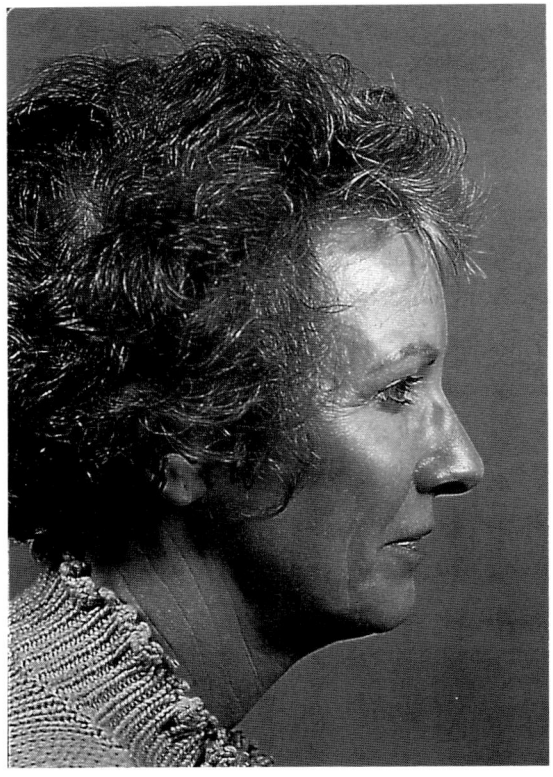

FIGURE 10.21. Four-foot, right lateral view, vertical position.

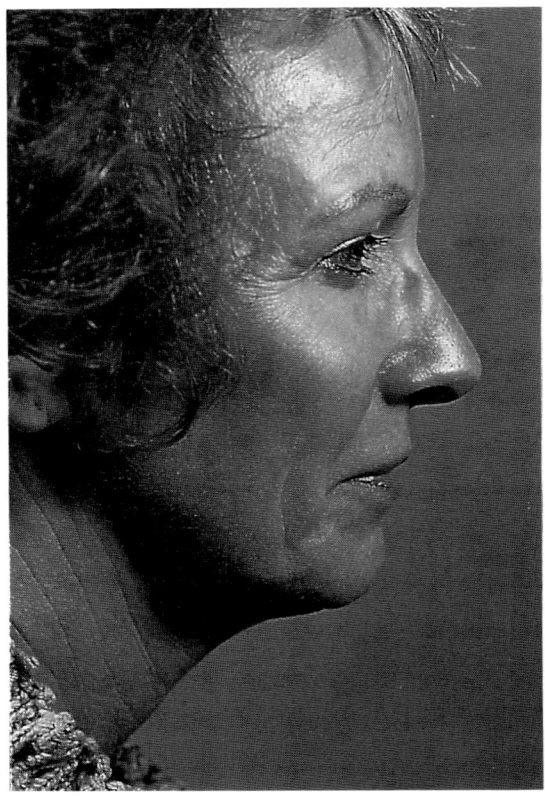

FIGURE 10.22. Three-foot, right lateral view, vertical position.

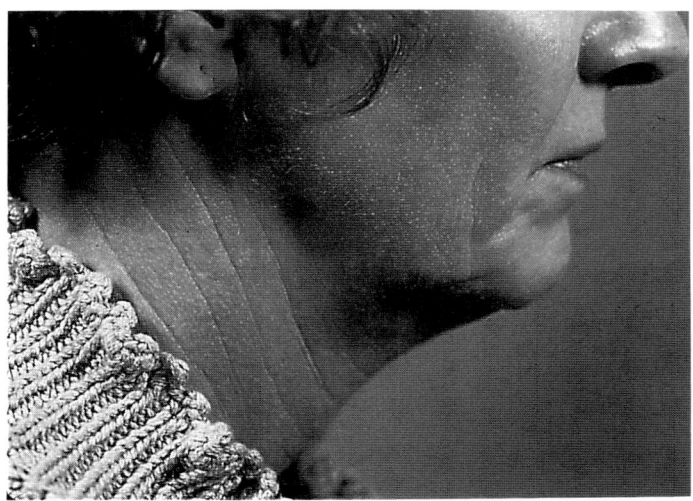

FIGURE 10.23. Two-and-a-half foot, right lateral view, vertical position from tip of nose, including chin and neck.

have been no changes in medications or the patient's physical status from the first history obtained at the original consultation (Table 10.5). The laboratory and physical examination are reviewed again with the anesthesiologist or anesthetist. Any final questions are reviewed with the patient and family at this time.

Planning and Marking

The patient is gowned, and the face, neck, and shoulders are prepped with Techni-Care surgical scrub for a minimum of 3 minutes. Using gloves, a ruler, and a gentian violet marking pen, all of which are sterile, the incision lines, extent of undermining, and areas of anterior cervical liposuction are outlined (Figures 10.24 through 10.29).

There are numerous methods to perform a facelift, with hundreds of variations in the incisions. For flap techniques there is the minilift, the short flap, the long flap, and the subperiosteal flap, to name just a few. The scope of this chapter is not to address all or even the major types just mentioned; each reader should review the literature and choose the method that best suits his or her needs. The following describes the method that we have employed over the past 20 years, a method that provides safety with effective, long-lasting results.

This method may be called the *modified Webster short flap technique.* Webster has written and lectured extensively on the short flap technique.[16-24] Webster performed a series of cases on which one side of the face was undermined extensively using the long flap technique and the opposite side was undermined more conservatively to a level no greater than 5 cm from the preauricular incision line. Evaluation revealed that there was no greater improvement in long-term effects on the side that was extensively undermined. Thus the long flap that produced the larger sheet of favorable fibrosis did not provide any advantage.[25] Extensive undermining was performed in which

TABLE 10.5. Interim medical history.

Interim medical history

Please answer the following questions and explain any YES responses:

YES	NO	
_____	_____	Have you had any recent change in your general health? Explain
_____	_____	Have you had any recent localized infection? Explain
_____	_____	Do you have any known drug allergies? Explain
		Have you recently had any of the following:
_____	_____	Diagnosed medical condition
_____	_____	High blood pressure
_____	_____	Diabetes
_____	_____	Heart condition
_____	_____	Sugar in urine
_____	_____	Accutane treatment for acne Explain
_____	_____	Are you taking any medications at the present time? (Please include those medications prescribed for you by Dr. Alt.) If so, please list: _____ _____ .

Address and phone number where you may be reached postoperatively:
_____
_____
_____

Date: _____ _____
               Signature

1/94

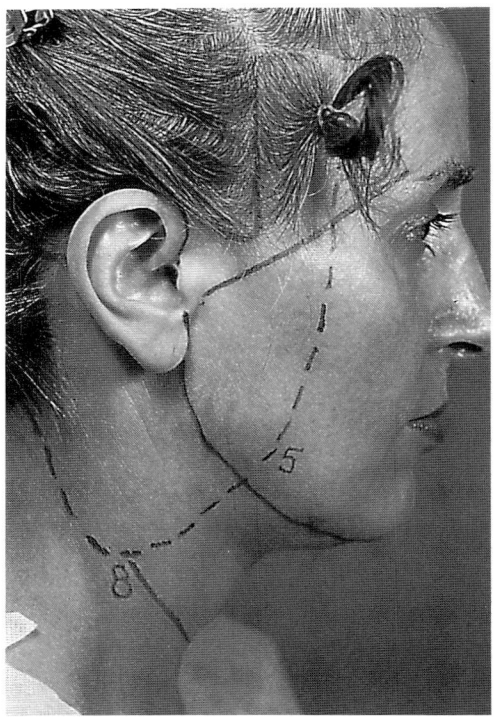

FIGURE 10.24. The extent of undermining is noted by the broken line, which is measured from the inferior border of the lobule to the mandibular ramus. This length is 5 cm. The inferior border of the lateral cervical flap is measured from the inferior border of the lobule to the midbelly of the sternocleidomastoid muscle and measures 8 cm.

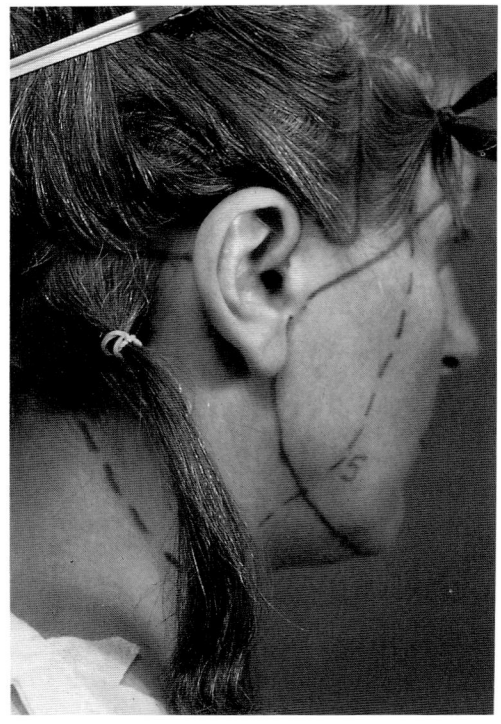

FIGURE 10.25. The flap is extended posteriorly 7 to 8 cm from the posterior border of the auricle. The inferior border of the mandibular ramus is marked as the superior limitation of the cervical liposuction.

the extent of the flap was carried to the lateral canthus, to the malar prominence, to the buccolabial fold, to the mental foramen, and into the neck at the level of the thyroid cartilage. Limited undermining was defined as dissection that was carried to one-half the distance. Patients were randomly selected for a short flap procedure or a long flap procedure or a procedure that combined a long flap on one side with a short flap on the opposite side. All patients had SMAS plication performed. Measurement of the excised tissue by weight showed that only 15% more skin was removed when extensive undermining was employed. Of greatest importance was that 80% of the complications occurred on the extensively undermined side. He also concluded that there was no significant difference between the aesthetic results of the long flap as compared with the short flap.

Plication vs. Imbrication of SMAS

The earliest known use of buried suspensory sutures was reported by Aufricht in 1961.[25] Mitz and Peyronie described the superficial musculoaponeurotic system (SMAS), which they believe to be responsible for the long-term effects of these suspension sutures.[26] The surgeon has two methods in which the SMAS can be advanced. Plication is the technique in which the SMAS is folded upon itself and fixed by buried sutures. Imbrication is the method in which the SMAS is undermined, advanced over the underlying tissues with the excess being trimmed and the edge fixed with the buried sutures. Webster has shown that imbrication has no advantage over plication.[19,23] Since imbrication requires more time and is more prone to postoperative complications, it is reasonable for the surgeon to use plication. The SMAS

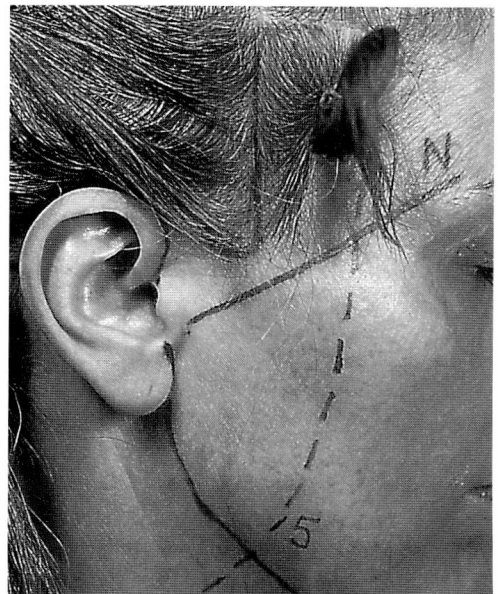

FIGURE 10.26. The superior portion of the temporal incision is horizontal to the temporal peak of scalp hair and measures 2 to 3 cm. The vertical portion is placed at midpoint or at the frontal two-thirds of the temporal tuft including the sideburn. The undermining is extended two-thirds of the distance from the anterior border of the pinna to the lateral portion of the orbital rim. The straight line from the inferior border of the tragus to the lateral aspect of the eyebrow labeled *N* is the approximate course of the temporal branch of the facial nerve.

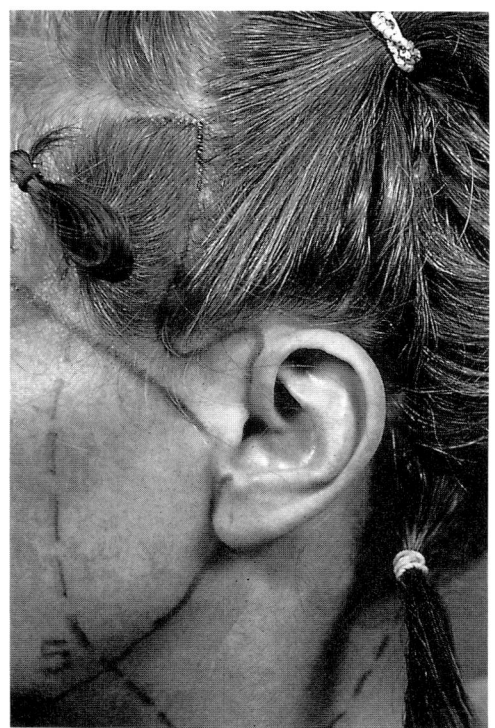

FIGURE 10.27. The inferior portion of the temporal incision curves around the inferior border of the sideburn and traverses superiorly and posteriorly over the glabrous skin for approximately 2 cm. It then curves downward and follows the anterior border of the auricle. Note that the hair has been combed and secured with rubber bands to eliminate an obstruction in the operative site.

plication provides improved long-term effects. In a study in which only one side of the face received SMAS plication, evaluation more than 10 years later showed that the improvement was more evident on the side that received the SMAS suspension.[22,23] Correction of the platysmal banding was improved and the preservation of the cervicomental angle was retained, as was improvement in the jowl on the plicated side.

Marking

The extent of undermining is outlined by measuring 5 cm from the lobule to the mid-ramus of the mandible and a second segment of 7 to 8 cm from the lobule to the mid-portion of the belly of the sternocleidomastoid muscle (Figures 10.24, 10.25, and 10.26). The anterior border of the undermining over the zygomatic process is two-thirds of the distance of a line measured from the anterior border of the pinna to the lateral aspect of the orbital rim (Figures 10.24, 10.25, and 10.26). A curved line connects these 3 points from the sternocleidomastoid muscle to the mandibular ramus and the zygomatic arch. Superior to this, the anterior border of the flap follows a vertical line from the zygomatic arch to a point level with the temporal peak of the scalp hair (Figures 10.26 and 10.27). The posterior cervical portion of the flap is bounded by a curved line running from the mid-portion of the sternocleidomastoid muscle to the posterior extent of the horizontal retroauricular incision line (Figures 10.24, 10.25, and 10.28).

The incision line begins with a 2 to 3 cm horizontal segment at the level of the temporal

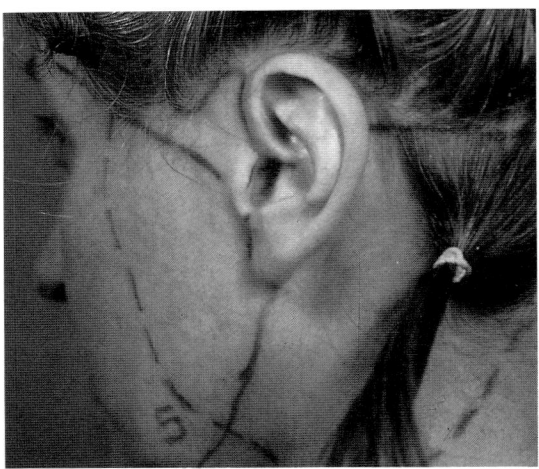 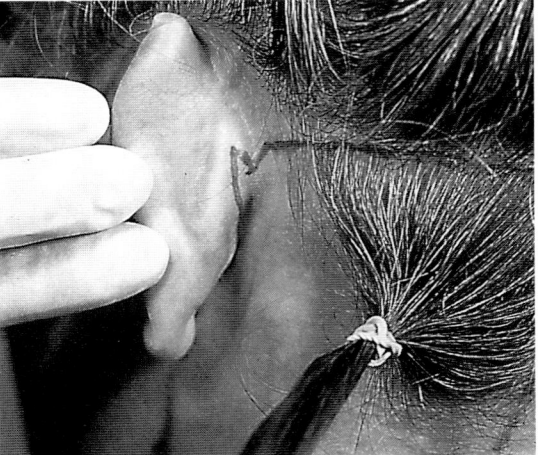

FIGURE 10.28. The postauricular incision measures 7 to 8 cm. and is 1 cm above the level of the external auditory meatus. The extreme posterior portion curves to form a 90° angle to allow correction for a dog-ear defect.

FIGURE 10.29. The postauricular incision is placed three to 5 mm onto the posterior surface of the cartilaginous external ear. A V-shaped incision is placed with the inferior position at the postauricular sulcus to eliminate a bridging scar as normal contraction occurs.

peak (Figure 10.26). At its posterior extent, the incision turns 90° and descends vertically through the temporal hair to include the posterior one-half to two-thirds of the temporal hair (Figures 10.26 and 10.27). As the incision reaches the inferior border of the temporal hair, it curves posteriorly to encompass all the hair and then traverses posteriorly and superiorly at a 45° angle, then curves approximately 165° and continues parallel to the anterior border of the pinna (Figures 10.26 and 10.27). When the incision reaches the superior border of the tragus, it takes a 90° angle posteriorly for several millimeters until it is posterior to the crest of the tragus. A second 90° angle is taken with the incision traversing inferiorly at the posterior border of the crest of the tragus, so that the incision line will be hidden. When the inferior border of the tragus is reached, the incision takes a 90° angle anteriorly until the anterior border of the lobule is reached. The incision then takes another 90° turn and traverses inferiorly in the crease created by the anterior border of the lobule. It curves around the inferior border of the lobule and continues in the crease created by the posterior border of the lobule. When the superior limit of the lobule is reached, the incision is displaced 3 to 5 mm onto the pinna until it reaches 1 cm above the superior border of the external auditory meatus (Figures 10.28 and 10.29). The incision then makes a 45° turn and traverses inferiorly and posteriorly to the base of the retroauricular sulcus. It then turns 45° to create a V over the sulcus with the posterior limb equaling the anterior limb (Figure 10.29). A 135° angle is created as the incision traverses posteriorly in a horizontal fashion for 6 to 8 cm, depending upon the size of the patient. The posterior portion of the horizontal limb is completed by curving the incision downward at a 90° angle until the end of the excision is approximately 2 cm below the level of the horizontal limb (Figures 10.28 and 10.29). A precautionary line is drawn from the inferior border of the tragus to the lateral aspect of the eyebrow to denote the approximate course of the temporal branch of the facial nerve (Figure 10.26). Another line is drawn on the inferior border of the mandibular ramus to denote the superior aspect of the anterior cervical liposuction. If fat is removed superior to this line, a ridge may be formed when the flap is redraped posteriorly and superiorly at the conclusion of the procedure (Figure 10.24, 10.25 and 10.26). Another line is drawn from the most inferior portion of the proposed flap as it overlies the belly of the sternocleidomastoid to the thyroid cartilage or the area inferior to this site where the anterior cervical skin and subcutaneous fat attains its thinnest measurement (Figure 10.24). This represents the inferior border of the cervical liposuction.

The hair of the temporal tuft is trimmed to 1 cm wide along the vertical and horizontal limbs of the temporal incision. Rubber bands are placed on the hair to avoid obstruction of the site during the surgery (Figures 10.24 through 10.29). The hair is trimmed slightly below and to 1 cm above the horizontal incision of the postauricular site (Figures 10.28 and 10.29). Pictures of the preoperative marking are taken, and the patient is then accompanied to the operative suite, where an intravenous line containing lactated Ringer's solution is placed for the administration of the preoperative, intraoperative, and postoperative medications. The table is draped so that both the headrest and entire surface of the upper half of the table is covered with sterile drapes. The patient is positioned on the table, and a full body drape is placed from the neck downward. A gas-sterilized nasal cannula is positioned and anchored with sterile tape to the forehead to provide a continuous flow of nasal oxygen during the procedure (Figure 10.30).

Marking a Pretragal Incision

The pretragal incision is commonly used with two conditions. First, males will usually obtain better results, because if the posttragal incision is used, advancement of the flap will displace whisker-bearing skin onto the anterior portion of the helix and tragus. Although this provides for better camouflage of the postoperative scar, male skin is thicker than female skin and is more difficult to redrape over the subtle contours of the tragal area. Also, whisker hair will grow on the tragus, which requires daily shaving or removal with electrolysis. Second, females with a protruding tragus that is angled greater than 45° from the plane of the face will have better results if the pretragal incision is employed. When the angle of the tragus protrudes to such a great extent, redraping of the preauricular skin is difficult.

In males the incision is placed approximately 1 cm anterior to the helix and passes vertically through the depression anterior to the tragus. The incision then passes in the crease on the anterior border of the lobule. By avoiding pressure on the skin edge, the incision can heal with an inconspicuous scar.

Intravenous Sedation

The facelift procedure can be adequately performed using general anesthesia, intravenous sedation, or local anesthesia alone. We prefer to avoid general anesthesia because of its slightly increased risk and the inconvenience of the endotracheal tube in the operative site. Local anesthesia alone can be used with oral or intramuscular sedatives; however, most patients prefer to be heavily sedated or unconscious during the procedure.

We prefer intravenous sedation because of its

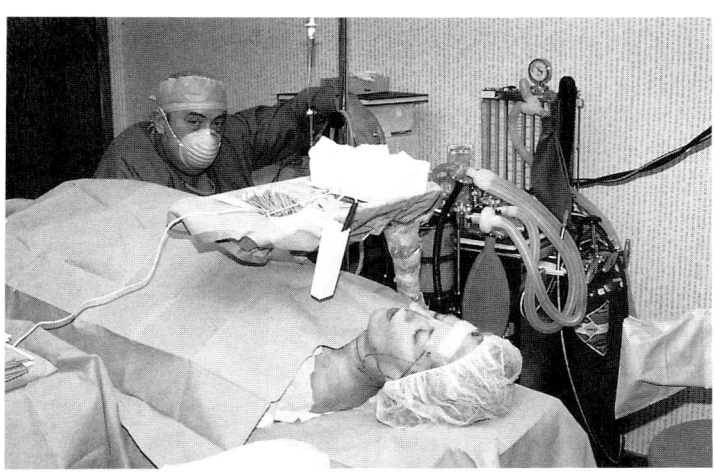

FIGURE 10.30. The patient is monitored with a pulse oximeter, an automatic blood pressure cuff, and an EKG. Intravenous sedation is used in combination with local anesthesia. A sterilized nasal cannula is used to continuously deliver oxygen. An emergency cart with medications, endotracheal tubes, an anesthesia machine, and a cardiac defibrillator are in the room.

safety, effectiveness, and decreased likelihood of postoperative nausea. As a rule, patients recover more rapidly and have less nausea from intravenous sedation as compared to general anesthesia. Sedation is initially achieved by the administration of 1 to 2 mg of midazolam hydrochloride and 50 micrograms of fentanyl citrate. The objective is to provide adequate sedation so that the patient does not recall the administration of the local anesthetic or any part of the surgical procedure. Once the local anesthesia has been infiltrated, the level of sedation may be decreased until the anesthesia is infiltrated on the second side. It is believed that many patients experience retrograde amnesia and, although they will sometimes talk during the procedure, most will not recall any of the events. Since this level of sedation does not paralyze the diaphragm or the accessory muscles of the thoracic cage, it is not necessary to assist the patient's breathing with an anesthesia machine. During the procedure the patient is monitored with a pulse oximeter, automatic blood pressure cuff, and cardiac monitor. An emergency cart is available, as are endotracheal tubes, a standard anesthesia machine, and a defibrillator.

Local Anesthesia

The areas of liposuction and the regions where the flaps will be created are infiltrated using Xylocaine® with epinephrine. Two solutions are used. A 1% solution of Xylocaine (10 mg/mL) with epinephrine 1:100,000 buffered with 8.4% sodium bicarbonate using a 10:1 dilution is administered with a 10 cc control syringe through a 25-gauge 1½-inch needle to the proposed incision lines. All other areas are anesthetized using 0.5% Xylocaine (5 mg/mL) with epinephrine 1:200,000 in a 10 cc control syringe with a 22-gauge 3½-inch spinal needle.

The anesthesia is begun in the anterior cervical area. A small submental incision is made after infiltrating the site with the 1% Xylocaine solution. The 0.5% solution is administered through this incision and from retrolobular incisions over the area of anticipated liposuction (Figure 10.31). The lines of incision are then infiltrated, using the 1% Xylocaine solution (Figures 10.32 and 10.33). Returning to the 0.5% Xylocaine, the postauricular and lateral cervical areas are infiltrated, followed by the administration of the anesthesia to the flap in the mandibular, preauricular, and temporal areas (Figure 10.34). Since the entire anterior cervical region is suctioned as a single segment, anesthesia must be administered to both the right and left sides. Because a considerable amount of time will elapse from the creation of the first flap on the right side to the flap on the second side, anesthesia is administered only to the right side of the face. The anesthesia is administered in the same sequence that the surgery will be performed. The liposuction of the anterior cervical region will commence 20 minutes after the area has been anesthetized.

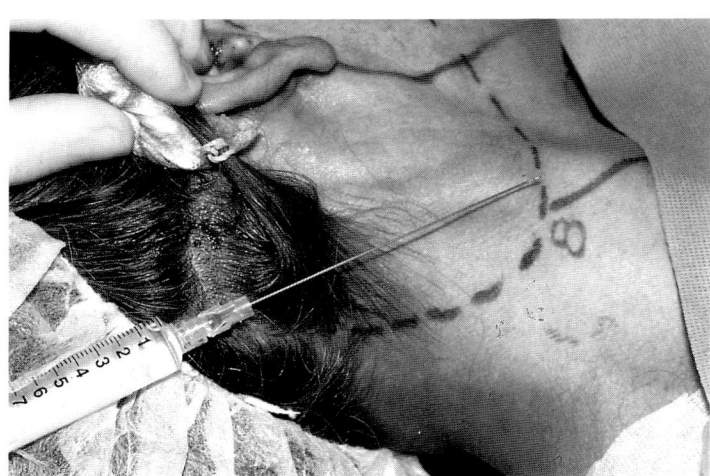

FIGURE 10.31. The flaps and liposuction sites are infiltrated using a 0.5% Xylocaine (5 mg per mL) with epinephrine 1:200,000, using a 22-gauge 3½-in. spinal needle on a 10-cc control syringe.

10. Facelift Surgery

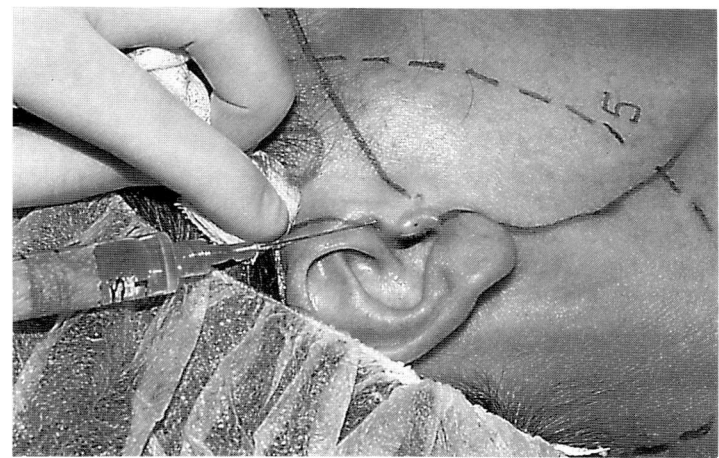

FIGURE 10.32. The incision lines are infiltrated with 1% Xylocaine (10 mg per mL) with epinephrine 1:100,000 buffered with an 8.4% sodium bicarbonate solution using a 10:1 dilution.

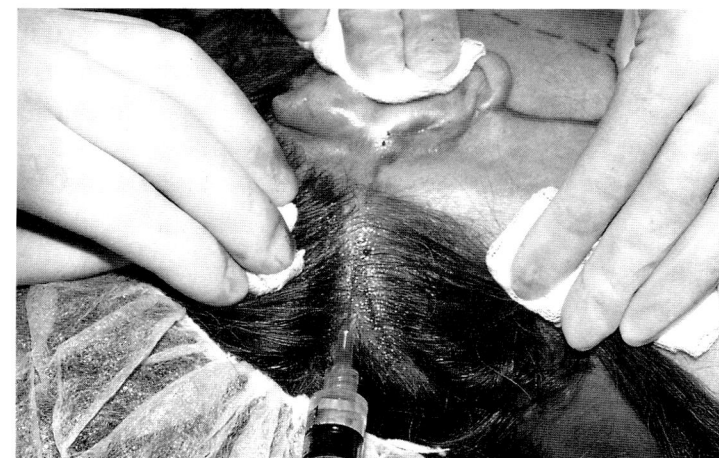

FIGURE 10.33. All incision lines are infiltrated using the 1% Xylocaine solution on a 5-cc syringe equipped with a 1½-in. 25-gauge needle.

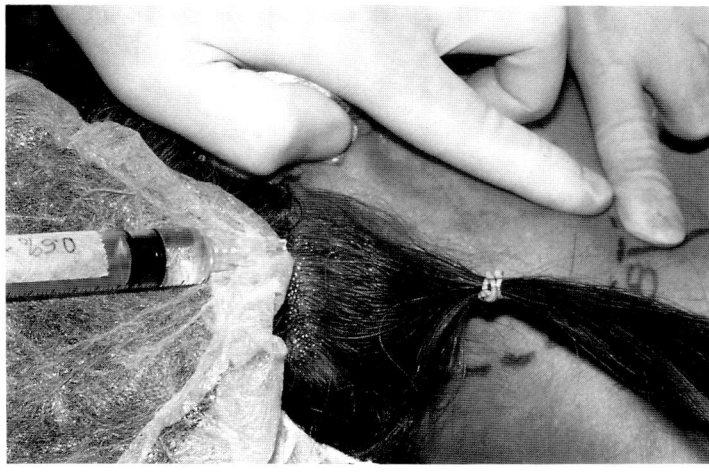

FIGURE 10.34. The 3½-in. 22-gauge spinal needle is very effective in allowing dispersion of anesthesia over a large field. The needle is introduced within the hairline and at the submental incision used for liposuction. This avoids puncture wounds through the skin of the flap.

Cervical Liposuction

The anterior cervical region is suctioned using a 15 cm length flat spatula cannula of 4 mm diameter with a single orifice. A standard liposuction machine is employed, using full negative pressure. The orifice of the cannula is directed away from the skin surface. If only a small area of fat is to be removed in the immediate submental area, a single submental incision will be adequate (Figures 10.35 and 10.36). If the patient has subcutaneous fat over the entire anterior cervical region, additional sites of entry in the postauricular area at the level of the lobule are made. Undermining through the thick fibrous tissue anterior and inferior to the lobular incisions is accomplished with a Ragnell scissors (Figure 10.37). Once the entire flap of skin has been elevated with the 4 mm cannula, a larger 6 mm spatula with a single orifice may be introduced to remove any remaining amounts of fat from the platysma (Figure 10.38). The introduction of this larger cannula is difficult at the onset of the liposuction, but the smaller 4 mm cannula can be introduced with ease.

If liposuction of the jowl is necessary, this can be done using a 3 mm cannula with a single small orifice following the creation of the flap. When the standard suction machine is used at full negative pressure of 27 to 28 inches of mercury, the small orifice is necessary to eliminate excessive extraction of fat over the jowl. An alternative method would be to use syringe-

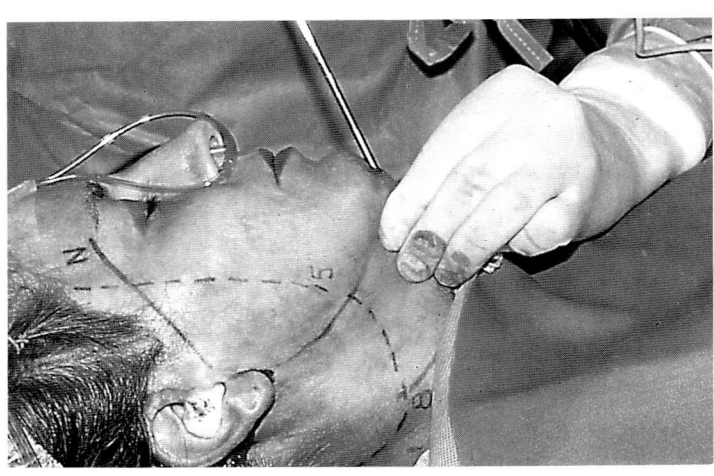

FIGURE 10.35. A 4-mm spatula cannula is introduced through the submental incision with the orifice facing away from the skin. The major portion of the fat is removed with this cannula in the entire anterior cervical region.

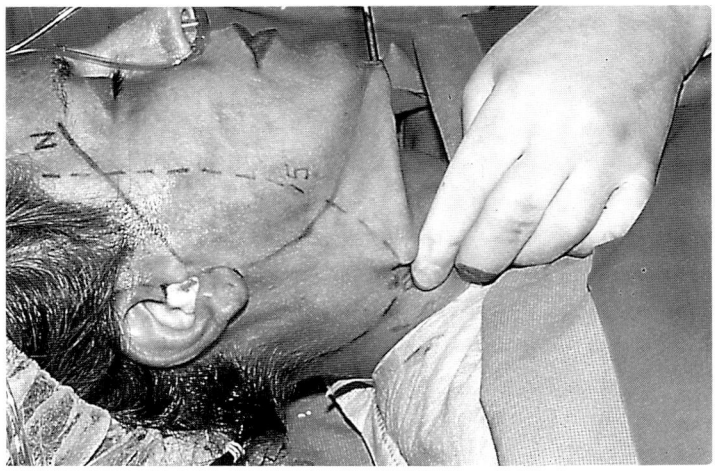

FIGURE 10.36. The 4-mm cannula can be easily introduced over the entire expanse of the anterior cervical region. Virtually all of the fat is removed to improve the final results of the anterior neck and the cervicomental angle.

assisted liposuction. Usually only a very small amount of fat extraction is necessary over the jowl and will often be less than 1 cc. Rapid extraction of fat using a larger cannula can result in formation of ridges in the area of the jowl. This defect is exceedingly difficult to correct postoperatively and should be avoided by careful intraoperative procedures.

Flap Creation

Retroauricular Flap

The retroauricular flap is the next area of attention. The lobule of the ear is grasped, and a small scratch is made in the inferior border of the lobule to identify its location when it is attached later to the redraped skin. An incision is made with a number 15 blade along the inferior and posterior border of the lobule. The incision then leaves the postauricular sulcus and rises to the level of 3 to 5 mm on the posterior portion of the auricle, to a level 1 cm above the superior border of the external auditory meatus (Figure 10.39). At this point the skin is notched in a V fashion over the sulcus with the apex of the V in the sulcus (Figure 10.40). This will minimize the likelihood of an elevated banded scar as the tissue contracts across this concave surface during normal healing (Figure 10.41).

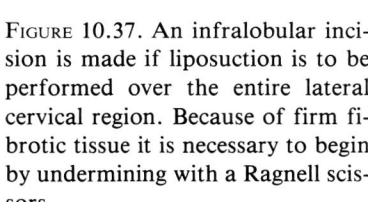
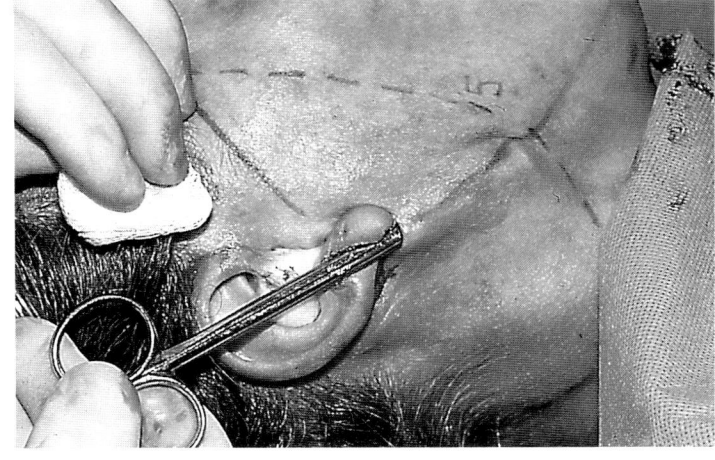

FIGURE 10.37. An infralobular incision is made if liposuction is to be performed over the entire lateral cervical region. Because of firm fibrotic tissue it is necessary to begin by undermining with a Ragnell scissors.

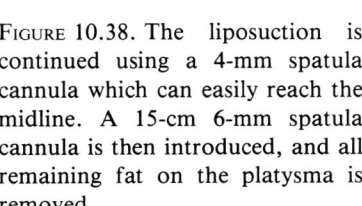
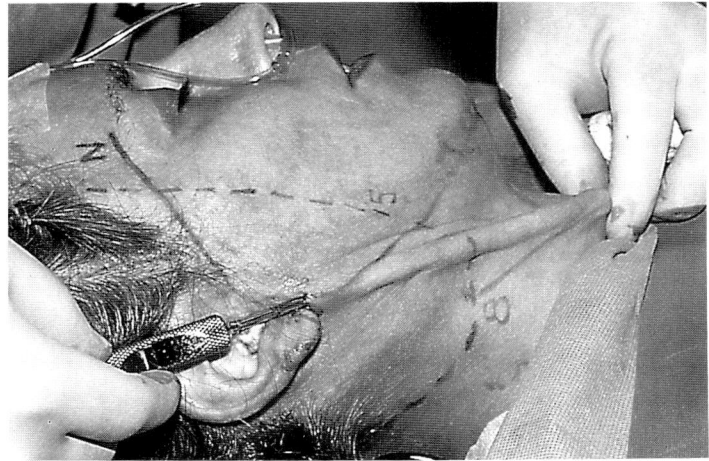

FIGURE 10.38. The liposuction is continued using a 4-mm spatula cannula which can easily reach the midline. A 15-cm 6-mm spatula cannula is then introduced, and all remaining fat on the platysma is removed.

The incision is then continued with the use of a number 10 blade in a horizontal fashion posteriorly for 7 to 8 cm and then curved downward, until it reaches a vertical position approximately 2 cm below the horizontal limb (Figure 10.42). This incision is made perpendicular to the skin, not parallel to the hair follicles, to increase the number of hairs that can potentially grow through the resulting scar. The depth of this incision is through the subcutaneous fat that is below the hair follicles but above the fascial plane of the temporoparietalis and occipitalis muscles. If any significant bleeding occurs, it should be cauterized, since a small arteriole can cause significant bleeding during the ensuing creation of a flap. Thirty cc of normal saline are instilled with a 25-gauge spinal needle to the area of the retroauricular flap, paying particular attention to that region over the mastoid area and the sternocleidomastoid muscle (Figure 10.43). This creates a plane of dissection, which will facilitate the creation of the flap. Asken prefers chilled dilute Xylocaine with epinephrine, noting that the decreased temperature will increase vasoconstriction.[27].

While an assistant holds the skin under tension below the inferior extent of the flap, the surgeon grasps the cut edge with a forceps and, with a 7-inch Gorney straight facelift scissors or a 7½-inch Gorney-Freeman straight facelift scissors begins the undermining with sharp dissection for the first 1 to 2 cm. Once the flap is raised to this extent, it can be quickly com-

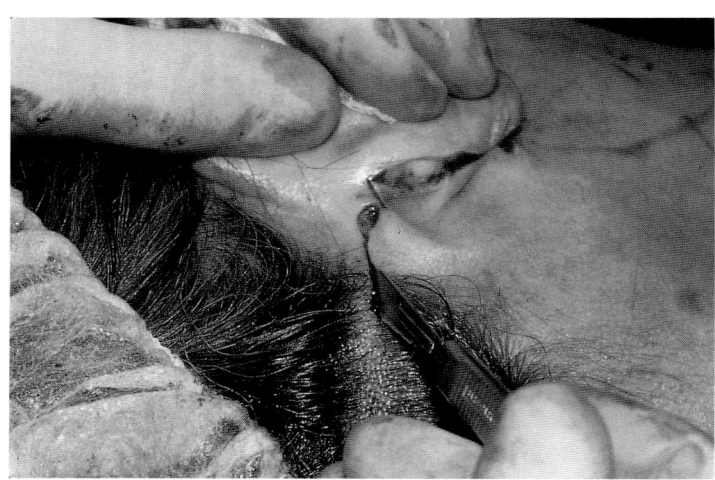

FIGURE 10.39. The vertical portion of the retroauricular incision is placed 3 to 5 mm anterior to the retroauricular sulcus as it traverses over the cartilage of the external ear. When the incision reaches the level of the posterior portion of the lobule, it is placed into the postauricular sulcus.

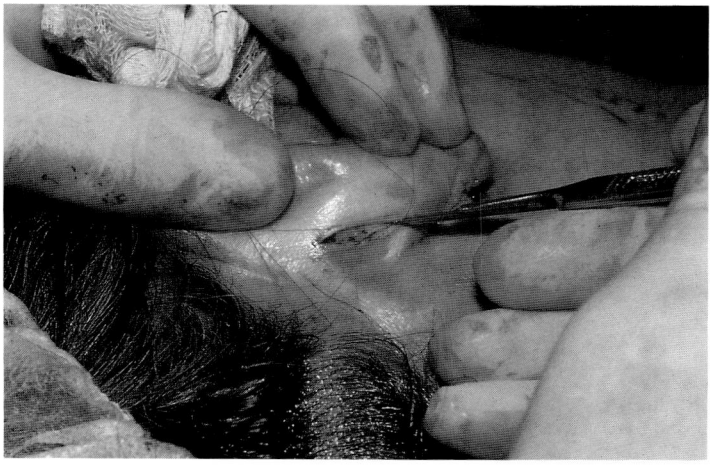

FIGURE 10.40. A V incision is placed at the retroauricular sulcus to diminish the likelihood of an elevated band of scar, which can occur if a straight line scar passes over a depression.

10. Facelift Surgery

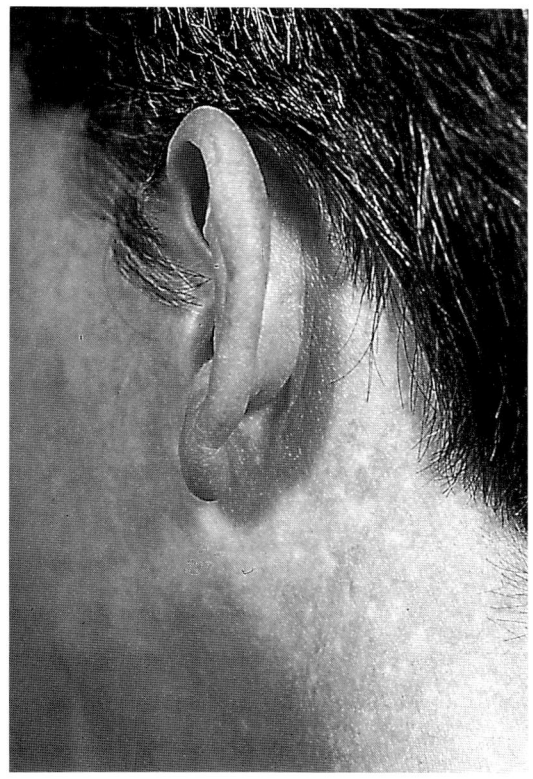

FIGURE 10.41. If an incision is made across the retroauricular sulcus using a broken line, a contracted elevated scar will not be produced, resulting in a natural appearing retroauricular sulcus.

pleted by opening the scissors slightly and advancing the scissors in the subcutaneous fatty plane to the inferior extent of the proposed undermining (Figure 10.44). The scissors may have to be opened and closed at the far extent of the flap, since mere advancement of the open scissors is generally not possible. This allows for a very rapid elevation of the flap, which can usually be completed in less than 2 minutes. Care should be taken over the sternocleidomastoid muscle to avoid injury to the great auricular nerve which lies superficial to the belly of this muscle, where it is posterior and parallel to the external jugular vein. It is in this area where the infiltration with the saline will be particularly advantageous to the surgeon. This area will usually bleed temporarily. The placement of 3 gauze pads into the site will act as a tamponade facilitating coagulation of the vessels while the preauricular flap is created (Figure 10.45).

Temporal Flap

The surgeon's attention is now focused on the temporal area, where the horizontal incision is made in the temporal hair (Figure 10.46). The incision then makes a right angle at its posterior end and is carried vertically through the middle of the preauricular tuft of hair. The horizontal incision is made perpendicular to the skin to cut across hair shafts, thereby incorporating more hairs that may grow through the scar. The

FIGURE 10.42. The horizontal segment of the retroauricular incision is placed approximately 1 cm superior to the level of the superior aspect of the external auditory meatus. It travels posteriorly a total of 7 to 8 cm. At its posterior segment, a curve of 90° is made for approximately 2 cm vertically to allow for correction of the dog-ear that will result from the rotation of the flap.

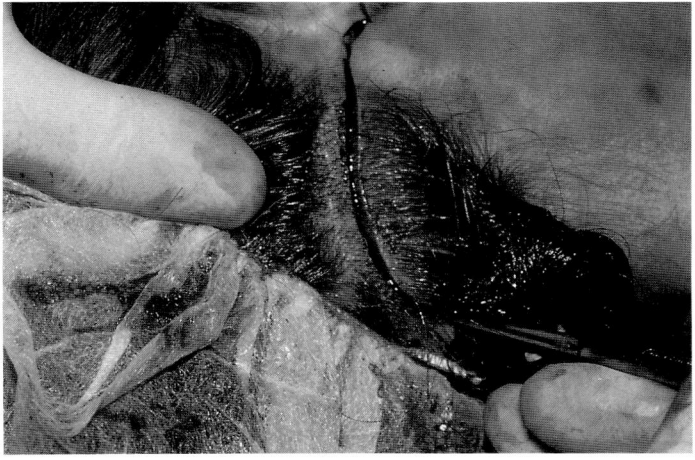

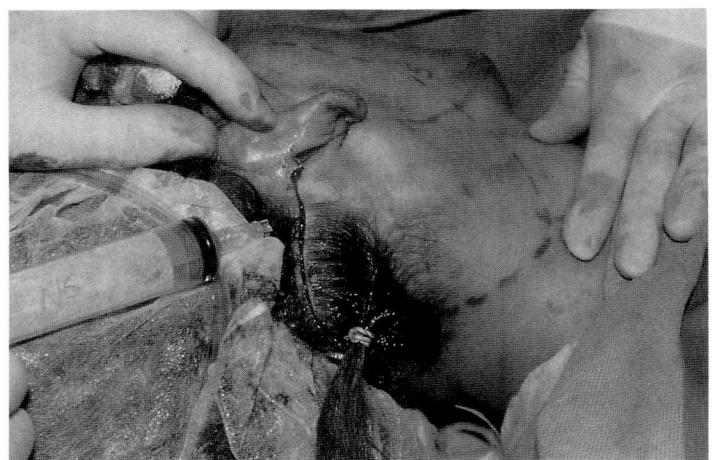

FIGURE 10.43. Thirty cc of normal saline is infiltrated over the postauricular flap to widen the plane of dissection. Particular attention should be focused on the mastoid process and the belly of the sternocleidomastoid over which more of the saline is placed since these areas are fibrotic and several important nerves traverse the body of the sternocleidomastoid muscle.

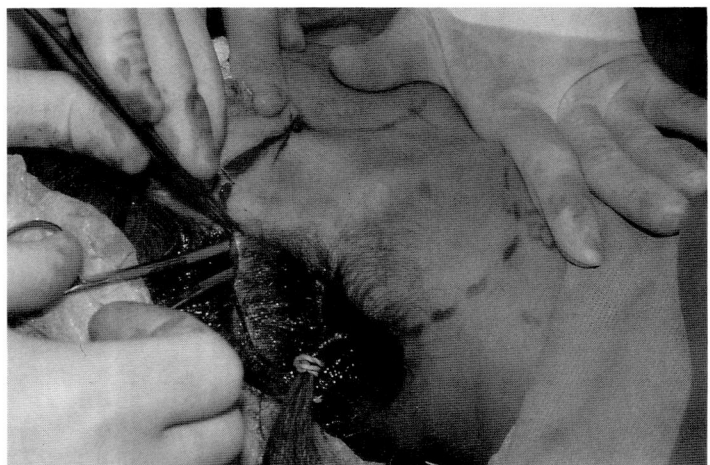

FIGURE 10.44. A Gorney–Freeman straight facelift scissors is used for the sharp dissection of the postauricular and lateral cervical flaps. The dissection must be below the level of the hair follicles and can proceed rapidly when proper tension is placed at the inferior border of the flap by the surgical assistant. The scissors are held open approximately 1½ cm while the scissors are advanced without closing the jaws. This will allow for very rapid and efficient dissection.

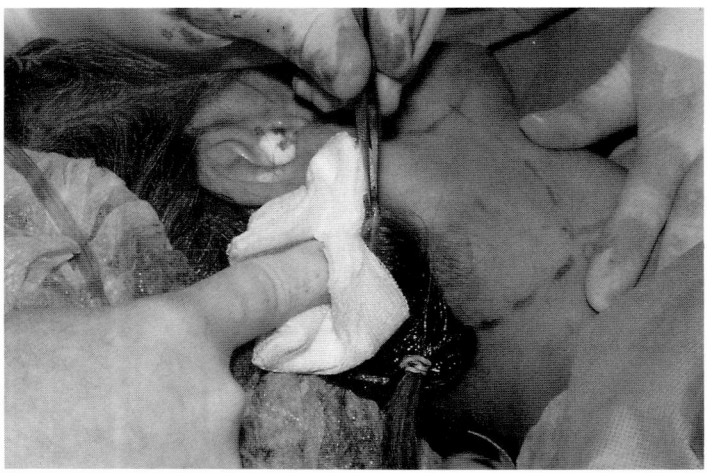

FIGURE 10.45. Three sterile gauze pads are placed into the pocket formed by the postauricular and lateral cervical flap. This will provide a tamponade which will promote coagulation in this area while the preauricular and temporal flaps are being created.

FIGURE 10.46. The horizontal incision of the temporal flap is made at the level of the temporal peak in the scalp hair. It is approximately 2 to 3 cm in length and is cut perpendicular to the skin to cut across hair shafts, thereby incorporating more hairs which may grow through the scar.

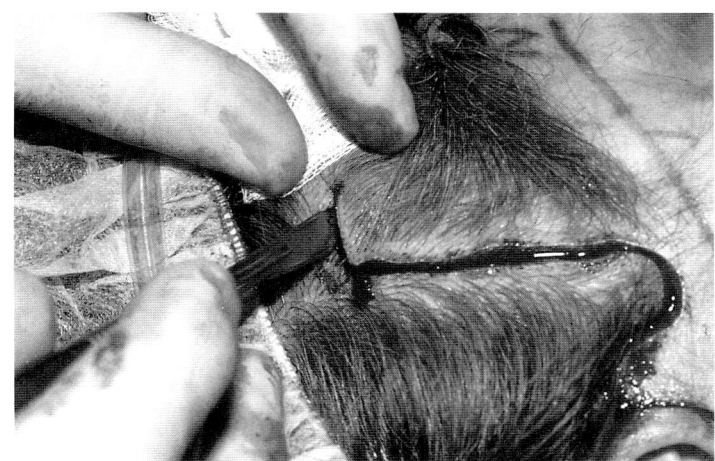

FIGURE 10.47. The vertical incision in the temporal area is made with either a no. 15 or no. 10 blade and is carried to the level of the underlying fascia. This incision is cut parallel to the hairs. The temporal incision is enlarged by using the back of the blade handle to facilitate carrying the incision to the underlying fascia. The hair follicles will be apparent and easily identifiable.

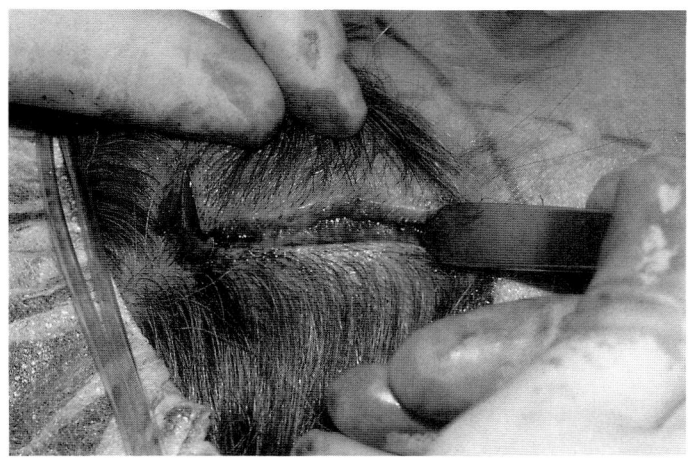

vertical incision is made parallel to the hair to decrease any loss of hair postoperatively. The incision can be made with either a number 15 or 10 blade. The end of the blade handle is used to separate the tissue down to the superficial temporal fascia (Figure 10.47). At the inferior portion of the sideburn, the number 15 blade is used to make a curvilinear incision at the bottom of the sideburn or at an area where the hair becomes sparse. The incision then follows the posterior edge of the sideburn to encompass a small area of preauricular skin. It is then curved back upon itself as it reaches the anterior portion of the auricle (Figure 10.48).

The undermining of the temporal skin begins at the superior portion of the flap. The right angle of the flap is raised and the hair follicles identified. A 7-inch curved Matarasso facelift scissors with blunt tips (Stille) is used for the elevation (Figure 10.48 and 10.49). The dissection should be deep to the hair follicles until the anterior border of the sideburn is reached, where it then becomes superficial to avoid the temporal branch of the facial nerve. Creation of the flap can be continued, using either sharp dissection with the Matarasso scissors or blunt dissection with the handle of a Bard-Parker blade (Figure 10.49). The flap is continued anteriorly for a total distance of 2.5 to 3 cm. The superficial temporal vein frequently is accidentally incised during the process of making the initial temporal incision. This can be cauterized without any permanent damage to the temporal nerve. Usually, there is no

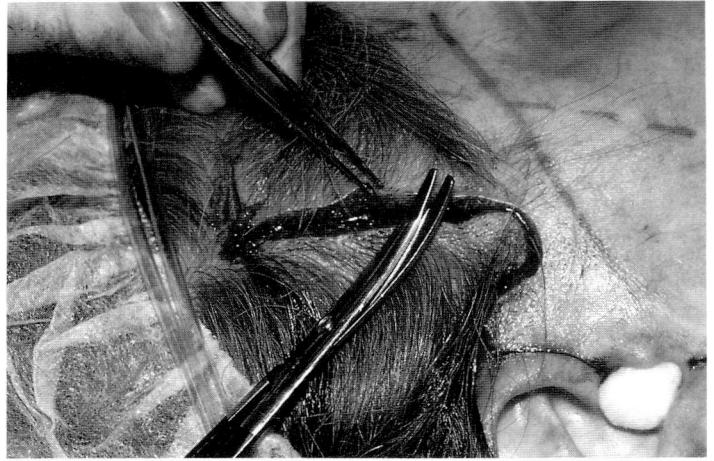

FIGURE 10.48. The anterior portion of the incision is grasped and placed under tension. The temporal flap can be elevated by blunt dissection using the back of the blade handle or with a curved Matarasso facelift scissors with blunt tip, as shown.

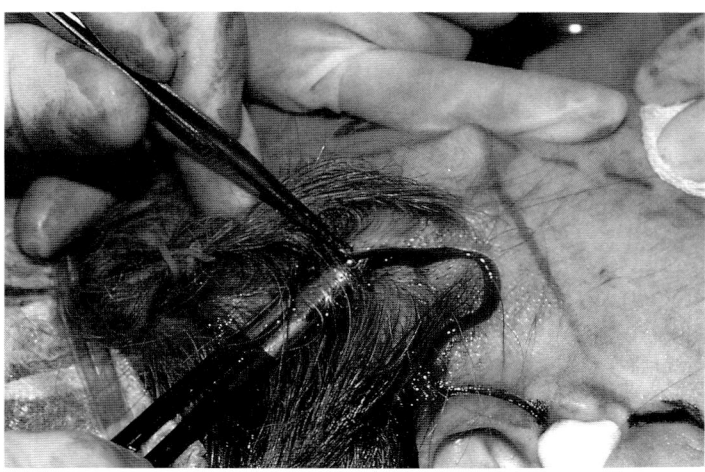

FIGURE 10.49. The initial dissection is placed below the hair follicles, then raised to a superficial level in the area immediately anterior to the temporal hair to avoid injury to the temporal branch of the facial nerve.

additional bleeding in this area, with the exception of those vessels that are on the skin edges.

Preauricular Flap

Attention is now focused on the preauricular flap, which is begun by incising along the anterior border of the lobule to the area anterior and horizontal to the inferior portion of the cavum (Figure 10.50). The incision makes a right angle and proceeds posteriorly in a horizontal fashion immediately inferior to the tragus for several millimeters until it reaches the concha. When the posterior border of the tragus is reached, a second right angle is produced, and the incision follows superiorly in a vertical pattern along the posterior border of the crest of the tragus (Figure 10.51). Care should be taken not to place this incision too far posteriorly, in order to avoid the necessity of draping the skin over the entire crest of the tragus.

At the superior border of the tragus, another right angle is made as the incision passes anteriorly in a horizontal plane for several millimeters until it reaches the anterior border of the helical crus. Here it turns upward 90° and follows the anterior border of the crus until it reaches the temporal hair. The incision then curves along the border of the temporal hair to meet that incision which was made previously for the temporal flap (Figure 10.52). Undermining superior to the tragus is extended to meet the undermining that has been completed from the temporal flap, and it is also extended inferiorly over the mandibular ramus to meet

10. Facelift Surgery

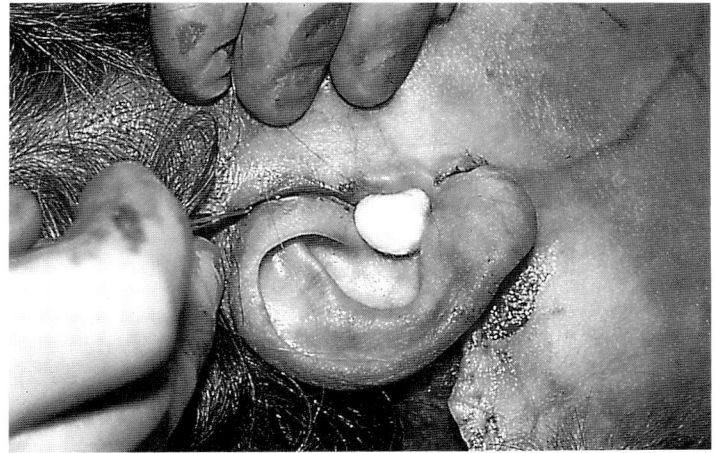

FIGURE 10.50. The preauricular incision is made beginning at the inferior border of the lobule and is carried superiorly along the anterior border of the lobule, where it makes a 90° angle posteriorly at the base of the tragus. The second portion of the incision is made superior to the tragus, where it follows the anterior border of the helix.

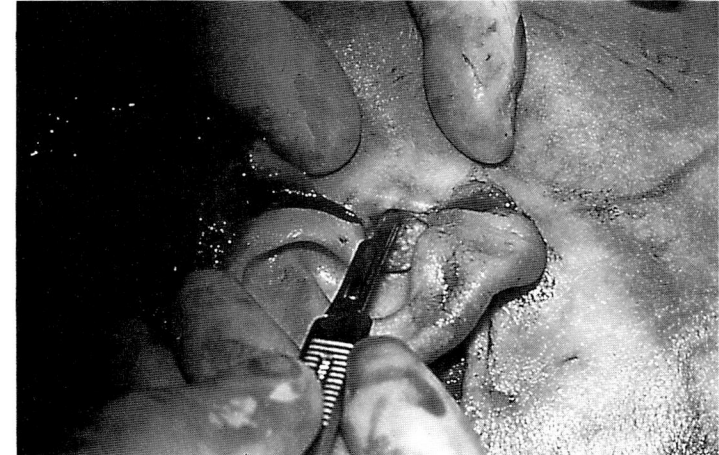

FIGURE 10.51. An incision is made on the posterior portion of the crest of the tragus where it courses superiorly to the superior border of the tragus, where it makes a 90° turn anteriorly to meet the superior portion of the preauricular incision.

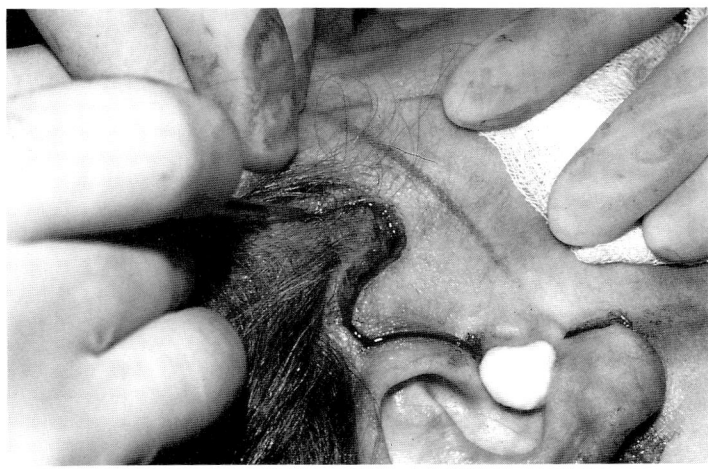

FIGURE 10.52. The incision curves anteriorly and inferiorly to encompass the glabrous skin that is present between the sideburn and the pinna. The incision then curves along the inferior border of the sideburn and meets the inferior portion of the temporal incision.

the undermining that has been completed in the retroauricular and lateral cervical regions (Figure 10.53).

Caution is advised to produce a thick flap in the preauricular and jowl area, since the flap will be longer than in the temporal area and thus its blood supply will be more precarious. The skin of the retroauricular flap is thicker and lends itself to adequate undermining. Since the skin of the preauricular flap and jowl area is quite thin on most patients, it is possible to undermine too superficially, causing a disruption of the dermal plexus and subsequent ischemia. Since the facial nerve is protected by the parotid gland in the preauricular area, the undermining can proceed at a deeper level than that of the temporal region. We prefer a long, curved scissors such as the 7-inch Matarasso facelift scissors or Ragnell scissors, with their broad, blunt tips, to avoid cutting through to the surface of the skin. This flap undermines quite easily and is usually accompanied by little bleeding. The superior portion of the flap is raised initially from the temporal site, followed by an approach from the surgical incision anterior to the lobule. Once the flap is raised, the only remaining attached skin is that which overlies the tragus. This area is infiltrated with a small amount of saline to assist in elevating the skin off the cartilage (Figure 10.54). A 6-inch Ragnell scissors is used to create the flap, carefully avoiding any injury to the cartilage that could result in a chondritis (Figure 10.55). This completes the undermining of the entire flap complex, including the retroauricu-

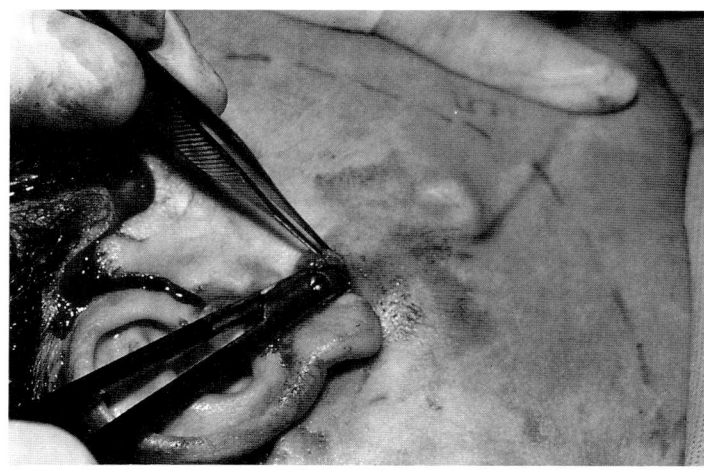

FIGURE 10.53. With tension applied to the distal aspect of the flap, undermining is completed from the lobule to the midmandibular region. The undermining of the preauricular flap is completed by extending dissection from the temporal flap to the mandible.

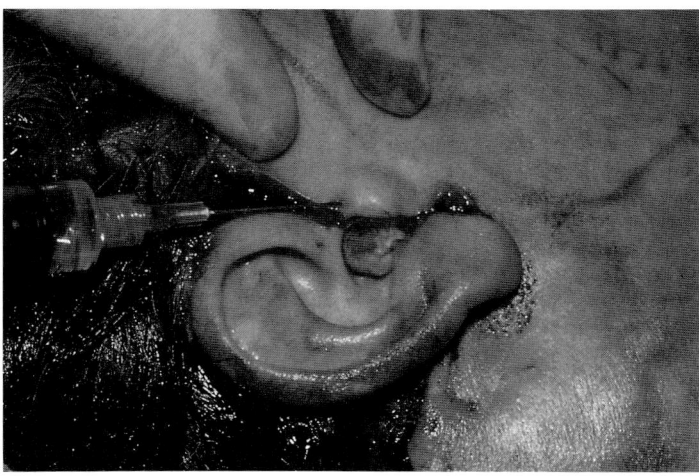

FIGURE 10.54. The only tissue that has not been elevated is that over the tragus. Saline is injected to provide hydrodissection.

10. Facelift Surgery

lar, temporal, and preauricular regions (Figure 10.56). With skill and experience, the creation of the incisions and elevation of the 3 areas of the flap complex will require between 8 and 12 minutes, depending upon the amount of bleeding incurred.

Facial Liposuction

A fatty layer will be present over the cheek from the malar area inferior to the mandibular ramus. Since the parotid fascia underlying this fat will be folded upon itself and plicated, it is necessary to remove this fat thoroughly. Prior to the development of liposuction, this was done by sharp dissection, which required close attention to detail to avoid injuring the parotid fascia and the parotid gland. By using the number 6 flat spatula cannula with a large orifice, liposuction employing a standard machine will very rapidly and safely remove this overlying fat, with no injury to the parotid gland and very little disruption of the venous complex (Figure 10.57 and 10.58). It is at this point that coagulation of any bleeding vessels should be done (Figure 10.59). If coagulation is performed while elevating the flaps, the time for the procedure will be unnecessarily extended and bleeding will recur during liposuction of the fat. The 3 gauze pads are removed from the retroauricular flap and the cannula is introduced if any blood has accumulated (Figure 10.60). Hemostasis is accomplished with cautery until the field is absolutely dry.

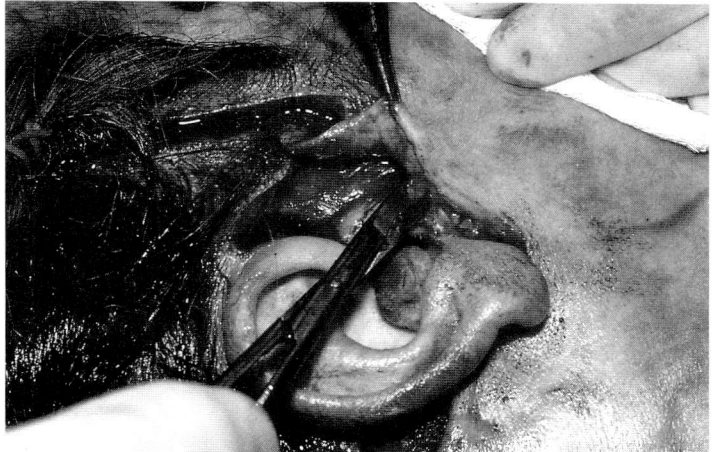

FIGURE 10.55. With infiltration of the saline, the flap is easily raised over the tragus. Care is taken to avoid injury to the tragal cartilage that may result in a persistent chronditis.

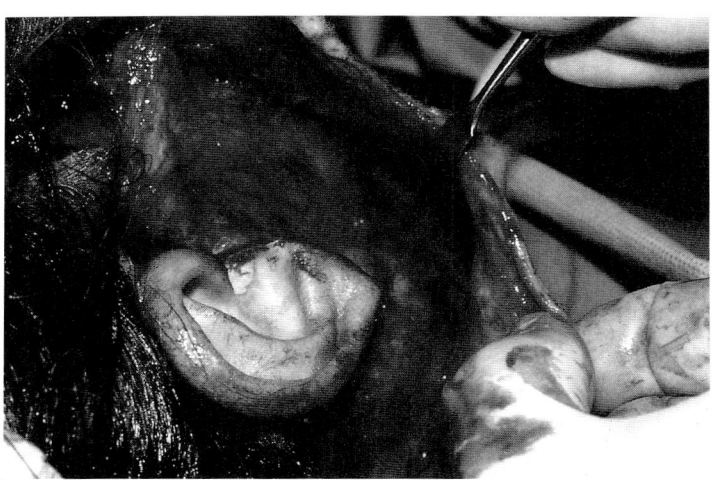

FIGURE 10.56. The entire flap complex is now complete and extends from the temporal region through the preauricular area, the mandibular region, the lateral cervical area, and the retroauricular region.

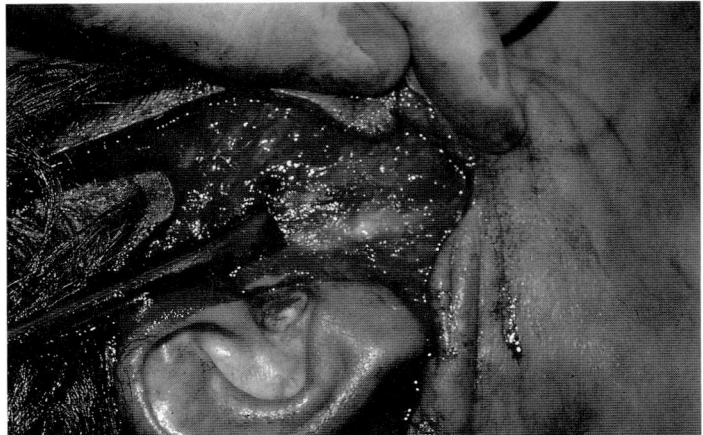

FIGURE 10.57. A 15-cm no. 6 liposuction spatula cannula is used to remove the fat over the parotid fascia.

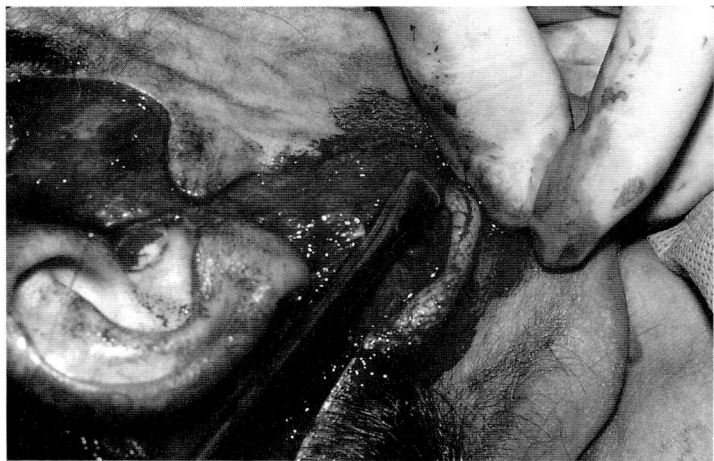

FIGURE 10.58. The cannula is then directed to the remaining fat overlying the mandibular region.

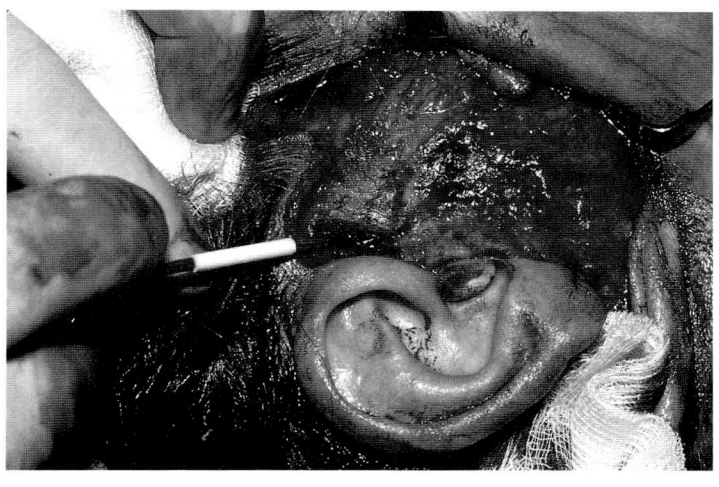

FIGURE 10.59. Hemostasis is accomplished using cautery. Only essential cautery of significant arterials are done prior to this time as a time-saving maneuver.

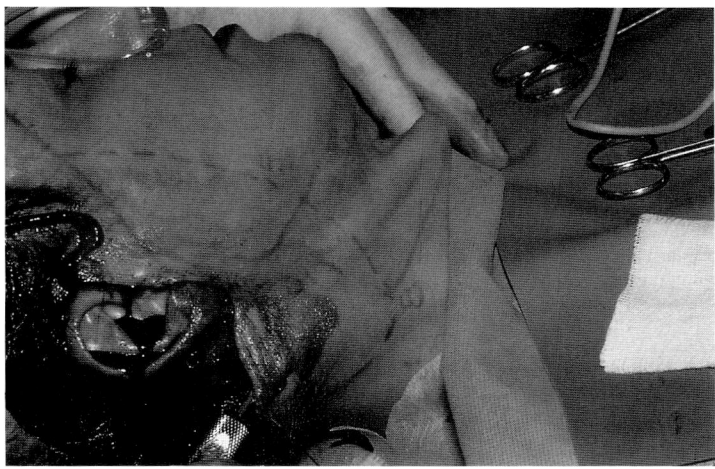

FIGURE 10.60. A no. 6 spatula is introduced into the inferior portion of the lateral and anterior cervical flaps to remove any blood that may have accumulated during the operation.

Bleeders are usually found at the distal end of the flap over the sternocleidomastoid muscle and in the posterior cervical triangle. It is important to extend the epinephrine-containing anesthetic beyond the planned extent of the undermining particularly in this lateral cervical region, since this is an area that is difficult to access and will frequently develop mild to moderate bleeding during the operative procedure. By obtaining adequate vasoconstriction, this situation can be avoided or diminished significantly.

Plication of the SMAS

It has been shown that plication or imbrication of the superficial musculoaponeurotic system can significantly improve the long term results of facelift surgery.[16-26] Since there is no significant difference between the ultimate results of plication versus imbrication, the former method is used because it requires less time and creates less injury and bleeding of the tissues. A stout, braided, synthetic suture, Ethibond 2.0, is used for plication. Unlike many surgeons who place only 1 or 2 plication sutures to elevate the jowl and anterior cervical region, we prefer to place 12 to 15 buried sutures along the anterior border of the sternocleidomastoid muscle and extending upward from the lobule of the ear anterior to the preauricular incision line and into the temporal area. This provides for even distribution of the tension on the SMAS and avoids the multiple depressions at the site of each buried suture that may occur when only several sutures are used. There are several key sutures placed during plication, their direction is as follows:

1. From the inferior border of the tragus toward the mentum.
2. From the superior border of the tragus toward the oral commissure.
3. From the mastoid process toward the cervicomental angle.
4. From the juncture of the horizontal and vertical incisions of the temporal flap toward the lateral portion of the orbital rim.

Each key suture correspondingly elevates the jowl, the angle of the mouth, the cervicomental angle, and the lateral periorbital region. All the sutures are placed paying very close attention to proper laying of the knot. Each knot contains 3 loops, with the exception of the key suture between the mastoid and the cervicomental angle, where 5 loops are used, since this is the most critical suture and tension will be great. The surgeon should be aware of the significant difference between the proper and improper tying of these knots. Surgeons frequently lay multiple half-hitches for these knots rather than alternating the laying of each loop in the fashion of a square knot. A half-hitch creates an unstable knot that will readily come undone regardless of the number of loops tied. By contrast, a properly laid knot employs the principles of a square knot, which provides stability and will not readily come undone.

The first plicating suture extends from a point slightly anterior to the inferior border of the tragus to a point approximately 5 cm inferior and anterior in the direction of the mentum (Figures 10.61 and 10.62). A large amount of tissue can be plicated, providing support to the SMAS and eliminating the laxity in the jowl area. All knots should be buried to avoid spontaneous postoperative extrusion.

An adequately tied knot should be cut on the knot so that fraying of the braided suture is minimized, decreasing the likelihood of postoperative infection. The use of the Laschal suture scissors facilitates the rapid automatic cutting of these sutures (Figure 10.63). The second suture anchors the tissues between the superior border of the tragus and the angle of the mouth (Figure 10.64). The distance that this suture travels is considerably less than the first suture and will probably be less than 2 cm prior to its tightening. The third key suture is placed high in the temporal region, immediately anterior to the skin incision. The distal portion of the suture is directed toward the lateral orbital rim (Figure 10.65). This will elevate the lateral aspect of the eyebrow and the malar area.

The fourth key suture has its posterior position inferior to the mastoid process, where it is anchored in the thick, fibrous tissue of the origin of the sternocleidomastoid muscle (Figure 10.66). Depending upon the laxity of the neck, a very large bite is possible and may measure up to 5 cm in length. The anterior bite is directed toward the cervicomental angle

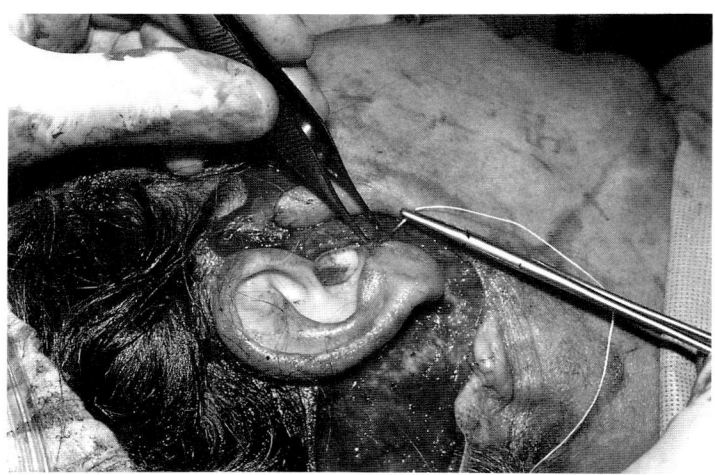

FIGURE 10.61. The first key suture of the plication is placed with its posterior bite at a level slightly anterior to the inferior border of the tragus.

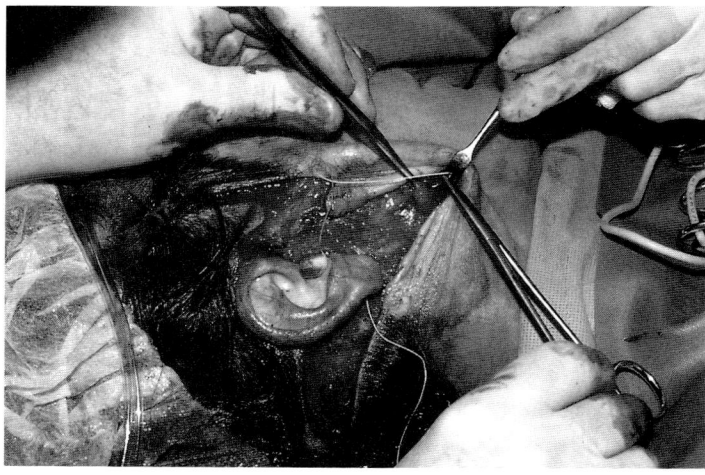

FIGURE 10.62. The distal bite of the first key suture of plication is taken approximately 5 cm inferior and anterior in the direction of the mentum.

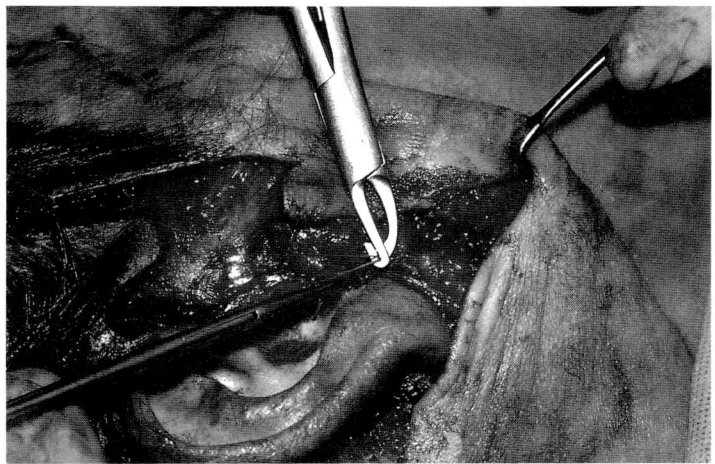

FIGURE 10.63. The knots are cut using Laschal scissors, which automatically cuts on the knot.

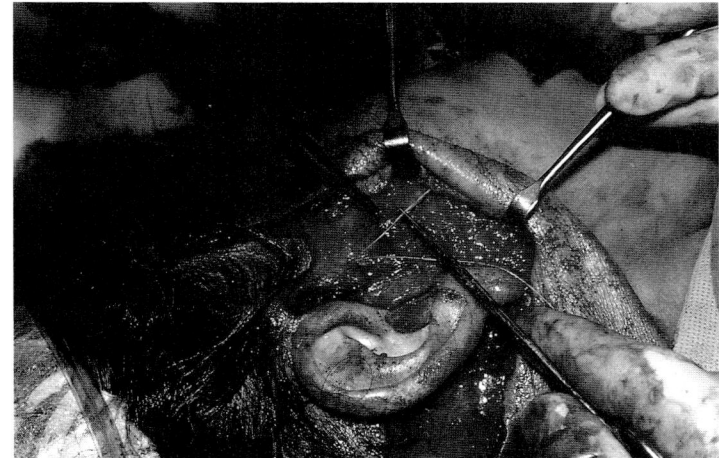

FIGURE 10.64. The posterior bite of the second key suture is placed immediately anterior to the superior border of the tragus and is directed at the angle of the mouth. Only a length of 2 to 3 cm can be plicated.

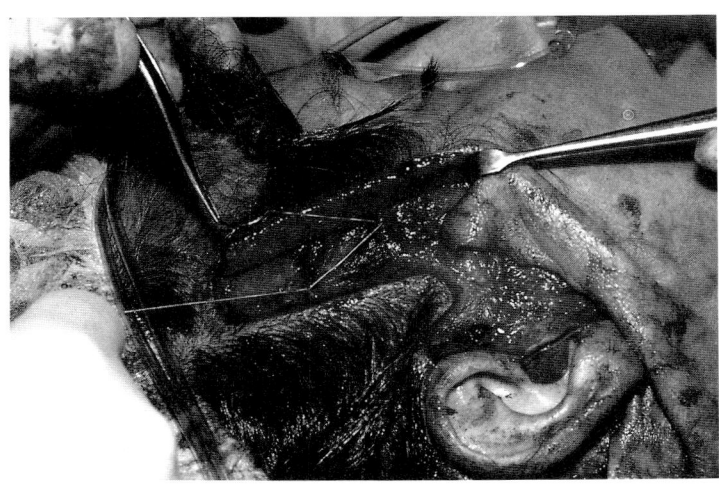

FIGURE 10.65. The third key suture is placed high in the temporal region several centimeters inferior to the horizontal temporal incision and immediately anterior to the skin incision. The suture is directed anteriorly and inferiorly toward the lateral orbital rim. A length of between 2 to 3 cm is possible to elevate in this area.

(Figure 10.67). Since this is the most critical suture in creating elevation of the cervicomental angle, considerable pressure is placed on this suture. Five loops are laid rather than the 3 that may be used in the other key sutures and the 2 loops that are used for the less critical sutures. To maintain pressure on each of these knots, a small needle holder with smooth jaws is clamped on the initial loop during the tightening and cinching of the second loop (Figure 10.68). Only in the fourth key suture is a surgeon's knot used; all other knots are laid in a square knot fashion. Generally this fourth suture remains exposed for a small distance superficial to the sternocleidomastoid muscle at the completion of the tie.

Additional sutures are placed superior and inferior to this key suture, which then may be left partially exposed or may be removed by the surgeon to be replaced with a suture that is not exposed. This region may be pulled so tight that a groove passing between the mastoid process and the cervicomental angle is formed; this groove will continue to be present even with redraping of the skin and may result in some concern for both the patient and the physician. With the diminution of postoperative edema and the subsequent relaxation of tissues, this groove always resolves, leaving a very well-defined cervicomental angle. Additional sutures are placed inferior to the mastoid process, with the posterior anchor being the anterior border of the sternocleidomastoid muscle. Bites in this area usually are about 2 cm in length in

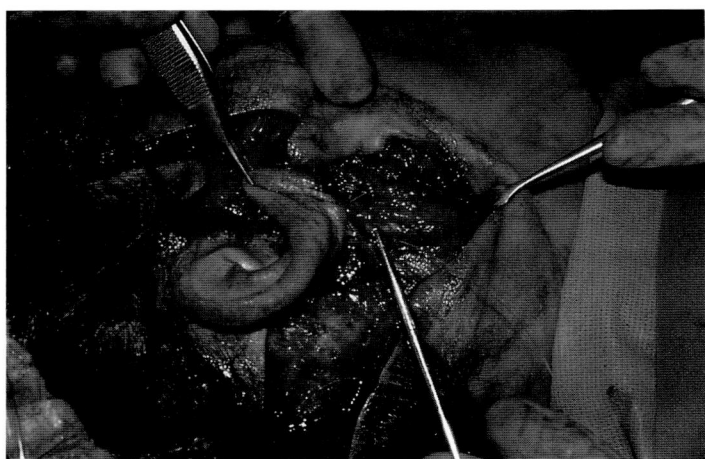

FIGURE 10.66. The fourth and most important key suture is placed inferior to the mastoid process, where it is anchored in the thick fibrous tissue of the origin of the sternocleidomastoid muscle.

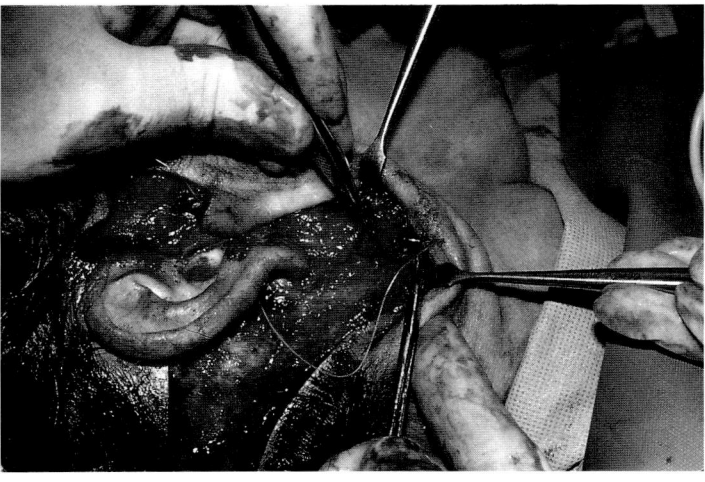

FIGURE 10.67. The inferior portion of the fourth key suture is directed toward the cervicomental angle. Depending upon the laxity of the underlying tissues, the length of this bite may be up to 6 cm.

FIGURE 10.68. The fourth key suture is tied under considerable tension and, therefore, a surgeon's knot rather than a square knot is used. To prevent the suture from loosening prior to the placement of the second loop, the first loop is held securely with a needle holder having smooth jaws. Because of the importance of this key suture, five loops are placed in the knot. All knots are buried to decrease the likelihood of postoperative extrusion.

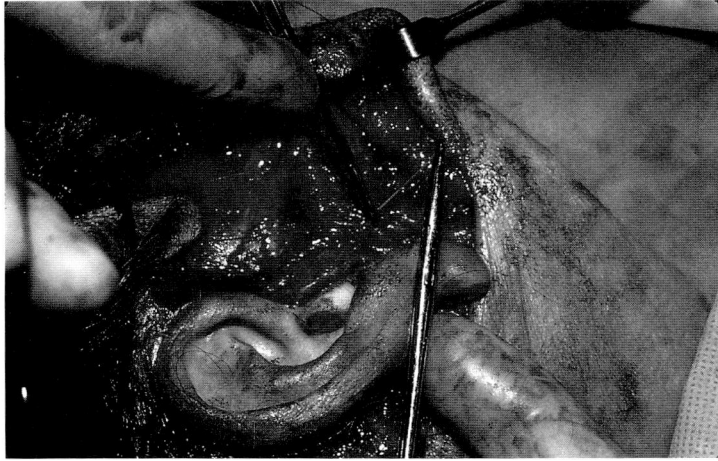

the superior portion and decrease to approximately 1 cm at the inferior portion of the lateral cervical area. If the bite is too long at the inferior portion, a bunching of tissue will appear that is apparent postoperatively, despite the fact that the overlying skin flap has been properly redraped. The purpose of these sutures is not only to give support to the anterior cervical region but also progressively to distribute the tension on the underlying sutures so that unnecessary bulges will not be apparent.

Additional accessory sutures are placed between the key sutures to provide support and to avoid depressions alternating with elevations, which occur when too few sutures are used. The point at which a suture is necessary is easily determined by grasping the SMAS with a forceps and placing tension on it to see if any movement superiorly and posteriorly is possible. If so, a suture should be placed at that site. The placement of each suture in the temporal and preauricular areas is approximately 1 cm anterior to the incision line.

Redraping of the Skin Flap

Following the placement of the plication sutures, which is the most important portion of the operative procedure, the skin is redraped (Figure 10.69). Moderate tension on the flap is placed in the retroauricular area and the temporal region. Only minimal tension is placed on the regions superior and inferior to the tragus and no tensions is placed on the flap in the area of the tragus.

FIGURE 10.69. After the suspension of the SMAS with plication sutures, the flap is advanced superiorly and posteriorly and temporarily redraped. Note that even with no tension, there is considerable amount of excess skin created by the suspension of the underlying tissues.

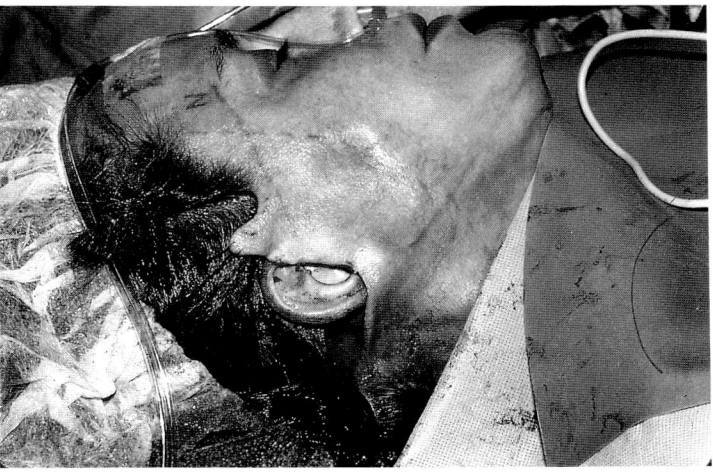

Retroauricular Flap

The skin is temporarily reattached at the region of the preauricular flap between the superior portion of the external ear and the remaining portion of the temporal hair tuft. The flap is advanced posteriorly and superiorly at approximately a 70° angle under mild tension (Figure 10.70). An incision is made in the flap using a number 15 blade. A staple is placed to secure the flap (Figure 10.71). Advancement of the flap in this region usually measures between 2 and 3 cm. The second area to be addressed is the retroauricular region, which is advanced at approximately a 60° angle from a horizontal position (Figure 10.72). The border of the flap that was originally at the inferior portion of the lobule can frequently be elevated to or slightly short of the level of the horizontal postauricular incision, yielding approximately 4 to 6 cm of excess skin (Figure 10.73 and 10.74). A temporary staple is placed 1 cm posterior to the retroauricular sulcus. These incisions are easily made by overlapping the flap under tension. A number 15 blade is placed on the skin at the level of the horizontal retroauricular incision line while slightly elevating the flap so that the indentation made by the blade can be seen in its relationship to the incision (Figure 10.72).

Additional portions of the retroauricular flap are placed under tension and advanced superiorly and posteriorly. Segments of skin 2 to 3 cm in width are cut (Figure 10.75). The middle section of the retroauricular flap may be advanced superiorly without any posterior displacement to improve the alignment of the

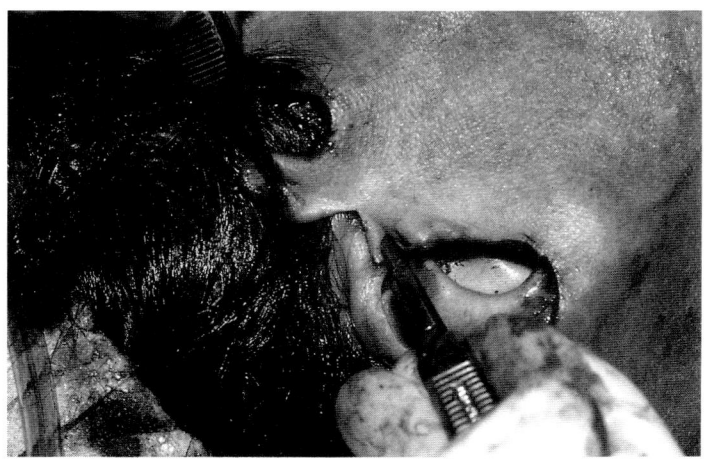

FIGURE 10.70. The flap is redraped under minimal tension at the superior portion of the external ear. An incision is made equal to the length of the overlapping skin. The direction of pull is approximately 70° from the horizontal.

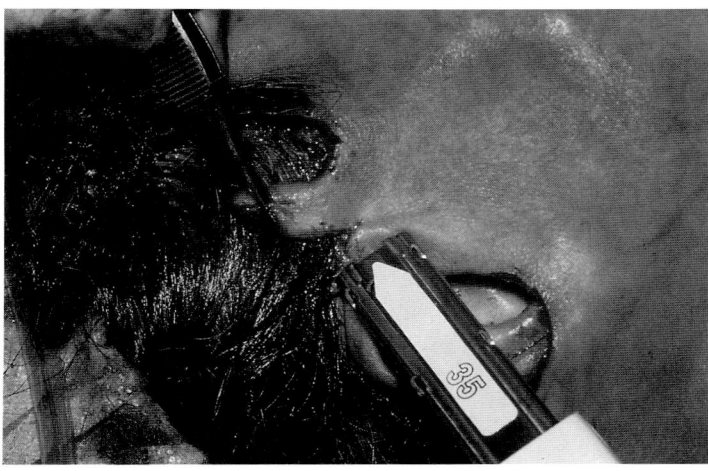

FIGURE 10.71. A temporary staple is placed between the skin flap and the glabrous skin immediately superior to the top of the external ear.

10. Facelift Surgery

FIGURE 10.72. The retroauricular flap is elevated in a superior and posterior direction approximately 60° from the horizontal. Moderate tension is placed on the flap to accentuate the improvement of the cervicomental angle and the jowl area.

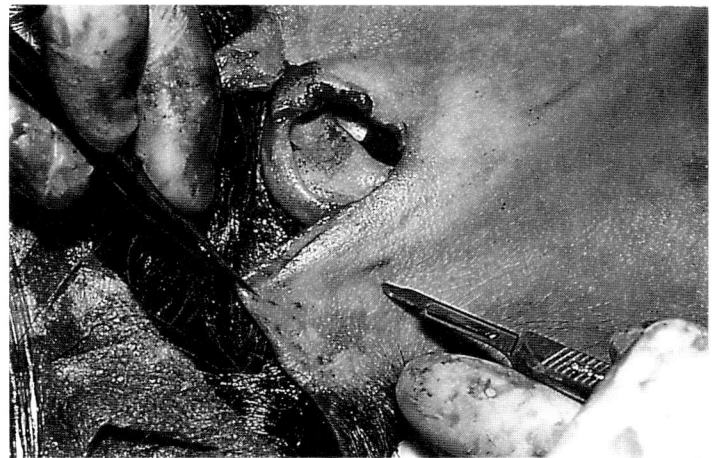

FIGURE 10.73. The flap is incised approximately 1 cm posterior to the retroauricular sulcus. The incision is carried to the full extent of the overlapping present on the flap.

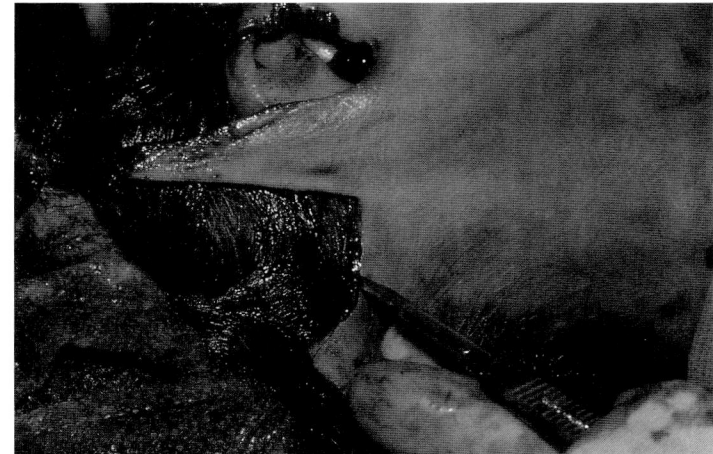

FIGURE 10.74. This is the area of greatest tension over the entire flap complex. It is not unusual to advance the flap 4 to 6 cm in this region, as seen on the ruler.

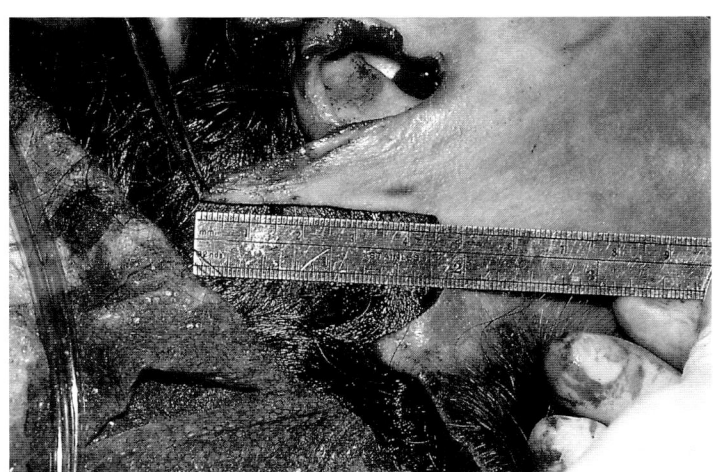

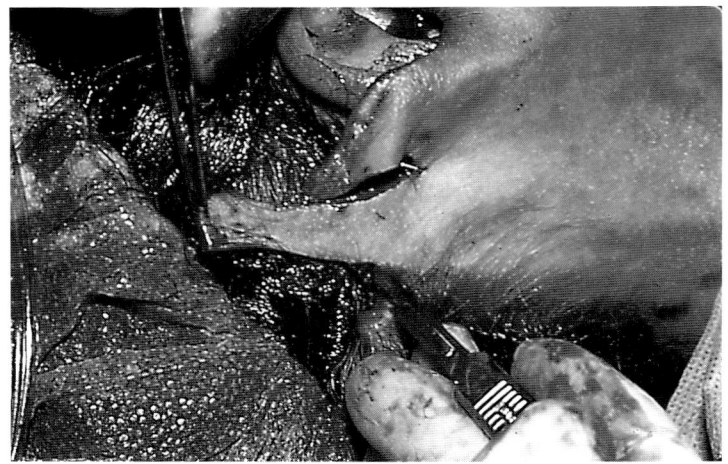

FIGURE 10.75. The central portion of the postauricular flap is advanced superiorly without any posterior displacement. This will improve the appearance of the occipital hairline by decreasing the step formation that occurs with advancement of the flap.

newly created retroauricular hairline. Some surgeons create an anterior and superior pull in an attempt to approximate the preoperative hairline. This eliminates posterior movement of the flap which is essential to obtain improvement in the cervicomental angle. Since this will create an excess of skin in the area of the lobule and will not place sufficient tension on the flap in the region of the cervicomental angle, this maneuver seems inappropriate. If given the option, most patients prefer to improve the cervicomental angle at the expense of a slight step in the postauricular hairline. If the retroauricular horizontal incision is placed high within the hair this step is inconsequential and is not visible even in patients who wear very short hair.

The remainder of the retroauricular flap is advanced in small segments, as described previously. Hand suturing with a running lock of 5.0 catgut is used in the areas of glabrous skin to avoid scarring from staples. In the areas of hair-bearing skin, staples are used. The 90° downward curve of the posterior end of the retroauricular incision greatly assists in eliminating a dog ear when the posterior segment of the flap is constructed (Figures 10.28, 10.29). The remaining segment of skin on the flap is usually longer than the remaining retroauricular incision line (Figure 10.76). By making a straight-line excision of the excess skin from the last staple to the farthest point of the incision as it curves downward, these lengths are equalized, eliminating a dog ear (Figures 10.77 and 10.78).

With the flap stabilized in the supra-auricular area and retroauricular areas, attention is focused on the lobule. The lower half and anterior portion of the external ear will be covered when advancing the flap (Figure 10.79). A 6-inch curved Peck-Joseph scissors is placed parallel to the posterior border of the external ear, and an incision is cut to a length 0.5 cm short of the attachment of the lobule. The lobule is delivered through this incision, the length of which is extended with the scissors until the lobule is snugly elevated by the flap without creating any redundant skin at the juncture of the flap with the inferior attachment of the lobule (Figure 10.80). The flap should not be cut so that the lobule will lie in its natural position because the large plane of scar created by the flap will contract anteriorly and inferiorly with normal healing causing a similar advancement of the lobule (Figure 10.81). All too often surgeons fail to recognize this important aspect of normal wound healing and complete the procedure by placing the lobule in its normal position. With the contracture of the flap, the lobule is pulled downward, causing a spread of the scar and elongation of the lobule, creating an elf's ear (Figures 10.1, 10.2, and 10.3) This defect, caused by poor planning, is grossly obvious from the anterior and lateral positions and can quickly lead to the identification of a patient who has undergone a poorly planned rhytidectomy.

The remaining anterior portion of the retroauricular flap is elevated, placed under mod-

10. Facelift Surgery

FIGURE 10.76. The remaining posterior portion of the flap will have an inferior limb which is longer than the superior limb. This will lead to dog-ear formation if no corrective measure is taken.

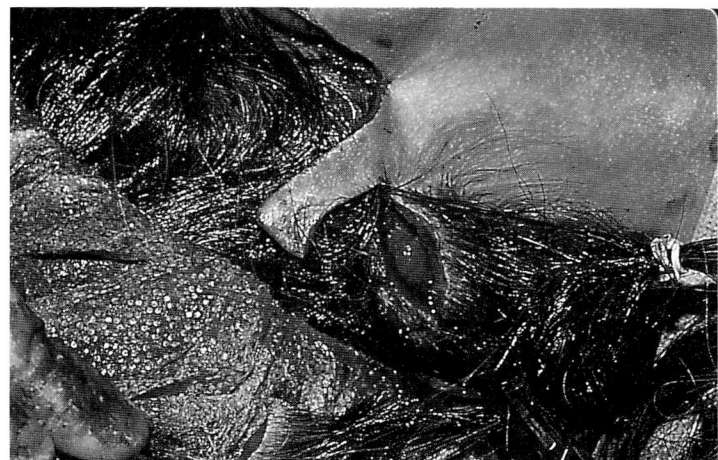

FIGURE 10.77. The flap is elevated under moderate tension, and the excess tissue is removed by incising a straight line from the middle portion of the flap to the inferior extension of the postauricular incision. Both the superior and inferior limbs become equal.

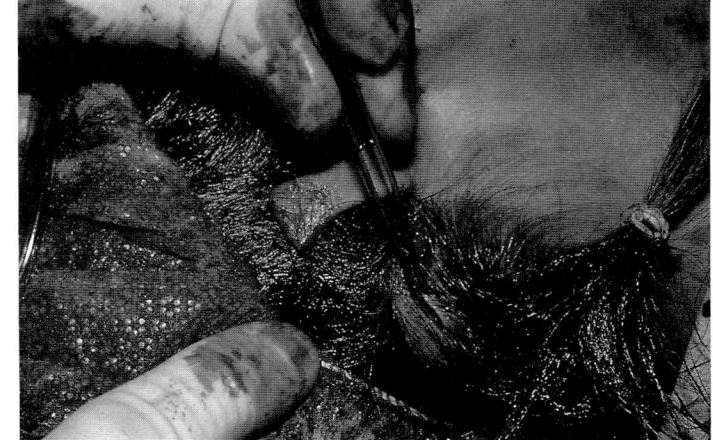

FIGURE 10.78. The incision on the flap is made parallel to the hair follicles. The hair-bearing skin is closed with surgical staples. The glabrous skin is closed by hand using 6.0 catgut suture employing a running lock closure.

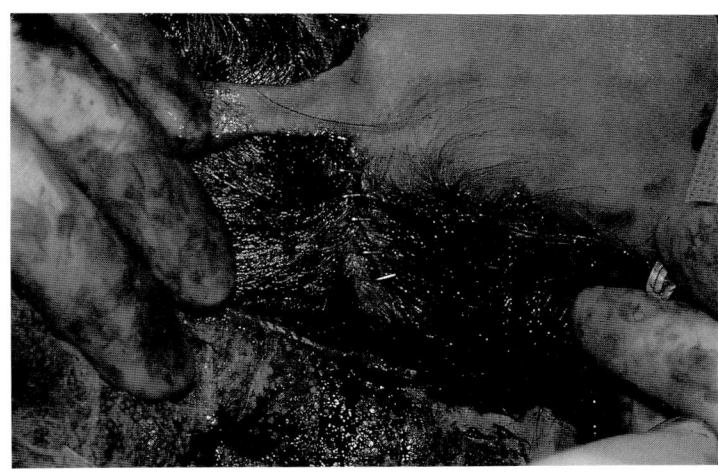

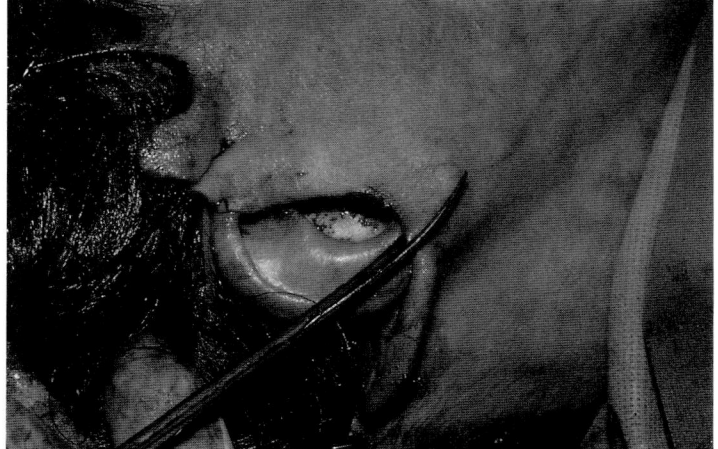

FIGURE 10.79. The excess skin of the flap covers the external ear. A 6 in. curved Peck–Joseph scissors is introduced to the area where the helix joins the lobule. An incision is made parallel to but slightly anterior of the posterior border of the auricle. This incision is extended to 0.5 cm short of the attachment of the lobule.

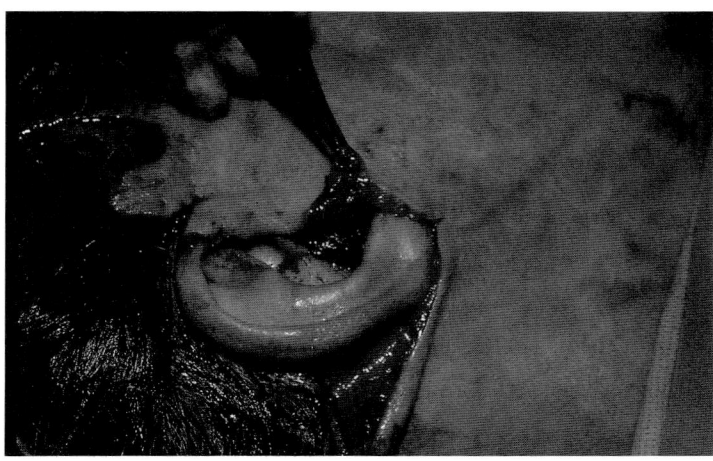

FIGURE 10.80. The lobule is delivered through the incision, which is lengthened until the lobule is snugly elevated by the flap without creating redundant skin at the juncture of the flap with the inferior attachment of the lobule.

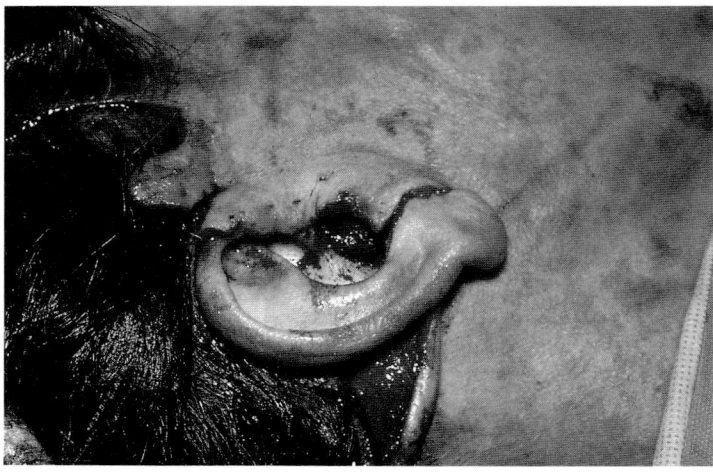

FIGURE 10.81. The position of the lobule should be superior and posterior to its natural position because contraction of the flap during normal healing will draw the lobule anteriorly and inferiorly.

FIGURE 10.82. The remaining anterior portion of the retroauricular flap is placed under moderate tension and excised.

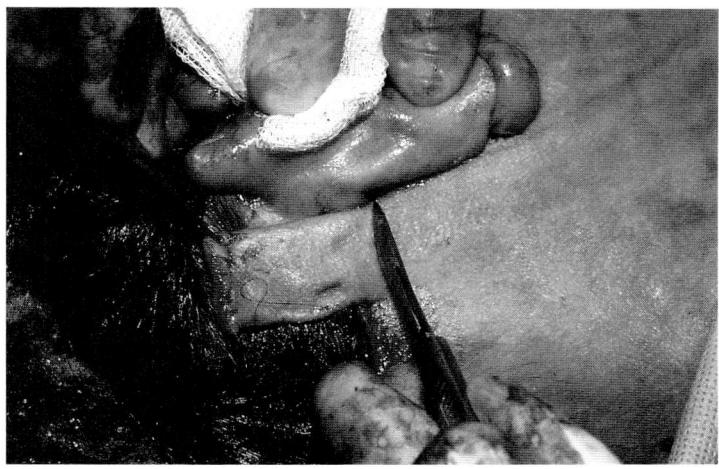

erate tension and excised (Figure 10.82). Since this is the longest segment of the flap and since the scalp hair may not fully cover this segment the surgeon should avoid excessive pressure particularly in the patient who is a smoker. Excess tension may lead to skin necrosis, scar formation and hypopigmentation. The excess skin is cut and the anterior segment of the horizontal postauricular flap is closed with suture to minimize the scarring seen with staples (Figure 10.83).

Temporal Flap

Attention is now redirected to the temporal flap, where the temporary staple may be removed or readjusted, if necessary. Since this is a short flap with excellent blood supply, a moderate amount of pressure is used. The excision is completed by rounding the newly created flap between its horizontal and vertical segments rather than cutting a right angle to correspond with these 2 segments (Figure 10.84). In so doing the surgeon can adjust this flap so that it can be rotated either superiorly or inferiorly without creating a dog ear (Figure (10.85). The vertical segment of the skin is trimmed and stapled. The surgeon should be cautious not to remove excessive skin, since a spread of the scar in this region will be quite obvious. Very little tension should be placed on the lower portion of this segment as it courses inferiorly on the newly constructed anterior border of the temporal hair tuft and as it curves around the inferior portion of that tuft (Figure 10.86). If a small amount of

FIGURE 10.83. The glabrous area of the retroauricular flap skin is hand sutured to minimize scarring, which is more evident when staples are used.

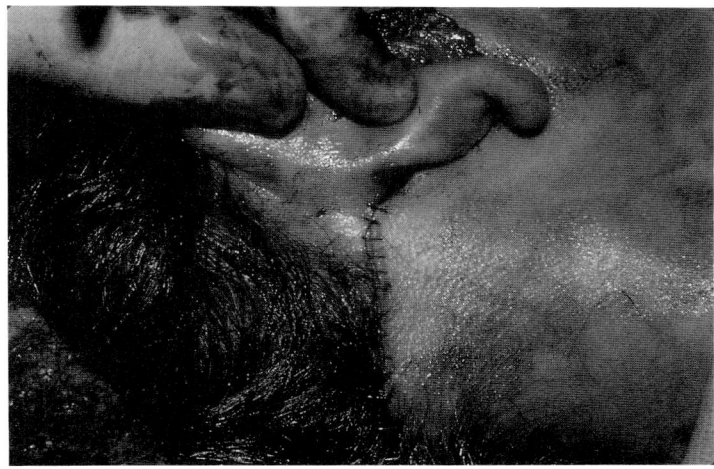

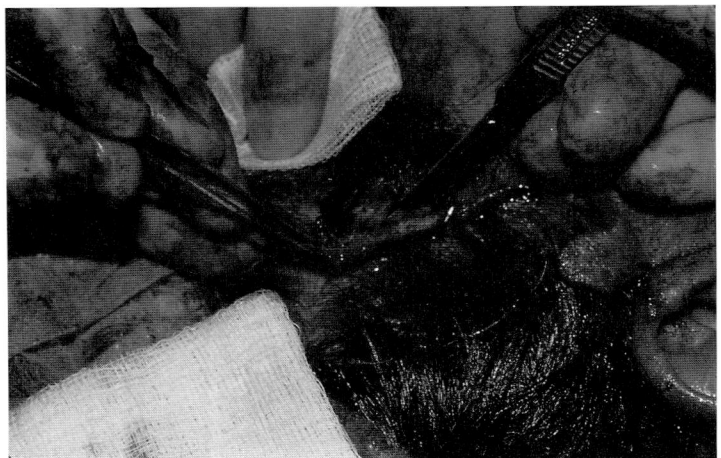

FIGURE 10.84. The temporal flap is trimmed superiorly in the shape of a curve, eliminating the right angle that was present. The flap may then be moved superiorly or inferiorly without creating a dog ear. The anterior portion of the horizontal incision is stapled first to avoid a dog ear in the temporal peak of the scalp hair.

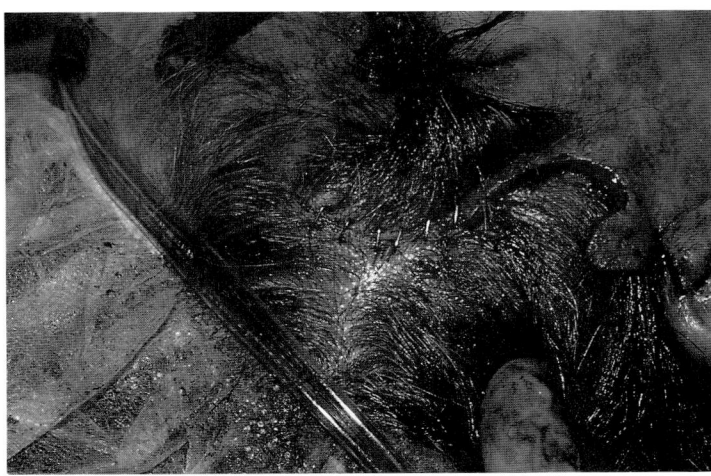

FIGURE 10.85. The verticle portion of the temporal flap is trimmed under moderate tension in the upper half and mild tension in the lower half.

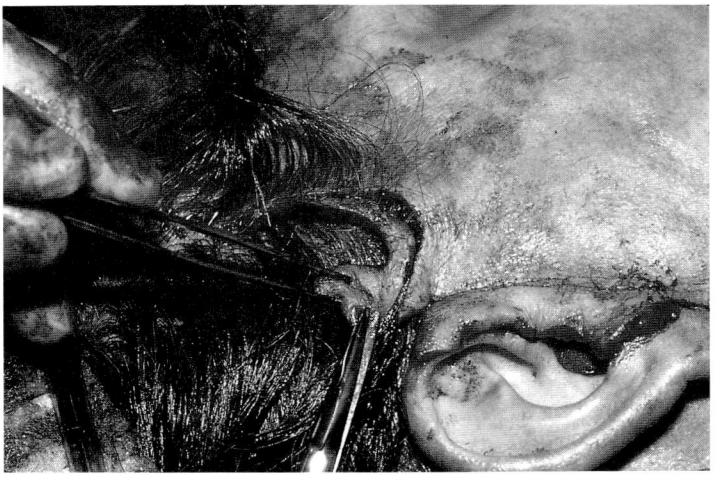

FIGURE 10.86. The excess skin is trimmed to correspond with the remaining temporal hair tuft. No tension should be placed on this portion of the flap to avoid a spread scar. This area is sutured with 5.0 catgut using a running lock suture.

10. Facelift Surgery

excess skin is inadvertently removed and the skin edges do not abut without tension, the surgeon can improve this by placing buried sutures to adjust the flap.

Preauricular Flap

A horizontal incision is made from the posterior edge of the flap to a position slightly superior to the tragus until the anterior border of the external ear is reached. A vertical incision is made parallel to the anterior border of the external ear and the excess skin is removed (Figure 10.87). A second horizontal incision is made several millimeters inferior to the tragus, and the excess skin anterior to the lobule is removed (Figure 10.88). Little or no tension is placed on the closure at the temporal hair tuft and the preauricular region, to avoid a spread scar. The segment of skin overlying the tragus is defatted, as one would do with a full thickness skin graft (Figure 10.89). This should be done reasonably aggressively so that the thin flap can follow the contour of the tragus. The inferior portion of the lobule is identified by the scratch made earlier in the procedure. An anchoring suture is placed at this location (Figure 10.90). In anticipation of migration inferiorly and anteriorly, the lobule should be placed in a position that is vertical to the external ear rather than its natural position, which is slightly anterior to the external ear. The suture is continued anterior to the lobule and stops at the level of

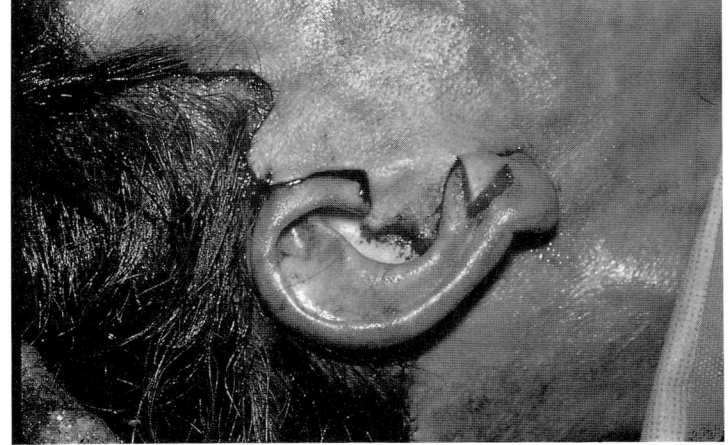

FIGURE 10.87. A horizontal incision is made until the superior portion of the tragus is reached. A vertical incision anterior to the auricle completes the excision of the excess skin in the superior portion of the external ear. A second horizontal incision is made to the inferior border of the tragus.

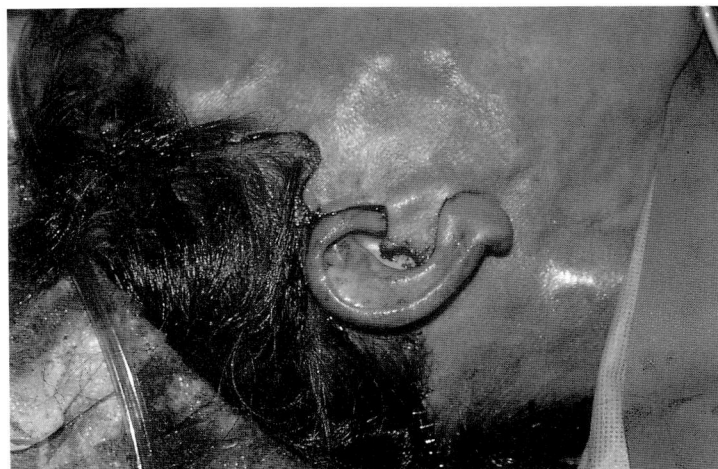

FIGURE 10.88. Excess skin overlying the lobule is excised leaving an incision line that will be closed under no tension. A running lock suture of 5.0 catgut is used.

the tragus (Figure 10.91). The incision line superior to the tragus is also sutured.

The remaining segment of untrimmed flap overlying the tragus is raised (Figure 10.92). Any additional trimming of subcutaneous fat is done, and preliminary excision of the posterior portion of the excess skin on the flap is completed. Sufficient excess skin should be left to accommodate for two factors. First, since there is a normal depression in the segment anterior to the tragus, proper redraping of the flap will move the flap anteriorly. The redraping and fixation of the flap in the pretragal area is completed by using 3 interrupted sutures, leaving at least several millimeters of skin between each suture to allow for adequate capillary filling of the tragal segment (Figure 10.93). These sutures are usually removed on the fifth day, but they may be removed earlier if the flap overlying the tragus receives inadequate blood flow. The second reason for providing excess skin for the tragal flap is that normal postoperative scar contraction will rotate the tragus anteriorly if the skin is draped snugly. This anterior displacement alters the normal appearance of the external ear and can be another tell-tale sign of a poorly planned rhytidectomy. The flap should be trimmed so that about 1 to 2 mm of excess skin remains when the flap is draped over the crest of the tragus. An incision slightly posterior to the crest of the tragus will camouflage the scar better than an incision and suture line that is

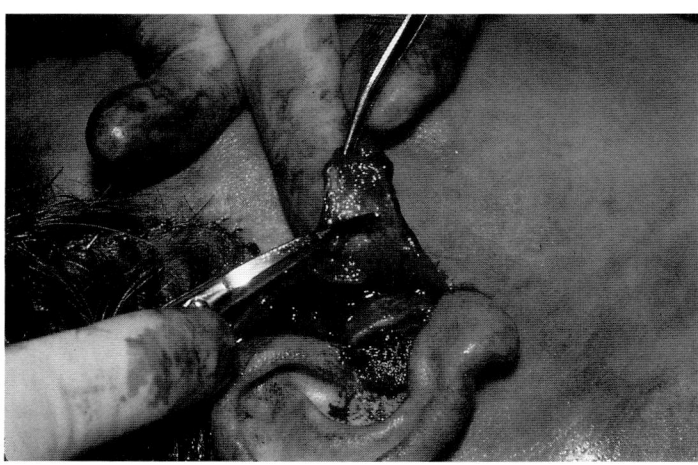

FIGURE 10.89. The skin flap overlying and adjacent to the anterior border of the tragus is aggressively defatted so that the thin flap will conform to the subtle contours of the tragus.

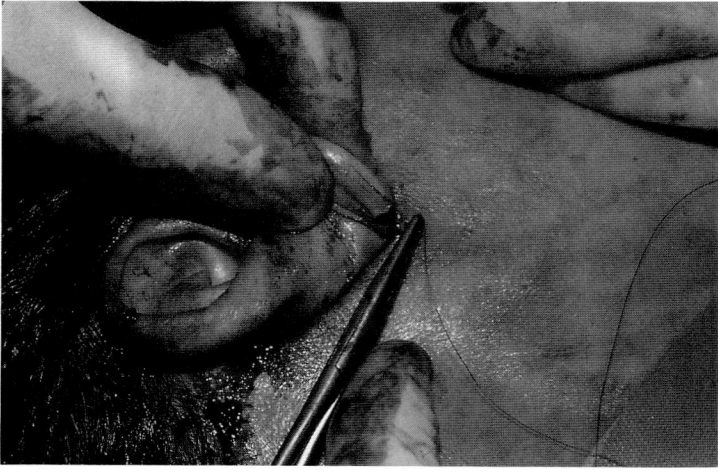

FIGURE 10.90. The inferior border of the tragus can be identified by the scratch which was placed on it when making the initial incision. A suture is placed between this point the superior portion of the flap.

10. Facelift Surgery

FIGURE 10.91. The anterior portion of the lobule is sutured to the preauricular flap with a running lock suture of 5.0 catgut.

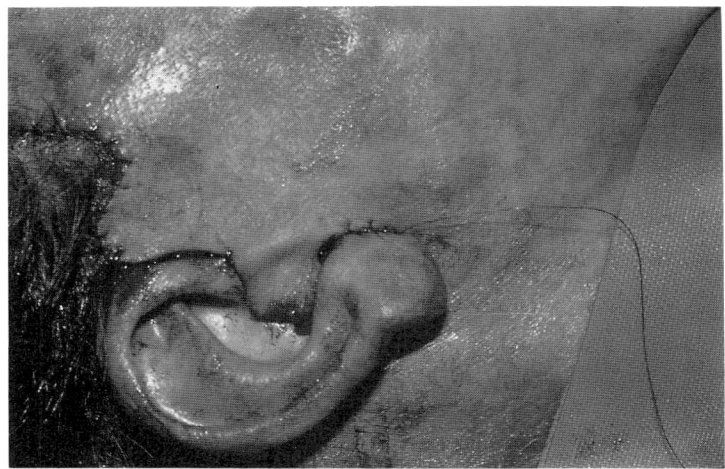

FIGURE 10.92. The pretragal flap is raised and any additional fat is trimmed. The posterior segment of the flap is excised to leave a modest amount of excess skin to readily cover the tragus.

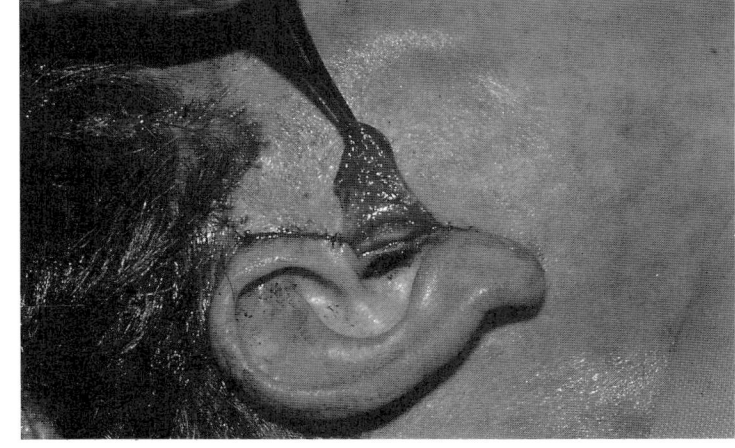

FIGURE 10.93. Three interrupted sutures of 5.0 catgut are placed in the depression immediately anterior to the tragus to duplicate the preexisting natural contour.

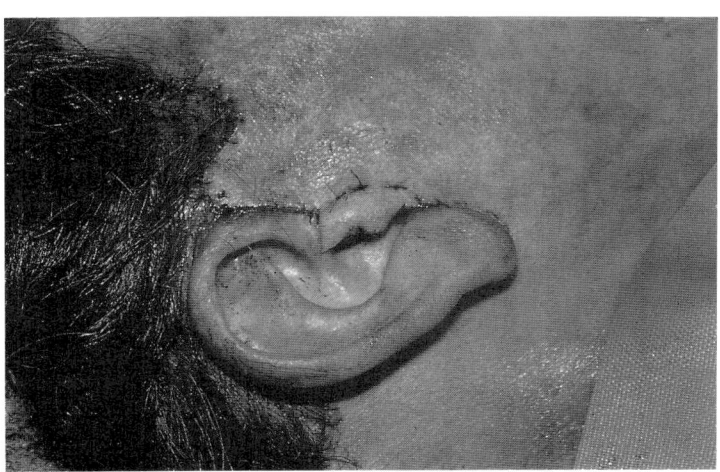

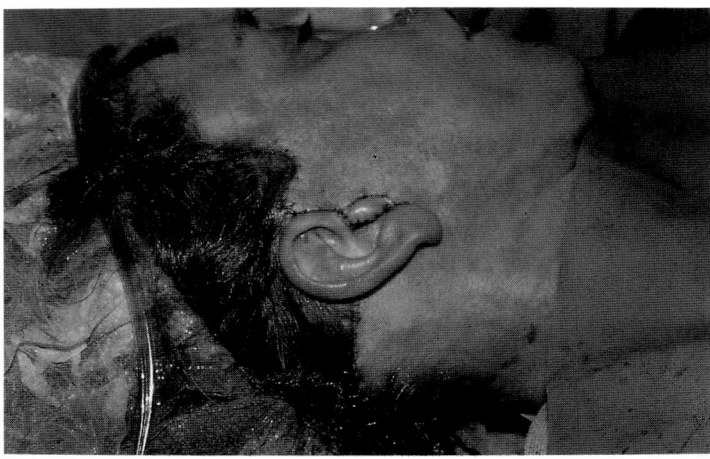

FIGURE 10.94. The tragal flap is trimmed to allow for a 1 to 2 mm excess of skin. The incision line is placed slightly posterior to the crest of the tragus so that the suture line will be camouflaged. Excess skin is provided to avoid anterior displacement of the tragus during subsequent scar contraction.

placed on the crest of the tragus. This incision line is closed with interrupted sutures of 5.0 cat-gut suture. The appearance of the external ear both at the tragus and the lobule will be slightly abnormal at the conclusion of the procedure (Figure 10.94). Subsequent scar contracture will provide an excellent long-term result.

Retroauricular Sulcus

The closure is completed by suturing the vertical portion of the retroauricular skin flap to the retroauricular sulcus. The flap is trimmed with a small V at the juncture of the horizontal and vertical incisions as the flap abuts the external ear posteriorly (Figures 10.95 and 10.96). This broken-line closure of the postauricular incision will decrease the likelihood of scar contracture over the retroauricular sulcus. A length of 1 to 2 cm is left unsutured at the superior portion of the flap as it attaches to the external ear (Figure 10.97). This provides an inconspicuous opening that can be used to evacuate any intraoperative or postoperative bleeding. Fresh blood or clots may be evacuated through this opening by the use of a small liposuction cannula or with gentle pressure being placed over the flap to direct the blood through this orifice. In addition to the postauricular openings, the sub mental incision may also be left unsutured to provide for an avenue of drainage. Some surgeons use a Jackson-Pratt drain during the first 24 to 48 hours. We have not found this to be necessary, since very little blood or serum should accumulate postoperatively if cautery has been sufficient. These suction drains add to cost and introduce a foreign body into the surgical site, which can be a nidus of infection.

Anesthesia for the second side should be administered 15 to 20 minutes prior to commencing surgery on that side. We prefer to administer this prior to the final trimming and suturing of the preauricular flap on the first side.

Postoperative Dressing

A large compression dressing is placed over the cheek and neck. It consists of sterile absorbent 12-inch cotton batting that overlies Telfa strips and Polysporin ointment on the lines of incision. The cotton batting is secured by 3 rolls of sterilized 4.5-inch Kerlix. Three rolls of 4-inch Coban bandages are then applied to provide light to moderate pressure to the surgical site. This dressing is carried onto the anterior cervical region as far as possible (Figure 10.98). If pressure is too tight over the hyoid bone, a vertical mid-line incision may be placed through the dressing.

Special attention should be paid to the ears to avoid excessive compression to the cartilage. Cotton or gauze is fashioned as a support and placed in the retroauricular sulcus to counteract any displacement of the cartilage. The dressing does not usually reach the inferior border of the

10. Facelift Surgery

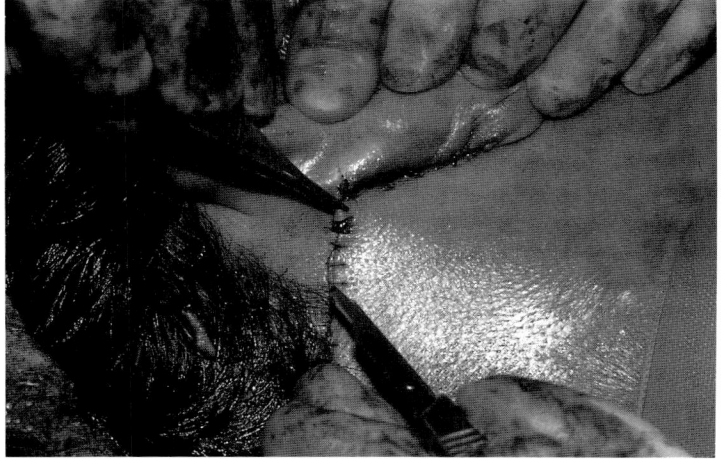

FIGURE 10.95. A V is excised from the retroauricular flap corresponding to that segment of skin which was created at the retroauricular sulcus during the initial incision.

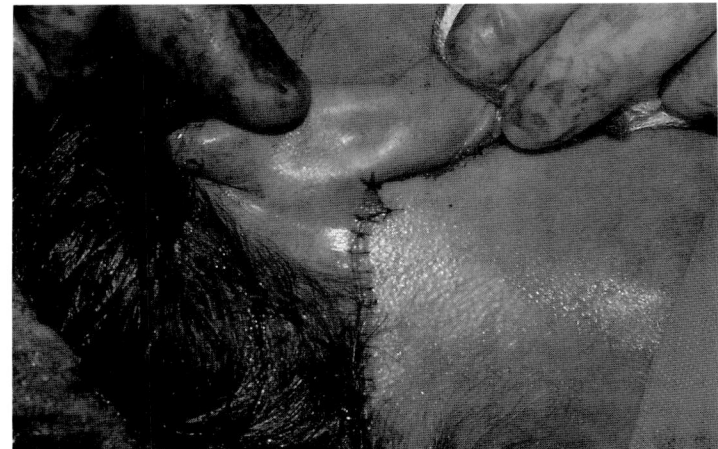

FIGURE 10.96. This broken line closure will avoid the formation of a contracture scar, which frequently occurs when an incision line crosses a concave surface.

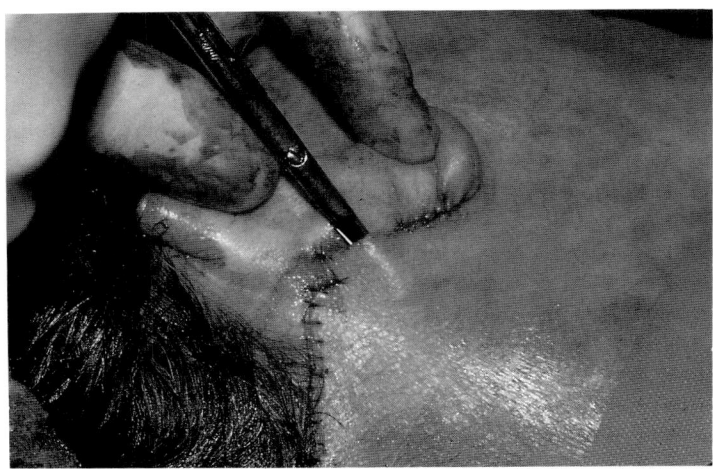

FIGURE 10.97. A length of flap measuring 1 to 2 cm is left unsutured at the superior portion of the flap as it attaches to the external ear. This provides an inconspicuous opening that can be used to evacuate blood.

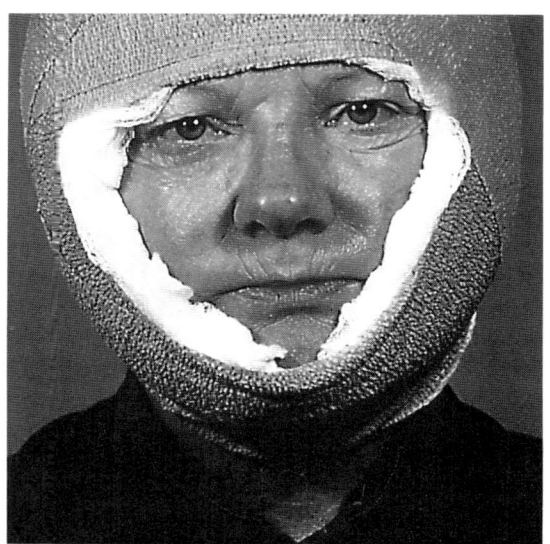

FIGURE 10.98. A large compression dressing consisting of sterile cotton batting Kerlix bandages and Coban dressings are applied to the surgical sites to provide moderate pressure. Support to the cartilage of the external ear should be provided with cotton batting in the retroauricular sulcus to prevent distortion which leads to considerable discomfort. This dressing is removed at the first postoperative day and reapplied for a second 24 hours.

undermined area in the lateral cervical region. Ecchymosis will usually form over this area and the inferior portion of the anterior cervical region. (To diminish the motion of the head and neck, the patient is encouraged not to talk or to eat a regular diet; a liquid diet that can be administered through a straw or a squeeze bottle is encouraged.) This dressing does not obstruct the view of the eyebrows or mouth, allowing the surgeon to evaluate the function of the temporal and marginal mandibular nerves, which may be areas of temporary paralysis as a result of infiltration of anesthesia. Although the flaps may not be readily viewed, they can be palpated through the anterior and posterior portions of this dressing. The dressing is removed the following morning and the patient is carefully examined. A similar dressing is reapplied for the second 24 hours to provide moderate compression and limitation of motion. This bulky dressing is advisable since many patients have minimal discomfort and may become too active, which can lead to bleeding. On the second postoperative day, the large dressing is replaced with a facial support garment, which is worn continuously for the following 12 days (Figures 10.99 and 10.100).

Postoperative Instructions

The immediate postoperative care consists of very limited activity, a liquid to soft diet, elevation of the head and chest on 2 pillows for the first 3 days, continuation of the perioperative antibiotics, and analgesics for relief of discomfort. The patient should have a responsible adult in attendance the first 24 hours so that if there is any need for assistance, advice, or transfer to the surgeon's office or hospital, this can be readily accomplished. (A list of the postoperative instructions is provided in Table 10.1).

Patients will experience mild to moderate discomfort primarily over the mastoid process and the sternocleidomastoid muscle where the plicating sutures have been anchored. This discomfort is usually relieved with the use of mild analgesics such as acetaminophen and codeine 0.5 grain or acetaminophen (Tylenol) in double-strength dosages. Because of the discomfort, large dressing, and need for elevation of the head, many patients have difficulty sleeping during the first 4 to 5 days. A mild hypnotic such as temazepan is provided. Refills on analgesics and hypnotics are not granted, to emphasize to the patient that minimal activity is important. Discomfort occurring after the fourth or fifth day is usually the result of overactivity. Most patients are up and about on the second day and can enjoy very limited activity. Following the first 48 hours, there is little likelihood that postoperative bleeding will occur, and activity may be liberalized to allow the patient to take short walks without raising the heart rate. Any exercise is strictly prohibited during these first 2 weeks.

The patient is seen daily for the first 2 postoperative days for dressing changes and evaluation. The patient returns on the fifth day for removal of the sutures in the areas that are visible, i.e., the temporal hair tuft, the pre-

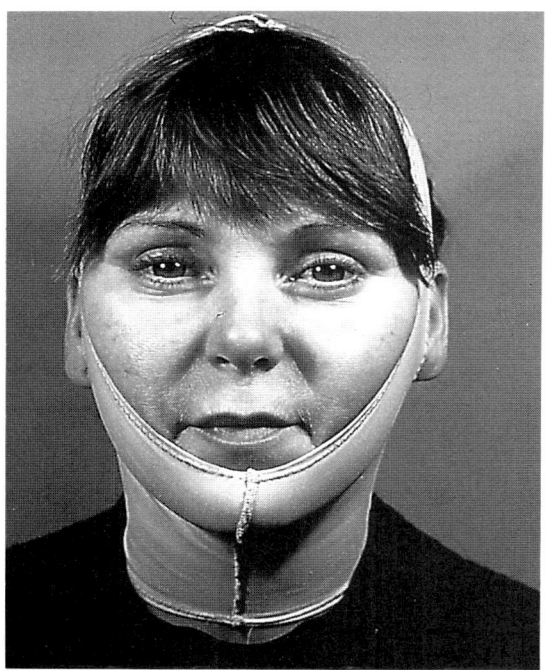
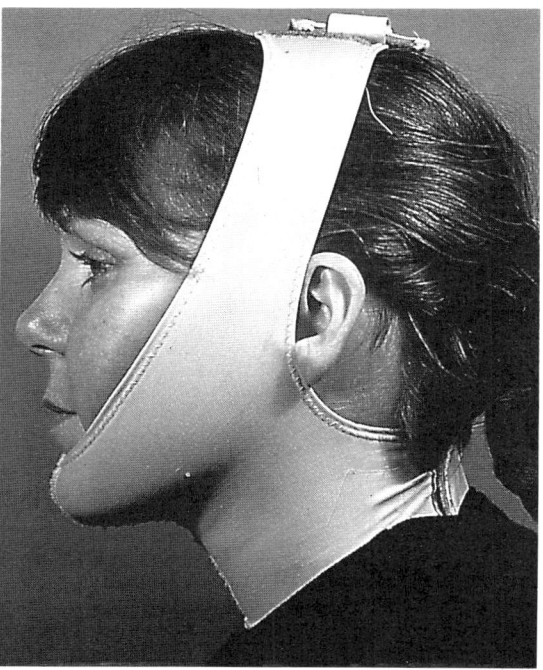

FIGURE 10.99. An elastic facial support garment is used continuously from the third to the fourteenth postoperative day to apply additional support. After returning to work the patient is encouraged to use the facial support garment while at home for the following three months.

FIGURE 10.100. The facial support garment provides moderate pressure to the anterior and lateral cervical regions, the cervical mental angle and to the preauricular and temporal regions, all of which were undermined. Since the maturation of a scar takes many months to be completed the use of the garment for the first three months while at home will improve long term results.

tragal region, and the preauricular area. On the seventh day, half the staples are removed, along with the sutures in the retroauricular sulcus. Patients are asked to remain in the local vicinity for the first 5 days.

During the second week, patients are not required to remain in the local vicinity, and activity is liberalized, allowing them to have limited activity and travel. This is a good opportunity for them to spend a sedentary week away from work and physical activity. They are instructed not to drive during the first 2 weeks, in order to avoid excessive motion of the head and neck. The patient may drive on the postoperative visit of the 14th day at which the remainder of the staples are removed.

It is expected that edema and ecchymosis will occur in areas of the liposuction and flap creation. Ecchymosis of the anterior cervical region is usually increased if the patient has a considerable amount of fat that must be suctioned since it is difficult to place a compression dressing on this area. A similar situation occurs in the inferior portion of the lateral cervical flap that lies over the middle and inferior portions of the sternocleidomastoid muscle. The plicating sutures will cause temporary distortion of the cervicomental angle, the mandibular outline, and the preauricular area. The patient's face will appear drawn tight during the first week; this gradually diminishes over the following 2 weeks.

Hypesthesia is expected over all areas of flap creation and regions that have undergone liposuction. The areas of liposuction should regain normal sensation within the ensuing 2 to 4 months. However, areas that have been undermined by sharp dissection will probably have permanently altered sensation, although most patients are unaware of this subtle change. Hypesthesia in the preauricular area will be appreciated by some patients during the immediate postoperative phase, requiring explanation and reassurance by the surgeon.

Although some surgeons allow their patients to return to work and normal activity at 1 week, we do not recommend this regime. Most of the ecchymosis and edema will have subsided by the end of 2 weeks; but patients in contact with the public will usually require 3 weeks before the ecchymosis and edema are resolved and the contour is close to that of a final result. At 3 weeks a casual observer would not be aware of the patient's recent surgery, although subtle changes will still be apparent to the patient. Edema will persist for 3 to 4 months.

Side Effects and Complications

Edema, ecchymosis, hypesthesia, and contour distortion are expected events following a rhytidectomy. These should all resolve spontaneously, with the exception of the subtle sensory changes in a flap that has been created by sharp dissection.

Postoperative Bleeding

Bleeding is the most common postoperative complication and is usually minor in extent. The most common site is the inferior portion of the flap overlying the sternocleidomastoid muscle or the retroauricular area overlying the mastoid bone. Most bleeding is less than 10 cc in amount and can be readily expressed through the retroauricular opening by applying gentle pressure with the hand. If the blood is no longer liquid and has clotted, extraction using a 4 mm liposuction cannula or a 16-gauge needle on a 5 or 10 cc syringe is quite effective. If other sites are involved and it is impossible to reach the area from this opening with a liposuction cannula, several sutures may be cut in the temporal or preauricular flap, or the submental incision may be reopened to allow introduction of the cannula. It is extremely rare following the expression of the liquid blood or clot that bleeding will recur and require further evacuation. Inspection with the flap open to allow for additional cautery is very rare but may be necessary in some patients. Following the evacuation of the blood, a compression dressing applying moderate pressure should be reapplied and the patient reexamined within a reasonable time period. Early postoperative bleeding is usually the result of vasodilatation following the cessation of the epinephrine effect on the vascular tree. It may also be caused by overactivity of the patient.

Late bleeding occurring during the second week may be caused by factors such as vomiting, overexertion, the consumption of alcohol, or bleeding and lifting. Any activity that will create a Valsalva maneuver is likely to produce bleeding. Evacuation of any palpable clot is important to avoid the weeks of induration and distortion that occur during the natural organization of the clot. Ultrasonic treatments can assist in resolution of these organizing clots.

Nerve Damage

Although it is uncommon, nerve damage is the most feared complication, since it can lead to permanent disability and deformity. In the procedure explained, there are 4 nerves that are susceptible to damage. These are the marginal mandibular nerve, the temporal branch of the facial nerve, the great auricular nerve, and the lesser occipital nerve. Other nerves that may be affected when more extensive undermining is used are the zygomatic and buccal branches of the facial nerve and the spinal accessory nerve.

Since the introduction of liposuction, the marginal mandibular nerve is probably the most susceptible to damage. As the cannula passes over the platysma in the area of the mandibular ramus, this nerve may be injured, resulting in a temporary paralysis of the depressor muscles of the lower lip. Duration of motor dysfunction varies but can last up to 3 or 4 months, during which time this weakness will prevent patients from pursing their lips and accomplishing normal articulation. Since liposuction involves blunt dissection, the patient can be assured that this defect will be temporary. The marginal mandibular nerve exits from the parotid gland near the angle of the jaw and overlies the masseter muscle. Along the mandibular ramus it is vulnerable to injury, since it is covered only by skin, subcutaneous fat, and the platysma muscle. This is a highly variable muscle that may be very thin and, in some people, totally absent.

The temporal branch of the facial nerve traverses an area that is centered over a line from the inferior border of the tragus to the lateral aspect of the eyebrow (Figure. 10.26). Careful attention should be taken when undermining the temporal flap in this area. The undermining should be immediately below the follicles of the temporal hair tuft and then brought to a very superficial level as the dissection advances anteriorly to avoid injury to this nerve. The temporal branch of the facial nerve is at its greatest risk as it crosses the zygomatic arch. The approximate location of the nerve can be identified by drawing a line from 0.5 cm below the tragus to a point 1.5 to 2.0 cm above the lateral aspect of the eyebrow. Alternately, the point of greatest vulnerability lies between a superior line that connects the superior border of the tragus to the most superior wrinkle on the forehead and an inferior line from the superior border of the earlobe to the lateral aspect of the eyebrow.[28]

The temporal nerve enervates the frontalis muscle, which, if injured, will prevent elevation of the eyebrow and affect normal animation of the forehead. The absence of wrinkling on one side of the forehead and an eyebrow that is displaced inferiorly are the clinical signs of frontalis muscle paralysis. It is not uncommon for this nerve to be affected with the infiltration of the operative anesthetic. When Xylocaine is combined with epinephrine, which is the recommended method, there may be temporary paralysis for up to 6 or 8 hours. This will cause concern to the surgeon until the normal muscle function is apparent on the following morning. A similar condition can exist in the muscles enervated by the marginal mandibular nerve.

The great auricular nerve may be injured as it passes along the anterior border of the sternocleidomastoid muscle. Because of its superficial location, careful dissection is necessary over the anterior border of the middle third of this muscle. Another cause of injury is placement of the plicating sutures into the anterior border of the sternocleidomastoid to elevate the platysma. This will usually result in only a temporary injury to the nerve, with full recovery expected. Cautery is usually not necessary in this area and, therefore, is not the usual cause for nerve damage. The great auricular nerve exits from the posterior border of the mid-portion of the sternocleidomastoid muscle and courses anteriorly and superiorly on the body of this muscle toward the external ear. It lies underneath the fascia of the muscle and is protected unless the fascia and the fibers of the muscle are interrupted during dissection. Its location can also be identified by its parallel and posterior position to the external jugular vein.[29] This nerve provides sensory perception for the skin of the inferior third of the external ear, lateral neck, angle of the jaw, and the postauricular region.

The lesser occipital nerve also emerges from the posterior border of the sternocleidomastoid muscle, which it parallels as it courses superiorly to enervate the neck and the scalp skin posterior to the external ear.

The zygomatic branch of the facial nerve may be injured if sharp dissection is extended along the zygomatic arch. The buccal branches of the facial nerve may also be severed if the dissection is extended to the oral commissure. The described method above does not create a flap that extends into either of these two regions, so injury to these two nerves should not occur.

The spinal accessory nerve is the remaining motor nerve that can suffer injury during facelift surgery. It is found in the posterior cervical triangle, where it exits the mid-position of the posterior border of the sternocleidomastoid muscle then passes inferiorly and posteriorly and enters the trapezius muscle. The nerve is exposed in this triangle and can be damaged, resulting in a weakness of the trapezius muscle leading to chronic aching of the shoulders, paresthesia of the arm, shoulder drop, and an inability to abduct the shoulder to more than

80°. This will present as a flaring of the wing of the scapula.

Infection

With proper sterile technique and the use of preoperative, intraoperative, and postoperative antibiotics, this is an exceedingly rare complication.

Skin Necrosis

Necrosis of the skin flap is rare but, when present in the preauricular area, can be cosmetically devastating. Smokers are believed by some to be at high risk for this complication because of their impaired vascular flow. The greatest length of the flap is at the retroauricular site where the horizontal and vertical incisions meet in the retroauricular sulcus. In addition, this skin is usually thin and placed under the greatest amount of tension in order to improve the cervicomental angle to the greatest extent. It is this area that is most susceptible to postoperative ischemia and subsequent scarring. When capillary filling is absent in this region, the sutures in the horizontal incision should be removed to decrease tension on the flap.

A spread horizontal scar in this area can be readily corrected postoperatively, as opposed to a linear vertical scar that has its origin at the horizontal incision line and extends inferiorly down the retroauricular flap. A vertical scar in this region is exceedingly difficult to correct and will always leave a visible scar, even when the correction has been successful. A full-thickness skin slough occurring in the preauricular flap is extremely rare but disastrous when it occurs. This can be the result of excessive tension placed on the anterior flap, overzealous thinning of the flap resulting in damage of the dermal capillary plexus, and unrecognized postoperative hematoma placing excessive tension on the flap. Using the method described above, we have never experienced this complication. If the involved area is moderate to large in size, correction of this defect is impossible. When small and adjacent to the preauricular incision, expanders may help to remove the scar.

Alopecia

Alopecia can result from undermining the flap at a level superficial to the hair follicles. This can occur in either the temporal flap or the retroauricular flap. Since the follicles are readily visualized when the flap is raised, this would be an uncommon complication. By contrast, the common absence of hair in the temporal tuft occurs when surgeons extend the vertical preauricular incision superiorly into the temporal area without preserving any of the temporal tuft of hair. In our experience, this is the most common method used by surgeons who perform rhytidectomy. Since the method described above will eliminate this cosmetic alteration, avoidance of this result merely requires appropriate planning. Temporary alopecia resulting from anagen effluvium caused by a compromise of the vascular supply is theoretically possible.

Abnormal Scarring

Hypertrophic scarring can occur, particularly in areas where the flap is placed under increased tension, such as the horizontal retroauricular scar. Since this area is covered by hair, a spread or elevated scar does not create the cosmetic defect that would occur if these changes were visible in the preauricular area. By avoiding any tension in the preauricular and lower temporal regions, the likelihood of hypertrophic scarring is decreased markedly and the occurrence of a spread scar is unlikely. An elevated band of scar can occur where the retroauricular scar crosses the sulcus. The method described diminishes the likelihood of this scarring.

Contour Irregularities

Irregular contouring and ridging can result from placing too few plication sutures to create a flat surface. A sufficient number of these sutures must be present over the preauricular area to avoid elevations and depressions. Inappropriate liposuction, particularly when a large caliber cannula is used, can occur over the jowl and preauricular area. Correction of this defect should be attempted with the use of lipotransfer, although results may be limited.

Intractable Pain

Postoperative pain of long duration is very uncommon and usually subsides within 6 months. Rees reports 2 cases in his extensive experience.[30] Both patients were judged to be disappointed with their cosmetic results, although the surgeon found the results to be excellent. No reasonable explanation could be found for this discomfort. Conway has encountered a similar case and suggests either trauma or surgical resection of the branches of the cervical sensory nerves as a potential cause.[31] Theoretically, these nerves may be severed as they exit from the posterior border of the sternocleidomastoid muscle.

Suture Extrusion

Rarely, the buried permanent sutures used for plication will extrude. We have had 2 cases over the past 20 years. A 57-year-old male presented with crusted keratotic lesions in the right preauricular area. The visit was 25 months after his rhytidectomy. He stated that he had noted inflammatory papules 3 months earlier. The inflammatory response continued and increased in size. The patient presumed that these were malignant lesions and was fearful of the diagnosis; consequently, he delayed medical examination. Because they were linear in nature and in the area that the plicating sutures were placed, a presumptive diagnosis of inflammatory response secondary to extrusion of permanently buried sutures was made. With further examination the sutures were found at the base of each of the 3 inflammatory and keratotic lesions. These were removed and a topical antibiotic was applied. The patient developed no perceptible scarring and has not experienced any more extrusion of sutures in the ensuing 4 years.

Postoperative Results

The following figures are of patients on whom we have performed the above described rhytidectomy (Figures 10.101A–D through 10.104A–D).

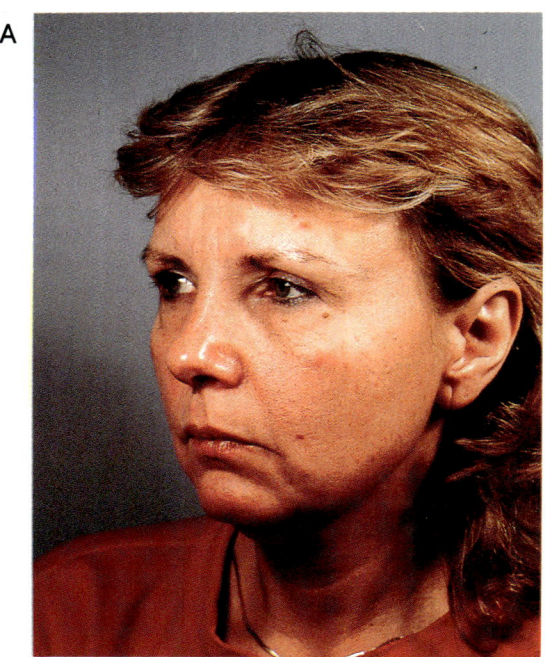

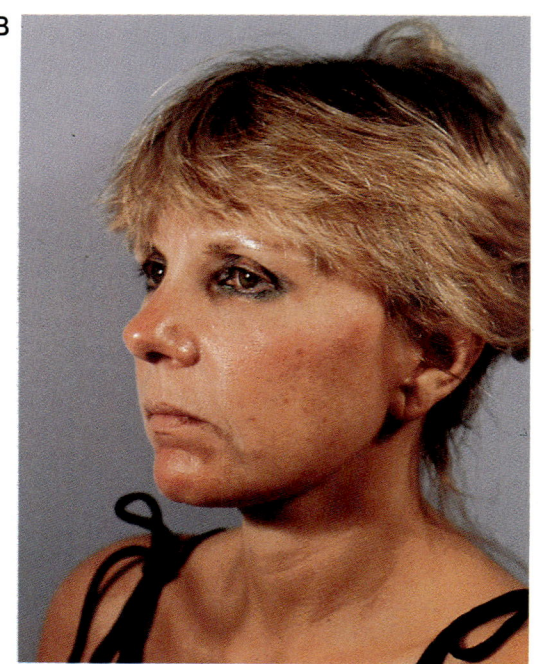

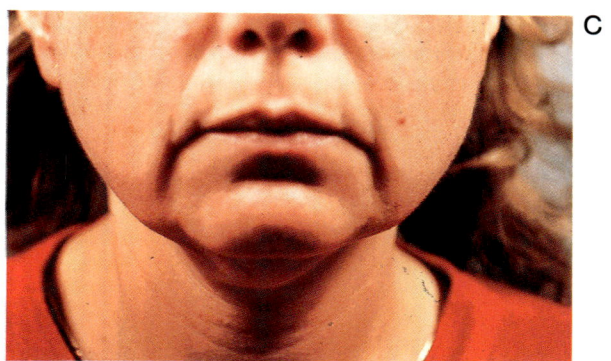

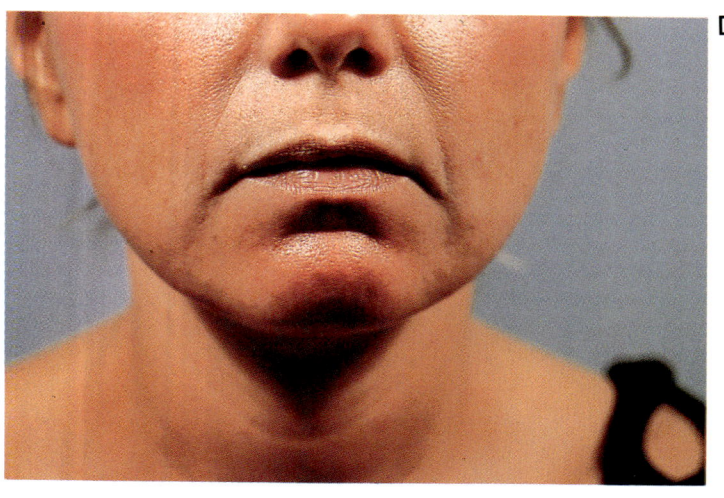

FIGURE 10.101. This patient is 44 years old. A and C are preoperative views. B and D are six month postoperative views.

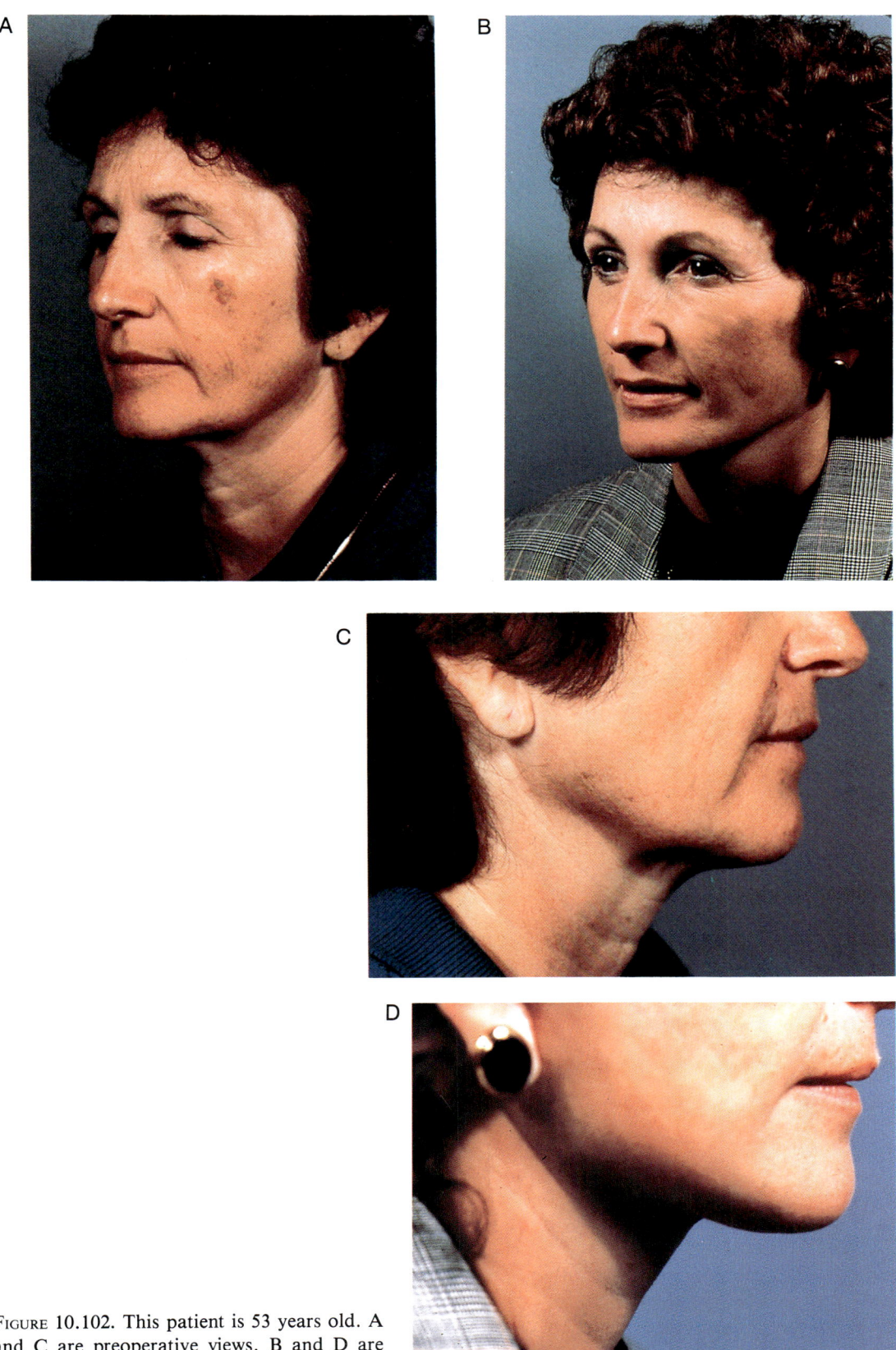

FIGURE 10.102. This patient is 53 years old. A and C are preoperative views. B and D are postoperative views.

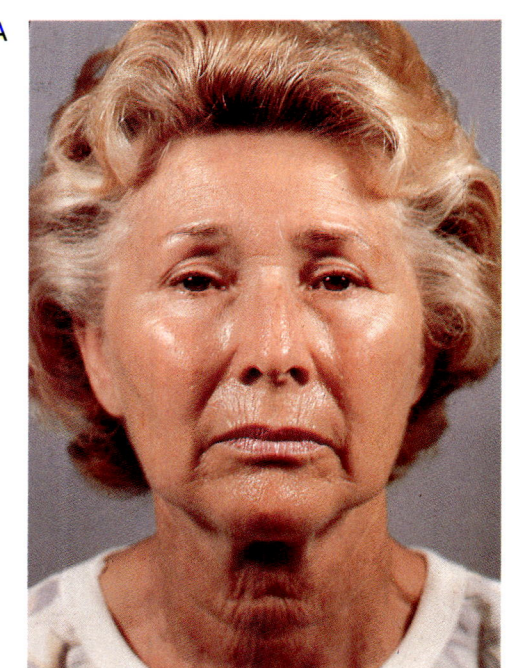
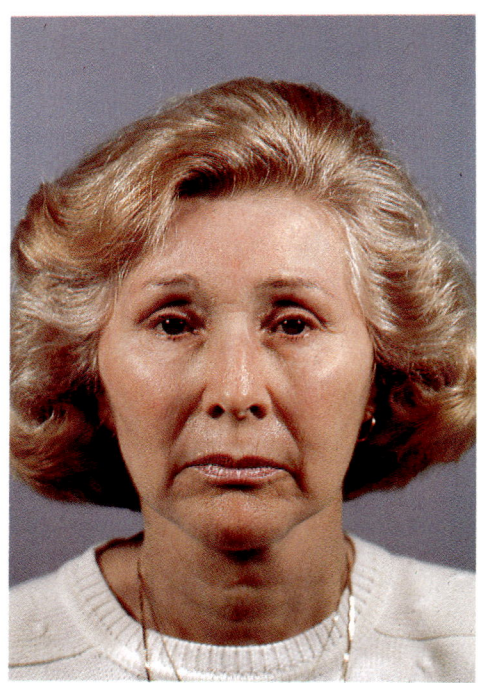
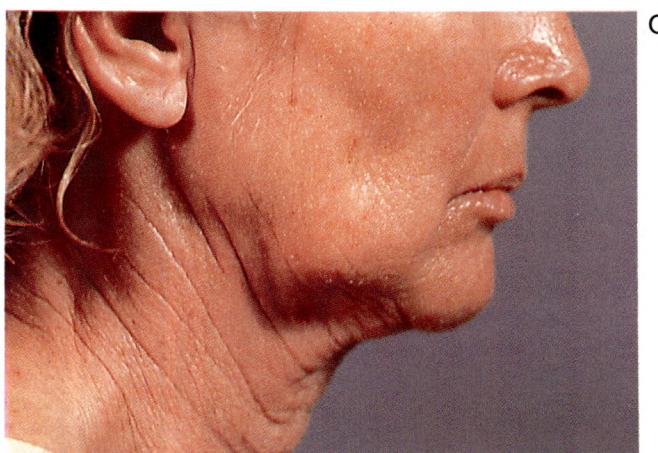
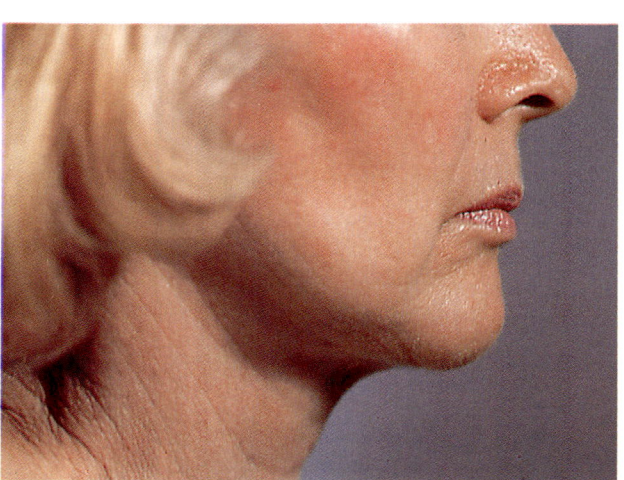

FIGURE 10.103. This patient is 63 years old. A and C are preoperative views. B and D are 12 month postoperative views.

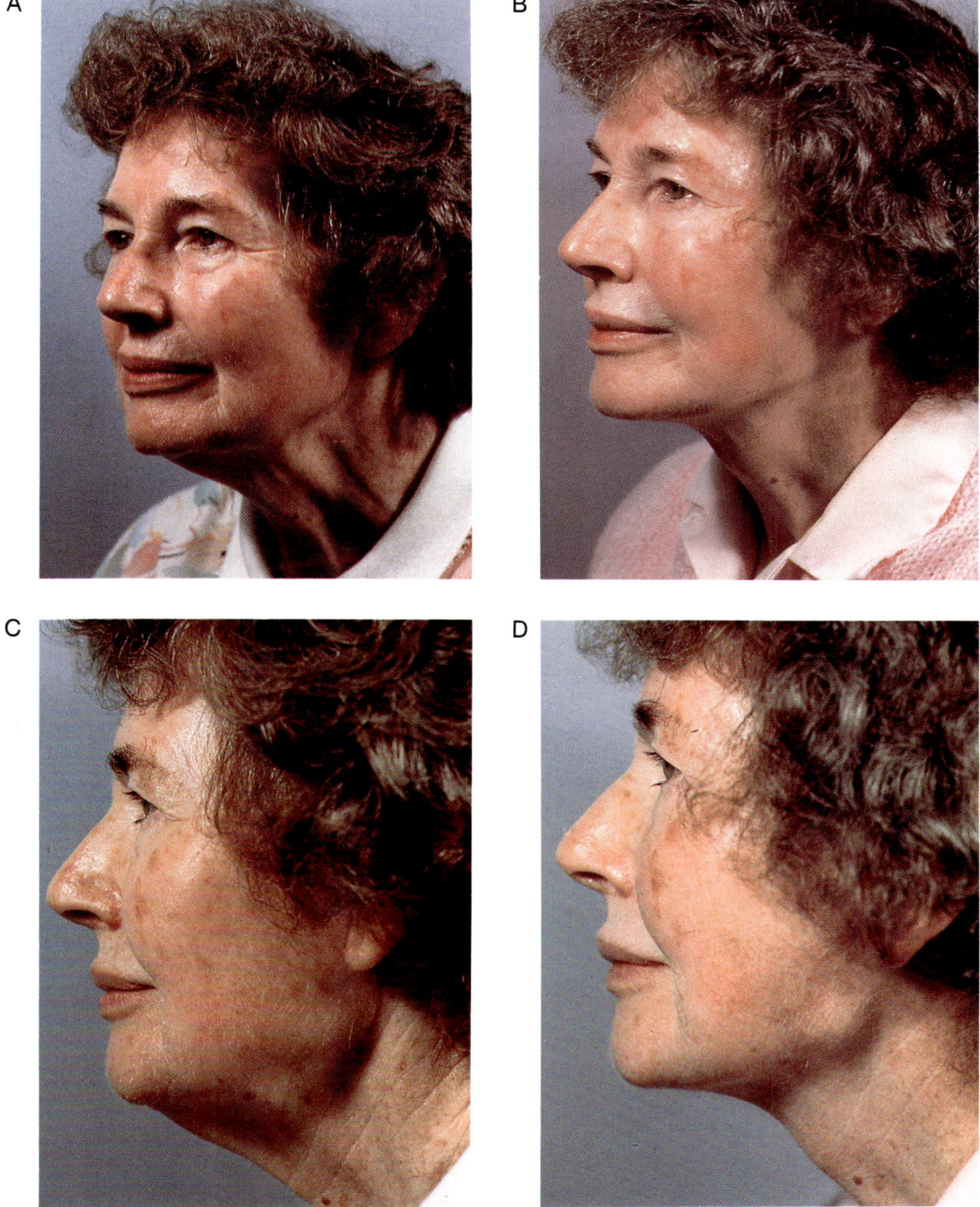

FIGURE 10.104. This patient is 73 years old. A and C are preoperative views. B and D are 15 month postoperative views.

References

1. Noel A. *La Chirurgie Esthetique, Son Role Social.* Masson & Cie, Paris, 1926.
2. Noel A. *La Chirurgie Esthetique.* Thiron & Cie, Clermont (Oise). 1928.
3. Passot R. La chirurgie esthetique des rides du visage. Presse Med. 1919; 27:258.
4. Joseph J. Plastic operation on protruding cheek. Dtsch Med Wochenschr. 1921; 47:287.
5. Lexer E. *Die Gesamte Wiederherstellungs-Chirurgie,* Vols. 1 and 2. Johann Ambrosius Barth, Leipzig, 1931.
6. Bames HO. Truth and fallacies of face peeling and face lifting, MJ & Rec. 1927; 126:86.
7. Bettman AG. Plastic and cosmetic surgery of the face. Northwest Med. 1920; 19:205.
8. Booth FA. Cosmetic surgery of face, neck and breast. Northwest Med. 1922; 21:170.
9. Bourguet J. La disparition chirurgicale des rides et plis du visage. Bull Acad Med Paris. 1919; 82:183.
10. Lagarde M. Cirurgie estetique du visage. Cron Med Lima. 1921; 38:321.
11. Hunt H L. *Plastic Surgery of the Head, Face and Neck.* Lea & Febiger, Philadelphia, 1926.
12. Miller CC. *Cosmetic Surgery,* 2nd ed. Oak Printing and Publishing Co., Chicago, 1906, 1908.
13. Stein RO. New methods in cosmetic face lifting (face tightening). Wein Klin Wochenschr. 1927; 4:83.
14. Wright MR. Psychological evaluation of a cosmetic surgical patient. In: *Cosmetic Surgery of the Skin: Principles and Techniques,* WP Coleman, CW Hanke, TH Alt, S Asken, eds. B.C. Decker, Philadelphia, 1991, pp. 373-397.
15. Lewis CM. Should face lifts be performed before the age of 40? Aesthet Plast Surg. 1985;9:47.
16. Webster R, Davidson T, White M. Conservative facelift surgery. Arch Laryngol. 1976; 102:657-662.
17. Webster R, Smith R, Smith K. Facelift, part I: extent of undermining of skin flaps. Head Neck Surg. 1983; 5(6):525-534.
18. Webster R, Smith R, Smith K. Facelift, part II: etiology of platysmal cords and its relationship to treatment. Head Neck Surg. 1983; 6(1): 590-595.
19. Webster R, Smith R, Smith K. Facelift, part III: plication of the superficial musculaoponeurotic system. Head Neck Surg. 1983;6(2):696-701.
20. Webster R, Smith R, Smith K. Facelift, part IV: use of superficial musculoaponeurotic system suspending sutures. Head Neck Surg. 1984; 6(3):780-791.
21. Webster R, Smith R, Smith K. Facelift, part V: suspending sutures for platysma cords. Head Neck Surg. 1984; 6(4):870-879.
22. Webster RC, Hamdan US, Smith RC. The considered and considerate facelift. Part I: conservative underminding, role of limited redraping, and choice of direction of pull. Am J Cosmet Surg. 1985; 2(3):1.
23. Webster RC, Hamdan US, Smith RC. The considered and considerate facelift. Part II: SMAS plication vs imbrication, theory of SMAS anatomy and dynamics, and conservation of platysma. Am J Cosmet Surg. 1985;2(4):65.
24. Webster RC, Beeson WH, McCollough EG. *Facelift in Aesthetic Surgery of the Aging Face.* Beeson and McCollough eds. C.V. Mosby Company, 1986, pp. 71-128.
25. Aufricht G. Surgery for excessive skin of the face. In: Transactions of the Second Congress of the International Society of Plastic Surgeons. A.B Wallace, ed., Williams & Wilkins, Baltimore, Maryland 1961.
26. Mitz D, Peyronie M. The superficial musculo aponeurotic system (SMAS) in the carotid and cheek area. Plast Reconstr Surg. 1976; 58:80-88.
27. Asken S. The facelift-cervicofacial rhytidectomy. In: *Cosmetic Surgery of the Skin: Principles and Techniques,* WP Coleman, CW Hanke, TH Alt, S Asken, eds. B.C. Decker, Philadelphia, 1991, pp. 335-354.
28. Pitanguy I, Ramos, AS. The frontal branch of the facial nerve: The importance of its variations in face lifting. Plast Reconstr Surg. 1966; 38:352.
29. Salasche SJ, Bernstein G, Senkarik M. *Surgical Anatomy of the Skin.* Appleton and Lange, Norwalk, 1988.
30. Rees TD. Facelift. In: *Cosmetic Facial Surgery,* TD Rees, Wood-Smith, eds. WB Saunders, Philadelphia, 1973, pp. 134-212.
31. Conway H. Factors underlying prolonged pain following rhytidectomy. Transactions of the 4th International Congress of Plastic and Reconstructive Surgery. Excerpta Medica Foundation, Amsterdam, the Netherlands, 1969, pp. 1120-1122.

11
Blepharoplasty

Laurence M. David and Sterling S. Baker

Blepharoplasty is performed for either functional or cosmetic reasons or a combination of these. Relatively few blepharoplasties are performed because of aging alone. Genetics does not always deliver the pleasing appearance desired or the functional structure that is desirable. Blepharoplasty should be an attempt to restore normal structure. Even though many patients relate a history of having recently developed "eyebags," careful inspection of past photographs and family members, including their own children, speaks to a genetic origin and a long-time existence of their eyebags. Eyelid changes commonly related to aging are actually those of sun-induced skin degeneration, those related to gravitational effects on the face and brow, and those genetically predetermined.

Recent years have seen important changes in blepharoplasty. Popularization of the transconjunctival approach and the modification of technique to include lasers are ongoing and exciting changes. Our understanding of structural abnormality and our concepts of an acceptable surgical result are more sophisticated today than in the past. Our patients are also more sophisticated and more demanding than they once were. It is necessary that any surgeon attempting contemporary blepharoplasty have a thorough understanding of normal eyelid structure and the ability to effect those changes needed to restore normal structure.

Aesthetic Considerations

There was a time when blepharoplasty was little more than removing excess skin from the eyelid. For some patients this was all that was needed, and there was considerable improvement. But there was another large group of patients who did not do as well. With our present-day concepts, it is easily understood why the simple removal of skin from an eyelid does not improve the appearance of most people.

Patients seeking consultation for blepharoplasty frequently try to demonstrate what they want by pulling backward and upward with a finger placed laterally on the lower lid. Others will lift their eyebrows for the desired upper eyelid effect. While beauty is geography-, culture-, and gender-related, there must be a representation of the ideal eyelid for each patient. In other words, how do we want our patients to look after surgery? For the answer to this question we need only go to our neighborhood magazine stand and purchase a few of the many magazines devoted to the movie stars and "the beautiful people." Clip out pictures of these idols. Take only the most beautiful and the most handsome. You can even collect those stars of yesteryear, as most of the features are enduring. What you will find is that there are certain features that most of these male movie stars have in common, and a separate list of features that most of the female stars have in common, with reference to the eye and the surrounding areas. There is little that the men share with the women when it comes to eyes and eyelids. Let us take a close look at this "ideal" so that we can try to define those features considered desirable by our patients. These features are listed in Table 11.1. Again, it is important to realize that there are certain limitations of anatomy and certain considerations of culture and race that must be taken into account. But if you keep these features in mind, at least you will know where you want to go (and where you do not want to go) for the majority of Caucasian patients.

Figure 11.1 illustrates the heavy upper male eyelid with little or no lid showing. The brow is heavy and prominent. It is flat and almost horizontal. "Crow's feet," lower lid creases, and horizontal brow creases may also be prominent. Indeed, these features even add to a masculine appearance. The eyes themselves are not at all prominent. It is as if they yield to the surrounding structure.

In contrast, the female eye is very prominent, with a light and delicate appearance of the upper lid (see Figure 11.2). A well-defined upper lid crease having ample lid exposed provides a good platform for makeup application. Makeup can be seen even when the woman's eyes are opened widely. The crease is not more than one-third of the lash-to-brow distance up from the lash line (see Figure 11.3). Lateral creases and prominent lower lid creases are not as well tolerated as on her male counterpart. Her brow is high and arched. The center of the brow is the high point of the arch and is located on a vertical line drawn through the lateral limbus. More contemporary women frequently

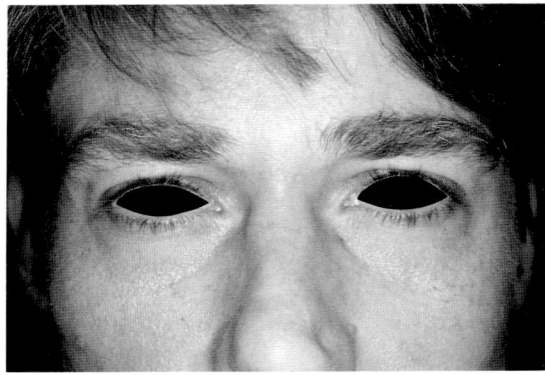

FIGURE 11.1. Prominent and flat eyebrows and heavy upper eyelids give a masculine appearance.

allow their brows to grow out thick and somewhat more prominent as compared to the beauties of yesterday (perhaps a contribution to the unisex look), but forehead creases are absent.

In neither male nor female are lower eyelid bulges with their accompanying shadows permitted. These shadows result from overhead lighting illuminating the top of the bulge but not the skin underneath. This gives a tired, dull, or "hangover" appearance, which is not attractive on either male or female. Figure 11.3 also illustrates the desired relationships between the various structures for the female. Note that the lower lid is elevated so that the central portion forms a tangent to, and is slightly above the inferior limbus, when the patient is in neutral gaze. Remember, nothing looks worse than a lower lid retracted below the inferior limbus.

You may conclude that upper lid blepharoplasty for the male patient is rarely performed for cosmetic purposes in our practices. This is

TABLE 11.1. Gender-related aesthetic considerations in eyelid surgery.

	Male	Female
Brow	Lower, heavier, flatter and more prominent	Higher, more arched, and less prominent
Upper eyelid	Heavier with little or no actual lid visible	Lighter and more delicately sculptured, with ample lid visible for makeup display
Lower eyelid	Creases are tolerated but not bulges or related shadows	Creases less tolerated, no bulges or shadows
Periorbital	Lateral creases are tolerated or even desirable	Lateral creases not well tolerated
Eyes	Not a prominent part of the face yielding to surrounding structures	Very prominent

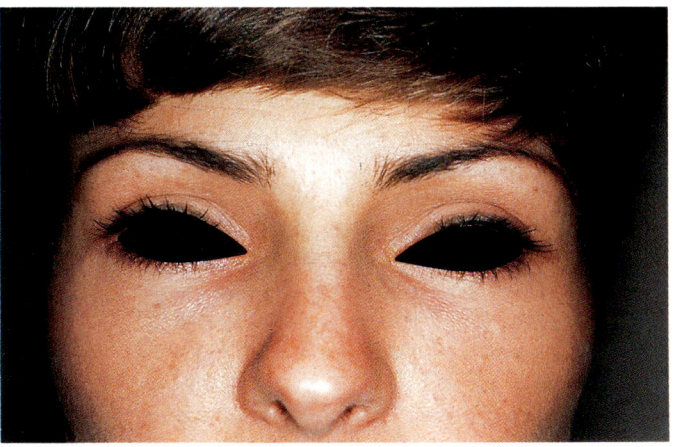

FIGURE 11.2. A prominent eye with delicate contours and high arched brow gives a feminine appearance.

correct. Almost all our upper lid cosmetic patients are women. Men are operated for lash ptosis or other functional reasons. Figure 11.4 shows a male patient after aggressive upper blepharoplasty. The resulting prominent upper eyelid and prominent eyes feminizes his appearance.

So, now that we have defined our "ideal normal," careful evaluation of our prospective patient and definition of his or her deviation from our ideal will allow us to develop a plan to restore normal structure, which we can now define as *beauty*.

Another important aesthetic consideration is the difference between quantity and quality problems. As an illustration, let us consider the patient with chronic sun exposure and wrinkles of the lower lids—otherwise structure of the lids is normal; there are no undesirable bulges or shadows. Excision of a portion of this skin will not only fail to solve the problem but will probably result in lower lid retraction to some degree. The error is the failure to recognize that wrinkles represent alterations of collagen and other elements located in the dermis. Removing a small portion of the skin does nothing to improve the quality of the remaining skin. Confusing a quality problem with a quantity

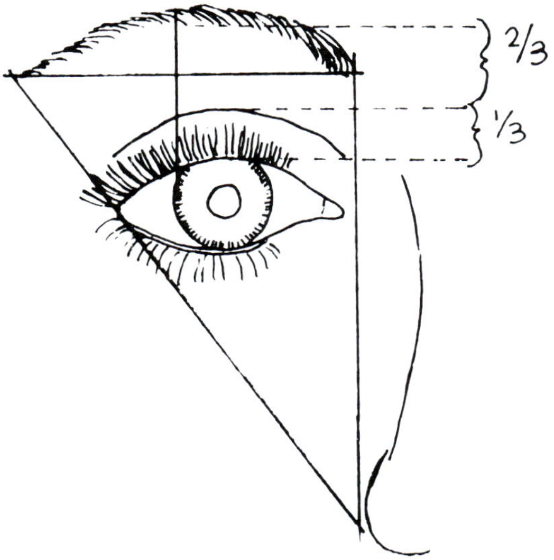

FIGURE 11.3. Topographical relationships of structure and the rule of one-third.

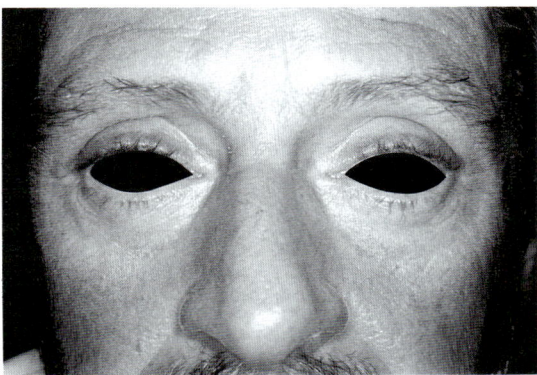

FIGURE 11.4. A male upper eyelid has been overcorrected to give a feminized appearance to the eyes.

solution dooms that solution to failure. Only those procedures designed to improve skin quality can help our patient. No resurfacing procedure involves skin excision. This illustration is a frequent and important reason for a poor cosmetic result.

If you keep in mind that wrinkling of the skin is a problem of poor skin quality and is not improved by cutting the skin, you will be well served. As surgeons we can only cut or remove skin, but we can not improve the quality of that skin. The patient who pulls lower eyelid skin to the sides and up must be told that surgery cannot, and will not, effect those changes. Whenever skin is excised from the lower eyelid, the lid is pulled down. Whenever skin is removed from the upper eyelid, the brow is pulled down.

We consider lower lid blepharoplasty to be a contouring procedure and not a skin procedure. By *contouring* we mean a surgery that designs a bed or platform to support skin. Skin is able to conform to the bed on which it lies and normally does not need to be excised. Considering the high incidence of resultant complications after lower lid surgery, it is hard to justify cutting lower lid skin for any reason other than for lateral canthotomy and tumor removal. In our considerable experience, providing a normal structure for the skin to lie on through transconjunctival fat removal almost always gives the best cosmetic result and only rarely leaves "excess" skin. This concept is difficult for those trained to other beliefs, but we advise that they try it and see for themselves.

Figures 11.5A and B illustrate the ability of lower lid skin to conform to the underlying muscle and fat bed. Even sun-damaged eyelid skin can do this, as can be seen in these photographs. Eyelid skin can do this very quickly, even older skin. It is rare in our experience to need skin excision after transconjunctival fat removal if adequate fat has been removed. Figures 11.6A and B show a

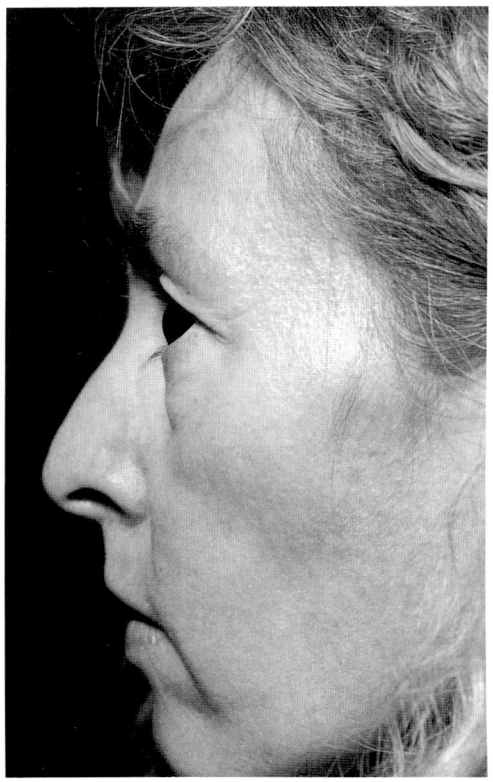
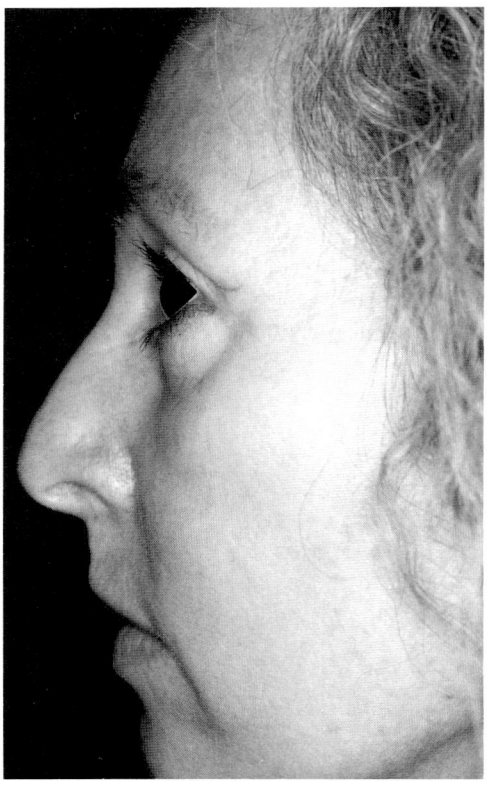

A   B

FIGURE 11.5. A. Before transconjunctival fat is removed. B. The skin of the lower eyelid will quickly conform to the bed created after fat removal.

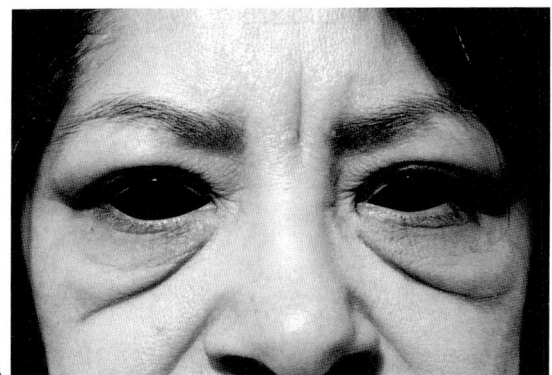 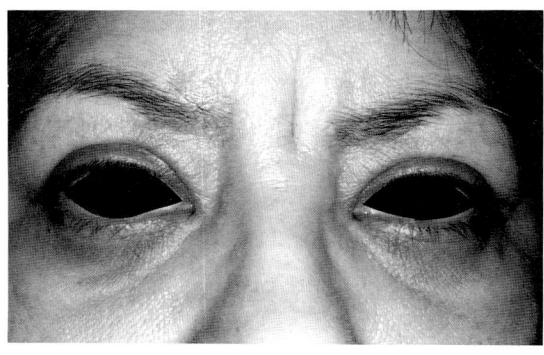

FIGURE 11.6. A. Before transconjunctival fat removal in a patient with obvious excess skin. B. After photo. No skin was removed.

patient who has "excess" skin. After transconjunctival fat removal, no skin was removed. For some patients several weeks may be required for the desired result, but given the complications of the alternative, it is worth the wait. If in the rare case there is remaining real excess or redundant skin, it can easily be directly and conservatively excised without lower eyelid retraction.

To reduce the aesthetics of eyelid surgery to a few simple rules is difficult, because it is not a simple matter. Indeed, it could be the subject of an entire volume. But let us try a few "rules of eye":

1. Upper blepharoplasty for men is often better left undone if cosmesis is the only consideration. Heaviness is not only acceptable but is often desirable.
2. Upper blepharoplasty for women should remove enough skin, muscle, and fat so that makeup can be applied to the lid and be seen even when the eye is widely open.
3. Lower blepharoplasty in both men and women should be limited to the removal of fat in order to prepare a proper bed on which the skin can lay. It should remove sufficient fat to eliminate bulges and the resultant shadows but must not remove enough to produce a hollowed-out appearance.
4. Wrinkles of the lower lid skin should never be surgically approached. Only resurfacing procedures can improve skin quality and remove wrinkles. Removing skin will pull the lid down.
5. Brow position is important and is sometimes preferred to blepharoplasty for upper eyelid cosmesis.
6. Nothing looks as bad as lower eyelid retraction. Do not trade shadows and bags for scleral show.
7. For every surgical complication there is a surgical correction that can result in a more serious complication.
8. Any surgery of the upper lid will pull the brow down to some degree. Any surgery of the lower lid will pull the lower lid down to some degree. An "eyelift" should not become an "eyedrop."

From the above discussion you can conclude that the surgeon must have several different procedures to offer. Upper eyelid blepharoplasty is a different operation from lower lid blepharoplasty, and men require different procedures than women. Add to those procedures a few brow, forehead, and reconstructive procedures, and it is easy to see how eyelid surgery has become a subspecialty requiring extra knowledge, training, and experience.

Surgical Anatomy

Knowledge of the eyelid anatomy is necessary for the blepharoplasty surgeon to achieve the desired cosmetic result. We will approach the anatomy in the order in which it is encountered during surgery. Upper and lower lids will be

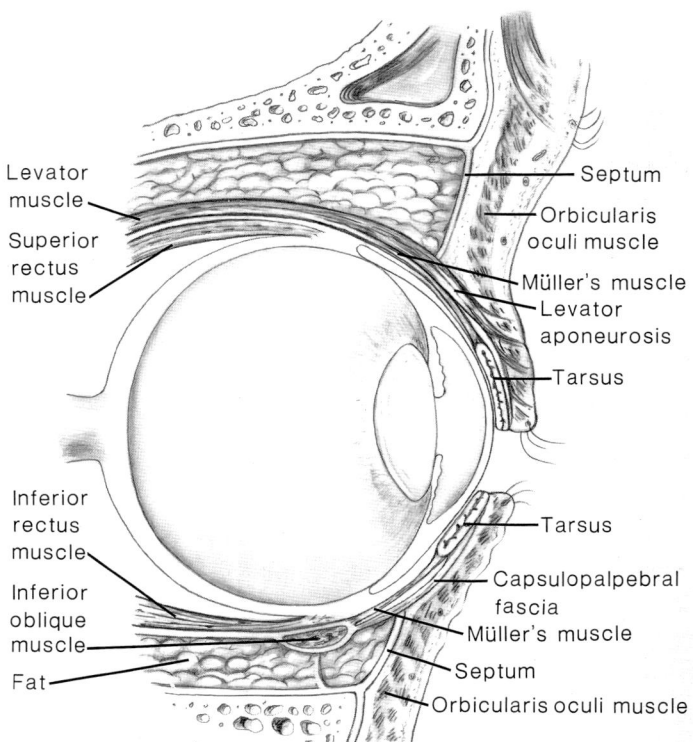

FIGURE 11.7. Cross-section of the upper and lower lids.

discussed separately. Layers of the lids will be divided into anterior and posterior lamellae. This promotes an understanding of structure as well as function. A detailed cross-section of the lids is shown in Figure 11.7. Table 11.2 contains the layers of the upper lid.

TABLE 11.2. Layers of the upper lid.

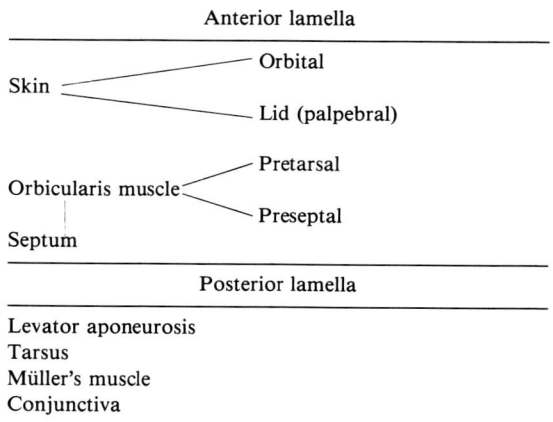

Upper Lid Skin

The orbital skin blends smoothly but perceptibly into the thin skin of the lid. The lid skin is among the thinnest in the body; it is comparatively devoid of fat. A guiding principle in lid surgery is to resect only the thin lid skin from areas that are mobilized during blinking (*i.e.*, above the lid margin). The incision, however, can be extended medially and laterally into the thick orbital skin to achieve optimal cosmetic results. Lid skin is fairly tightly attached to underlying orbicularis, especially in that portion adjacent to the lid margin and overlying the tarsal plate. Care should be taken to minimize the removal of this skin above the tarsus to avoid lid and lash eversion.

A near constant finding in non-Asians is a lid crease lying approximately 10 mm above the lashes at the lid apex. The lid crease roughly follows the upper edge of the tarsus and is produced by the insertion of an anterior division of the levator aponeurosis. Blepharoplasty closure should ideally be placed in the lid crease. This placement serves to minimize the cosmetic significance of the surgical scar, because the scar is concealed in the lid crease when the eye is open and because a normal blink is too rapid to reveal details in the lid crease during closure.

Orbicularis Muscle

Unlike the skin, the orbital orbicularis muscle (see Figure 11.8) blends imperceptibly into the palpebral orbicularis. Palpebral orbicularis can be further separated into the pretarsal portion adjacent to the lid margin and the preseptal portion superior to the tarsus. The orbicularis is well vascularized and is the chief source of bleeding encountered during surgery on the anterior lamella.

The palpebral orbicularis muscle is attached to the medial orbital wall, with the major attachment being adjacent to the medial canthal tendon. A physiologically important portion of the medial attachment is to the lacrimal sac, which lies deep to the medial canthus. The lacrimal pump is driven by this attachment. Laterally, the pretarsal orbicularis blends with the lateral canthal ligament in its attachment to the lateral orbital wall, while the preseptal orbicularis sweeps around the lateral orbital

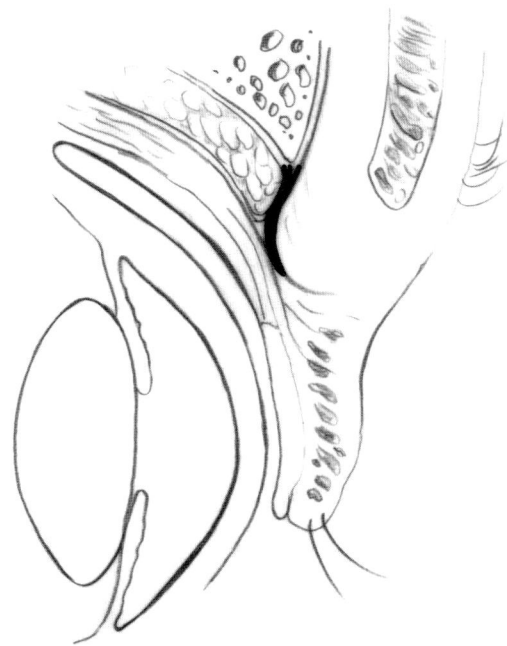

FIGURE 11.9. Septum orbitale—upper lid.

rim and blends with its counterpart from the lower lid. There is no distinct lateral raphe. The pretarsal orbicularis is tightly adherent to the tarsus, while the preseptal portion is loosely adherent to the septum. Normally, skin resected during blepharoplasty is from that overlying the septum and not the tarsus. The most easily found surgical plane in this area of the anterior lamella is between the orbicularis and the septum. Therefore, most blepharoplasties will include at least some preseptal orbicularis as part of the resected tissue.

Septum Orbitale

The septum is an avascular translucent structure separating the anterior and posterior lamellae (refer to Figure 11.9). It extends from an attachment at the superior bony orbital rim toward the tarsus, where it blends into the levator aponeurosis 6 to 10 mm above the tarsus. Immediately below the septum lies the preaponeurotic fat pad of distinctly yellow fat. During the surgical dissection, the fat pad

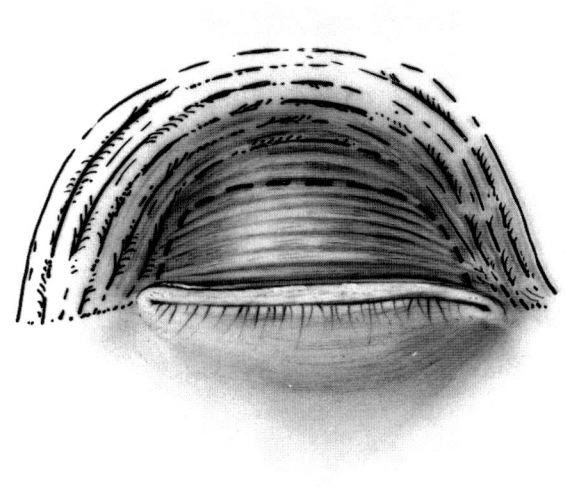

FIGURE 11.8. Orbicularis muscle—upper lid.

is located by closing the eyelid to put the septum on stretch and placing gentle digital pressure on the globe. The yellow fat is seen bulging through the septum at the mid-portion of the upper edge of the field. Medial to the preaponeurotic fat lies the nasal fat pad, which is white in comparison. Laterally lies the pinkish lacrimal gland, which may have a significant anterior prolapse. The septum is the most important anatomical landmark in the upper lid, because it can be used to identify the levator muscle and its aponeurosis. Damage to these structures can produce ptosis.

Levator Aponeurosis

The levator palpebral oricularis muscle lies in the superior orbit above the superior rectus muscle (see Figure 11.10). It originates at the orbital apex and extends anteriorly to the orbital outlet, where its muscular fibers fan out beneath the preaponeurotic fat pad to blend into the tendinous aponeurosis. The aponeurosis lies beneath the septum and has three major insertions: into the superior anterior tarsus; into the anterior tarsal fascia; and into the palpebral skin roughly overlying the superior margin of the tarsus and thereby creating the lid crease. Damage to the superior aponeurosis can be avoided by limiting deep dissections to the septum overlying the preaponeurotic fat pad, as described above. Another surgical landmark lying deep to the inferior edge of the aponeurosis is a transverse plexus of vessels 1 to 2 mm above the superior margin of the tarsus. These vessels are not normally seen in blepharoplasty surgery, which is presumptive evidence that the opaque aponeurosis overlying them is intact. During closure of the blepharoplasty wound, deep skin sutures passed through the aponeurosis will enhance reformation of the lid fold.

Tarsus

The tarsus is a relatively thick elastic tissue that extends horizontally across the lid margin. Its greatest vertical dimension is about 10 mm at the lid apex. The tarsus lies deep to structures encountered during blepharoplasty surgery but is an important landmark in establishing the lid crease. Significant removal of orbicularis and skin superficial to the tarsus is normally avoided in order to prevent lash and lid eversion.

Muller's Muscle

Muller's muscle is a thin layer of vertically oriented muscle fibers lying deep to the levator aponeurosis. Muller's muscle is enervated by the sympathetic system, and its function is to augment lid elevation. Its major significance is during preoperative evaluation to exclude Horner's Syndrome (unilateral pupillary miosis, ptosis, and facial anhidrosis).

Conjunctiva

The deepest layer of the lid is palpebral conjunctiva. This mucous membrane is a continuation of the bulbar conjunctiva. It has little significance in blepharoplasty surgery.

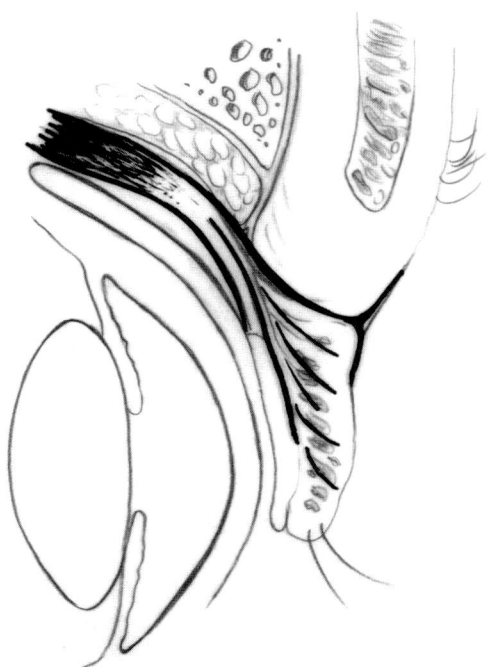

FIGURE 11.10. Levator palpebrae muscle and aponeurosis—upper lid.

Lower Lid

Table 11.3 contains the layers of the lower lid. The lower lid skin covers the entire lower lid, from the orbital rim to the lashes. This skin is thin and structurally similar to that found in the upper lid. It is usually tightly attached to the underlying orbicularis, especially that overlying the tarsus. While significant damage can occur to this skin from many causes, including aging and sun exposure, there is rarely the same degree of redundancy that can exist in the upper lids.

Vigorous excision of apparently excess skin during blepharoplasty can produce marked vertical shortening. From a cosmetic perspective, this vertical shortening, results at a minimum in an unpleasant rounding of the lateral canthal angle and, at its most florid expression, produces a frank ectropion that exposes mucosal surfaces. From a functional perspective, the lower lid is in a "tethered" position, which restricts complete lid closure during blinking. The resulting uneven distribution of tear film over the ocular surfaces can lead to exposure keratoconjuntivitis—a chronic, often debilitating, and sometimes sight-threatening complication.

Lower Lid Orbicularis Muscle

The orbicularis is divided into the pretarsal and preseptal portions. The lower lid tarsus is

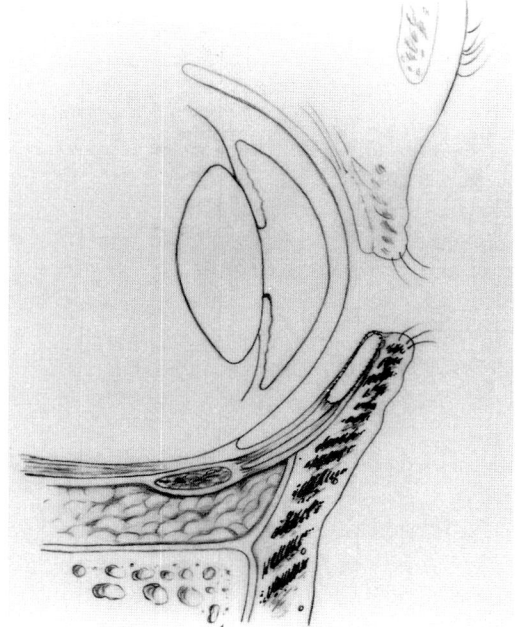

FIGURE 11.11. Orbicularis muscle—lower lid.

smaller than its upper lid counterpart. Therefore, most of the orbicularis in the lower lid is preseptal. The pretarsal muscle basically attaches with the medial and lateral canthal ligaments to the orbital walls, while the preseptal portion attaches medially to the orbital wall and laterally blends with the preseptal orbicularis of the upper lid. Thus, there is not an anatomically distinct lateral raphe (see Figure 11.11).

Septum Orbitale

The septum extends from the orbital rim to the lower margin of the tarsus (refer to Figure 11.12). It is avascular and translucent. Lower lid "bags" are produced by prolapsed orbital fat bulging the septum anteriorly. The external surgical approaches to blepharoplasty divides the septum horizontally. In the retroseptal transconjunctival approach to blepharoplasty, the septum is not transected. Closure of the septum as a separate layer should be avoided, since such an effort almost certainly produces a postoperative cicatricial ectropion.

TABLE 11.3. Layers of the lower lid.

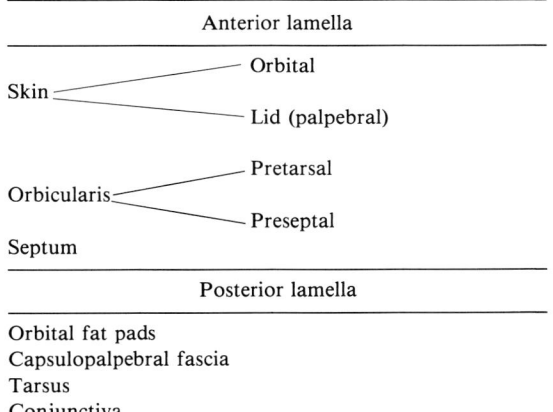

Orbital fat pads
Capsulopalpebral fascia
Tarsus
Conjunctiva

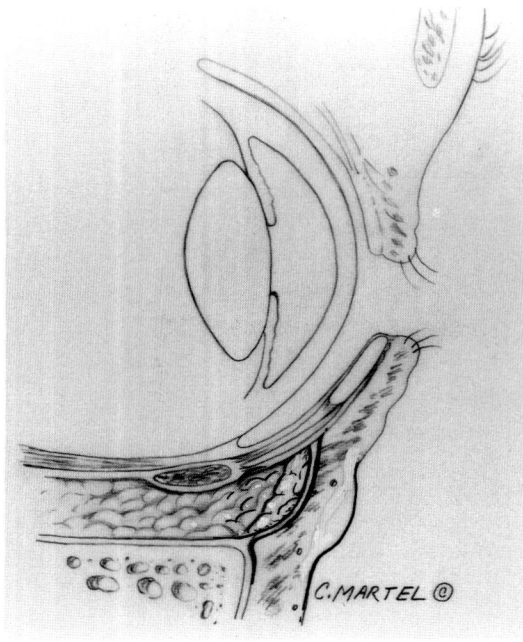

FIGURE 11.12. Septum orbitale – lower lid.

Posterior Lamella Lower Lid

The most important component of the posterior lamella in blepharoplasty is the orbital fat pads. The fat pads are separated into anatomically indistinct nasal, medial, and lateral groups. Removal of the prolapsed fat is the major goal of lower lid blepharoplasty. This fat is well vascularized, and care must be taken to achieve absolute hemostasis during its resection.

The most serious complication of blepharoplasty is blindness. The most probable cause of this complication is retrobulbar hemorrhage combined with postoperative edema to produce increased intraorbital pressures sufficient to occlude the central retinal artery. Vision should be routinely checked during the postoperative period in each eye separately to assure early and rapid recognition of this complication.

The capsulopalpebral fascia extends from the inferior rectus extraoccular muscle to the inferior border of the tarsus. It serves to retract the lower lid on down gaze and is analogous in function to the levator aponeurosis of the upper lid. There is no separate levator (or more logically retractor) muscle of the lower lid.

The tarsus of the lower lid is similar in structure and function to its counterpart in the upper lid. Both are elastic tissue, and both serve as horizontal stabilizers—the "ribs" of the eyelids. However, the lower lid tarsus is about 5 mm in its greatest vertical dimension, as compared to about 10 mm of greatest vertical height of the tarsus in the upper lid.

The deepest layer of the lower lid is the conjunctiva. This mucous membrane reflects off the globe and onto the lid in the inferior cul-de-sac. A prominent horizontal plexus of vessels occurs just to the lid side of the inferior cul-de-sac. Transconjunctival incisions for lower lid blepharoplasty should be placed toward the lid side of this plexus of vessels.

Upper Lid Blepharoplasty

Hooding of the upper lids can be both a cosmetic and functional disturbance that commonly prompts patients to seek consultation. A puffy, drooping appearance of the upper eyelids not only gives the patient a tired, sad appearance, it may also produce a worried one, as it causes horizontal furrowing of the forehead as the patient attempts to raise the eyelids out of the way. To a certain extent, this is an aging phenomenon, but there is certainly a genetic element involved, with quite young people being affected if their pedigree is not as kind as it could be.

Hooding, puffiness, heaviness, and drooping of the upper eyelids can be due to redundant skin, thick muscle, prolapsed orbital fat, or any combination of these factors. One or more of these structures may require alteration for an improved appearance.

Selection of patients who are appropriate while omitting those who are inappropriate along with intelligent preoperative planning are important to obtain a successful result. A good candidate for upper lid blepharoplasty is one who will be made happy by the restoration of normal structure and in whom you are able to alter structure toward normal. Keep in mind that our definition of *beauty* means "normal structure." This will usually be a patient who requires the removal of skin, muscle, fat, or some combination of these three elements.

Brow position and its role in the deviation from normal upper lid structure must be considered. Keep in mind that the male brow can be lower and not arched, while the female brow should be higher and arched.

True blepharoptosis will not be corrected by skin excision but requires shortening of the levator aponeurosis or Muller's muscle.[1,2] One should test for this preoperatively by lifting the brows to the normal position and noting the position of the upper eyelid margin. Normally, they should lie 1 to 2 mm below the upper limbus.

Evaluate the prospective patient for medical conditions, such as thyroid disease, and for ophthalmologic disease, which might interfere with surgery. Visual acuity is tested to establish a baseline for comparison postoperatively. Internal medical or ophthalmologic consultation is sometimes recommended. Check for medications, particularly for anticoagulants such as aspirin or ibuprofen, which will increase hemorrhage and bruising. These medications should be discontinued at least 2 weeks before surgery. Table 11.4 is the list of medications we give to our patients that are to be avoided for at least 2 weeks before surgery. Be sure to go over the specific possible complications of blepharoplasty. Table 11.5 is the consent form that we use for blepharoplasty patients.

Preoperative photography is always performed with the patient sitting. Views should include frontal, with upward and downward gaze, and in neutral position, as well as oblique and lateral. Mark the lower incision lines with the patient in the sitting position and the eyes closed. Whenever possible, follow a natural crease. For some patients, this is not possible. The upper line of excision is marked with the patient laying down and is usually the easier line to decide on. Fine-tip surgical markers are helpful. Thicker markers tend to smear during prep or during lower lid procedures and can be quite messy.

The crease selected can be from 6 to 12 mm above the lash line. The higher the crease selected, the more feminine the final appearance. But remember, it usually should not be higher than one-third the distance from lash to brow (see Figure 11.3). A high lid crease is not usually desired for males. Supratarsal fixation helps establish a deeper and more well-defined

TABLE 11.4. A list for patients of medications having anticoagulent effects. These medications should not be taken for at least 2 weeks prior to surgery.

Advil	Emprazil tablets
Alka-Seltzer tablets	Emprazil-C tablets en tab
Alka-Seltzer Plus Cold Medicine	Equagesic
Anacin capsules and tablets	Excedrin
Anacin Maximum Strength capsules and tablets	Extra-Strength BufferinFeldene
APC tablets	Fiorinal with Codeine
APC with Codeine, Tabloyd Brand	4-Way Cold tablets
Arthritis Formula by the makers of Anacin tablets	Gemnisyn
Arthritis Strength Bufferin	Goody's Headache powders
Ascodeen-30	
Ascriptin	Ibuprofen
Aspirin	Indocin
Aspergum	Measurin
Aspirin Suppositories	Midol
Anaprox	Momentum Muscular Backache Formula
Bayer Aspirin	Monacet with Codeine
Bayer Children's Chewable Aspirin	Motrin
Bayer Children's Cold tablets	Naprosyn
Bayer Timed-released Aspirin	Norgesic/Norgesic Forte
BC powders	Norwich Aspirin
Buff-a-Comp tablets	Pabirin buffered tablets
Buffadyne	Panalgesic Percodan and Percodan-Demi tablets
Bufferin	Persistin
Butalbital	
Cama Inlay tabs	Quiet World Analgesic/ Sleeping Aid
Cetased, Improved	Robaxisal tablets
Cheracol capsules	Salsalate
Clinoril	SK-65 Compound
Congespirin	St. Joseph's Aspirin for Children
Cope	Sine-Aid
Coricidin D Decongestant tablets	Sine-Off Sinus Medicine tablets-Aspirin Formula
Coricidin for Children	Stendin
Coricidin Medilets tablets for Children	Stero-Darvon with A.S.A.
Coricidin tablets	Sulindac
	Supac
Darvon	Synalgos capsules
Darvon with A.S.A.	Synalgos-DC capsules
Darvon-N with A.S.A.	Tolectin
Dristan Decongestant capsules and tablets	Triaminicin tablets
Duragesic	Vanquish
	Verin
Ecotrin tablets	Viro-Med tablets
Empirin	Vitamin E
Empirin with Codeine	
Emprazil	Zorprin

TABLE 11.5. Consent form

SPECIAL CONSENT FOR BLEPHAROPLASTY

PATIENT: _____

DATE: _____ TIME: _____

1) I hereby authorize _____ , M.D., to perform a surgical procedure known as Blepharoplasty, or commonly called a plastic surgical operation on the _____ eyelids and surrounding structures, on:

_____
Patient's Name

2) The procedure in paragraph 1 has been explained to me by the above doctor, and I completely understand the nature and consequences of the procedure. The following points have been specifically made clear:
   a) Some of the possible complications of Blepharoplasty operations are bleeding, infection, abnormal discoloration or pigmentation of the skin of the eyelids, abnormal folding-in or folding-out of the eyelids, inflammation and disease of the cornea (the cornea is the outer "window" of the eye), and allergic or other bad reactions to one or more of the substances used in the operation.
   b) Some of the complications of eyelid surgery can cause prolonged illness, scarring, permanent disability and the need for further surgery. Very rarely, partial and even complete blindness has resulted from eyelid surgery. Allergic reactions have even been known to cause death.
   c) There, of course, are scars as a result of this surgery, and these scars are permanent. Every effort will be made to conceal them or to make them as inconspicuous as possible. Eyelid skin heals with an unusually fine scar and is hardly noticeable even on close examination. On occasion, a thickening or spreading of a scar may develop requiring surgical revision.
   d) That the incision lines usually are conspicuous early postoperatively and for an indefinite period of time.
   e) On occasion, following lower lid surgery, the eyelid may be pulled down. This is usually of a temporary nature and the lid returns to its normal position after the swelling subsides. Rarely, this condition may require further surgery for correction.
   f) That there will be discoloration about the eyes for several days, and that in some cases this can persist for considerably longer.
   g) The eyes may tear for an indefinite period of time following surgery. This is due to swelling of the tear drainage ducts and usually returns to normal after the swelling subsides.
   h) Rarely, because of tightness of the lids, there may be dryness of the eye itself at night after retiring. This is temporary and corrects itself at night after the lid skin loosens. Ointments resembling artificial tears may be used to correct the temporary dryness.
   i) On occasion, the eye may have a sensation of a foreign body present. This is of a temporary nature and not serious. Occasionally an antibiotic ointment may be prescribed until the condition is corrected.
   j) Due to the nature of the procedure, an exact end-result cannot be predicted, and I have not been given any guarantee of specific results.
3) I am aware that the practice of medicine and surgery is not an exact science, and I acknowledge that no guarantees have been made to me as to the results of the operation or procedure.
4) I consent to be photographed before, during, and after the treatment; that these photographs shall be the property of the above doctor and may be published in scientific journals and/or shown for scientific reasons.
5) I agree to keep the above doctor informed of any change of address so that he can notify me of any late findings, and I agree to cooperate with the above doctor in my care after surgery until completely discharged.
6) I have read the above consent and fully understand the same and do authorize the above doctor to perform this surgical procedure on me.

The operation has been explained to me, and I fully understand the nature of the procedure and the risks involved. I acknowledge and understand that no expressed or implied warranty has been given to me.

PATIENT'S SIGNATURE: _____

WITNESS: _____ DATE: _____

(OVER)

(Continued)

TABLE 11.5 (Continued)

IF THE PATIENT IS A MINOR, COMPLETE THE FOLLOWING:

The patient is a minor _____ years of age, and we, the undersigned, are the parents or guardian of the patient and do hereby consent for the patient.

SIGNATURE: _____
(Parent or Legal Guardian)

WITNESS: _____

lid crease. It may be desirable in women and in the Asian eye but unwanted for blepharoplasty in men if a masculine look is desired.

The line should not be drawn medial to the punctum, as excisions into the area of the medial canthus are prone to postoperative webbing or banding. If there appears to be too much medial laxity, a burrows triangle may be taken, base down, but the incision should be ceased at the medial punctum. This may also be taken as a secondary or delayed procedure.

Laterally, it is important to carry the incision line out far enough to remove all redundant skin and to hide in a skin crease the lateral excision whenever possible. Try to keep all lateral incisions within the orbital area in younger patients. In our experience it is almost impossible to remove too much skin from the upper lid of female patients as long as thin eyelid skin is sutured to thin eyelid skin and not to the heavier brow skin. Lagophthalmos is more likely to result from pulling down of the lower eyelid than from pulling up of the upper lid. The same is true for dry eyes.

The upper incision line is drawn with the eyes closed gently. The skin is grasped with fine-toothed forceps and the redundant skin folded over the lower line; this determines the desired amount to be removed, and the upper incision line is marked. This has been variably said to be when the eyelids now lie in a natural position,[3] or until one is just opening the eye,[4] or when there is 1 to 2 mm of eyelid opening.[1] The most important thing to remember about marking (and about upper lid surgery in general) is to keep it symmetrical. Symmetry hides a multitude of errors, while asymmetry will destroy an otherwise perfect surgical result.

After intravenous sedation, lidocaine 1% with epinephrine is infiltrated using a 30-gauge or smaller needle. Inject 2 cc of this solution just under the skin laterally and milk the anesthetic across the eyelid using Q-tips or fingers.[5] Inject the local beneath skin that is marked for excision so that any hematoma produced will be excised during surgery. One to 2 ml of anesthetic is all that is usually required to produce adequate effect. If sedated, the patient should be adequately monitored, and sufficient time (about 10 minutes) should be allowed for the epinephrine to exert its effect if a scalpel is to be used for excision. When a laser is used instead of the scalpel, this becomes irrelevant, because of the photocoagulation effect of the laser.[6-9] The patient is draped and prepared. If eye shields or other protective devices, such as a David-Baker clamp,[10] are used, they are positioned at this time (see Figures 11.13A and B). When using a laser, eye shields must always be in place.[5,8,10]

With an assistant or the David-Baker clamp providing downward traction, which allows the levator aponeurosis to be relatively protected during the skin muscle flap elevation, make an incision with a scalpel or the laser through the skin and muscle. Using blunt-tipped scissors or laser and a fine-toothed forceps, undercut and remove the skin and orbicularis muscle, thus exposing the septum.

After careful hemostasis has been achieved (not usually needed for laser procedures), apply pressure on the globe to make the retroseptal fat pad prolapse and become more obvious. Incise and open the entire length of the septum to expose the fat. Gently grasp the fat with fine-toothed forceps and use a cotton bud to gently dissect away the surrounding tissue. Do not clamp fat or pull vigorously. Use the laser to excise this fat after draping it over wet cotton tips or sponges, or cut and electrocoagulate for

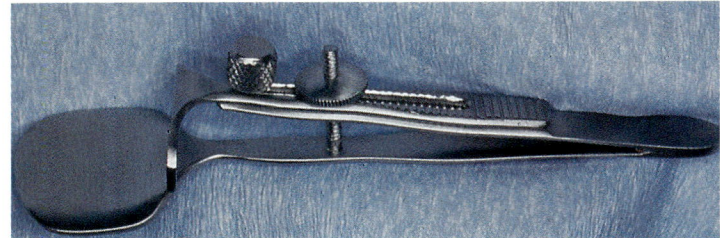

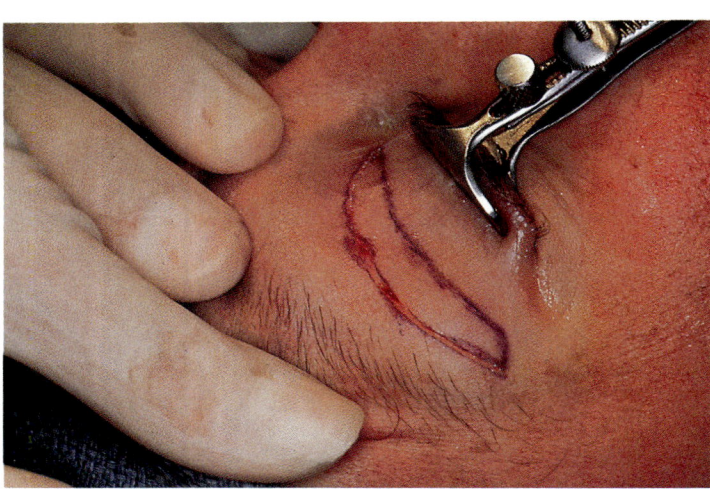

FIGURE 11.13. A. The David-Baker eyelid clamp. B. The David-Baker eyelid clamp in proper position, protecting the eye while it provides traction on the levator and upper eyelid skin.

hemostasis if a scissors is used. Fat of the medial compartment is whiter in color than the yellow middle compartment. Apply pressure at the lateral canthus directed toward the glabella to prolapse the medial portion of the fat pad. It is important in this area to ensure that the tendon of the superior oblique muscle has not been caught up in the fat pad or clamp, and cautious coagulation is important here. If a laser is used, the anatomy is easily visualized and no additional hemostasis is needed.

We feel that clamping of retroseptal fat is best avoided for an additional reason: It may place too much traction on the posterior orbital blood vessels and be a cause of postoperative hemorrhage. We prefer to excise the fat without clamping. Wound closure is performed with or without supratarsal fixation; 6-0 or 7-0 absorbable or nonabsorbable running or interrupted stitches all have proponents, and it probably matters little what specific stitch is used. It does, however, matter that the bite taken on each edge of the wound is at the same depth.

Usually, if nonabsorbable stitches are used they are removed at or around 3 days. For the past several years, we have used a few 6-0 mild chromic sutures for skin positioning and then cyanoacrylate glue. We are most pleased with this method of closure.

Lower Lid Blepharoplasty

This procedure may be performed via a transcutaneous or transconjunctival approach. This latter technique may be performed via a preseptal or retroseptal approach. Each will be discussed in turn.

Transcutaneous Blepharoplasty

Possible complications and their correction must be discussed with the patient. Lower lid retraction including ectropion, scleral show and lateral canthal deformity[11] is the most common complication of lower eyelid surgery.

The muscle skin flap commonly employed so often produces lower lid retraction, including scleral show, and especially at the inferolateral section of the eye,[4] that for many years, even in the best of hands, "good" before and after photos presented at meetings and published have tended to show this deformity. A certain "surgical," almost startled, look is obvious. This avoidable complication results from either overzealous skin or muscle excision or septal shortening as the healing scar after septal penetration contracts, or from a combination of these. We believe that lower lid retraction is most commonly due to contraction of the septal scars after penetration. This shortens the vertical dimension of the lower lid and pulls the lower lid margin down. It is unfortunate that the lateral canthus is poorly supported by the lateral canthal tendon in comparison to its medial counterpart and tends not to cope well with any stress imposed by surgery in this region.

As these problems are so frequent with this approach, two clinical tests become important to assess the capabilities of the lower lid to withstand the proposed surgery. These include the snap test and distraction test. The snap test is easily performed. With the patient staring straight ahead, grasp the lower eyelid and retract it away from the globe, then release it. The time taken for the lid to rebound to its normal position should be about 1 second. The distraction test involves pulling the lower eyelid out from the globe as far as is comfortable and measuring the distance from globe to lid. It should not exceed 7 mm. Patients who fail either or both of these tests are at great risk for postoperative lid retraction. In fact, even patients who do not fail these tests may end up with postoperative lower eyelid retraction.

Protuberance of the globe must also be evaluated. No matter what the cause (exophthalmos, shallow orbits, etc.) the patient with protuberance of the globe is at risk for postoperative retraction.[3]

Lagophthalmos must also be assessed. With the eyebrows in the normal position and the eyes lightly closed, if the eyelids do not totally close, any lower lid retraction will add to the problem and may not be coped with by the cornea.

Dry eyes are evaluated by performing a Schirmer's test. With the strip placed in the inferior cul-de-sac, both reflexive (without local anesthetic drops) and basal (with local anesthetic drops) tests are performed. Less than 5 mm of wetting signifies inadequate tear production. Patients with this condition should be informed that they may require a tear supplement postoperatively.

Orbicularis function may need to be assessed in those with a history of Bell's palsy or other cause of nerve or muscle dysfunction. This may be assessed reasonably by trying to open the patient's eyes against their maximal contraction. A difference between the two sides signifies a weakness that may make one again more prone to postoperative normal exposure.

Visual acuity testing is addressed as in the previous section on upper lid blepharoplasty and is of similar importance.

Skin quality needs to be discussed with the patients. They must understand that this surgery will not correct poor quality of lower lid skin. If the skin quality is indeed the major complaint, skin treatments should be instituted (resurfacing, sunblocks, etc.), not blepharoplasty. Collagen can temporarily fill wrinkles and resurfacing can be useful. Attempted correction of wrinkles using a scalpel near an unsupported lower lid is fraught with danger and ill-conceived.

General medical considerations remain the same as for the upper eyelid, but thyroid-induced eye disease and sicca syndrome are even more important for lower eyelid surgery, because of the risk of ectropion. The same drug contraindications apply as for the upper lib surgery. Avoidance of anticoagulants is even more important than in upper eyelid surgery, because of the possibility of retrobulbar hemorrhage.

Preoperative photography is done with the patient looking straight ahead and with the patient looking up. Lateral and oblique views are also useful. Polaroids are useful for intraoperative guidance.

Markings are usually placed at about 2 to 3 mm distance from the ciliary margin, and the visible fat pockets are often also marked. Incision lines begin inferior to the punctum and extend to the lateral canthal angle, then take a 10° inferolateral turn and hopefully will be hidden in one of the periorbital rhytids. This extension usually tracks for about 10 mm.

Local anesthetic is infiltrated using 2% xylocaine with 1:100,000 epinephrine and a number 30 needle. Wydase is sometimes added to aid in the spread of the local anesthetic, as it is preferable to use only 1 injection in this area. Topical anesthetic is used to anesthetize the conjunctiva. Corneal protectors, if they are used, are placed at this time.

Incision through skin only will expose the orbicularis muscle. Blunt scissors are used to cut through the muscle, and the septum is now seen. This should be done with the direction of the scissors parallel to and not directed toward the orbit.

A 4-0 vicryl or silk stitch is placed through the superior margin of the incision through the orbicularis, and the stitch ends are clamped and drawn cephalad back over the head of the patient to protect the eye if shields are not being used. It also provides the necessary traction to allow undermining of the skin muscle flap from the septum, which is performed with blunt scissors.

The orbital septum is now on view, and the fat can be seen bulging beneath it. This bulging can be exaggerated by pushing on the orbit. The septum is then incised over the maximal bulging area, and the fat pads are teased up. This fat is commonly coagulated. As is the case with upper lid blepharoplasty, we do not like to clamp the lower lid fat, since traction on these pads may cause bleeding or hemorrhage during or postoperative. We prefer to excise unclamped fat using a scissors and use coagulation as needed for hemostasis.

The cephalad traction suture is cut and the flap is draped back to fill the new concavity left after the fat has been removed. This is held in position with a wet-tipped Q-tip applicator, and the patient is asked to open his or her mouth and look up, which will retract the flap maximally. The redundant skin is excised in a crescent fashion and, last, the upper edge of the flap has some orbicularis muscle trimmed.

The wound is then sutured with continuous or interrupted sutures, and ice-cold saline-soaked gauze or a dental roll is placed over the concavity of the lower eyelid. The wound is then dressed after being sure that hemostasis is adequate.

The other eye is operated on in the same fashion.

Transconjunctival Blepharoplasty

This approach is fast becoming the technique of choice for lower eyelid blepharoplasty.[4,5,8,9] We have successfully used this method for the past several years to the exclusion of transcutaneous lower lid blepharoplasty. If the patient is considered to be at risk of postoperative ectropion or retraction or has poor orbicularis function, you and your patient are much safer using this approach. It also eliminates a scar on the skin.

The main criticism of this transconjunctival approach is the inability to trim redundant skin or hypertrophic orbicularis. However, it is likely that this aspect of the surgery may have been given too high a priority in the past and that the redraping of the lower eyelid onto its newly reformed concave bed may take up a surprising amount of "redundant" skin and muscle. Given the difficulty and side effect profile of the transcutaneous procedure, it is not surprising that the transconjunctival approach continues to gain in popularity.

Visual acuity testing is, of course, mandatory, and other testing, as suggested under the transcutaneous section, should be done but does not assume quite the same importance.

The Retroseptal Approach

Preoperative photography remains the same as with the transcutaneous approach. A local anesthetic mixture of 1% xylocaine 1:100,000 epinephrine with or without 1:10 diluted Wydase, similar to that employed in other blepharoplasty procedures, is injected below the orbital septum into the fat pads directly through the conjunctiva. Use a Jaeger plate (stainless steel) to apply light pressure to the globe after retracting the upper eyelid inferiorly. Fat will bulge under the conjunctiva and will allow injection of the conjunctival surface while the globe is protected by the stainless steel plate. If a CO_2 laser is to be used, Wydase is not needed, since the spread of energy is greatly restricted when compared to the use of electricity for coagulation. Also, no intraoperative reinforcement of local anesthetic will be needed if the CO_2 laser is used.

Markings are usually made only to remind oneself where the fat pockets are maximal clinically on the skin surface. No markings are used on the conjunctival surface.

If a sharp instrument is to be used for incision, waiting 10 to 15 minutes at this point is very important to ensure that the full vasoconstrictive effect of the epinephrine is experienced. If the CO_2 laser is to be used, there is no need to wait.

If scleral shields are to be used, they are lubricated and inserted after topical anesthetic drops have been instilled. The protective Jaeger plate serves as adequate protection for the globe as well as enabling you to apply pressure to the globe; it is the better choice in this procedure.

The lower eyelid is retracted with an eyelid retractor, and the upper eyelid may be brought down to protect the eye if shields are not being used and to allow a vehicle for gentle pressure to be applied to the globe. When using a CO_2 laser, an eye shield, preferably the Jaeger plate, is always used.

Incise the conjuctiva with sharp scissors, cutting cautery, or CO_2 laser, from the lateral end of the fornix to its medial end. The choice of hot cautery, unipolar or bipolar diathermy cold steel, or CO_2 laser will vary from surgeon to surgeon, but the same end point of meticulous hemostasis is required here. Deepen the incision until fat is visible. The three fat pads will come into view and they are dealt with differently by various surgeons. Many tease out the fat, clamp, and cauterize. Again, we do not advocate clamping of the fat for the same reason as given previously. The conjunctiva may be sutured or not sutured. We prefer to use no sutures. The eyelid is pulled up into its correct position and the orbital rim felt through the skin to ensure that the fat has been removed. Preoperative photos are reexamined and if content, cold saline packs are placed on the lower eyelid. Then the other eye is begun.

Preseptal Approach

Utilize photography is as for the other types of blepharoplasty. Local anesthesia is similar to the retroseptal approach, except the injection is made into the plane below the orbicularis muscle. Apply a little pressure, then inject throughout the lower lid, producing a hydrodissection of the preseptal plane.[4] Topical anesthetic eye drops are inserted into the eye and supplemental palpebral conjunctival injections may be performed. Eye shields may be inserted.

After everting the lower eyelid, a vicryl stay stitch is inserted into the palpebral conjunctiva about 2 mm anterior to the fornix and is retracted cephalad, and a retractor is inserted anterior to this stitch and retracted inferiorly, revealing the septum. Often the fat will be seen bulging through the septum. From now on the procedure resembles the transcutaneous approach.

Postoperative Care

After the procedure "ice is nice" and is used continuously as compresses or packs for the first day. We give oral antibiotics but no oral or IV steroids. Electrocautery is a major cause of postoperative swelling. This is usually slight if the CO_2 laser is the cutting tool used, and antiinflammatory agents are not needed.

The patient is given an emergency contact phone number, especially if a transcutaneous lower lid blepharoplasty has been performed, and instructed to call if there is pain, excessive swelling, or bruising. Rubbing the eyelids is to be avoided. Instruct the patient not to pull down the lower lid looking for the incision if the transconjuctival approach was used, as this can open the healing incision and cause bleeding. Routine followup is usually begun with an appointment at 3 days, when cutaneous stitches may be removed.

Contact lenses can go back in at the end of the first week. Local heat may help with any bruising after the third day postoperative.

Complications

Many of the complications of blepharoplasty relate to the transcutaneous lower lid blepharoplasty and have been discussed previously.

The most dreaded complication is retrobulbar hemorrhage, with the potential for loss of vision. Excess pain, swelling, and eccymosis should alert the surgeon to this possibility and the patient seen as an emergency case. An occuloplastic surgeon should be alerted. If diagnosis is confirmed, lateral canthotomy may be performed as an emergency procedure. This is an emergency situation, and immediate attention is required.

Lower lid scleral show or ectropion can be avoided by good choice of technique and proper patient selection.

Dry eyes will be aggravated by any scleral show or lagophthalmos and may require supplemental artificial tears. Lagophthalmos may contribute to dry eyes, corneal irritation, and corneal ulceration. In the presence of normal orbicularis function, it is unusual for this to be more than a transient postoperative concern. Gravity is our ally in upper eyelid surgery but our foe in lower eyelid surgery.

Asymmetry of the upper lids is critically examined by the patient and, if produced, can usually be repaired at a secondary procedure.

Euophthalmos from excessive periorbital fat removal will produce a sunken eye appearance; if recognized immediately, some may be able to be replaced at the time of the procedure. But, like lower eyelid retraction, this side effect is best dealt with by avoiding it rather than curing it.

Secondary procedures for scleral show, retraction, or ectropion may need to be considered but are not the purpose of the discussion.

Summary

Blepharoplasty is a very popular and successful cosmetic technique and, properly performed, provides one with very patients. The upper lid requires careful planning of the incision lines to ensure symmetry and that the proper amount of skin is taken. The transcutaneous lower lid approach has to be very carefully performed so that lid retraction, ectropion, and scleral show do not come to haunt the surgeon. The transconjunctival approach may be a preferable one where no skin or muscle removal is needed.

References

1. Perman KI. Upper eyelid blepharoplasty. J Dermatol Surg Oncol. 1992;18:1096–1099.
2. Wilkins RB, Papita M. The recognition of acquired ptosis in patients considered for upper eyelid blepharoplasty. Plast reconstr surg. 1982;70:431–434.
3. Shorr N, Enzer YR. Considerations in aesthetic eyelid surgery. J Dermatol Surg Oncol. 1992;18:1081–1095.
4. Asken S. Cosmetic eyelid surgery—blepharoplasty. In: *Cosmetic Surgery of the Skin*, WP Coleman, CW Hanke, TA Alt, S, Asken eds. B.C. Decker Inc., 1991, Philadelphia, pp. 267–293.
5. David LM, Abergel RP. CO_2 laser blepharoplasty. In: *Cosmetic Surgery of the Skin,* WP Coleman, CW Hanke, TA Alt, S Asken, eds. B.C. Decker Inc., 1991, Philadelphia: pp. 295–301.
6. Baker SS, Muenzler WS, Small RG, Leonard JE. Carbon dioxide laser blepharoplasty. Opthalmology. 1984;91:238–244.
7. David LM, Sanders G. CO_2 laser blepharoplasty: a comparison to cold steel and electrocautery. J Dermatol Surg Oncol. 1987;13:110–114.
8. David LM. The laser approach to blepharoplasty. J Dermatol Surg Oncol. 1988;14:741–746.
9. Morrow DM. CO_2 laser blepharoplasty. A comparison with cold steel surgery. J Dermatol Surg Oncol. 1992;18:307–313.
10. David LM, Baker SS. David-Baker eyelid retractor. Am J Cosmet Surg. 1992;9:147–148.
11. Neuhaus RW. Lower eyelid blepharoplasty. J Dermatol Surg Oncol. 1992;18:1100–1109.

12
Skin Lesions of Aging

C. William Hanke and Lisa A. Francis

A whole array of skin conditions, including many benign and malignant tumors, occur with increasing frequency as we enter middle age (Table 12.1). Some of the conditions are due to chronic ultraviolet light exposure (photoaging), while others are part of the natural aging process (chronologic aging) (Tables 12.2 and 12.3). In this chapter we will review and illustrate many of the skin conditions related to aging.

Benign Tumors

Angiokeratoma of the Scrotum

Angiokeratomas of the scrotum (angiokeratoma scroti, angiokeratoma of Fordyce) appear in mid- to late life as 2 mm to 4 mm red papules on the scrotum (Figure 12.1). The papules are soft and compressible at first but later become bluish and hard. Treatment is not necessary unless bleeding occurs.

Cherry Hemangioma

Cherry hemangiomas (senile hemangioma) are domed-shaped papules exhibiting bright red or purple color (Figure 12.2). They range in size from 1 to 3 mm in diameter and may occur alone or, more commonly, in groups.

Although more frequently seen in the elderly, the hemangiomas begin appearing in early adulthood, usually on the trunk. Cherry hemangiomas are benign and treatment is usually not necessary. They may be removed with laser or by electrodesiccation if desired.[1]

Chondrodermatitis Nodularis Helicis

Chondrodermatitis nodularis helicis is characterized by small, painful nodules on the helix of the ear. The lesions occur mainly in elderly men (90%), less often in women (10%). The etiology is unknown, but repeated trauma may be contributory. The lesions may appear crusted and ulcerated (Figure 12.3). Rarely do they exceed 1 cm in diameter.

Treatment is usually begun with topical or intralesional corticosteroids. Surgical excision is also used, but recurrence is not uncommon.

Portwine Stain

Portwine stain (or portwine hemangioma) is a congenital capillary vascular malformation. Usually present at birth, a portwine stain begins as a pink or red macular patch. The lesion grows in proportion to the growth of the individual and generally gets darker and thicker throughout life. During mid-life the lesion may become purple, exhibit a raised, warty appearance, and become prone to bleeding following minor trauma (Figure 12.4).

Portwine stains are caused by an increased number of blood vessels in the skin. Red blood cells are trapped in the blood vessels, giving the lesion its characteristic appearance.

Until recently treatment options were limited to relatively unsuccessful excisions, skin grafts,

TABLE 12.1. Skin conditions associated with aging.

Benign tumors
Angiokeratoma
Cherry hemangioma
Chondrodermatitis nodularis helicis
Portwine stain ectatic nodules
Sebaceous hyperplasia
Seborrheic keratosis
Skin tags/acrochordons
Solar lentigo
Spider angioma
Venous lake

Malignant tumors
Angiosarcoma of the face and scalp
Atypical fibroxanthoma
Basal cell carcinoma
Lentigo maligna melanoma
Merkel cell carcinoma
Mycosis fungoides
Squamous cell carcinoma

Premalignant conditions
Actinic keratosis
Actinic cheilitis
Arsenical keratosis
Bowen's disease
Chronic radiation dermatitis
Extramammary Paget's disease
Lentigo maligna

Dermatoses/infections
Contact dermatitis
Decubitus ulcer
Favre-Racouchot syndrome
Granuloma fissuratum
Herpes zoster
Neurodermatitis
Perlèche/angular cheilitis
Poikiloderma of Civatte
Reactions to drugs
Rosacea/rhinophyma
Scabies
Senile purpura
Stasis dermatitis/ulcers
Telangiectasia
Tinea pedis/onychomycosis
Xerosis/asteatotic dermatitis/eczema Craquelé

TABLE 12.2. Skin disorders and tumors associated with chronic ultraviolet light exposure.

Actinic cheilitis
Actinic keratosis
Basal cell carcinoma
Bowen's disease
Lentigo maligna
Malignant melanoma
Squamous cell carcinoma
Solar lentigines
Favre-Racouchot syndrome
Poikiloderma of Civatte
Solar telangiectasia
Venous lakes
Senile purpura
Cutis rhomboidalis nuchae
Premature wrinkling
Dyspigmentation

and tattooing. Tattooing of lesions was abandoned because of the inability to match the color of the surrounding skin. With the advent of the argon laser and the pulsed-dye laser (PDL), treatment options have dramatically improved.[2] The PDL is tuned to a wavelength of laser light that is absorbed selectively by hemoglobin in the red blood cells in the blood vessels. The blood vessels are destroyed, but the surrounding tissue is left virtually unharmed. The incidence of scar formation and adverse effects following PDL is less than 1 percent.

Sebaceous Hyperplasia

Sebaceous hyperplasia occurs in middle-aged or elderly individuals as soft, yellow papules on the face (Figure 12.5). These 2 to 3 mm lesions are often multiple. The center of the papule is a

TABLE 12.3. Skin manifestations of chronologic aging.

Increased laxity of eyelid skin
Protruding upper and lower eyelid fat pads
Sleep creases
Crow's feet
Hereditary hair loss
Severe wrinkling
Gravitational sagging
Easy bruisability
Loss of natural hair color
Fragility of nails
Deepening of facial furrows

12. Skin Lesions of Aging 189

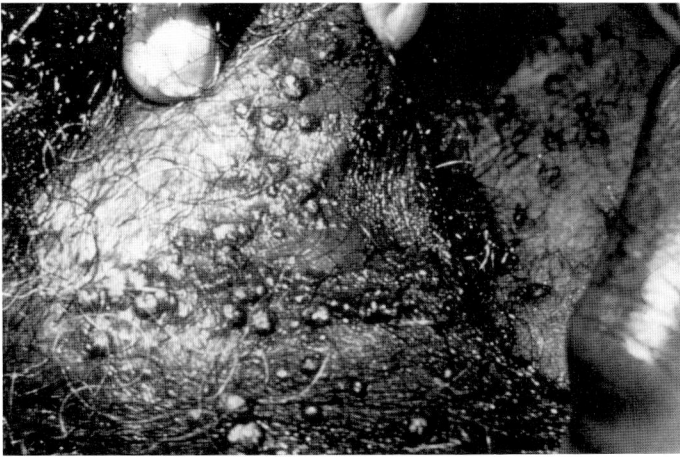

FIGURE 12.1. This 79-year-old man has multiple angiokeratomas on the scrotum. (Used with permission, C. William Hanke, M.D.)

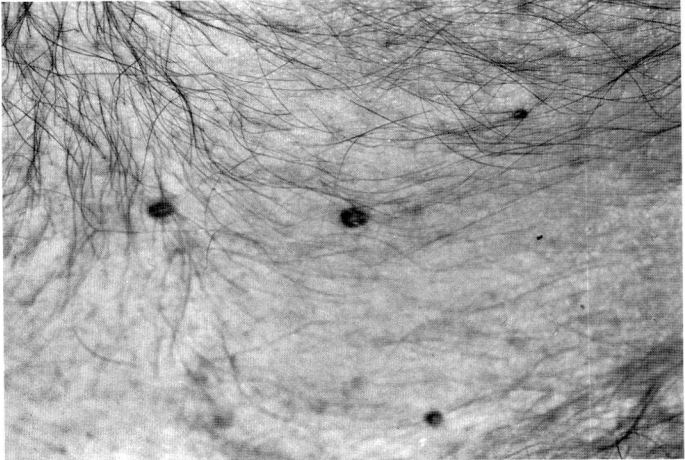

FIGURE 12.2. A 70-year-old man has characteristic cherry hemangiomas on the chest. (Used with permission, C. William Hanke, M.D.)

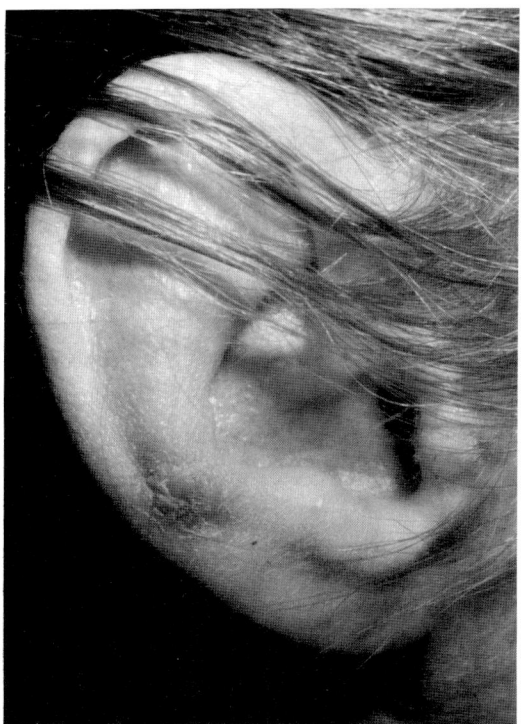

FIGURE 12.3. Chondrodermatitis nodularis helicis chronicus is seen as a tender papule overlying the auricular cartilage. (Used with permission, C. William Hanke, M.D.)

single enlarged sebaceous gland with many lobules grouped around a common duct. Telangiectasia may be present and may mimic basal cell carcinoma.

Some of the lesions will resolve spontaneously but may recur. Treatment methods include superficial scissors excision, shave excision, electrosurgery, and topical acid.

Seborrheic Keratosis

Seborrheic keratosis (SK) is a common benign tumor that begins as a sharply defined, light-brown papule. With time the tumor becomes thicker and darker. It has a greasy surface scale, giving it a pasted-on appearance (Figure 12.6). SK is the most common tumor seen in elderly individuals and ranges from less than 1 cm to several centimeters in diameter. SKs usually appear on the trunk, face, and extremities but do not occur on the palms or the soles.

Histologically, there are five types of seborrheic keratosis. These are classified as acanthotic, hyperkeratotic, clonal, irritated, and reticulated. Effective treatments include curettage and cryosurgery with liquid nitrogen.[3] Deep excision and suture of these lesions are not necessary.

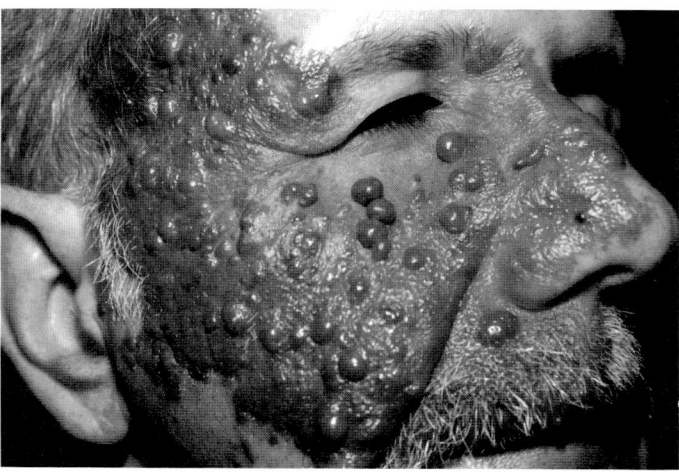

FIGURE 12.4. A 56-year-old man has developed multiple papular ectasias in a portwine birthmark. (Used with permission, C. William Hanke, M.D.)

12. Skin Lesions of Aging

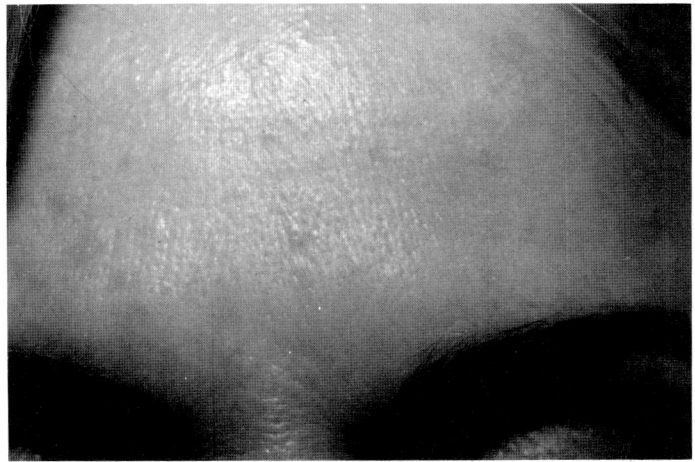

FIGURE 12.5. A 57-year-old woman has sebaceous hyperplasia on the forehead. (Used with permission, C. William Hanke, M.D.)

Skin Tags/Acrochordons

Skin tags are flesh-colored or light brown papillomas consisting of extraneous skin that commonly appear on the neck, upper chest, or axillae. Although they appear in both sexes, they are more common in women. Most skin tags range from 1 to 5 mm in size and have an irregular or pedunculated appearance (Figure 12.7).

Treatment modalities include superficial surgical removal, cryotherapy, or electrodesiccation. Treatment is simple and curative—rarely do the lesions reappear.

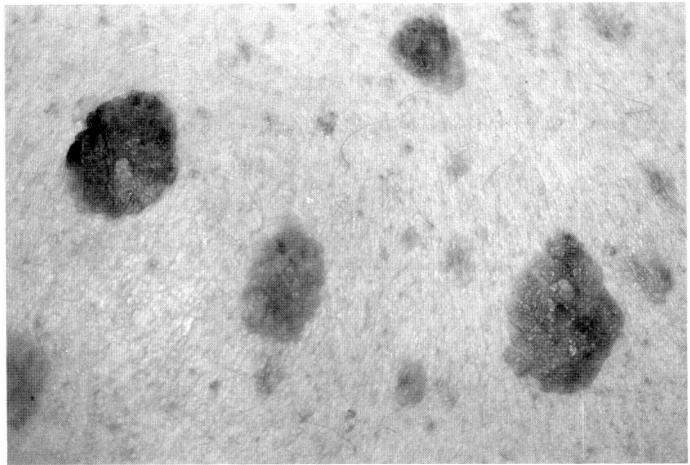

FIGURE 12.6. Seborrheic keratoses are superficial brown papules and plaques that often appear on the trunk after age 40. (Used with permission, C. William Hanke, M.D.)

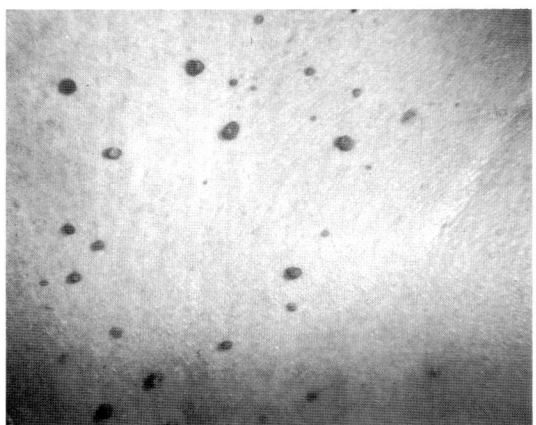

FIGURE 12.7. Elderly individuals may develop multiple skin tags on the neck or axilla. (Used with permission, C. William Hanke, M.D.)

Solar Lentigo

Ninety percent of Caucasians develop solar lentigines (lentigo senilis, liver spots) by age 70. These dark brown macules have an irregular outline and usually occur in multiples on sun-exposed areas. These lesions, although much more common in people over 40, can occur at any age after prolonged sun exposure.

Treatment involves superficial removal of the lesion. Freezing with liquid nitrogen, curettage, and treatment with ruby laser have been shown to be effective (Figures 12.8 and 12.9).

Spider Angioma

Spider angioma (spider ectasia, nevus araneus) is characterized by a central punctum. Surrounding the punctum are many dilated branches of the angioma, resembling spiders' legs. They occur at all ages but are common on the noses of women after age 40. Treatment alternatives include electrosurgery and laser (refer to Figures 12.10 and 12.11).

Venous Lakes

Venous lakes are dilated veins filled with blood. The lesions may occur singly or in multiples. The lakes may be interconnected by channels. They are most common on the exposed skin of the elderly and occur on the ears, lips, face, and neck (Figure 12.12). Venous lakes range in size from 1 mm to several millimeters in diameter and with pressure can be emptied of their blood. Venous lakes probably occur because of severe solar elastosis and loss of stromal support around weakened blood vessels. Electrosurgery or laser provides effective treatment.[4]

Malignant Tumors

Angiosarcoma of the Face and Scalp

Angiosarcoma is a rare, aggressive, malignant tumor. It is characterized by edema, erythema, and changes in the skin that resemble bruises. Nodules and plaques may be present (Figure 12.13). The clinical borders are indistinct. Angiosarcoma usually occurs on the scalp in patients in their seventh or eighth decade. Because of its aggressive behavior, it may invade cervical lymph nodes, metastasize to major organs (i.e., lungs, liver), or grow into the orbit or calvarium.

Treatment is surgical excision, but because the tumor extends far beyond the clinically visible margins, Mohs micrographic surgery is sometimes warranted.[5] Radiation is often given in patients who are not surgical candidates.

Atypical Fibroxanthoma

Atypical fibroxanthoma affects fair-complected elderly individuals. The tumor appears as a rapidly growing, pale red nodule, usually on a sun-exposure part of the body such as the head and neck (Figure 12.14). The tumor may grow to a size of approximately 1 cm; it rarely grows larger than 2 cm. In rare cases metastases to regional lymph nodes have been reported.

Surgical excision is usually curative.

Basal Cell Carcinoma

Basal cell carcinoma (BCC) is the most common type of skin cancer. It affects all

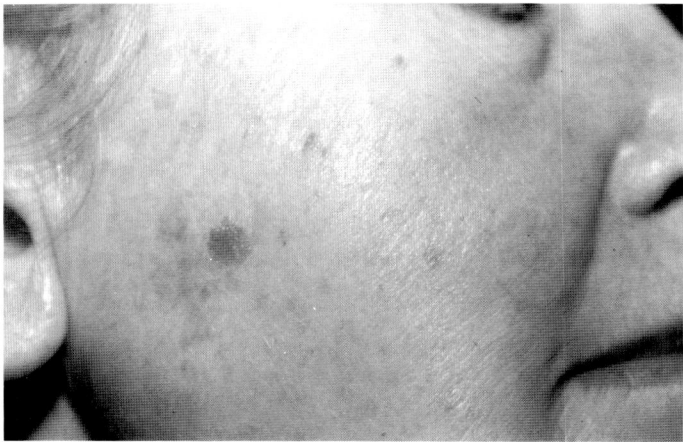

FIGURE 12.8. A 57-year-old woman has multiple unsightly brown solar lentigines on the cheek. (Used with permission, C. William Hanke, M.D.)

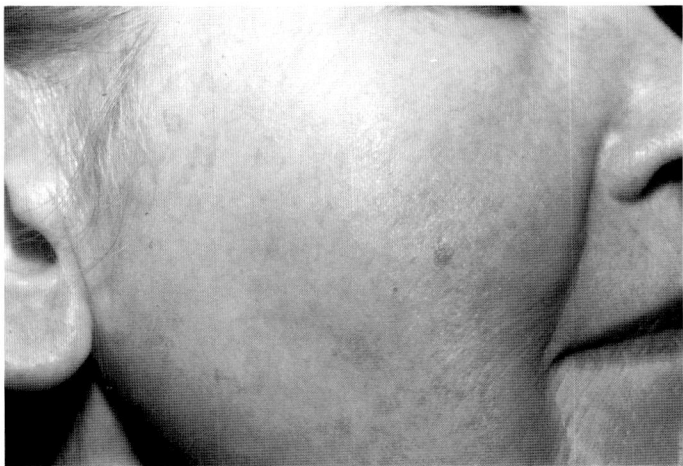

FIGURE 12.9. The solar lentigines on the cheek of the patient in Figure 12.8 have been removed with superficial curettage. (Used with permission, C. William Hanke, M.D.)

populations but is most common in fair-skinned Caucasians. Almost all BCCs occur on sun-exposed areas of the body. Greater cumulative sun damage in a given area of skin increases the chances that basal cell carcinoma will develop. Most BCCs are found in patients over age 50. Because of the popularity of sunbathing and outdoor sports, however, younger patients are being seen more often with BCC due to greater sun exposure at an earlier age.

Chronic sun exposure and ultraviolet damage is the leading etiologic factor for BCC. Arsenic exposure has been shown to cause BCC in some patients. Therapeutic x-ray treatments can lead to the development of BCCs in the treated area

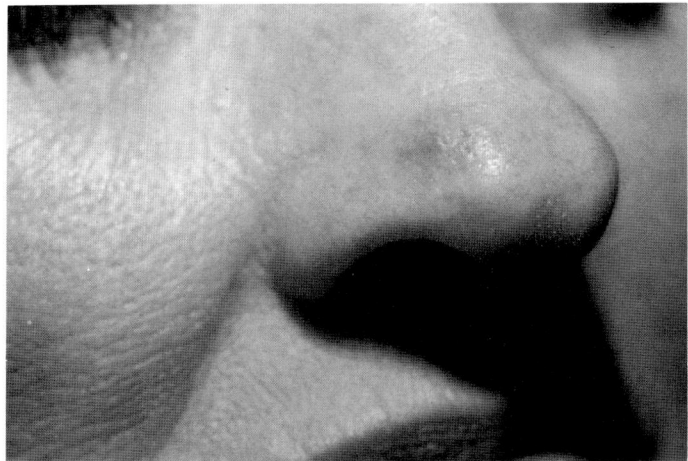

FIGURE 12.10. A 50-year-old woman has a spider angioma on the nasal tip. (Used with permission, C. William Hanke, M.D.)

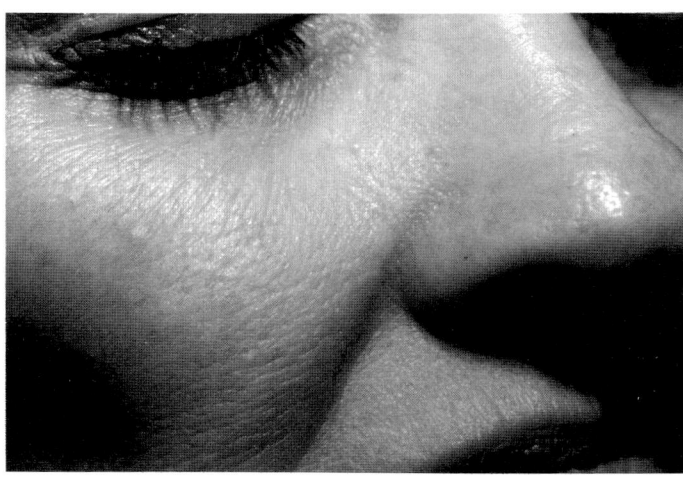

FIGURE 12.11. The spider angioma of the patient in Figure 12.10 has been removed with 1 pulsed dye laser treatment. (Used with permission, C. William Hanke, M.D.)

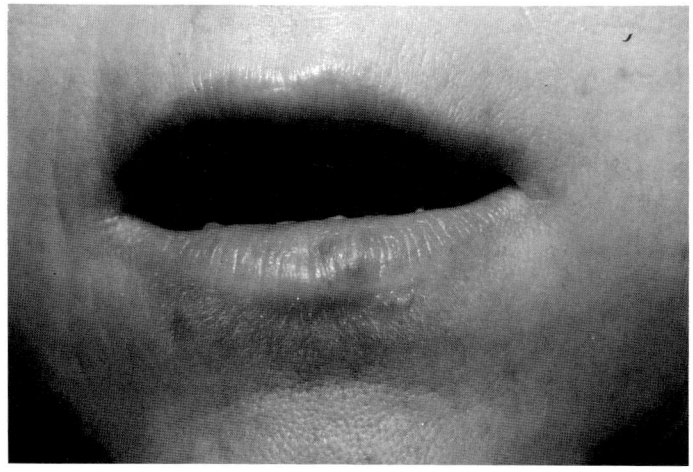

FIGURE 12.12. A blue venous lake is present on the vermilion of the lip. (Used with permission, C. William Hanke, M.D.)

12. Skin Lesions of Aging

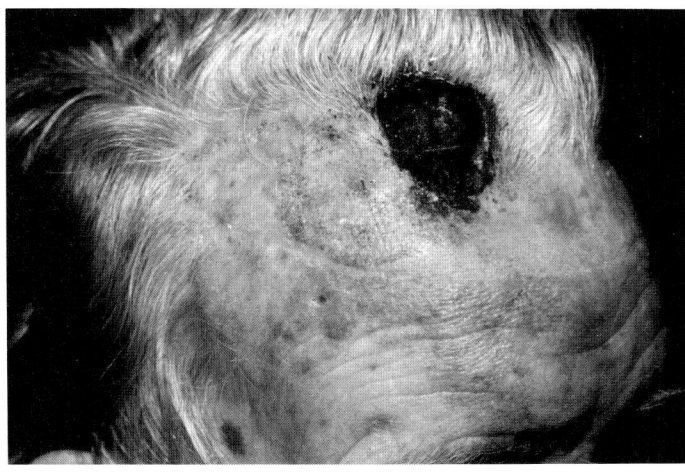

FIGURE 12.13. An elderly man has an ulcerated angiosarcoma on the scalp. (Used with permission, C. William Hanke, M.D.)

many years later. Certain genetic disorders also can predispose to BCCs.

Basal cell carcinoma appears clinically as a small, pearly nodule or papule with characteristic telangiectasias (Figure 12.15). As the tumor enlarges, it may bleed easily with minimal trauma. If left untreated the tumor may erode and invade bone or vital structures. BCCs only infrequently metastasize.

Treatments for BCC include surgical excision, cryosurgery, curettage, 5-fluorouracil, and radiation therapy. Mohs micrographic sur-

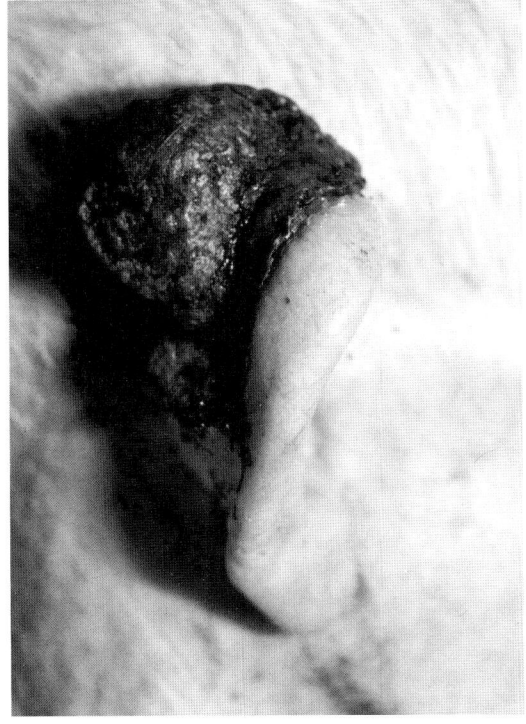

FIGURE 12.14. This elderly man has an atypical fibroxanthoma on his ear. (Used with permission, C. William Hanke, M.D.)

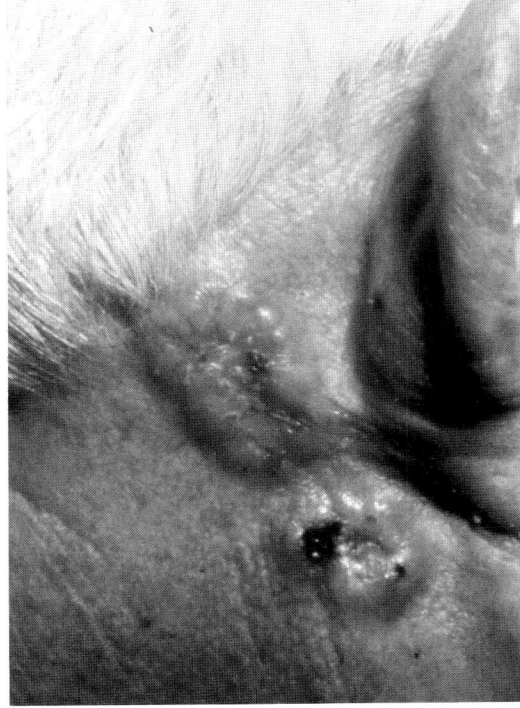

FIGURE 12.15. A 72-year-old man has 2 typical rodent-ulcer basal cell carcinomas on the neck. (Used with permission, C. William Hanke, M.D.)

gery is particularly effective for recurrent and other problematic BCCs.

Malignant Melanoma

Malignant melanoma (MM) is by far the deadliest form of skin cancer, because of its metastatic potential. Survival rates vary according to the anatomical depth of the tumor as measured by an ocular micrometer. A patient with a superficial, localized upper dermal melanoma may have a 90% or greater chance of surviving 5 years following excision. A patient with a deep dermal melanoma may live only a matter of months.

MM affects men and women equally. The incidence rate among whites is 6 to 7 times higher than that for blacks living in the same geographical area. Sun exposure is thought to be causative, since the incidence rate of MM increases in populations living closer to the equator.

The clinical signs of malignant melanoma are easily recognized. Any skin lesion with variation of color (*i.e.,* combinations of black, tan, light brown, blue, red, white), an irregular border, asymmetry, or rapid growth should be considered suspicious.

There are several types of malignant melanoma. Lentigo maligna melanoma is a large, flat, freckle-like patch with a variety of different colors within the lesion. This type is seen on the faces of elderly individuals. Superficial spreading melanoma is a smaller lesion characterized by an irregular border and a slightly raised surface (Figure 12.16). Nodular melanoma consists of a raised papule or nodule. Amelanotic melanomas are devoid of melanin and appear pink. Their benign clinical appearance may result in delay in diagnosis.

Early diagnosis often allows melanomas to be treated before deep dermal invasion occurs. The treatment of primary melanoma is surgical excision with margins of 3 cm or less, depending on microscopic depth of invasion. Once regional or distant metastases develop, the chance for cure drops precipitously. Immunotherapy and chemotherapy are only minimally effective.

Merkel Cell Carcinoma

Merkel cell carcinoma (MCC) belongs to a class of tumors known as the amine precursor uptake and decarboxylation (APUD) tumors. MCC occurs in elderly people as a pink, red, or blue firm solitary tumor on the sun-exposed areas of the arms, legs, neck, or head (Figure 12.17). The lesion is painless and has a high local recurrence rate following excision. The average age of patients with MCC is 70 years.

MCC is aggressive and grows rapidly, and it metastasizes to regional lymph nodes in approximately 50% to 79% of cases. In 25% to 33% of cases, the tumor will metastasize to the liver, lung, or brain.

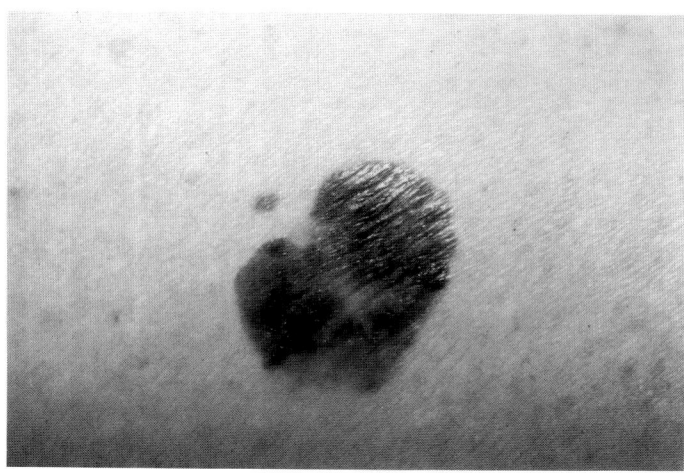

FIGURE 12.16. This superficial spreading malignant melanoma has been enlarging for 6 years on the back of a 60-year-old man. (Used with permission, C. William Hanke, M.D.)

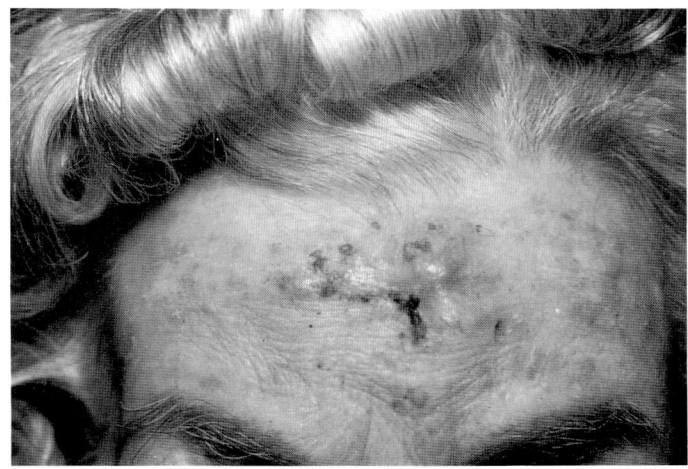

FIGURE 12.17. Merkel cell carcinoma is an aggressive malignancy that most commonly develops on the head and neck area of elderly persons. (Used with permission, C. William Hanke, M.D.)

Treatment alternatives include wide excision of the lesion with regional lymph node dissection, chemotherapy, radiation therapy, and Mohs micrographic surgery.[6]

Squamous Cell Carcinoma

The etiology of squamous cell carcinoma (SCC) is not as clear as that of basal cell carcinoma. In Caucasian patients the majority of the SCCs occur on sun-exposed areas of the body (head, neck, and upper extremities), while in other populations (Black, Asian, Indian) the ratio between sun-exposed and non-sun-exposed areas is approximately 1:1 and the most common sites are the lower limbs. The incidence in fair-skinned people is dramatically higher than in darker-skinned people. Solar radiation, x-rays, and arsenic exposure have been found to be causative in the development of SCC.

SCC usually begins in sun-damaged skin or in a solar keratosis. It often appears as a nodule or ulcerated nodule on the skin (Figure 12.18). SCC is considered more serious than BCC because of its ability to metastasize in a minority of cases. The treatment is similar to that described for BCC.

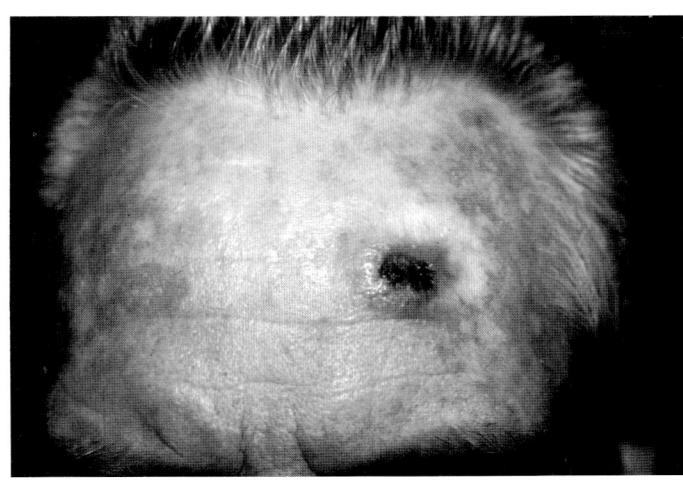

FIGURE 12.18. This 70-year-old man has an ulcerated squamous cell carcinoma on the forehead. (Used with permission, C. William Hanke, M.D.)

Premalignant Conditions

Actinic Keratosis

Actinic keratosis (AK) (solar keratosis, senile keratosis) affects almost the entire white elderly population. AK, the most common precancerous lesion, is found almost exclusively on sun-exposed areas of the body of middle aged or elderly people. Fair-skinned individuals with a history of excessive sun exposure may develop AK at a young age. Bald-headed men may develop hundreds of hypertrophic AKs on the scalp after many years of sun exposure.

AK can range in size from 1 mm to several centimeters. It commonly appears as a scaly reddish-brown or yellowish-black papule or macule (Figure 12.19). Bendl and Graham[7] and Montgomery and Dörffel[8] report that 20% of patients with AK develop squamous cell carcinoma.[9]

There are five histologically distinct types of actinic keratosis. These include hypertrophic, atrophic, bowenoid, acantholytic, and pigmented. Bowenoid actinic keratosis is a type of in situ squamous cell carcinoma. The lesion may progress to a locally aggressive, invasive SCC. Large amounts of melanin are found in pigmented actinic keratosis. AKs are treated with superficial destructive methods such as curettage, topical acids, or cryosurgery (Figures 12.20, 12.21, and 12.22).

Actinic Cheilitis

Actinic cheilitis (solar cheilitis, actinic keratosis of the lip) occurs predominantly on the lower lip of elderly men. In the acute form, actinic cheilitis appears after prolonged sun exposure, often during the summer. Symptoms include redness, swelling, and ulceration. The condition tends to improve in the fall and winter, but may recur during the following summer.

The wrinkled, scaly variety of actinic cheilitis is usually chronic (Figure 12.23). The border of the lip becomes white or gray, and erosion and ulceration may follow. The condition, if untreated, may evolve into squamous cell carcinoma.

Actinic cheilitis can be treated with topical 5-fluorouracil, surgical excision, or carbon dioxide laser.[10,11]

Arsenical Keratosis

Arsenical keratoses are most common on the palms and soles and develop many years after arsenic ingestion. The hard, yellow nodules may coalesce to form verrucous plaques, which may also appear on other parts of the body (Figure 12.24). Arsenical keratoses can be a clinical sign of potential internal cancer.

Some arsenical keratoses develop into Bowen's disease and then into invasive squamous cell carcinoma. Treatment usually involves surgical excision.

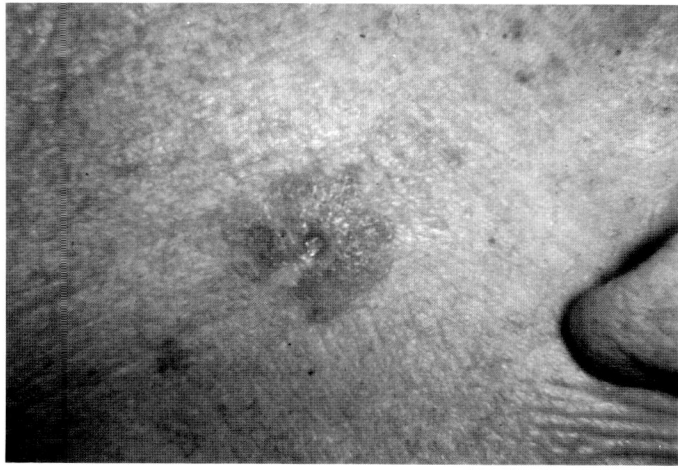

FIGURE 12.19. Actinic keratosis is a localized area of premalignant change that develops on sun-damaged skin. (Used with permission, C. William Hanke, M.D.)

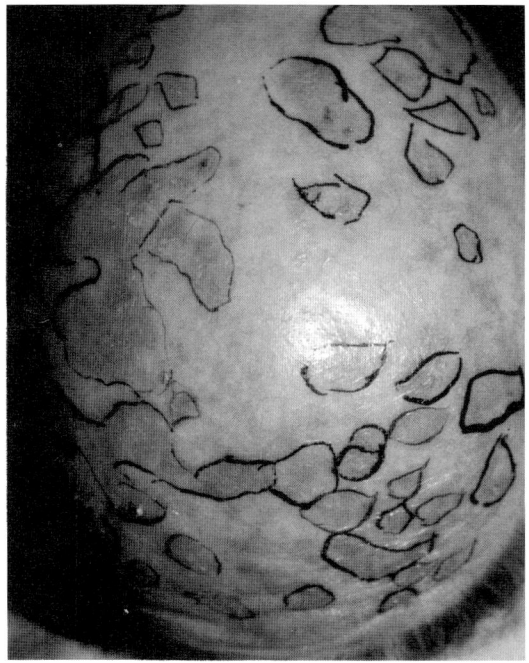

FIGURE 12.20. A 61-year-old bald-headed man developed multiple hypertrophic actinic keratoses on the scalp. (Used with permission, C. William Hanke, M.D.)

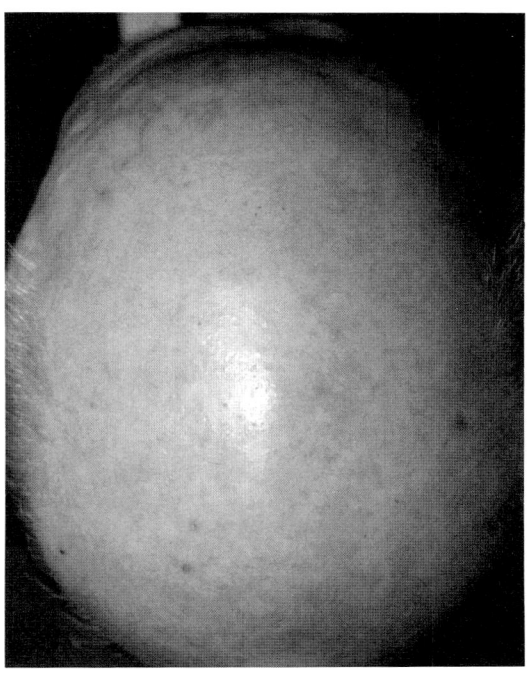

FIGURE 12.22. Four weeks later, the scalp has healed with a good result (the same patient as in Figures 12.20 and 12.21). (Used with permission, C. William Hanke, M.D.)

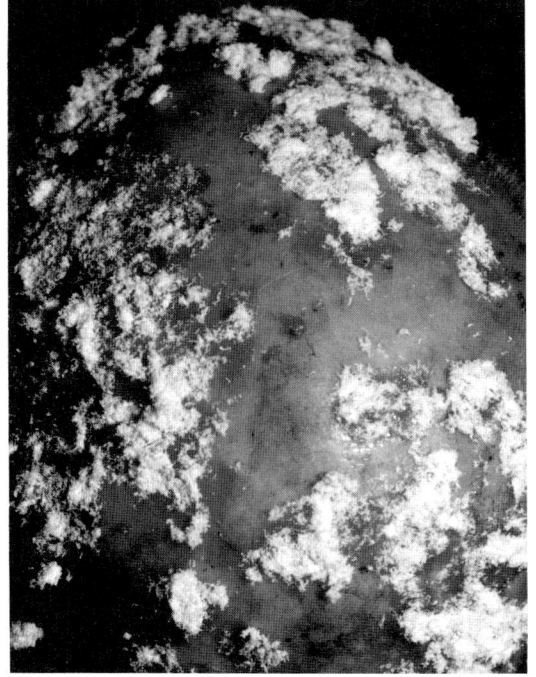

FIGURE 12.21. The scalp of the patient in Figure 12.20 is seen immediately following removal of actinic keratoses with superficial curettage. The white material is hemostatic collagen. (Used with permission, C. William Hanke, M.D.)

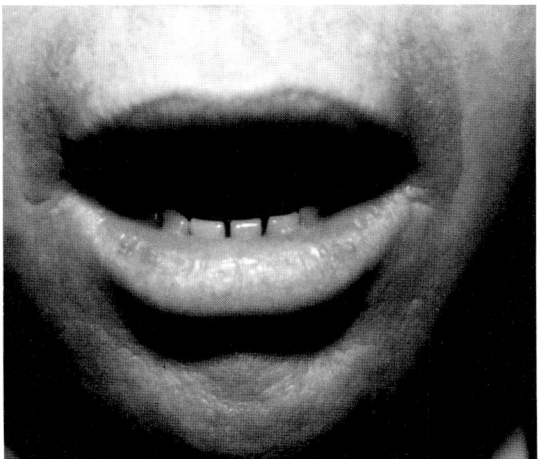

FIGURE 12.23. This 60-year-old golfer has developed actinic cheilitis on the vermilion of the lower lip. (Used with permission, C. William Hanke, M.D.)

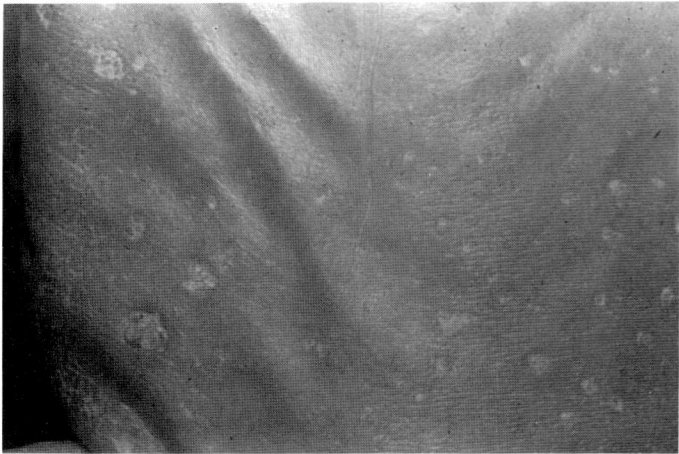

FIGURE 12.24. Arsenical keratoses are thickened punctate papules that occur in individuals who have been exposed to arsenic. (Used with permission, C. William Hanke, M.D.)

Bowen's Disease

Bowen's Disease is a premalignant form of squamous cell carcinoma. About 80% of cases affect Caucasian men, and the onset is often in the fourth or fifth decade. Equal numbers occur on exposed and covered areas of the body, with one-third occurring on the head and neck. One-third of patients have multiple lesions. If given enough time, Bowen's disease will evolve into invasive squamous cell carcinoma.

Bowen's disease appears clinically as a scaly, erythematous, fissured plaque and usually is distinct from the surrounding normal skin (Figure 12.25). There is controversy regarding a possible association between Bowen's disease on non-sun-exposed areas and extracutaneous malignancies; however, exposure to arsenic has not been ruled out as a causative factor.

Treatment for Bowen's disease is like that for any carcinoma in situ. Surgical excision, cryosurgery, electrodesiccation/curettage, or Mohs micrographic surgery are modalities used in treating these lesions. Bowen's disease can involve hair follicle epithelium and penetrate to the level of the subcutaneous fat.

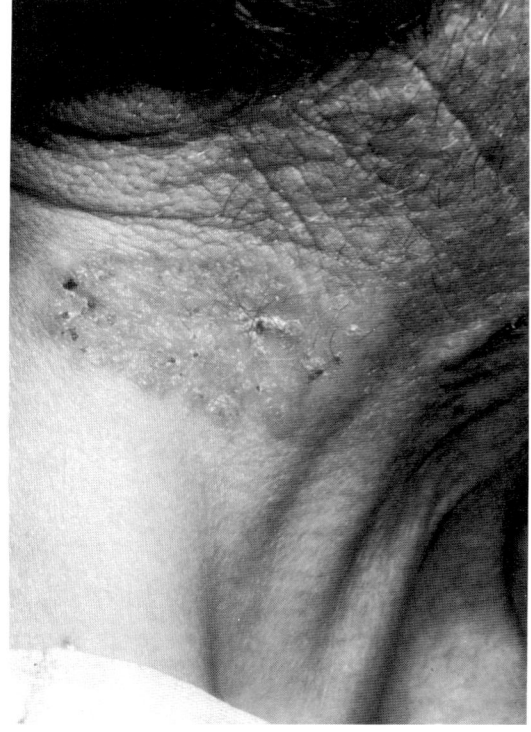

FIGURE 12.25. A fair-skinned 65-year-old man developed an area of Bowen's disease on the neck. (Used with permission, C. William Hanke, M.D.)

12. Skin Lesions of Aging

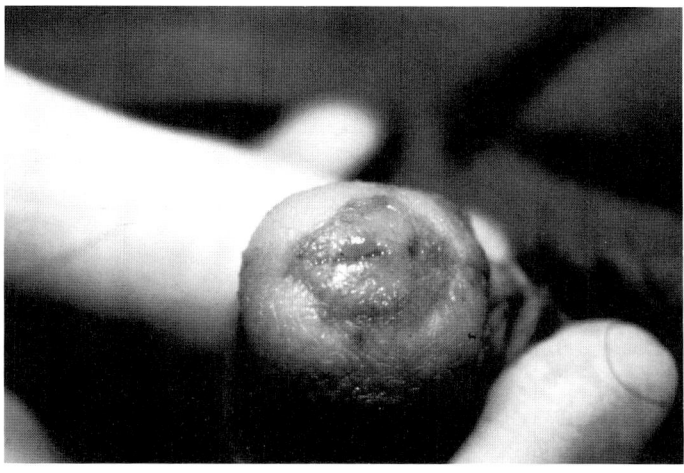

FIGURE 12.26. An uncircumcised 70-year-old man developed erythroplasia of Queyrat on the glans penis. (Used with permission, C. William Hanke, M.D.)

Erythroplasia of Queyrat

Erythroplasia of Queyrat (EPQ) is the designation given to Bowen's disease of the glans penis. It occurs as a bright red plaque that can be accompanied by scaling and crusting (Figure 12.26). EPQ occurs almost exclusively in uncircumcised males as young as 20 years or older than 70. The treatment is surgical.

Chronic Radiation Dermatitis

Until the early 1970s, low doses of radiation were used to treat various benign dermatologic disorders (*(e.g,* teenage acne), primarily on the face and neck. Chronic radiation dermatitis develops long after exposure to fractional doses of radiation. Patients with skin Type I or II are especially vulnerable. Clinical signs of chronic radiation dermatitis include skin erythema, atrophy, hyper-and hypopigmentation, telangiectasia, and ulceration (Figure 12.27). Many patients are asymptomatic for 20 to 30 years, then develop multiple basal cell or squamous cell carcinomas in the radiation-treated areas.[12]

Patients with chronic radiation dermatitis should be examined at regular intervals for premalignant or malignant changes in the affected area. Subsequent exposure to ultraviolet light is to be avoided, as is trauma to the area.

Extramammary Paget's Disease

Unlike Paget's disease, which occurs on the breast, extramammary Paget's disease (EMPD) usually occurs in the anogenital region, most frequently on the vulva, and less commonly on the male genitalia.

The condition presents as a reddish-brown, moist, eroded plaque much like eczema (Figure

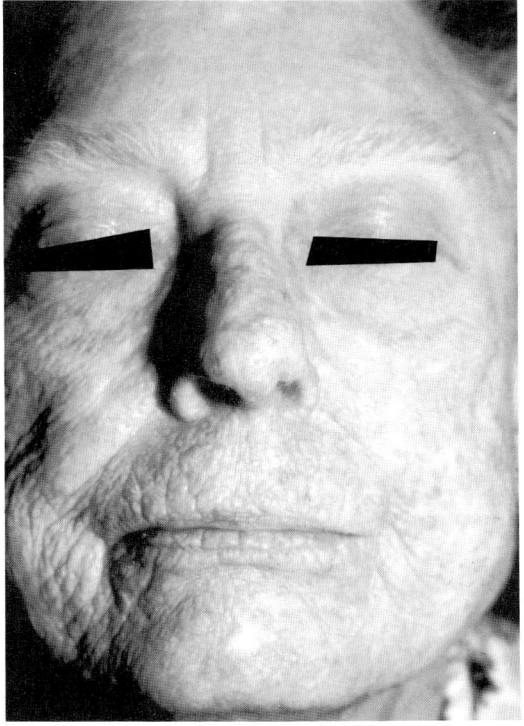

FIGURE 12.27. A 67-year-old woman had x-ray treatments for acne at age 15. She now has chronic radiation dermatitis and has had many basal cell carcinomas treated on the face. (Used with permission, C. William Hanke, M.D.)

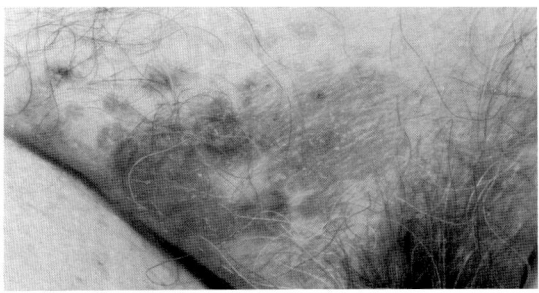

FIGURE 12.28. Extramammary Paget's disease is a refractory premalignant condition that affects the anogenital area of elderly individuals. (Used with permission, C. William Hanke, M.D.)

12.28). EMPD can be painful and pruritic. The tumor is classified as a primary intraepidermal apocrine carcinoma. EMPD is occasionally indicative of an internal malignancy. It grows slowly and usually spreads well beyond the clinically apparent margins. Surgical excision of the tumor often results in regional recurrence. Margin control is important, and some success with Mohs micrographic surgery has been reported.[13]

Lentigo Maligna

Lentigo maligna (Hutchinson's freckle, senile freckle) occurs almost exclusively on sun-exposed areas of the face in elderly patients. It presents as an unevenly pigmented, light brown or dark brown macular patch. The growth is very slow (Figure 12.29). It may spread to involve an area of several centimeters or more. One-third of lentigo malignas that grow to a size of 4 to 6 cm will eventuate in lentigo maligna melanoma.

Conservative removal of the lesion is usually all that is required. This may be achieved by electrodesiccation/curettage or surgical excision.

Dermatoses/Infections

Contact Dermatitis

Contact dermatitis is caused by an allergic reaction to any number of items or by contact with a primary skin irritant. Some of the most common causes of allergic contact dermatitis include metals (especially nickel), plants (e.g., poison ivy), and cosmetics. Symptoms and signs of contact dermatitis include pruritus, erythema, and vesiculation (Figure 12.30). Elderly individuals may develop prolonged episodes of contact dermatitis due to decreased immune function. Primary irritant contact dermatitis can be especially severe. Treatment includes avoidance of the allergen and allowing the dermatitis to resolve naturally. In some cases topical or systematic steroids may be necessary.

Favre-Racouchot Syndrome

Favre-Racouchot syndrome is characterized by nodular elastosis with cysts and comedones on the upper lateral cheeks. Thickened yellow plaques are also present (Figure 12.31). It is the result of profound ultraviolet damage and is found predominantly in men. Favre-Racouchot syndrome can be prevented by avoiding exposure to ultraviolet radiation. Treatment with retinoids is currently being investigated and appears promising.

Granuloma Fissuratum

Granuloma fissuratum (acanthoma fissuratum) is caused by the constant pressure of the nose- or earpiece of eyeglasses in elderly individuals. Skin that is constantly traumatized develops into a small nodule with a fissure or furrow in the center. It may mimic a basal cell carcinoma clinically (Figure 12.32). The correction of poorly fitting eyeglasses is usually curative.

Perlèche/Angular Cheilitis

Perlèche is caused by both physical and biological factors. The microorganism *Candida albicans* is responsible for the actual physiological condition known as perlèche. However, the microbe alone cannot cause the condition. In elderly patients oftentimes the skin sags at the corners of the mouth. This is the result of gravitational effects of aging or to poorly fitting dentures, which can lead to overclosure of the mouth. The corners of the mouth develop furrows that can trap saliva. The saliva accumulates and erodes the skin, creating a moist

12. Skin Lesions of Aging

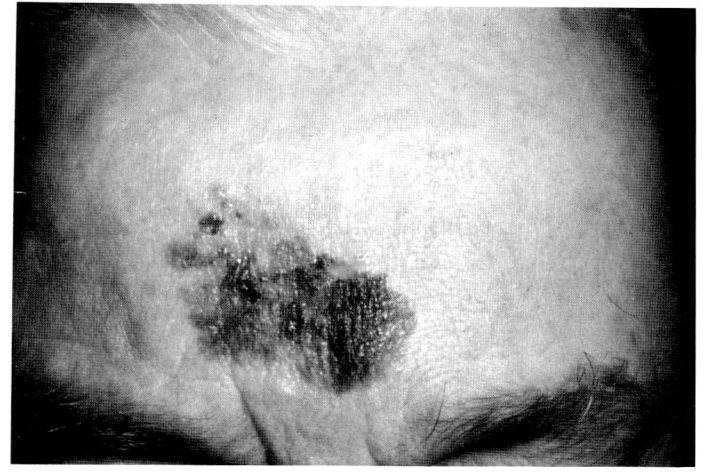

FIGURE 12.29. A 75-year-old man has had an enlarging lentigo maligna on the forehead for 8 years. (Used with permission, C. William Hanke, M.D.)

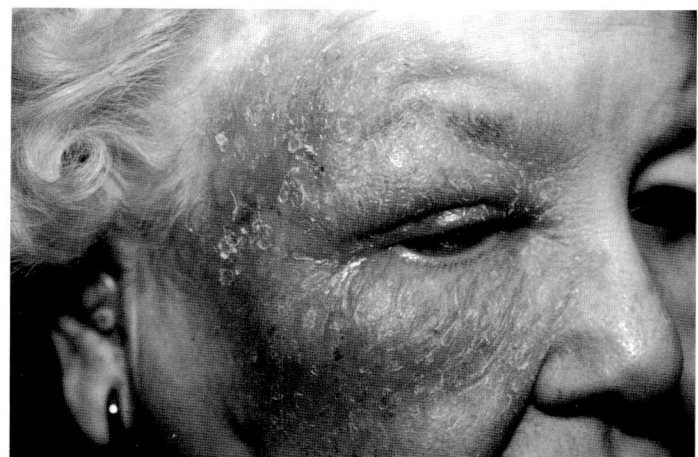

FIGURE 12.30. This elderly woman developed allergic contact dermatitis to a topical antibiotic. (Used with permission, C. William Hanke, M.D.)

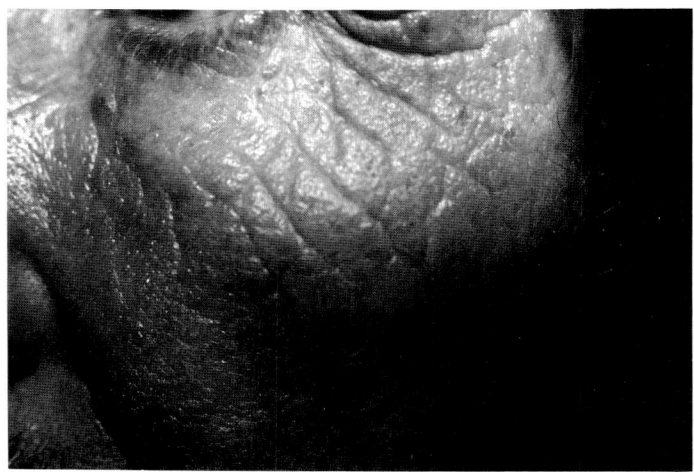

FIGURE 12.31. Favre-Racouchot syndrome is characterized by deep solar damage and comedones on the upper cheek. (Used with permission, C. William Hanke, M.D.)

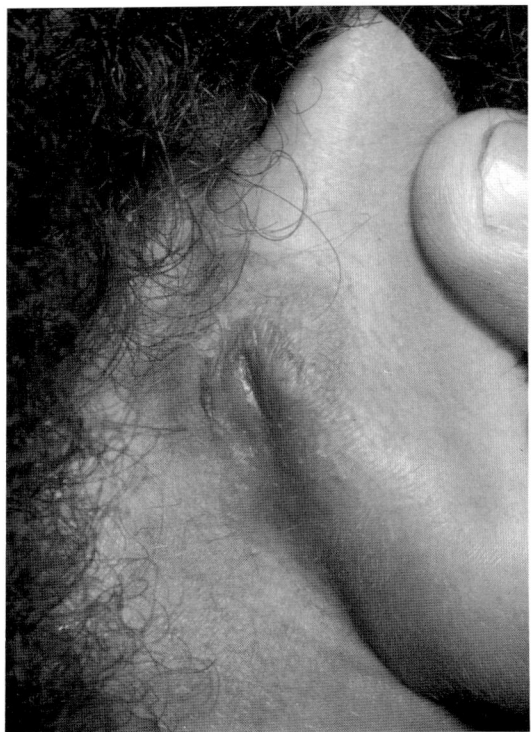

FIGURE 12.32. Granuloma fissuratum is often seen as a tender fissure in the postauricular sulcus of elderly individuals. It is caused by pressure from eyeglasses. (Used with permission, C. William Hanke, M.D.)

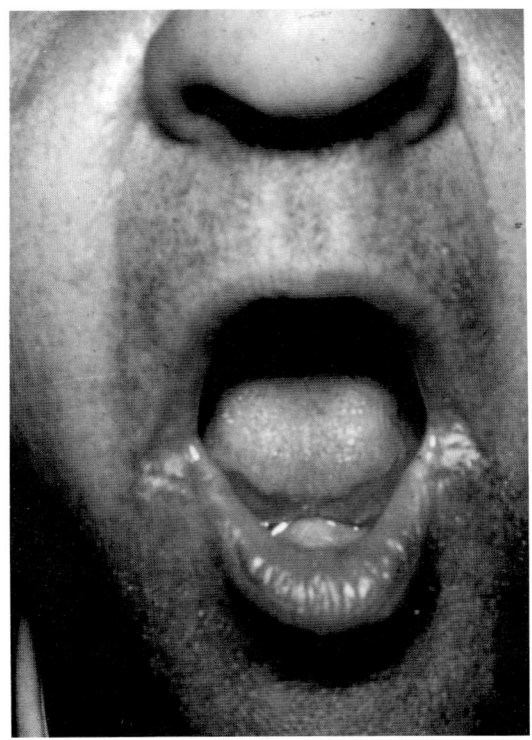

FIGURE 12.33. Perlèche is an overgrowth of *Candida albicans* that occurs in sagging skin folds adjacent to the mouth in elderly individuals. (Used with permission, C. William Hanke, M.D.)

environment that is ideal for the growth of *C. albicans* (Figure 12.33).

Perlèche is treated by the application of clotrimazole cream to the corners of the mouth and the use of clotrimazole lozenges dissolved in the mouth to combat the growth of *C. albicans*. It is also important to supplement the antifungal treatment with vitamins, zinc, and iron, since poor nutrition often underlies the disease.

Poikiloderma of Civatte

Poikiloderma of Civatte commonly occurs in middle-aged women on the sides of the face and neck after many years of sun exposure. This condition is characterized by blotchy, reddish-brown hyperpigmentation, hypopigmentation, telangiectasia, erythema, and atrophy (Figure 12.34). It has been suggested that a photodynamic substance in cosmetics may be a causative agent for some cases of poikiloderma of Civatte. Pulsed dye laser has recently been advocated as effective treatment.

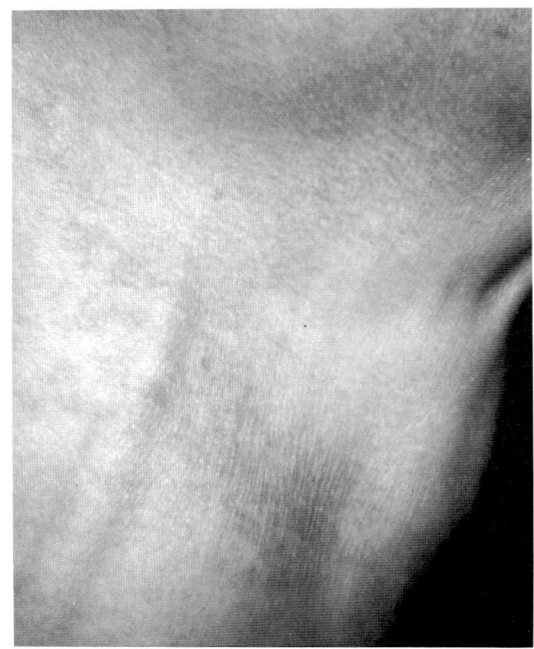

FIGURE 12.34. A 55-year-old woman with a history of heavy sun exposure has developed poikiloderma of Civatte on the neck. (Used with permission, C. William Hanke, M.D.)

Rosacea/Rhinophyma

Rosacea is a condition characterized by chronic erythema and telangiectasia involving the middle third of the face. The condition may be accompanied by edema, papules, pustules, and nodules. Although rosacea is more common in women between ages 30 and 50, it is usually more severe in men.

There are three types of acne rosacea, which may occur alone or in combination. The erythematous telangiectatic type is characterized by erythema, telangiectasia, and follicular pustules (Figure 12.35). The glandular hyperplastic type leads to the condition called rhinophyma and is characterized by variable enlargement of the nose and surrounding tissues (Figure 12.36). This variety is commonly seen beginning in the fifth decade of life. The papular type is characterized by raised papules measuring 1 to 3 mm in diameter.

The episodes of rosacea may begin sporadically, but as the disease progresses, the episodes become more frequent until the condition becomes constant. Only variations in the severity of the erythema distinguish major episodes.

Treatment for rosacea is nonspecific. Vasodilating substances should be avoided (*i.e.,* hot beverages, extremes of heat and cold, spicy food). The pustular component of the disease may be treated by any of the treatments used for acne.

The treatment for severe rhinophyma is surgical excision of the redundant nasal tissue. This is accomplished using a variety of methods including dermabrasion, CO_2 laser ablation, and electrosurgical excision.[14] The cosmetic results are usually good, although recurrence of the redundant tissue is possible.

Senile Purpura

Senile purpura occurs on sun-damaged skin in the elderly. The most common locations are the backs of the hands and the forearms. With age the dermis thins, thereby reducing support for dermal blood vessels. The subcutaneous fat layer also undergoes progressive atrophy with age in many individuals. Imperceptible minor traumatic events can result in fairly large areas of senile purpura (Figure 12.37).

Stasis Dermatitis

Stasis dermatitis results from inadequate venous circulation in the legs. Scaling, swelling, erythema, oozing, and crusting are characteristic of this disorder. Ulceration of the skin may occur, especially near the medial malleolus.

Treatment includes the use of pressure garments, emollients, and topical antibacterial agents. Local wound care and systemic antibiotics may be required if ulceration occurs.

Telangiectasia

Telangiectasia is the proliferation and dilation of dermal blood vessels, which result in the characteristic fine, wirelike red or blue vessels that are visible on the skin surface. The causes of telangiectasia are numerous. They are commonly seen on the noses and cheeks of middle-aged and elderly individuals and are more common in women. Oftentimes these individuals have fair skin and have had significant sun exposure.

The telangiectasias can be removed easily with electrosurgery or laser (Figures 12.38 and 12.39).

Tinea pedis

Tinea pedis, a dermatophyte infection on the feet, is most commonly caused by *T. rubrum*, *T. mentagrophytes*, or *E. floccosum*. The dermatophyte causes scaling, maceration, and ulceration of the skin in the webs between the toes, and occasionally on the sole or instep of the foot. An inflammatory variant can exhibit pustules, vesicles, or bullae and may be confused with other types of dermatitis. A diagnostic potassium hydroxide wet mount from the roof of a vesicle will reveal hyphae.

The incidence of tinea pedis in populations that wear closed shoes is much higher than that of barefoot or sandled populations. The dermatophyte is spread easily in warm, moist environments such as are found in pools and locker rooms. Topical antifungal agents are often sufficient for treating tinea pedis. Oral antifungal agents are often required to eradicate inflammatory dermatophyte infections.

Older individuals can develop refractory dermatophyte infections of the toenails (Figure 12.40). Current treatments for onychomycosis

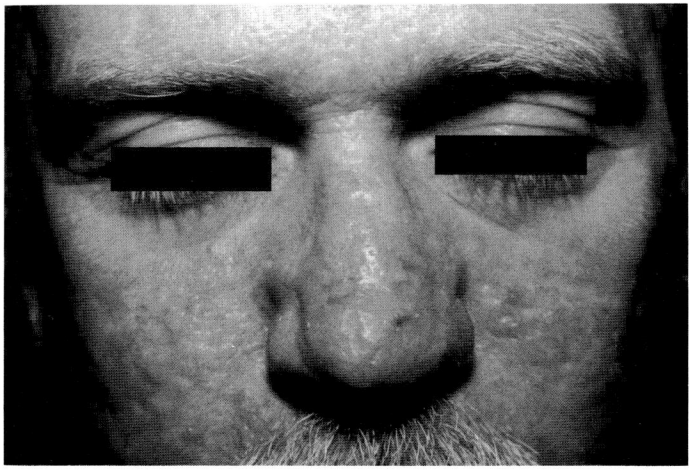

FIGURE 12.35. Acne rosacea is characterized by redness and acneform pustules that affect the central face. (Used with permission, C. William Hanke, M.D.)

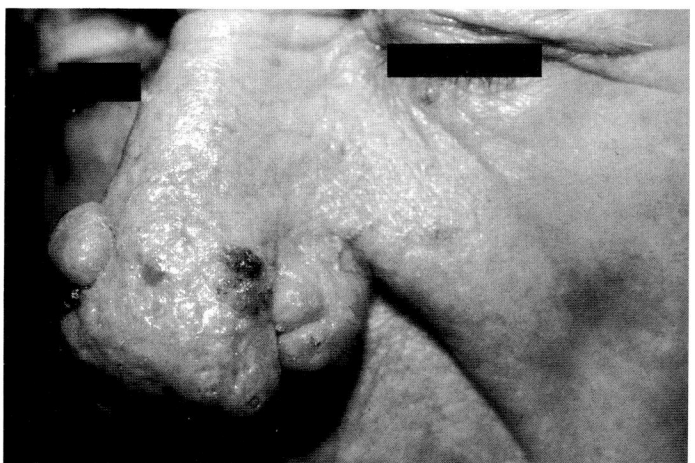

FIGURE 12.36. Rhinophyma is the glandular-hyperplastic form of acne rosacea that is seen in men over age 50. (Used with permission, C. William Hanke, M.D.)

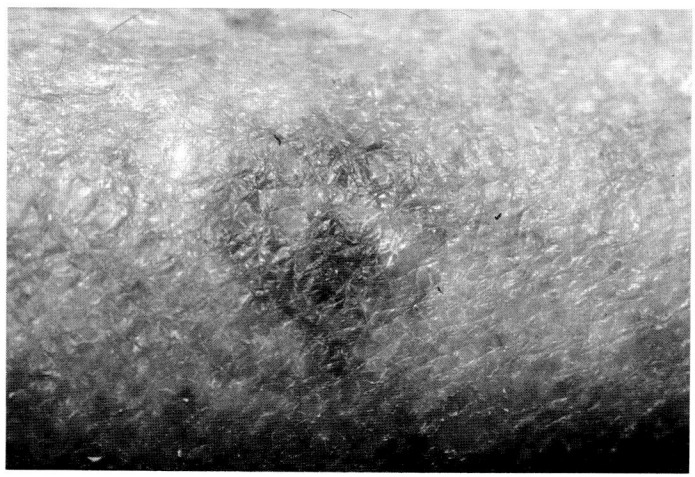

FIGURE 12.37. An elderly individual has developed a bruise on the dorsal forearm following imperceptible minor trauma. (Used with permission, C. William Hanke, M.D.)

12. Skin Lesions of Aging

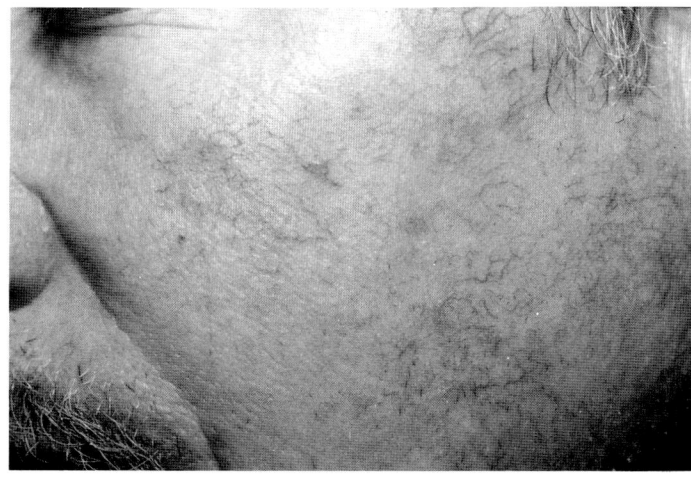

FIGURE 12.38. A 50-year-old man with a history of heavy sun exposure developed multiple solar telangiectasias on the cheeks. (Used with permission, C. William Hanke, M.D.)

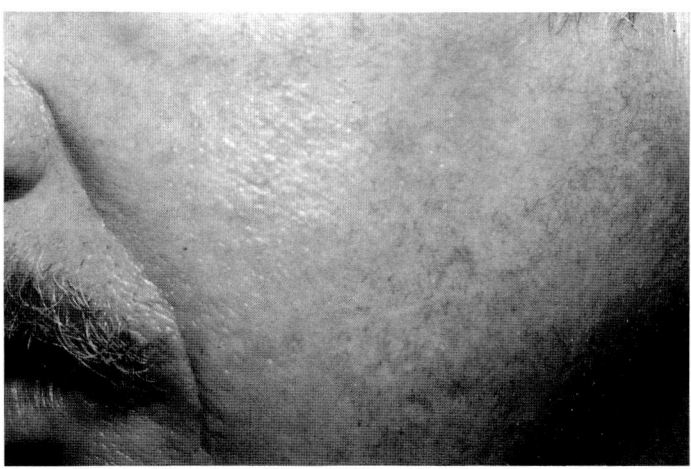

FIGURE 12.39. The patient in Figure 12.38 is seen 4 weeks following removal of the solar telangiectasias with argon laser. (Used with permission, C. William Hanke, M.D.)

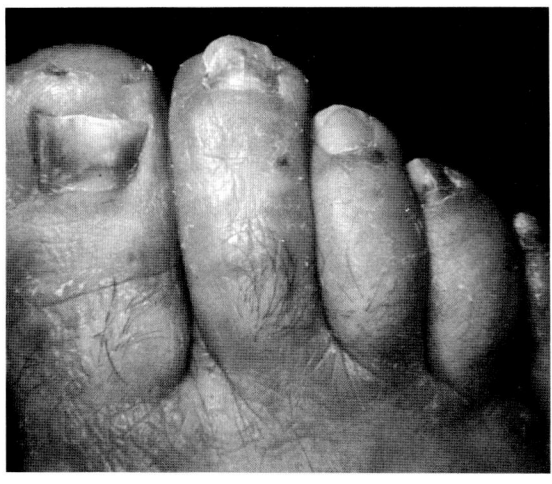

FIGURE 12.40. This 44-year-old man has scaling of the skin of the feet and opacity of the toenails. *Trichophyton rubrum* is causative. (Used with permission, C. William Hanke, M.D.)

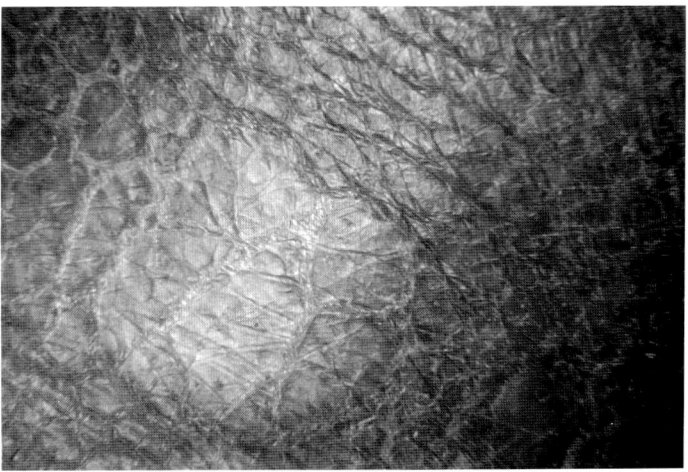

FIGURE 12.41. A 75-year-old black man has severe dryness of the skin (xerosis) on the leg. (Used with permission, C. William Hanke, M.D.)

are effective in only one-quarter of cases. Therefore, the physician may recommend that onychomycosis not be treated.

Xerosis/Eczema Craquelé/Asteatotic Dermatitis

Xerosis is a disorder of aging characterized by the dry, rough feel of the skin of the elderly. It occurs more often at times of the year when humidity is low. Histological studies show that the stratum corneum and epidermis of the elderly does not change appreciably from youth. Reduction in sebum output with age may be part of the cause of xerosis.

Eczema craquelé (asteatotic dermatitis) is characterized by extremely dry, scaled, and fissured skin accompanied by itching (Figure 12.41). It is most likely to affect the elderly but can also be indicative of HIV infection or the side effect of H2 antihistamine blockers. Many extrinsic factors may also be causative agents. These include degreasing agents, chemicals, deodorant soaps, and cold, dry air.

Treatment depends on the underlying cause of the condition. Symptoms may be relieved by eliminating drying soaps or adding humidity to the air in one's home. Some cases may require treatment with topical steroids and antipruritics.

Miscellaneous Aging Changes

Crow's Feet

Crow's feet are the fine lines that radiate out from the lateral corners of the eyes (Figure 12.42). They are caused by facial animation and

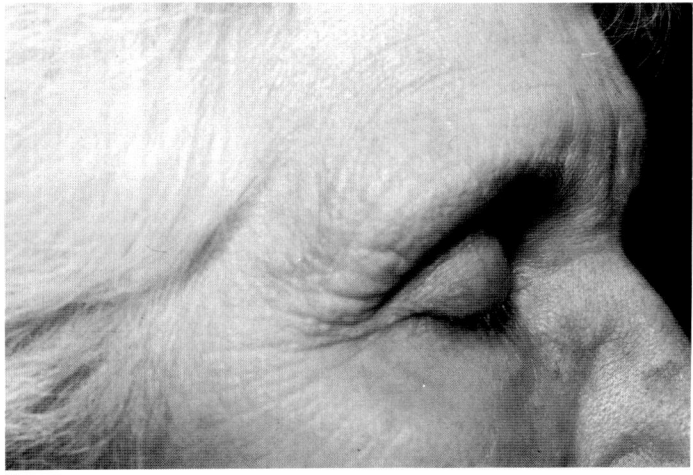

FIGURE 12.42. Crow's feet are wrinkles at the lateral aspect of the eye. (Used with permission, C. William Hanke, M.D.)

12. Skin Lesions of Aging

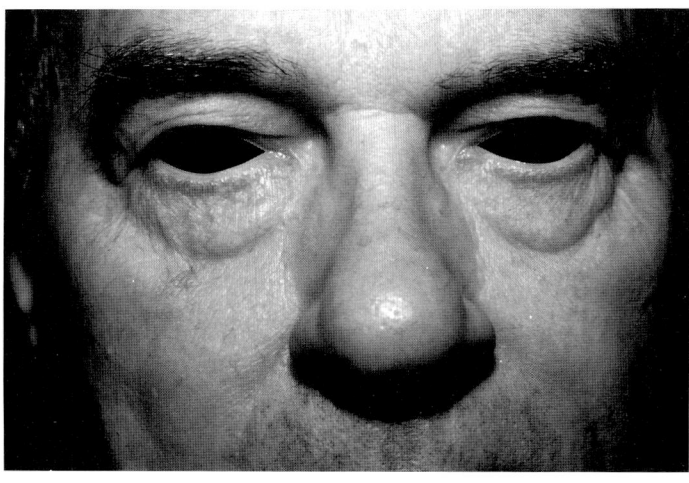

FIGURE 12.43. A 66-year-old man has pronounced lower lid fat pads. (Used with permission, C. William Hanke, M.D.)

become more pronounced with age. These lines, if they are not deep, can give the face the pleasant appearance reminiscent of a smile. Deep creases can be treated with collagen injections. However, the thin dermis in this area of the face predisposes to "beading" or lumpiness following injection. Tretinoin, chemical peel, dermabrasion, and other dermal fillers are additional therapeutic alternatives.

Increased Laxity of Eyelid Skin and Protrusion of Intraorbital Fat

The skin of the eyelids becomes redundant with age (dermatochalasis). Visual fields can be obstructed by sagging upper eyelid skin, especially at the temples. The orbital septum is a fascial sheet that holds the intraorbital fat in place. As the septum weakens with age, the intraorbital fat can produce obvious bulges on the eyelids (Figure 12.43). Redundant skin and fat pads can be excised from the upper and lower lids using blepharoplasty techniques.[15]

Hereditary Hair Loss

Hereditary pattern hair loss (androgenetic alopecia) is the most common type of hair loss and occurs in both males and females. Androgenetic alopecia is a hormonally influenced, inherited trait. Males may develop considerable hair loss by the early twenties and baldness by age 25 or 30 if family history is strong. Because of minimal androgen production, females rarely experience balding but may develop considerable thinning of the hair (Figure 12.44).

Treatment options are limited and depend on the extent of the hair loss. Success has been minimal with topical minoxidil. Surgical hair transplantation is effective in properly selected candidates.

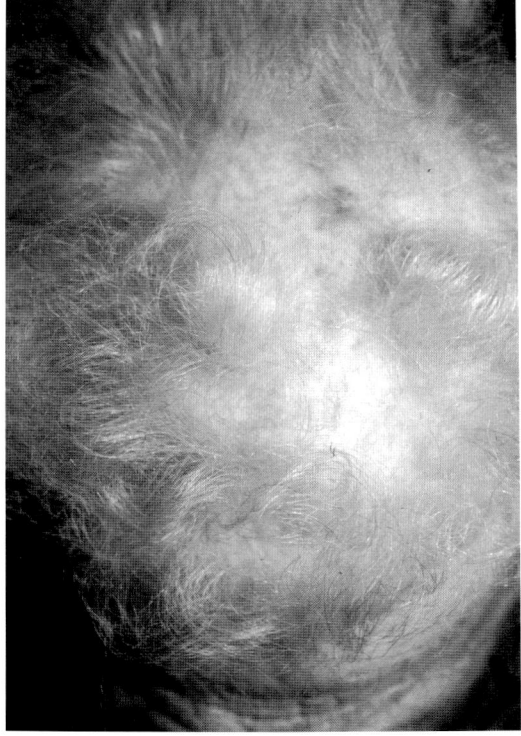

FIGURE 12.44. Hereditary hair loss in an elderly woman is characterized by thinning rather than baldness. (Used with permission, C. William Hanke, M.D.)

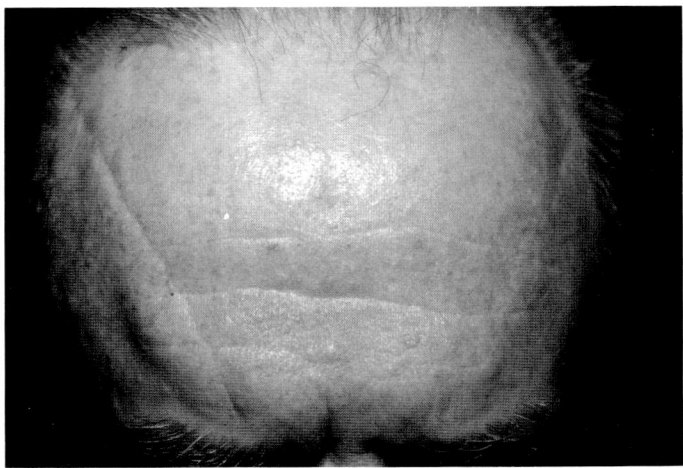

FIGURE 12.45. Sleep creases are unilateral vertical lines that can develop on the forehead of elderly men and women who prefer to sleep on one side of the face. The creases can also been seen on other areas of the face. (Used with permission, C. William Hanke, M.D.)

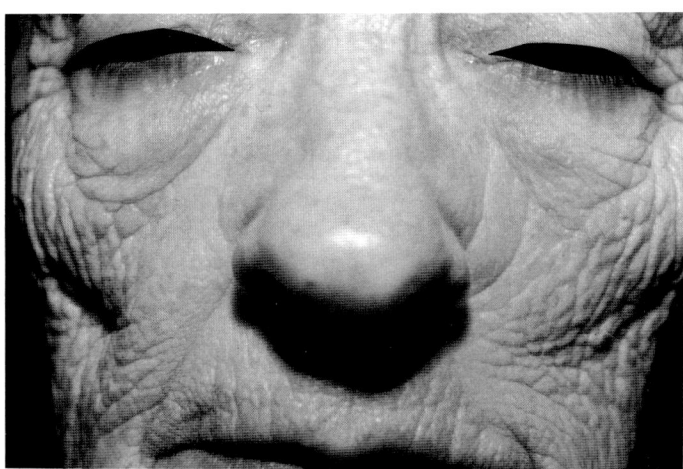

FIGURE 12.46. A 72-year-old woman with a history of heavy sun exposure has severe wrinkling of the facial skin. (Used with permission, C. William Hanke, M.D.)

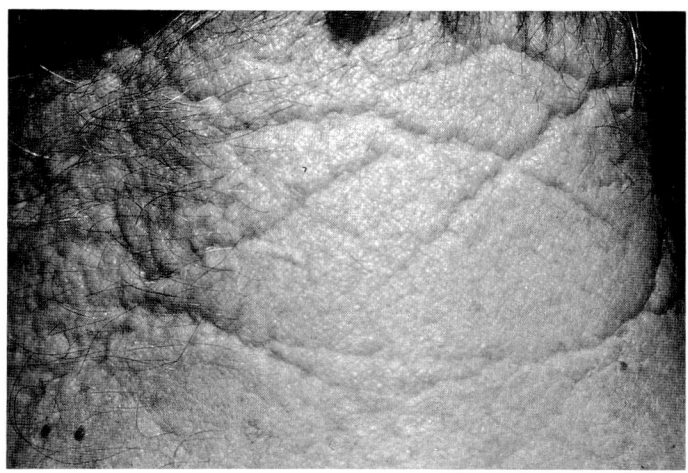

FIGURE 12.47. A 50-year-old farmer has severe sun damage on the posterior neck (*i.e.,* cutis rhomboidalis nuchae). (Used with permission, C. William Hanke, M.D.)

Sleep Creases

Sleep creases are caused by prolonged mechanical pressure from a bed pillow against the skin during sleep. The creases usually occur on only one side of the face such as the forehead (Figure 12.45). This asymmetric distribution distinguishes them from other movement-related lines. In men the creases are usually deep, straight, and vertical. In women the lines are usually less deep.

Patients can be instructed to alter their sleep positions to alleviate the sleep creases.[16] Filler-substances are not very effective if the causative mechanical pressure is repeated each night.

Severe Wrinkling

Severe wrinkling (solar elastosis, actinic elastosis) is the result of many years of sun exposure. Clinically, the skin appears leathery and has a yellowish tint (Figures 12.46 and 12.47). The sun-damaged skin is dry and atrophic. Telangiectasias may appear in the skin on the head, neck, and extremities. These changes are histologically distinct from those of chronological aging. Aged skin loses elastic fibers only. Actinically damaged skin shows thicker, curled, and tangled elastic fibers and also degeneration of collagen fibers. Fair-skinned individuals, in contradistinction to darker individuals, are less resistant to actinic damage from solar exposure.

Treatment for sun-damaged skin includes the use of topical tretinoin, topical alpha hydroxy acids, chemical peels, dermabrasion, and injectable filler substances.[17-20] "Sags and bags" (gravitational changes) can be treated with excision (i.e., facelift, blepharoplasty) or liposuction.

References

1. Arndt KA. Argon laser therapy of small cutaneous vascular lesions. Arch Dermatol. 1982;118:220.
2. Morelli JG, Tan OT, Garden J, et al. Tunable dye laser (577nm) treatment of port wine stains. Lasers Surg Med. 1986;6:94.
3. Mohs FE. Seborrheic keratoses. JAMA. 1970;212:1956-1958.
4. Landthaler M, Haina D, Waidelich W, et al. Laser therapy of venous lakes (Bean-Walsh) and telangiectasia. Plast Reconstr Surg. 1984;73:78.
5. Mikhail GR, Kelly AP. Malignant angioendothelioma of the face. J Dermatol Surg Oncol. 1987;3:181-183.
6. Hanke CW, Conner AC, Temofeew RK, Lingeman RE. Merkel cell carcinoma. Arch Dermatol 1989;125:1096-1100.
7. Bendl BJ, Graham JH. New concepts on the origin of squamous cell carcinoma of the skin: solar (senile) keratosis with squamous cell carcinoma—a clinico-pathologic and histochemical study. Proceedings of the National Cancer Conference 6:471, 1971. New York, New York.
8. Montgomery H, Dörffel J. Verruca senilis und Keratoma senile. Arch Dermatol Syph (Berlin). 1932;166:286-296.
9. Marks R, Rennie G, Selwood TS. Malignant transformation of solar keratoses to squamous cell carcinoma. Lancet. 1988;1:795.
10. David LM. Laser ablation for actinic cheilitis. J Dermatol Surg Oncol. 1985;11:605-608.
11. Robinson JK. Actinic cheilitis: a prospective study comparing four treatment methods. Arch Otolaryngol Head Neck Surg. 1989;115:848-852.
12. Davis MM, Hanke CW, Zollinger TW, Montebello JF, Hornback NB, Norins AL. Skin cancer in patients with chronic radiation dermatitis. J Am Acad Dermatol. 1989;20:608-616.
13. Coldiron BM, Goldsmith BA, Robinson JK. Surgical treatment of extramammary Paget's disease. Cancer. 1991;67:933-938.
14. Clark DP, Hanke CW. Electrosurgical treatment of rhinophyma. J Am Acad Dermatol. 1990;22:831-837.
15. David LM, Sanders GH. Carbon dioxide laser blepharoplasty: a comparison to cold steel knife methods. J Dermatol Surg Oncol. 1987;13:110.
16. Stegman SJ. Sleep creases. Am J Cosmet Surg. 1987;4:277.
17. Kligman AM, Grove GL, Hirose R, Leyden JJ. Topical tretinoin for photoaged skin. J Am Acad Dermatol. 1986;15:836-859.
18. Brody HJ. Variations and comparisons in medium depth chemical peeling. J Dermatol Surg Oncol. 1989;15:953.
19. Monheit GD. The Jessner's and TCA peel: a medium depth chemical peel. J Dermatol Surg Oncol. 1989;15:945.
20. Millikan LE. Long-term safety and efficacy with Fibrel in the treatment of cutaneous scars—results of a multicenter study. J Dermatol Surg Oncol. 1989;15:837.

13
Hair Restoration

D. Bluford Stough and Craig S. Schauder

Androgenetic alopecia, or common baldness, occurs widely in both women and men, basically through the same underlying mechanisms. Circulating androgens enter susceptible cells of the hair follicle and are transported through the cytosol to the nucleus, where combination of androgen with the cell's genetic material takes place.[2] The net effect is an eventual slowing or inhibition of hair growth, possibly through interference with the cell's high-energy transfer systems, which are critical to rapid protein production.[3] Continued androgen action over time and through repeated hair growth cycles results in a shrinkage or miniaturization of the hair follicle, and the hair that is elaborated by the follicle becomes fine and eventually almost invisible.

The specific action of androgens at the follicle level has been under investigation for some time. Testosterone is the principal circulating androgen in males. In women, proandrogens and androgens are secreted by the adrenals and the ovaries. Some testosterone is normally present in the circulation in females. The major ovarian proandrogen is 4-androstenedione, while the primary adrenal proandrogen is dehydroepiandrosterone. However, it is generally accepted that it is not testosterone or dehydroepiandrosterone or androstenedione that is the active androgen in androgenetic alopecia but, rather, dihydrotestosterone (DHT), in both sexes. The enzyme systems necessary for the conversion of testosterone, dehydroepiandrosterone, and androstenedione to DHT are known to be present and operative in the skin, in hair follicles, and in particular in sebaceous glands, which together constitute one of the body's major sites for androgen metabolism.

Mechanisms of Androgenetic Alopecia

Current research on the hair follicle's functional activity indicates that hair "loss" may actually be better understood by viewing it as a failure to regrow in addition to taking the measure of the more readily apparent failure to retain. Shedding or falling out of hair is a normal event in the hair cycle, whereas failure to regrow hair is not. In androgenetic alopecia it may be primarily the regrowth mechanism that fails. Recent studies are shedding new light in this area. One study reports finding slow-cycling stem cells, capable of being activated by dermal papilla cells but located in the bulge area of the hair follicle.[4] Cells of this type have long been presumed to exist but were believed to be located in the matrix cell area, lower in the follicle. A bulge activation hypothesis has been proposed as a model for at least part of hair regrowth initiation processes,[5] and studies are continuing.

Heredity

Common baldness is an inherited trait,[6] with susceptibility at the cellular, nuclear level in the individual hair follicle under genetic control.

13. Hair Restoration

Clinical manifestation of alopecia is also linked, in some as yet unknown way, to a chronicity factor that is itself genetically controlled but which apparently proceeds independently of androgen action—that is, the biological clock for baldness keeps on ticking even when androgens are absent. If androgens then become available or are introduced, as in the treatment of eunuchs with testosterone, baldness will ensue and will rapidly establish a pattern of loss commensurate with life-long androgen exposure.[7]

Women

The implications of the catch-up phenomenon for the medical treatment of women should not be overlooked. Women who are subjected to compounds or influences possessing androgenic activity may be made vulnerable, depending on the extent of their genetic predisposition, to a rapid alopecic process in much the same way as eunuchs who are treated later in life with testosterone.

In most women androgenetic hair loss is less severe overall than in men and results in a more diffuse and less obvious pattern of loss, usually with sparing of the frontal hair line. There is some indication that biochemical differences at the hair follicle level may ultimately explain the lessened severity of androgenetic alopecia in women. High levels of aromatase have been found in the spared frontal hair follicles of women.[8] Aromatase is an enzyme that converts androstenedione and testosterone to the aromatized metabolites estrone and estradiol, thus making the androgen precursor forms unavailable for conversion to the potent dihydrotestosterone. Nevertheless, studies suggest that the prevalence of androgenetic alopecia in women is no lower than in men. Female alopecia becomes more apparent following menopause, when there is waning estrogen production and the concomitant loss of its antiandrogen effect.

Incidence

The high incidence of androgenetic alopecia in the population is common knowledge,[9] even though a definitive study has yet to be done. Studies in Caucasian males generally support approximation to a 10% rule: 10% affected in their teens, 20% in their twenties, 30% in their thirties, and so on, with a somewhat higher incidence from age 65 on.[10] Other races, specifically Japanese, Chinese, American Indian, and some blacks, are relatively unaffected by androgenetic alopecia.

Hair on the sides and back of the head is generally spared from the processes of androgenetic baldness, in the vast majority of individuals. Cells of the hair follicles in these "safe hair" areas are impervious to androgen action, protected by some as yet unknown mechanism. The cells may have receptors on their surface that deny rather than facilitate the entry of androgen into the cell, or there may be a barrier in the intracellular, cytosolic transport system normally responsible for carrying androgens through the cell and into the nucleus. It may also be that the molecular-level recognition sequences in cell genetic material are structured so as to thwart androgen linkage. Whatever the mechanism of protection, the innate growth characteristics of "safe" occipital region hair render it suitable for transplantation to areas of baldness, since it will continue to grow according to its own genetic character and will remain unaffected by surrounding baldness.

The History of Hair Restoration

Micrografting was the first technique of transplantation to be developed. It was initially devised for the replacement of eyebrow hair, however, and was applied only much later to cosmetic hair restoration procedures. It was the introduction of flap procedures as well as round punch grafting that supported the first hair transplantation performed on a comprehensive scale. Round graft use gave rise to cornstalking and scarring. Minigrafting and micrografting came into use first as a means of camouflaging round grafts and were subsequently used to produce cosmetically superior hairlines.

Scalp reduction was developed as a means of removing bald scalp in order to decrease the total size of the area to be treated with transplantation. Scalp reduction has undergone numerous modifications and improvements, most aimed at maximizing the amount of scalp removed in each procedure and at camouflaging the resultant scar. A more detailed history of each major individual hair restoration technique appears below.

Round Punch Grafts

Although autografts of hair-bearing tissue were first reported in the early 1800s, the first published report of round punch grafting as we know it today appeared in the Japanese literature in 1939,[11] and described the treatment of cicatrical alopecia with small autografts bored out with a trephine. War intervened, and Okuda's work was not widely appreciated until many years later. In the West round punch grafting was first reported by Orentreich in 1959.[12] Orentreich described the procedure in detail and, perhaps more important, demonstrated conclusively the validity of the principle of "donor dominance." This principle dictates that hair transplanted to a new region retains its own characteristics of growth and appearance and does not take on attributes of the new surroundings; in particular, it does not become vulnerable to baldness when placed in a bald area.

Based on the work of Okuda and Orentreich, round punch grafting became a mainstay of hair transplantation procedures, first as a means of harvesting donor tissue grafts and transplanting them without further division and later as a means of harvesting tissue for dissection into smaller grafts, following the introduction of minigrafting and micrografting techniques. Round punch grafting is still an important component in hair transplantation procedures. It is used most often in combination with other approaches to hair restoration, including micrografting, minigrafting, linear grafting, and scalp reduction.

Micrografts and Minigrafts

As with round punch grafting, early developments in micrografting were first reported in the Japanese literature. Sasagawa reported single hair grafting in 1930,[13] and in 1959 Fujita described the use of small dissected grafts to repair eyelash, eyebrow, and other deficits.[14] However, in the West it was Marritt's 1980 report on single-hair grafting for eyelash repair[15] that was the prelude to the expanded, and soon widespread, use of micrografts and minigrafts.

The significance of these small grafts of 1, 2, 3, or up to 8 hairs lies in the fact that they provide the tool with which to achieve a high degree of visual blendability in the overall transplant while at the same time allowing great versatility in the pattern in which grafts are placed within the recipient bed. These small grafts may be varied in size and shape and can be widely scattered or densely clustered, used to create zones of graded density. The use of small grafts thus provides the means to expand the concept of transplant design. The trend in future efforts to perfect the hair transplant will in our opinion be the development of superior patterns using the various sizes and shapes of small grafts.

Incisional Slit Grafting

The term *incisional slit grafting* refers to the placement of small grafts, *i.e.*, micrografts and minigrafts, into small slits that have been incised in the recipient bed. Incisional slit grafting came to prominence as a technique for minigrafting and micrografting in the late 1980s. It was further developed as a means for accomplishing entire transplantations.[16] The number of small grafts employed in the completion of a total or "finished" hair transplantation solely by this technique varies considerably but usually is in the several hundreds, accumulated over several sessions.

Advantages of the incisional slit grafting method include preservation of existing hair, less vascular compromise to the recipient area, and less scarring as compared to punch grafting. The use of this technique alone or in combination with other techniques has resulted in the development of new transplant design concepts.

Thin Strip Grafts

The first report of strip grafts appeared in 1964, when Vallis[17] described re-creating a frontal hairline through the use of 2 long and relatively wide (up to 8 mm) strips of hair-bearing donor scalp. Inconsistent growth patterns were associated with the Vallis strips, most likely secondary to their large size. In the 1970s use of a parallel-bladed knife was described in relation to the harvesting of square donor grafts of 4 mm on each side.[18] In these studies the knives were used to cut square donor grafts as well as the square recipient bed sites into which they were placed. In recent years the concept of a parallel-bladed knife has been combined with the concept of smaller strip grafts, and new knives have been developed.[19] The blades of the new knives are fixed at 2 mm or 2.5 mm apart; they make possible the harvesting of donor graft tissue in the form of thin strips that are many centimeters long and highly uniform. These strips are subsequently dissected to provide smaller grafts in whatever size wished. This technique for graft harvest and preparation can be much more rapid than methods that involve round graft harvest and dissection.

Linear Grafting

Linear grafting is a natural outgrowth of the ability to harvest hair-bearing donor tissue in long, thin strips, and is still a relatively new technique.[20] Linear grafting involves the use of strip grafts of 2 mm or 2.5 mm by 10 mm to 100 mm and inserting in appropriately sized incisional slits. These grafts may be used in the recipient area posterior to the frontal hairline as well as in the more central area of the scalp. Linear grafting provides an efficient means to achieve greater density, and it reduces the cornstalking appearance that may result from the use of individual minigrafts immediately posterior to the frontal micrograft zone.

Scalp Reduction

Scalp reduction for the treatment of baldness as we know it today was introduced in the mid-1970s. It has since been widely and successfully applied. The term *scalp reduction* refers to the surgical removal of relatively large segments of bald scalp. It is used to reduce the size of the area requiring transplantation.

The first report of scalp reduction appeared in French literature in 1976[21] and was later published in American literature in 1977.[22] The technique remained little known, however, until Stough and Webster presented their paper entitled "Esthetics and Refinements in Hair Transplantation" at the International Hair Transplant Symposium in Lucerne, Switzerland, in February 1978. Sparkhul, speaking at the same symposium, is generally credited with the first use of the term *scalp reduction*.

Unger and Unger had meanwhile conducted their own studies based on the concept of scalp reduction by surgical means, and they published their findings in 1978.[23] Bosley published details and results of a large study of sagittal mid-line reductions in 1979.[24] Significant contributions since then have been made by Alt,[25,26] who introduced the paramedian reduction, and by Norwood and Shiell,[27] Fleming and Mayer,[28] Nordstrom,[29] and also by Marzola,[30] who introduced a procedure for radical reduction, or total scalp lift. A modified version of the scalp lift procedure was described by Brandy.[31]

Flaps

Although scalp transposition flaps have a century-long history of use in reconstruction procedures, the first report of their use for cosmetic purposes was published by Lamont in 1957.[32] Later, procedures for long, twice-delayed temporoparietal-occipital (TPO) flaps were developed by Juri, who published a report of his work in 1975.[33] Elliott in 1977 reported on the use of bilateral, short, temporoparietal, nondelayed flaps;[34] while Nataf in 1979 reported the use of a long, postauricular flap dependent on microvascularization.[35] Ohmori described the application of microvascular surgery involving complex anastamoses to the creation of free, vascularized flaps.[36] Stough developed procedures for a long, horizontal, twice-delayed, temporoparietal-occipital flap that could be used in an office setting to create an entire hairline. The technique and results were reported in 1980 and 1985.[37,38]

Initial Patient Assessment

The assessment of patients for hair transplantation has been steadily changing, influenced both by widening experience and by the advent of micrografting and minigrafting. As a result of technical advances and the availability of multifaceted procedures, it is currently possible to offer treatment that will bring at least some improvement to virtually anyone who desires it. However, there are a few factors that may potentially contraindicate treatment with hair transplantation surgery, as discussed in this section.

Impaired Health

Each patient should provide a complete history. The presence of conditions that require the care of other specialists may require consultation. Hair transplantation is contraindicated in individuals whose state of health, either physical or psychological, indicates that the necessary surgical procedures would pose an unacceptable risk to their well-being. While few in actual number, these patients may include those with a range of disorders, including cardiovascular disease; uncontrolled hypertension; reactions to anesthetics, antiobiotics, or other substances; poorly controlled bleeding diatheses; and dermatologic conditions such as active lupus, morphea, and alopecia areata.

Psychological factors that contraindicate transplantation surgery include personality disorders and frank psychoneuroses, particularly paranoia. Fearfulness and anxiety of marked degree are also warning signs, as are goals and expectations that are unrealistic.[39]

Extreme Youthfulness

Some surgeons exclude the very young patient, i.e., under age 23. Early-onset hair loss can be an indicator for an eventually severe hair loss pattern, and in any case indicates that the course will be unpredictable. There is a risk that the pattern of growth created with transplanted grafts may be left isolated by a retreating native growth and that the donor hair mass in some cases will be insufficient to support ongoing corrective procedures. Most young patients who seek transplantation for very early and minimal hair loss may be advised to wait until their future pattern of hair loss can be better discerned.

Insufficient Donor Hair

Individuals do exist, although they are quite rare, who simply have an insufficient quantity or quality of hair to allow transplantation. Some patients in this category have an occipital donor area with very sparse, low-density, fine-caliber hair that achieves only marginal coverage of its own indigenous space. Some patients have occipital hair that exhibits good donor hair characteristics but is not present in sufficient volume. In patients who still have not experienced the major portion of their hair loss, the observation of severe recession or thinness in the temporal and parietal hair-bearing regions is an unfavorable sign. This pattern of early loss is an indicator that is associated with eventual severe hair loss. Another indicator of an eventually severe pattern of loss is the presence of whisker hair in the periauricular area, especially in young men. "Whisker hair" is short, curly hair resembling hair of the beard.

Poor Motivation

It is both the initial and the sustained motivation of the patient that determines to a large extent how successful hair transplant surgery will be in the patient's eyes after completion of all procedures. Patients who have difficulty accepting the long-term, multistage nature of hair transplantation are poor candidates. Similarly, patients who have unrealistic expectations are poor candidates—individuals who believe that hair restoration will culminate in cosmetic perfection or who expect happiness as a direct result of their surgery will inevitably be disappointed. Patients should be questioned closely and listened to carefully about their expectations and motivations. Nothing should be assumed. Younger patients should possess a clear, firm, and durable motivation that can sustain them through months or even years of periodic treatment.

Gender

Treatment of androgenetic baldness in women by hair transplantation can be very successful in carefully selected patients.[40] The major factor that renders treatment problematic is the fact that in women the hair of the entire scalp area may be diffusely affected by ongoing alopecia. Prediction of the eventual extent of the process is difficult, although family history may provide some indication. Thus, in women, donor grafts taken from the occiput and transferred to a new area may at a future time be subject to alopecia. In addition, women cannot be considered successfully treated by the creation of a naturally thinned look as can men, since a full head of hair is society's norm for female appearance.

Incisional slit grafting techniques allow enhancement to be undertaken in women without the need to remove any of the still viable existing hair. Small grafts may be placed among native hair in areas that are a cause of concern, to increase density and provide better coverage. Hair transplantation in women is also indicated for treatment of alopecia due to scarring as a result of burn injury, trauma, and certain disease processes. Micrografts and minigrafts may also be used to camouflage the scars resulting from surgical facelifts and browlifts.

Design Principles

Hair restoration design depends on the judgment, skill, and experience of the surgeon. It can be useful to remember that the primary purpose of the hairline in hair transplantation is to adequately *frame the face* of the patient, which means to place the correct visual limits to the forehead. Hairline height and lateral contours can be used to accomplish this goal. On the other hand, the purpose of central crown-area hair grafts is to provide coverage and to blend with and support the hairline. The purpose of the transplant as a whole is not to attempt to restore the lush growth of youth but to *break the visual impression of baldness*.

One of the most important aspects of design and planning involves the effective integration of the variety of hair transplantation techniques that are available. Each type of graft and recipient bed site has its own usage rationale. For example, very small micrografts are of greatest effectiveness in the frontal hairline, where they can be used to create a zone of graded density, while larger grafts are used more effectively in the central crown, where they can be used to enhance density. Usage concepts are discussed more fully in the later section on recipient bed management.

An almost infinite number of graft patterns for hair restoration can be devised, depending on patient needs. The sequence in which procedures take place is also open to variation. Figure 13.1 shows an idealized restoration se-

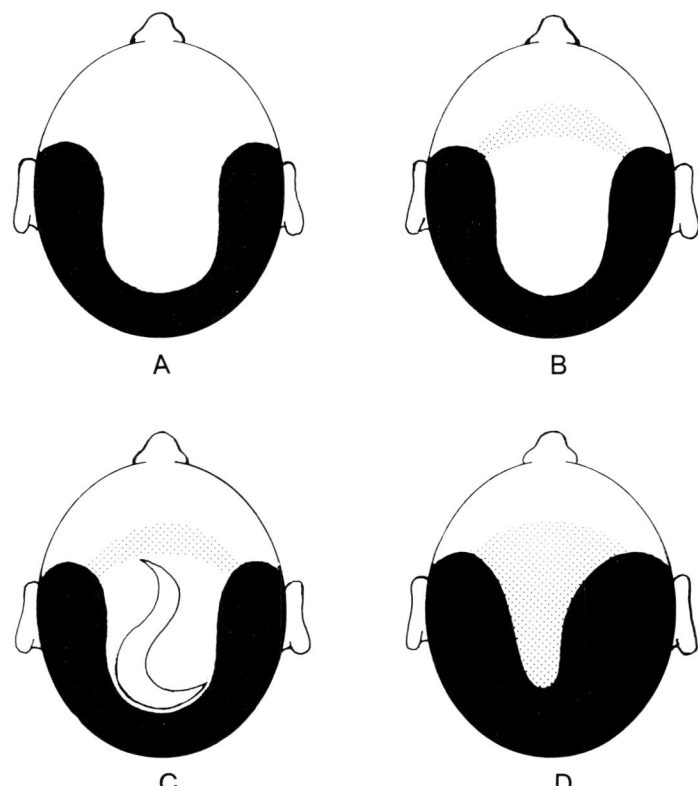

FIGURE 13.1. Idealized restoration sequence showing integration of scalp reduction and hair transplantation procedures.

quence that combines scalp reduction with hair transplantation. The contours and stages shown are not intended as actual treatment templates but, rather, as an illustration of the concept of sequencing and the integration of techniques.

In Figure 13.1, (A) represents the area of baldness seen in the incoming patient; (B) represents the early stages of treatment during which hairline creation is begun at the same time that initial reduction procedures are carried out; (C) represents intermediate stages of treatment involving enhancement of the hairline area combined with additional reduction procedures; and (D) represents the completed restoration, in which a well-established hairline blends with central area grafts that provide coverage of the bald scalp remaining after reduction.

Hairline Height Determination

A significant challenge facing the transplant surgeon is the matter of hairline design, in particular the determination of the hairline height on the forehead and the shape and contour of the hairline lateral arms. Lateral arms are defined as the bilateral (left and right) aspects of the hairline as it courses away from the frontal mid-point and toward the temporal area.

Early Greek and Roman aesthetic and artistic standards for beauty, particularly as expressed in studies of anatomic proportion and angulation by Leonardo da Vinci,[41] provided a basis for early hair transplantation standards for hairline height and, to a lesser extent, shape. Early transplant surgeons also drew on the experience of the makers of hairpieces for information concerning hairline height on the forehead.

Over the years since then, a standard approach to hairline design for hair transplantation has evolved. This approach includes the tripartite-face method for hairline height analysis; and the lateral canthus method for frontotemporal angle apex location, which largely determines lateral arm shape and position. These two methods have together provided a design technique that offers some measure of guidance and a fair certainty against unintentional medical oddities.

Tripartite-Face Analysis

The anthropometric-aesthetic facial analysis related most directly to hairline height determination is tripartite-face analysis. Tripartite-face analysis involves division of the face into three segments based on imaginary horizontal planes passing through anatomic markers. These markers consist of the hairline anterior limit, the glabella, the subnasale, and the menton (chin). This three-part division of the face was believed to provide an indicator for the "correct" vertical depth or width of the forehead and thus for the anterior limit for the hairline. These proportions pertain primarily to women.

It was subsequently recognized in men that the most advantageous and durably effective height for the transplant hairline lay some distance posterior to that indicated by strict tripartite-face analysis. It was observed that in most patients, excepting only those reaching maturity with a retained, well-defined widow's peak or an unregressed forelock, a moderately regressive placement of the hairline best simulated natural patterns that are appropriately mature and cosmetically effective on a permanent basis. A transplant hairline height that is excessively youthful, *i.e.,* too far forward or too low on the forehead, carries a very high risk of becoming inappropriate and unattractive within a few years.

The magnitude of the regression distance imposed between the tripartite-face–indicated hairline height and the actual transplant hairline height has always been a matter of judgment. Some have described the distance as being 2 finger-widths above the topmost brow wrinkle. Some have used a set distance of 7 cm to 9 cm above the glabella as the appropriate anterior limit of the hairline. And some have used a chin-to-nose measurement as an indication of correct forehead vertical depth. There is a maxim that the younger the patient to be treated for hair loss, the higher or more posteriorly the transplant hairline should be placed, because of the link between early-onset hair loss to late-severity hair loss and the magnified regression potential that it represents.

Physiognomy involving the forehead itself can play a part in hairline height determination. If the shape of the forehead is not well defined

13. Hair Restoration

by bony structure, and in particular if the slope of the forehead is such that its junction with the scalp is poorly distinguishable and appears as one long "backslope," then the hairline should be placed sufficiently anteriorly to interrupt the continuity of the slope and give definition to the forehead.

Hairline Shape Determination

Once the height of the transplant hairline has been determined, the shape of the lateral arms between the frontal midpoint and the junction with temporal area hair can be considered. In a standard design approach, the lateral arm shape is primarily determined by using the lateral canthus (the lateral terminus of the eye fissure) to locate the apex of the frontotemporal angle. The frontotemporal angle is formed by the junction of the hairline lateral arm with the superior fringe of the temporal area hair.

Lateral Canthus Indicator

A vertical line drawn through the lateral canthus in a frontal view of the patient is postulated to strike the position of the apex of the frontotemporal angle, even as the apex recedes and traces a path posteriorly (see Figure 13.2). Once the apices of the frontotemporal angle have been sited, the shape of the lateral arms of the hairline can be arrived at by drawing a symmetric and evenly curved line that encompasses all three marker points: the frontal hairline height at mid-point, and the apex sites of the left and right frontotemporal angle. The position of the contemplated transplant angle apex should then be regressed in proportion to expectations of future natural regression, much as the hairline height is regressed based on the same expectation. The effect that moving the angle posteriorly has on the lateral arms is shown in Figure 13.3. It should be noted that the lateral arm viewed in profile usually exhibits a horizontal, nonslanted orientation in the anterior-posterior course.

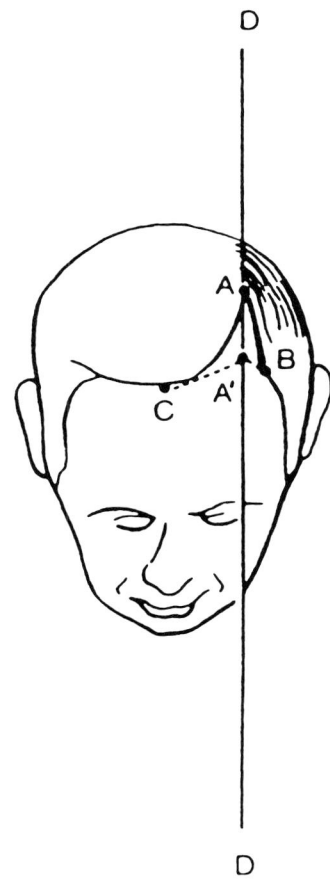

Front view

FIGURE 13.3. Positioning of hairline lateral arms in response to anticipated regression of the frontotemporal angle. Lateral arms generally appear horizontal when viewed in profile.

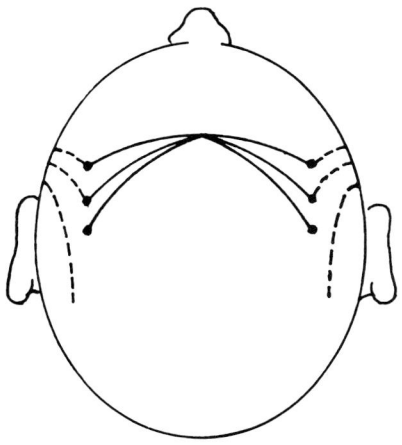

FIGURE 13.2. Lateral canthus indicator for the frontotemporal angle apex.

The temporal hair must also be considered in connection with hairline lateral arm design. If temporal hair is deeply regressed, either superiorly or at its vertical margin, or if it is thin and weak in nature, the proposed hairline lateral arms should be made less well defined as they approach the temporal area, and any merge with temporal hair should be softened and blurred. A definite V-shaped angle should not be attempted, since future loss in the junction area may be severe and may leave transplants stranded.

The proposed hairline height and lateral arm shape are assessed in profile as well as frontally. It has been axiomatic in hair transplantation that the hairline should not be allowed to angle below the horizontal as it courses anteriorly from the temporal area.

Individualized Contours

A key direction for hair restoration in the future is likely to be the development of techniques for highly individualized restoration design. There is an extraordinary variety in facial features and native hair growth contours, in the population at large and among patients. Standard design approaches may be clearly inadequate in some cases.

Temporal Area

Androgenetic hair loss with regression of temporal area hair typically occurs in the most superior and anterior portion of that area, along the inferior border of the frontotemporal angle or frontal gulf. In some patients the anterior point of the temporal fringe as well as some portion of the anterior vertical margin may also be lost. In transplants designed to remain effective over a long span of time, the frontotemporal angle, *i.e.,* the intersection of hairline with temporal area, is placed well posterior to its youthful location. This allows future regression to proceed without negation of transplant effectiveness. Transplantation in the temporal area itself is contraindicated except in cases of hair loss due to trauma, burns, quelled disease processes, and surgical scars for reasons related to high visibility.

In cases of severe baldness Norwood Class VI or VII, in which the superior margin of the temporal area hair is lowered substantially and accentuated regression of the vertical margin of the temporal fringe has occurred, hair transplantation may be problematic if not actually contraindicated in a very few. Donor hair may be insufficient to allow the creation of a natural appearance in the area where intersection of hairline with the temporal hair mass takes place. One approach in such patients is to restrict transplantation to the frontal forelock area, with no attempt made to re-create a frontotemporal angle or to transplant in the vertex (refer to Figure 10–12).

Crown/Vertex

The terms *crown* and *vertex* both mean, technically, the "top of the head." However, both terms have also been used to refer not only to the top of the head but also to refer selectively to the smaller, circular region toward the posterior of the top, where it begins to round off inferiorly toward the occiput. The smaller posterior region is the area of sworls in hair growth direction. It is also the site of the round, tonsure-like bald spot often referred to as "vertex baldness" or "crown baldness." In this discussion the term crown refers to the entire top of the head, more or less the area that might be encompassed by the rim of a royal crown placed squarely on the head; and the term vertex is used to signify the smaller posterior area where sworls occur. The crown may thus be at least partly inclusive of vertex area.

In hair restoration both of the areas signified by the terms crown and vertex are appropriate sites for scalp reduction procedures. Scalp reduction is the excision of bald scalp in relatively large segments. Reduction procedures are carried out on areas of complete and near-complete baldness and can achieve a striking diminution of the total area that requires transplantation. Reductions can usually be carried out concomitantly with transplantation, particularly transplantation to the hairline zone anterior to the reduction area.

Central Crown

The central crown region can, generally speaking, accommodate the transplantation of larger grafts in addition to smaller grafts. The use of larger grafts can achieve a desired greater density. Linear grafts that are 2 mm or 2.5 mm wide by 5 mm to 15 mm long can be used in this area, as can round punch grafts of up to 4 mm in diameter. Blending is accomplished by interspersing smaller grafts as necessary for good cosmetic effect. Transplantation to the central crown area must be integrated with any anticipated reduction procedures to be carried out in the area.

When baldness in the central crown/vertex region is not complete, *i.e.,* when viable hair is still present to an extent that renders it useful as a restoration component, and when the native hair can reasonably be expected to remain viable for some years (as when the patient is a younger man), then restoration may take the form of supplementation, with moderate to large numbers of grafts being interspersed among native hair. This represents a long-term treatment approach, since such patients can be expected to require periodic update procedures as the native hair growth slows. These patients should be counseled about this aspect of their hair restoration.

Vertex

If baldness occurs in the vertex region, transplantation as a remedial approach is a complex matter, and potentially unsatisfactory. This region has been aptly labeled a "bottomless pit," meaning that no reasonable quantity of grafts will suffice to achieve an adequate restoration. In many cases insufficient donor hair is present to even consider transplanting the vertex. Successful restoration by grafting in this area is hampered by a high visibility stemming from the greater curvature of the region and its near-vertical position. In addition, local sworls are difficult to reproduce. Most important of all, androgenetic alopecia is progressive and, therefore, following completion of restoration, a halo of bald scalp around the grafted area will occur with time (see Figure 13.4). For all these reasons, baldness in the vertex region is usually

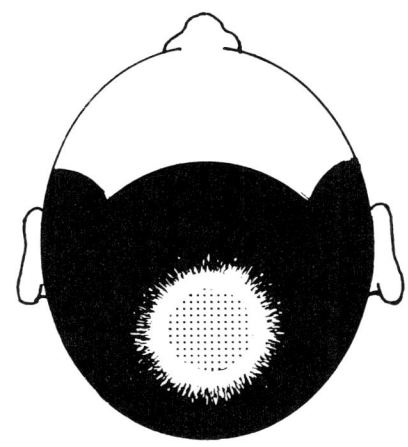

FIGURE 13.4. Ongoing alopecia may create a halo around a transplanted tonsure area.

treated preferentially with scalp reduction as a first approach. Grafting may follow completion of the reduction sequence if necessary.

Hair Characteristics

Hair transplantation today is no longer as dependent on the characteristics of the individual patient's donor hair for success as it once was. The ability to distribute hair in the bald area more effectively by means of very small graft use has opened hair restoration treatment to many candidates who might have been rejected in former times. The physical characteristics of hair, however, are still important in planning and design.

Color

Hair runs a range of colors, from pearl-white gray through auburns and reds, through light browns and dark browns, to jet black, and all shades in between. Skin also runs a range of colors, from pale white through ruddy, bronze, dark brown, to black, also with many shades in between.

The significance of skin and hair color in hair transplantation lies in their potential for promoting a blend-in effect on the one hand (sandy hair with light skin, black hair with dark skin); or, on the other hand, for bringing about a problematic, high-visibility, high-contrast effect (stiff, straight, black hair, and pale or white skin). The blend-in effect makes it possible to achieve a natural and compatible appearance and makes it possible to execute design options more easily. The high-contrast effect has the opposite result, requiring in some cases the use of additional micrografts and sometimes the use of extra-fine lower-occiput or temporal hair micrografts to bring about sufficient visual blending.

Curl

Curly hair is generally a boon in transplantation because of its cosmetic effectiveness in coverage. Curly hair gives a visual effect of increased hair volume, density, and body. Many surgeons advise their patients to have a permanent wave during the week preceding transplant procedures, to ensure that the appearance of the transplanted hair will have maximum effectiveness. This beneficial effect is seen also with extremely curly hair such as that found in many black people. However, extremely curly hair continues its curl beneath the skin and through the length of the hair follicle, so that the follicle itself is curled to the same degree. Harvesting of curly donor hair and the subsequent trimming out of individual grafts must be executed with a particular view to avoiding damage to curved follicles, e.g., by using a round punch that can be made to follow an arcing motion to follow the curve of the follicle. Although curly hair provides effective coverage at its location, it may not be trainable for grooming purposes and generally cannot be combed to cover nearby areas.

Caliber/texture

The significance of caliber and texture in hair transplantation is linked, as with other hair characteristics, to the issue of desirable visual blendability versus undesirable high-contrast visibility as well as to the issue of adequate coverage. Large-caliber, coarse, stiff-textured hair, especially if it is dark in color, has the potential to be highly visible, almost on a hair-by-hair basis, especially if it is transplanted into skin of a contrasting tone, as, for instance, black hair in white skin. In these cases transplantation can sometimes be given a more natural appearance by providing adequate micrografting of finer hair, taken for example from the inferior occiput, in order to bring about a blended look, especially in hairline and part areas.

At the opposite end of the spectrum, hair of small caliber and fine texture, especially if it is a sandy or mixed light-and-gray color, can be expected to provide an exceptional degree of visual blendability, but it may also require the transplantation of a relatively larger mass of donor hair to reach a given level of cover and effectiveness.

Density

The term *density,* as applied to hair, means the number of viable hair follicles in a particular finite area, *e.g.,* in a 4 mm diameter circle on the scalp. *High density* may be defined as approximately 20 hair follicles per 4 mm circle and *low density* as 6 to 10 hair follicles per 4 mm circle. Density of hair in donor tissue affects both coverage potential for the donor hair mass and for individual grafts of any particular size. It also affects the cosmetic visibility of hair transplanted as a single unit of tissue. High density hair can produce a "clumping" or "cornstalking" effect more readily, especially when used in large round grafts. On the other hand, high density hair can provide enrichment and superior coverage in areas posterior to the hairline and provide good comb-over volume.

Styling Considerations

Posttransplant styling preferences and possibilities should be carefully explored during transplant planning. Styling procedures can make the difference between an effective restoration and one that appears to fall short cosmetically. The patient's willingness and ability to maintain styling options should also be examined. Hair characteristics such as color, curl, caliber, texture, and density should be analyzed for their

Donor Grafts

Extent of Safe Hair

In most patients the occipital and temporal regions can be relied on for a sufficient quantity of donor hair to accomplish a cosmetically effective transplant restoration, except in the small number of individuals who suffer very severe patterns of baldness. When patients are also viable candidates for the removal of some portion of the bald scalp through reduction procedures, a given donor mass can cover a commensurately greater part of the original treatment area. Harvesting of uniform strips of tissue using multibladed knives has greatly simplified the process of assessing the extent of safe hair and the feasibility of transplantation. A single incision of 8 cm to 15 cm length by 0.75 cm width will generally provide several hundred trimmed grafts, or enough for 1 session. The individual patient's occiput can thus be easily assessed by simple visual inspection to determine if there is enough area present for the requisite number of sessions.

Graft Harvesting

The occipital region is harvested preferentially, because of its greater width and because of the heightened vascularity that may be encountered temporally. However, temporal region hair may be used if needed. Almost all graft harvesting for hair transplantation is currently accomplished with the use of multibladed knives. Some round grafts are still used in selected cases, primarily to increase density in the central vertex area posterior to the hairline.

Antibiotics

Perioperative antibiotics are routinely administered, beginning the evening prior to surgery and continued for several days postoperatively. Type and dosage may be changed as necessary; however, infection as a complication of hair restoration surgery is rarely seen.

Anesthesia

Local anesthesia may be accomplished with 10 cc 0.5% xylocaine with 1:200,000 epinephrine, followed by 10 cc 0.25% bupivacaine (Marcaine) with 1:200,000 epinephrine. Added injections may be necessary, particularly after several hours have passed during procedures.

Turgor

For all graft harvesting, heightened turgor is first imparted to the donor area by the injection of saline into the dermis and the subcutaneous fat layer. Heightened turgor has the effect of straightening hair follicles so that less damage occurs with knife passage. It also raises the scalp so that the incision can reach a depth that is below that of the follicle base but above the vascular plexus lying at slightly greater depth.

Saline injection takes place with simultaneous application of pressure using a plastic turgor plate (see Figure 13.5). This device was developed by the authors and is designed to confine the injected saline within a limited area. The turgor plate has a curved shape to approximate the occipital skull contour, and it contains a centrally placed slot or open space of 3 cm by 11 cm, which allows access to the injection area at the same time that pressure is being applied to perimeter tissues. Firm turgor is critical to the production of donor grafts of good quality.

Thin Strip Harvesting

Multibladed knives that are currently available have fixed distances between blades of either 2 mm or 2.5 mm and can mount either 2, 3, or 4 blades (see Figure 13.6). The 4-bladed knife is preferred because of its capacity to produce with 1 incision an amount of donor tissue sufficient for the completion of 1 transplant session.

The average incision length using the multibladed knife is approximately 12 cm but ranges from 8 cm to 16 cm. The yield of grafts from strips is somewhat density-dependent, since small bits of tissue that have no hair follicles will be discarded in the trimming process. If the space between knife blades is 2.5 mm rather than 2 mm, yields of graft per centimeter will be

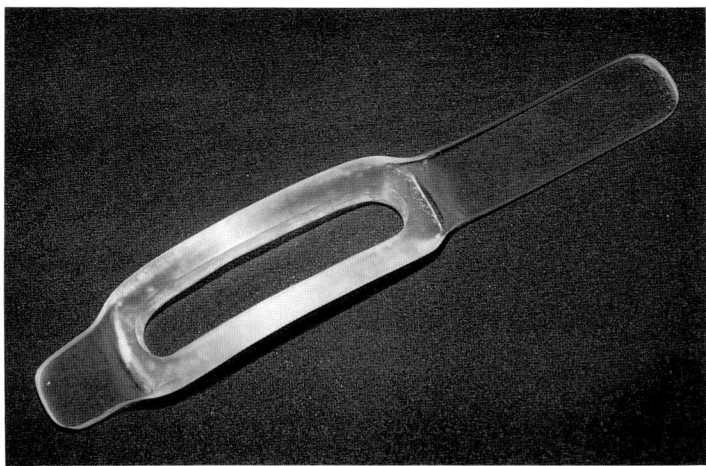

FIGURE 13.5. The turgor plate prevents infiltrated solution from diffusing throughout the scalp, so firm turgor can be maintained for strip harvesting.

greater. Nevertheless, yields can be dependably calculated for purposes of session planning (see Table 13.1). Minor adjustments or reconciliations to the plan can take place without difficulty following completion of graft trimming.

Since the nerve supply of the occiput follows an inferior-to-superior path in the scalp, the successive horizontal incisions made for sequential transplant sessions are placed at levels that also follow an inferior-to-superior course. That is, the first session horizontal incision (see Figure 13.7) is usually made in the most inferior portion of the occiput that is to be utilized. Subsequent incisions are then placed at successively higher levels, taking care that sufficient hair-bearing scalp to maintain good coverage of the donor scar is left intact between incision sites. Placing each incision above the previous one prevents scar formation from interfering with future anesthesia induction; moreover, the hypoesthesia that may occur superior to incisions can lessen the amount of anesthesia needed for future incisions. In younger patients a 2 cm zone should be left unharvested at the superior and inferior margins of the donor area.

A fair degree of skill is required to control the angle and depth of a multibladed knife. The plane of the incision should parallel hair follicle direction. To ensure that this occurs, the strips are periodically inspected for proper orientation parallel to the hair follicles as the incisions are being made. The incision should maintain a depth that is below the base level of the follicles but above the supragaleal vascular bed when possible. The depth of the incision is also

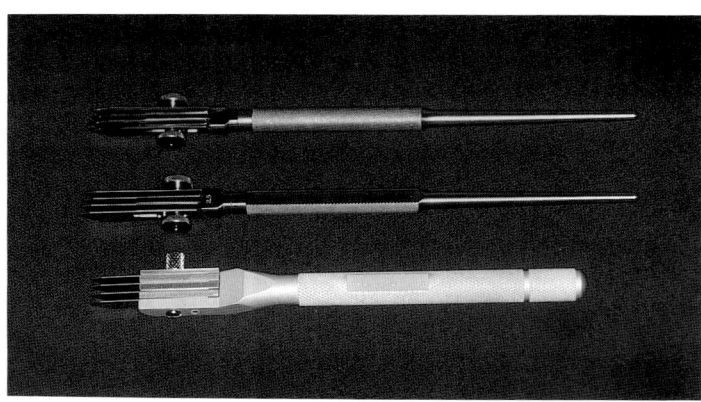

FIGURE 13.6. Multibladed knives.

13. Hair Restoration

TABLE 13.1. Calculations for a session size vs. yield, and totals vs. strip length.

Yield per 1 cm strip		Total strip length	
micros (1 to 2 hairs)	10	170 micros	17 cm
1.25 + mm	8	80 1.50+ mm	13 cm
1.50 + mm	6	60 2.00+ mm	15 cm
1.75 + mm	5	Combined length:	45 cm
2.00 + mm	4	Incision = 15 cm × 3 strips	

inspected periodically. Prior to removing the strips, each end of the incision is brought to a V-shape using an ordinary scalpel to avoid "dog ears." Incised tissue strips are freed from the donor bed using scissors to cut through the subcutaneous fat layer well below the base of the follicles. Strips are then placed in a petri dish of saline preparatory to trimming.

Strip harvesting of donor tissue using multibladed knives has several advantages. Harvesting itself is less lengthy and demanding on patient and staff. The donor site wound exhibits better approximation because of the clean, straight-line incision. The dissection of large numbers of micrografts and minigrafts remains a demanding process but may be slightly more rapid and efficient with strips than with large round grafts.

Round Graft Harvesting

If large regular round grafts are to be used, they can be harvested by means of manual or power-driven trephines ranging up to 4 mm in diameter. Large round grafts may be harvested in combination with strip harvesting, in which case they may be taken as a short, continuous horizontal row from the centermost portion of the multibladed knife incision site. Occipital hair density is usually greatest in mid-occiput.

Round graft harvest is indicated in patients with very curly hair. The trephine can be directed in an arcing motion during harvest, so that it follows the curvature of the follicle from skin surface to below the level of follicle bases. Trephines used to obtain round grafts should be maintained at surgical sharpness, since sharpness is a crucial factor in the production of grafts of good quality.

Graft Trimming

All grafts are maintained in a shallow bath of saline or Ringer's lactate solution, atop sterile gauze pads. Strict sterility is maintained throughout all trimming and dissection procedures as well as during the later implantation process. Manipulation of grafts is usually accomplished with fine microsurgical forceps of one type or another, and necessary trimming cuts are made with ultra-sharp scalpel blades, usually a number 10 Personna with a round edge. The round edge can be rolled as pressure is applied, to produce clean tissue severance. Sterile, moistened tongue depressors may be used as a cutting surface to stabilize the donor tissue momentarily. Trimmed grafts are placed

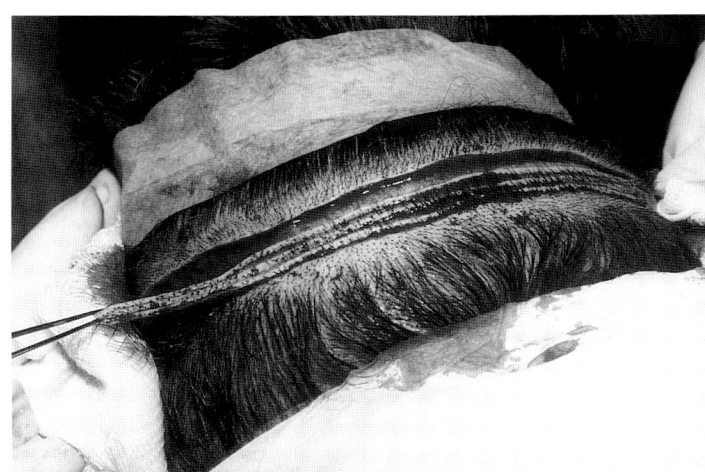

FIGURE 13.7. Strip harvesting. The 4-bladed knife produces 3 tissue strips with a single incision.

in fresh petri dish and saline environments, in sorted rows that denote size. A sorting scheme can also indicate grade or density characteristics of the prepared grafts.

The purpose of the graft trimming process is threefold. First, all transected hair follicles (see Figure 13.8) must be removed. These damaged follicles have the potential for aberrant growth (ingrown hair) if implanted and may cause cyst formation. Second, the subcutaneous fat layer must be trimmed to 1 mm of the follicle bulb. This retained layer acts as a shield during handling; however, retaining any more than 1 mm makes planting more difficult and decreases graft survival. Third, grafts must be trimmed to required sizes, following the plan for the transplant session.

Size and Yield

Table 13.1 shows a typical series of graft sizes that might be used in a transplant session and gives the expected yield per centimeter of donor strip for each graft size. The table also shows typical calculations that can be used to determine the requisite length of the incision for strip harvesting. It should be noted that the mix of graft sizes may change considerably from session to session and from patient to patient.

Individual grafts are cut a small amount larger than the designated size, as signified by the "+" beside the figures shown in Table 13.1. Upon placement in a hole cut by a trephine that is precisely the designated size, the grafts will fit snugly. Grafts that have been separated from strips and trimmed to size are transferred to fresh saline-filled petri dishes and lined up in rows of 20 (see Figure 13.9). Graft sizes are not mixed within rows.

Recipient Bed Management

The use of micrografts and minigrafts in a variety of formats and in combination with other components of hair transplantation and restoration, *e.g.*, with round grafts, linear grafts, reduction procedures, and flaps, has provided the stimulus for a productive and ongoing state of flux in hair transplantation techniques for a number of years. The progress and change continue as new combinations of grafts and new procedures are devised and tested. In the midst of change, however, it continues to be the skill of the operator, particularly in the judicious placement of grafts in patterns, that dictates the ultimate success of the hair transplant.

Hairline

The hairline is usually conceptualized as a zone or band of graded hair density in which the density increases anteriorly to posteriorly. The contour of the band or zone conforms to the hairline shape designed for the particular patient. The frontal hairline or leading edge of the zone is approximately 5 mm to 10 mm in

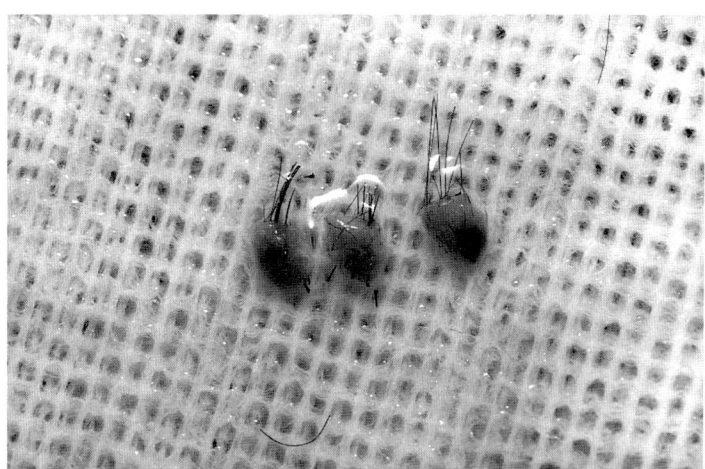

FIGURE 13.8. Transected hair follicle. If not trimmed it may grow abnormally and cause cyst formation or ingrown hair.

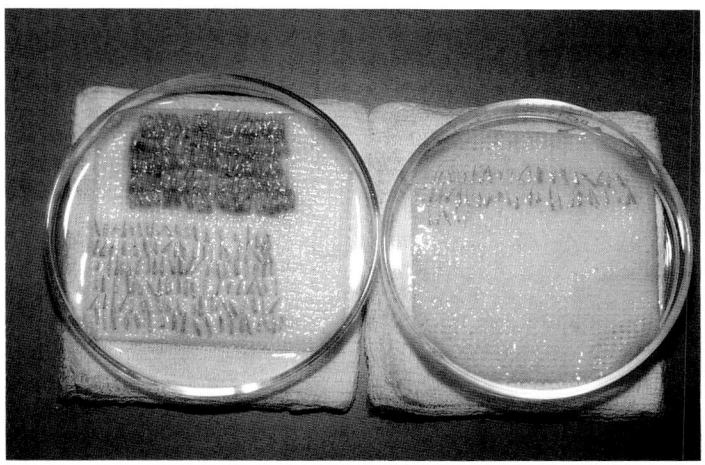

FIGURE 13.9. Petri dishes containing the total accumulation of grafts to be used in one session.

depth and contains only micrografts of 1 or 2 hairs. The micrografts are distributed in a deliberately random and staggered fashion, rather than being placed in a line that seems to be "marching in unison" on the forehead. Minigrafts are placed among micrografts in the posterior limit of the frontal hairline and increase in number and size moving posteriorly across the extended hairline zone. The extended hairline zone can be conceptualized as a bandlike area that is comprised of the frontal hairline anteriorly and extending posteriorly to the anterior limit of the scalp reduction area. In some cases, when donor tissue is available in sufficient quantity, round grafts up to 4 mm may be used in the extended hairline zone and camouflaged by smaller grafts. At its most posterior, the hairline band or zone is designed to merge with or otherwise blend with the grafts of the central area, and a match in density should occur.

Central Area

Transplantation of the central area may be delayed to accommodate reduction procedures in that area. The central area may be transplanted with virtually any type of graft that is available. If there is sufficient donor tissue, the interior of the central area may be grafted with a quantity of regular round grafts of up to 4 mm in diameter. This approach can be used to achieve greater density in the central area and a greater appearance of fullness in the overall transplant. Linear grafts may also be useful for increasing density in the central area. Linear grafts 2 mm or 2.5 mm wide, depending on the knife used for harvesting, and up to 15 mm long or longer, may also be useful for increasing density in the central area.

If donor tissue is limited, the central area may be transplanted with a less dense accumulation of minigrafts. The latter approach can be used successfully to modify and ameliorate the appearance of complete baldness, even though the final coverage achieved is sparse in comparison to the higher-density transplants.

Site Preparation

Recipient sites are made with either incisional slits or punch holes. The pattern of recipient bed slits and holes within the treatment area follows the plan prepared for the individual patient for that particular session. Typically, the growth direction of the new graft hair will correspond to the direction or angulation imparted to the recipient hole or slit at creation.

Micrografts

Micrografts contain 1 or 2 viable hair follicles. They are extremely blendable—that is, they tend not to stand out visually. Micrografts are used primarily in the crafting of the frontal hairline zone. Micrografts can also be placed in proximity to larger grafts to increase visual blending of the larger grafts. Relatively large numbers of micrografts are required to create normal levels of hair density.

Recipient spaces for 1-hair and 2-hair micrografts may be prepared using either a number 16 needle inserted for 10 minutes or by creating a slit using a NoKor-type injectables-vial needle. NoKor-type needles have a sharp triangular tip resembling a lancet that can be used repeatedly to incise slits in large numbers. No dilator is needed, and thus the slits can be placed very close together. This may be particularly useful in the frontal hairline zone, where numerous grafts must be placed very close together to create a graded-density effect.

The use of 16-gauge needles to create micrograft sites may limit somewhat the number of grafts that can be placed in a given area at one time, because of the space requirements of the needles while in place for the 10-minute waiting period.

Minigrafts

Minigrafts contain 3 to 8 viable hairs. Minigrafts are used to provide coverage in any part of the scalp posterior to the micrograft-only frontal hairline zone. Minigrafts are used extensively in the extended hairline zone and as needed in any location in the central and vertex areas. Although the density that can be achieved using minigrafts alone is not always high, adequate coverage is feasible if sufficient donor hair is available. The blendability of minigrafts is exceeded only by that of micrografts and is especially good in the lower size range.

Round hole sites for minigrafts are prepared using small round punches. Useful sizes for minigrafts of 3 to 8 hairs are punches of 1.25 mm, 1.50 mm, 1.75 mm, and 2.00 mm diameter. These small trephines are applied manually and provide a superior level of control of distribution of grafts and penetration of tissue in round hole site preparation. The incoming graft will have by design and planning been cut so that its size is actually larger by a very small amount than the trephine diameter. That is, grafts that are grouped under the designation "1.50 mm" are actually a very small amount larger than 1.50 mm and are so grouped because they will be placed in a site cut by a 1.50 mm trephine. The object is to routinely achieve a graft-to-site fit that is snug but not too tight so that the grafts pop out. Small-bore trephine site preparation removes bald scalp and replaces it with hair-bearing scalp. Minigraft round hole sites are generally given a scattered distribution, which nevertheless conforms in an overall fashion to the transplant design for the particular patient.

Incisional slit sites for minigrafts of 3 to 8 hairs can be prepared by making a single stab wound using a number 15 scalpel blade. This method of site preparation is particularly useful when conservation of existing native hair is of concern, since slits can be placed between hairs. The disadvantages of slits are compression of grafts and less achievable density, since no bald scalp is removed.

Round Punch Grafts

Large round punch grafts up to 4 mm in diameter may be used to provide enhanced density when donor hair is present in adequate quantity. These large round grafts are used primarily in the area posterior to the hairline and in other parts of the central area where indicated. A cornstalking effect may occur when round grafts are used; they should be placed so that visual shielding is provided by other grafts. Round hole sites for large round grafts are prepared with hand or power-driven punches.

Linear Grafts

Linear grafts of varying length are cut from the same narrow strips of donor tissue that minigrafts are prepared from. Linear grafts may be used directly behind the micrografts of the frontal hairline in some cases, to provide a more continuous appearance.[20] Linear grafts may also be placed in the central area to provide enhanced density. Sites for linear grafts are prepared as an incisional slit made with a number 10 round scalpel blade. The slit length is matched to graft length. The linear grafts are then stablized by an overlapping suture with plain gut.

Graft Placement

Grafts of all kinds and sizes are placed in their respective recipient bed sites by the same general procedure. The subcutaneous fat below the bulb is gently grasped, using jeweler's forceps. The forceps should be fine-tipped, preferably straight, and with a not-too-lengthy taper. (A lengthy taper promotes crimping and burr formation.)

Grafts are inserted at once in the appropriate orientation and attitude. If adjustment is necessary, particularly any involving rotation, the graft generally should be completely removed and reinserted. The grafts should not be grasped in such a way that the hair follicles are compressed, and care must be taken to see that no loose or extraneous hair makes it way into the site as the graft is being placed.

Cleansing

Hydrogen peroxide (1.5%) in a gentle spray is applied to the scalp frequently by means of a hand-pump spritzer, covering one small area at a time. The sprayed area is then blotted with sterile gauze pads. This removes any crusting that has developed.

Grafts prepared from tissue harvested in donor areas where the patient's hair is darker in color or has a greater degree of curl should be symmetrically dispersed rather than being allowed to concentrate and create an unevenness or a noticeable patch.

Aftercare

The grafted area is coated with antibiotic ointment and a pressure bandage is applied. After 24 hours the bandage is removed and the scalp is carefully shampooed. The patient is advised to refrain from strenuous activity for several days. Thereafter normal activity can resume.

Figures 13.10 through 13.13 show before, intraoperative, and after views of several patients who received a combination of various graft types and scalp reduction procedures. It should be noted that the intraoperative views each represent a single stage in sometimes lengthy treatment sequences. The photographs are thus not intended to portray an entire sequence of treatment for any of the patients but, rather, to illustrate the concept of integration of graft types and recipient bed preparation techniques within a treatment area. Before and after views are shown for the reader's convenience.

Scalp Reduction

The basic principles of scalp reduction are the same for all reductions, with differences between the various types related largely to incision configuration (see Figure 13.14) and the amount of tissue removed per procedure. All reduction procedures except the radical scalp lift involve ring block anesthesia. There is an initial incision, undermining of surrounding scalp, a second incision that detaches the tissue, and wound closure.

Repetition and Planning

Scalp reduction goals are usually reached in successive stages, with several reductions taking place, separated by periods of 2 to 6 months. Scalp reduction procedures are usually combined with hair transplant procedures. Transplant procedures, particularly those involving the hairline area, can often be carried out concomitantly with scalp reductions (refer to Figure 13.10).

Scalp Laxity

Scalp laxity and thickness are factors to be considered in planning reductions. Individual-laxity characteristics are such that a thick scalp may be found to exhibit a high degree of scalp laxity, while a thin scalp may be found to exhibit little scalp laxity. Thin scalp (0.5 to 0.7 cm) is in general physically easier to stretch, and thus may allow removal of a larger amount of bald skin in a single procedure. However, thick scalp (0.8 to 1.0 cm) may in general tolerate a larger total amount of tissue to be removed over several procedures. Either thick or thin scalp may be subject to postprocedure

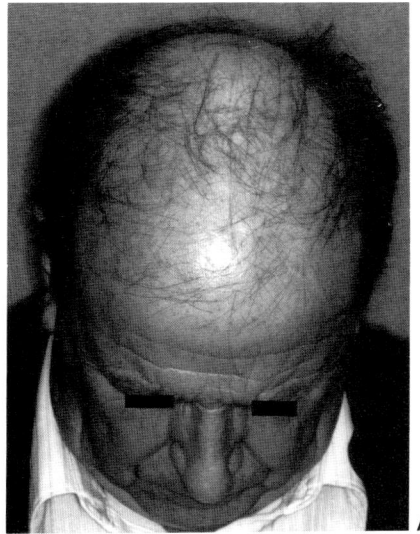
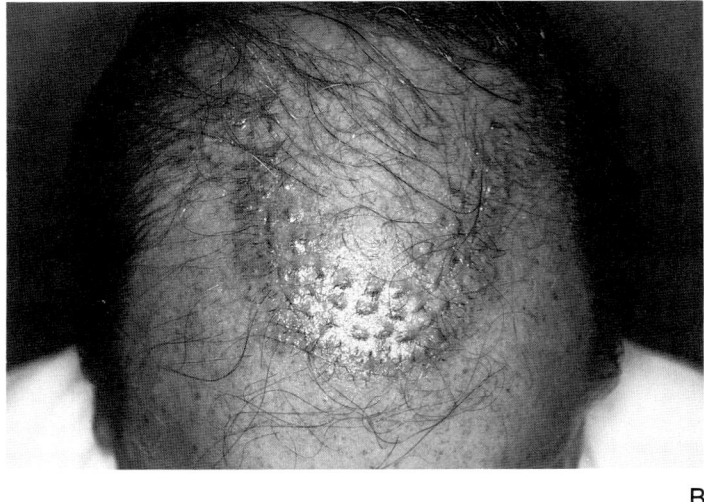
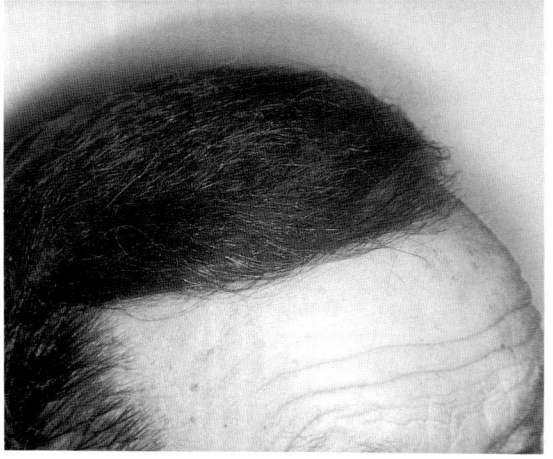

FIGURE 13.10. A. Patient A. B and C. The design of this transplant reflects the need to avoid a definite intersecting of the hairline with a still receding temporal fringe. Graft totals: 90 half-rounds, 800 minigrafts, 480 micrografts.

stretchback of the incision scar, depending on individual characteristics.

Sagittal Mid-line Reduction

The sagittal mid-line reduction technique described by Bosley[24] in 1979 rapidly became and still is the most widely used reduction technique, because of its relative ease and surgical simplicity. In mid-line reductions a symmetric ellipse of bald scalp is removed from the top of the head.

After anesthesia is established, the ellipse to be excised is marked out in its entirety on the scalp surface. The first incision comprises one complete side of the ellipse. This first incision provides access for the undermining, in which the scalp is loosened above the periosteum. Undermining is always carried out in the avascular subgaleal plane to the supraauricular areas laterally and the occipital ridge posteriorly and generally reaches 5 cm to 10 cm on both sides of the initial incision, depending on scalp laxity.

When undermining is complete, the loosened scalp is overlapped to determine accurately the position of the second incision. Wound closure tension is estimated and considered. The second incision is made and the ellipse removed. The

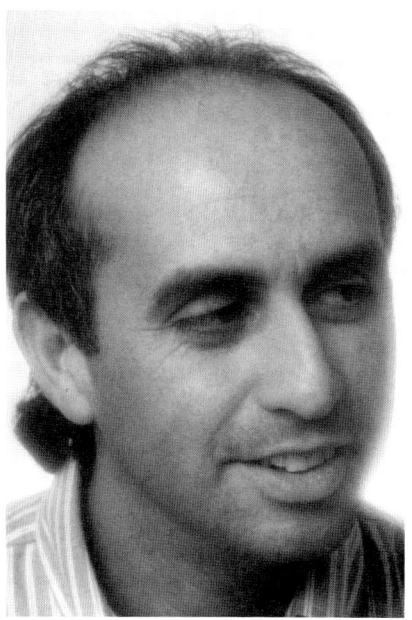
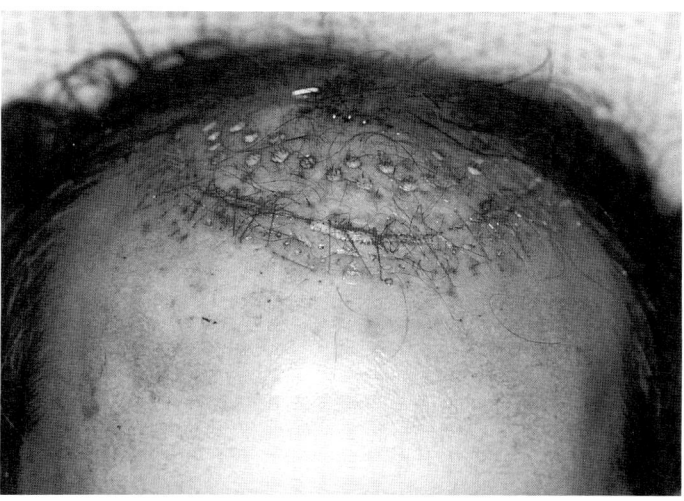
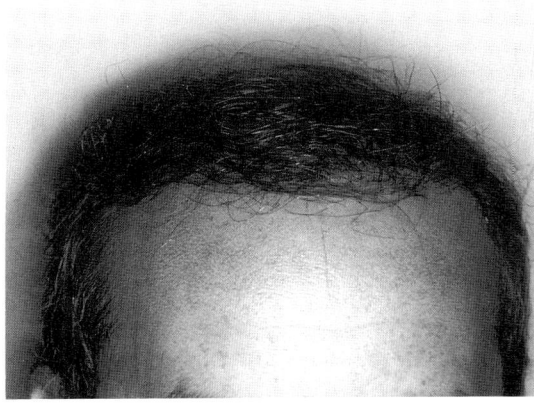

FIGURE 13.11. A. Patient B. B and C. Linear grafts in multiple sites immediately posterior to the frontal hairline micrograft zone are held in place by a fine suture which crisscrosses the linear graft area. Graft totals: 64 regular rounds (4 mm), 24 linear grafts of 1 cm length, 53 linear grafts of 3 cm length, 314 minigrafts, 490 micrografts. Four scalp reduction procedures were carried out.

wound is closed with an absorbable suture by approximating the edges of the tough fascial galea first, followed by closure of the skin with staples.

There are a number of well-described drawbacks to the sagittal mid-line approach.[26] The hairline is distorted anteriorly while the occipital fringe is displaced posteriorly, thus lowering the vertex alopecia. This pattern is more-susceptable to stretchback due to the unilateral tension vectors. Finally, with subsequent reductions, the slot defect occurs, which is a scar in the occipital hair fringe with the hair growing away from it, thus making it more noticeable. It is very difficult to camouflage.

Z-plasty

Procedures aimed at correcting the slot defect include the use of a Z-plasty or its variations at the posterior end of the mid-line incision.[42] In the Z-plasty procedure, small flaps are transposed relative to each other so that an appropriate downward direction in hair growth is imparted to the crucial vertex/occipital area and thus covers the scar. The Z-plasty can be used with other reduction procedures as well.

Paramedian Reduction

The paramedian reduction[25] offered some improvement over the sagittal midline approach,

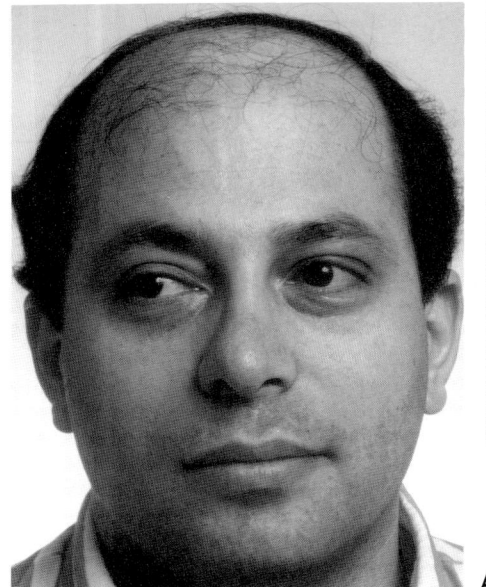
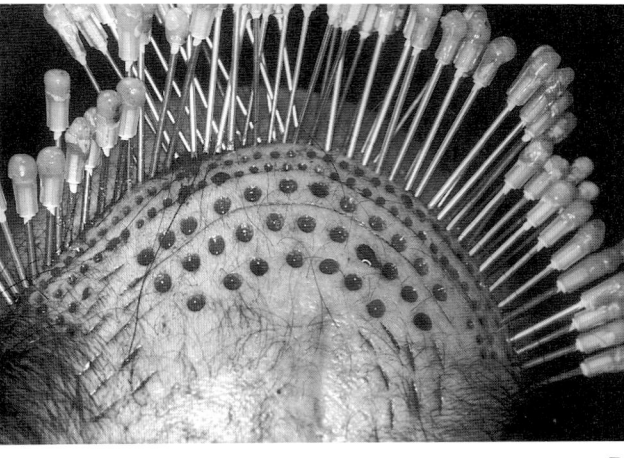
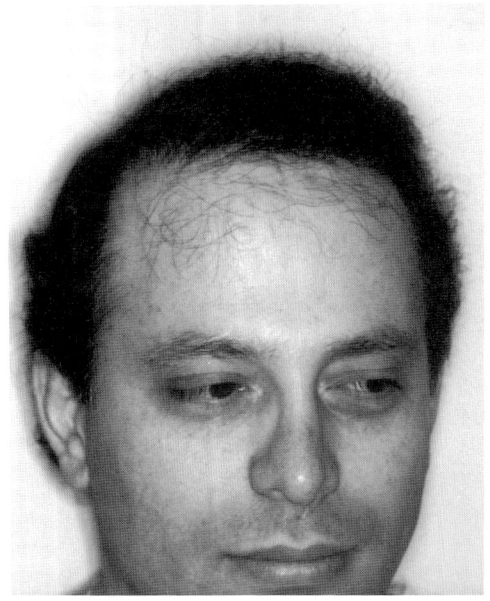

FIGURE 13.12. A. Patient C. B. Micrograft sites in the frontal hairline were created by needle insertion. C. The transplant hairline is placed several centimeters posterior to the original hairline. Grafts totals: 80 regular rounds (4. O mm), 62 half-rounds, 658 minigrafts, 470 micrografts. Seven scalp reduction procedures were carried out.

by introducing a curvilinear aspect to the reduction incision and by shifting the incision laterally, away from the mid-line. The paramedian thus avoids the limitations of the sagittal mid-line reduction, and it can be used in cases of extensive baldness, particularly those involving the occipital area. Advantages of the paramedian include elevating the occipital fringe superiorly, avoidance of a vertical scar (slot defect) in the occipital region, less stretchback, better camouflaging of the scar, and removal of relatively larger amounts of tissue than is possible in the sagittal mid-line approach. One limitation of the paramedian is the poor undermining access to the contralateral supraauricular area. Also, paramedians are usually alternated from side to side and thus 2 scars are present.

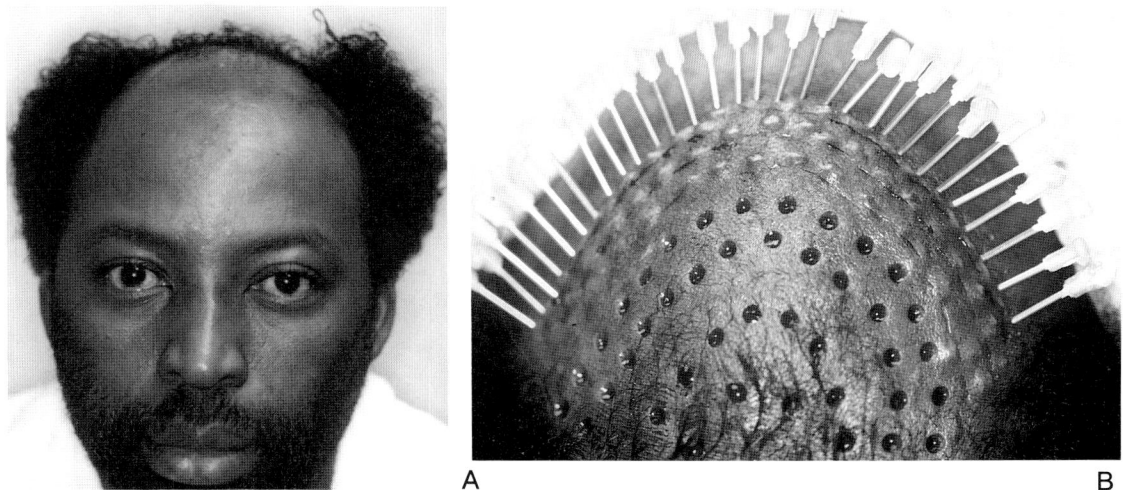

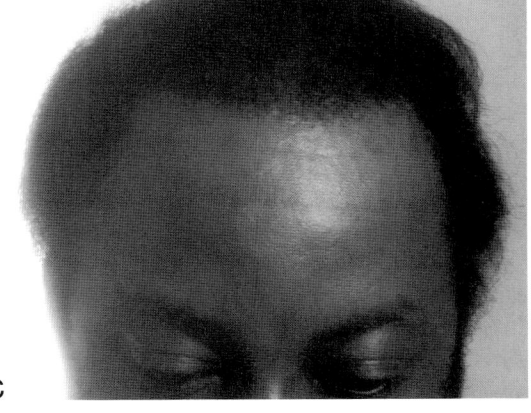

FIGURE 13.13. A. Patient D. B and C. The use of round donor grafts is indicated in patients who have very curly hair and thus highly curved hair follicles. The trephine can be manipulated to avoid follicle damage during harvesting. Other types of grafts may also be used, particularly in the hairline area. Graft totals: 44 regular rounds (4. 0 mm), 247 half-rounds, 374 minigrafts, 180 micrografts. Three reductions were carried out.

Modified-S Reduction

Following the introduction of the sagittal midline reduction technique, a number of other configurations for scalp reduction incisions were devised, most in an attempt to avoid the slot defect and to increase the amount of tissue that could be removed in a single procedure. One of the most effective of the non-mid-line reduction incision configurations is the modified-S.[43] The modified-S reduction incision is somewhat tightly curved at its anterior reach, which is slightly posterior to the hairline, then assumes a relatively more open and sweeping curve in its posterior course. The posterior course lies along the superior border of the occipital fringe. The outline of the segment to be removed is narrowed to a point at the anterior and posterior limits and is widened as it traverses the mid-scalp area.

There are a number of advantages to the modified-S configuration. The modified-S has a greater length, particularly in comparison to a mid-line incision, because of its curved shape. By its nature the longer length allows the removal of more bald scalp per procedure. The modified-S need not extend into the frontal hairline zone or into the posterior vertex-occiput region to gain length.

The overall contour of the modified-S reduction causes tension on the remaining scalp to be distributed evenly. This reduces the amount of stretchback of the anterior portion of the modified-S serves to remove anterior bald scalp

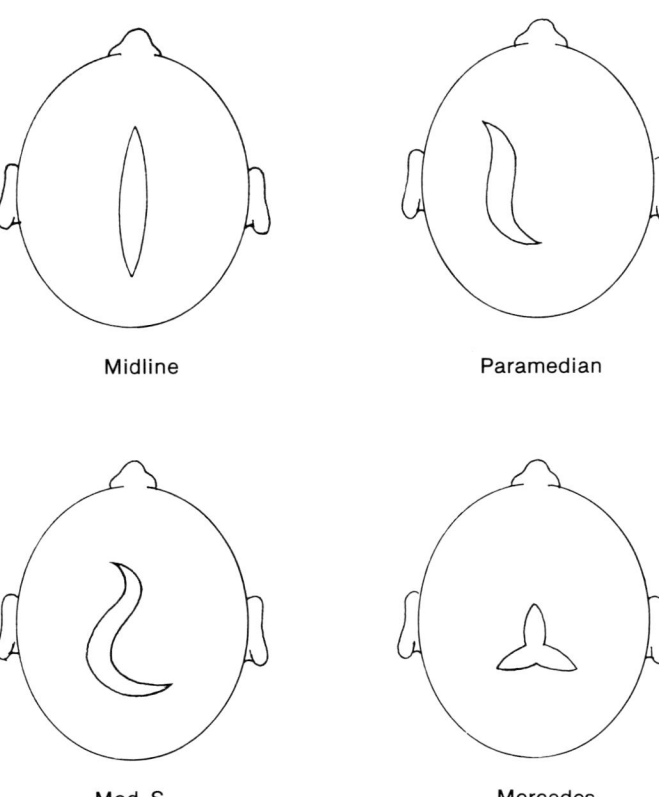

FIGURE 13.14. Basic shapes used in scalp reduction procedures: mid-line, paramedian, modified-S, and Mercedes.

without distorting the hairline. The posterior curve of the S tracks the superior occipital fringe, so the removal of scalp results in movement of the occipital scalp superiorly, with the great advantage of avoiding the slot defect. The geometry of the modified-S incision assures substantially greater visual and manual access in the undermining process. The scar of the modified-S procedure is camouflaged along the occipital fringe, which is the most critical area for cosmetic purposes. Figures 13.15 and 13.16 provide before and after views of a patient who underwent a total of 3 modified-S reductions.

Mercedes Reduction

The Mercedes reduction was designed for removal of bald scalp in the vertex region. The original design was subsequently modified to avoid placing a scar at the center of the region and to avoid the necrosis to which the original design proved vulnerable. The Mercedes procedure is still advantageous in some horizontal forms of vertex alopecia.

Scalp Lifts

Radical or massive reduction techniques have been employed. The procedure was developed by Marzola[30] and later modified by Brandy.[31] In this approach virtually the entire hair-bearing portion of the scalp is undermined, requiring surgical dissection down into the posterior neck region. the occipital artery and never are sacrificed in this procedure. The entire bald area is eventually excised in several successive procedures, until at completion the edges of the native temporal hair are joined at the mid-line of the top of the head. The results are impressive, but the difficulty of performing such surgery is considerable. There have been significant postoperative problems, particularly with necrosis due to inadequate perfusion. Recently, however, this complication has been

13. Hair Restoration

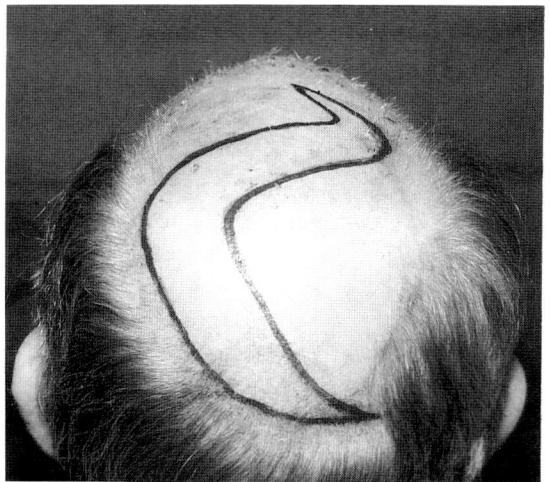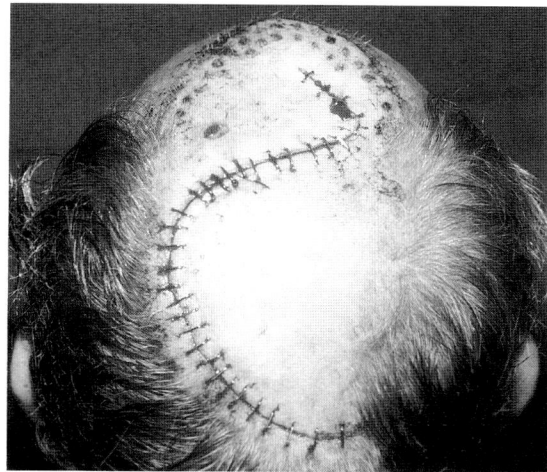

FIGURE 13.15. Before (A) and after (B) one modified-S scalp reduction.

dramatically reduced by occipital artery ligation 2 weeks prior to surgery. This more radical procedure can be very effective in selected patients.

Flaps

Flap procedures can be extremely effective in the correction of male pattern baldness, if the candidate is ideal and if surgical expertise is available. Two of the most troublesome aspects of flap procedures in the past, the inescapable scar at the anterior edge of the hairline and the posterior direction of growth of the hair forming the new hairline, can both now be modified and for the most part corrected, through the use of micrografting procedures. However, ideal candidates are not seen frequently, and the number of surgeons who have been trained in flap procedures is diminishing. The more desirable candidates are individuals who have reached a maturity level that allows their eventual pattern of baldness to be projected to lie between class III and class V in the

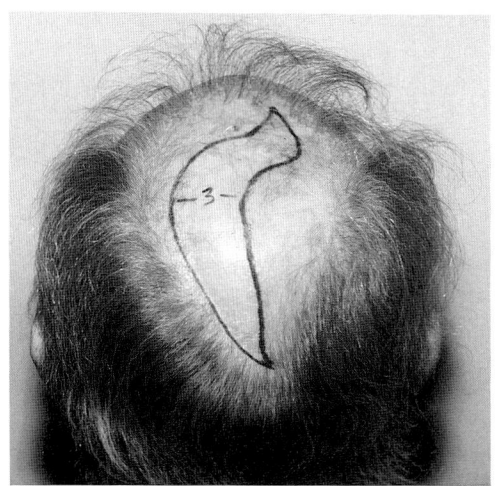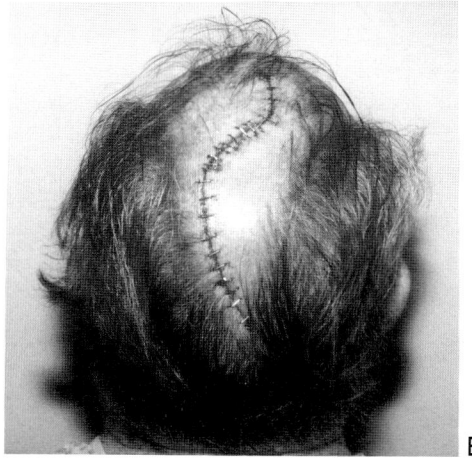

FIGURE 13.16. Before (A) and after (B) of the same patient after his third modified-S reduction.

Hamilton/Norwood system[44] and who possess an adequate quantity of good-quality hair. The length and width dimensions of the donor area must be adequate to provide for hairline recreation and still maintain an overall balance in appearance postoperatively.

Juri Flap

The Juri flap[33] has its pedicle-base in the temporal region and includes the posterior branch of the superficial temporal artery. It traverses smoothly upward and posteriorly, forming an arc that has its peak height near the anterior boundary of the hair-bearing parietal area. The Juri flap curves inferiorly and then gradually straightens as it continues and traces the occipital artery. The flap terminates near the inferior limit of occipital hair growth. This long flap can be transposed and repositioned, in a twice-delayed procedure, to form a new hairline that completely traverses the anterior portion of the bald scalp. The inferior occipital terminus of the Juri flap dictates that undermining prior to closure, already an extensive process, must often also be extended into the neck region in consideration of tension on closure. This is a disadvantage.

Juri also described two flaps of lesser length, one with its base-pedicle in the retroauricular area and one with its base in the occipital area. The retroauricular-pedicled Juri flap is used to augment the longer flap just described and is transposed to correct an area of baldness in a region posterior to the long frontal flap or flaps. The occipital-pedicled Juri flap has been used to replace bald scalp of the posterior crown or vertex region. However, many surgeons feel that scalp reduction and hair-bearing graft procedures are more suitable for correction of baldness in this region since they are safer, easier, and more reliable.

Stough Flap

The Stough temporoparietal-occipital (TPO) flap (see Figure 13.17)[38] is a long and largely horizontal flap that is a modified Juri flap. The pedicle-base is positioned so as to incorporate both the posterior branch of the superficial temporal artery and its counterpart vein. Inclusion of both vessels in the pedicle is considered critical to adequate perfusion of the flap itself, and Doppler studies[45] are mandatory in locating the artery definitively. The counterpart vein is located by visual inspection of the underside of the pedicle, with galeal scoring if necessary, and the pedicle location is changed if necessary to achieve inclusion. In a very small number of cases, perhaps 1 in 1,000, either the superficial temporal artery or the vein will be missing altogether; in these cases the risk of necrosis following a flap procedure is extremely high.

The pedicle location for the Stough TPO flap is also carefully planned to provide a pivot point that will establish a predetermined frontotemporal angle, i.e., one that is commensurate with esthetic hairline design and that takes into account the patient's facial shape. The narrow width of the pedicle acts to prevent "dog ear" formation. The flap is 2.5 to 3.0 cm in width at the pedicle, then gradually widens as it traverses an anterior path to the parietal area, where it angles 90° posteriorly and turns inferiorly for a short distance before assuming a horizontal direction through the mid-occiput. The flap reaches 3.2 cm as it traverses the parietal region and 3.4 cm as it traverses the occiput. The terminus of the Stough flap is located 2 to 5 cm beyond the occiput mid-line. The length of the flap is planned preoperatively according to the dimensions required for hairline creation. The procedure is usually performed in 2 stages, the second stage following 10 days after the first. Occasionally there are 3 stages, or delays, in the procedure. Figure 13.18A and B show before and after views of a patient who receive a Stough flap procedure.

Elliott Flap

The Elliott flap[34] is a relatively short, nondelayed, temporal-pedicle flap that traverses the temporo-parietal area, tapering posteriorly to its terminus in or near the occipital area. This flap is 12 to 15 cm long, 3 cm wide at its pedicle. In our opinion it is primarily of use in reconstruction procedures, although it has been used to create a hairline by joining a left-side flap

13. Hair Restoration

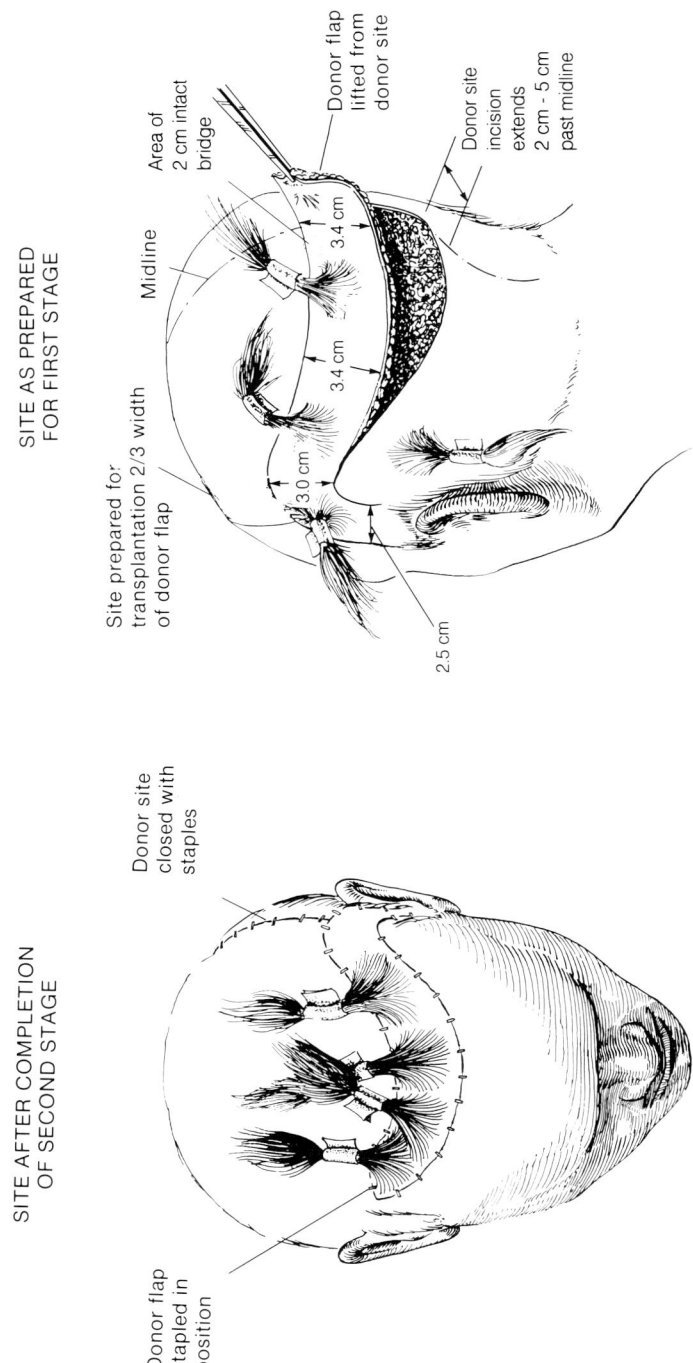

FIGURE 13.17. The Stough modification of the temporoparietal-occipital flap.

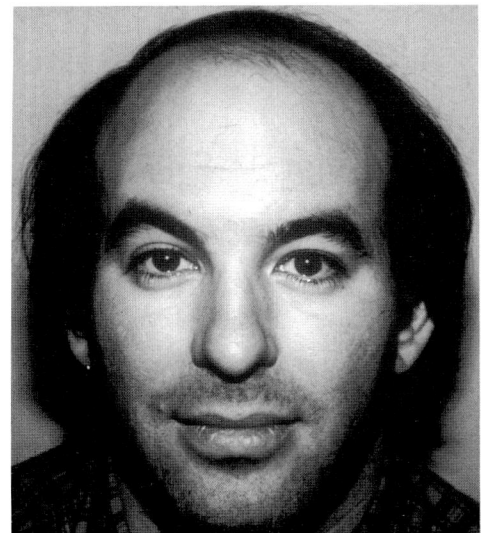 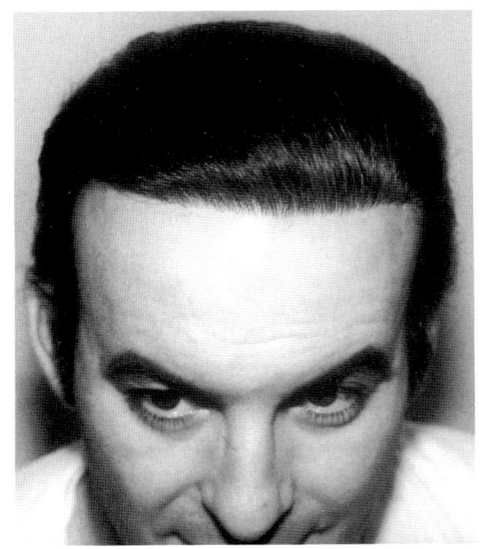

FIGURE 13.18. Before (A) and after (B) views of a patient who received a Stough TPO flap.

and a right-side flap at or near the middle of the forehead.[46] The two hairline flaps are preferably transposed in separate procedures.

Complications

There are very few complications with hair transplantation procedures. The same is true for scalp reduction procedures, with the exception of radical scalp lifts.

Bleeding

Bleeding is perhaps the most commonly encountered problem in hair transplantation; even so, it is seen infrequently. Prevention of excessive bleeding can be virtually assured by the preoperative cessation of medications that affect blood clotting or cause vasodilation, including aspirin and other antiinflammatory preparations, niacin, and vitamin E. In addition, patients should be carefully screened for the presence of or history of bleeding diatheses and appropriate control measures instituted preoperatively. Intraoperative copious bleeding from the infrequent severed arteriole is controlled by the placing of a suture. Anxiety, which can cause increased blood pressure and other hemodynamic changes, should be controlled with preoperative tranquilizers or other medication.

Scarring

Scarring associated with hair transplantation and scalp reduction procedures is minimal and is perhaps due more to individual healing characteristics than to inherent consequences of the procedures themselves. However, closure of a wide donor area defect under excess tension can lead to visible scar formation, which may need to be corrected in subsequent procedures. Keloid scar formation is rare and can usually be anticipated with adequate preoperative attention to history and old scars. Reduction procedures occasionally give rise to unusually large scar formation in some individuals. These scars can be improved in subsequent reduction procedures in which the incision may be closed with less tension, or in surgical procedures aimed specifically at scar removal.

Cobblestoning

The cobblestoning effect, in which transplanted grafts are slightly elevated above the level of the epidermal surface by factors related to incomplete graft trimming, insertion, or subgraft postoperative bleeding, usually resolves and flattens over a period of several months to several years. If the effect is severe, dermabrasion or other remedial procedures may be used. The divot effect, in which the donor graft surface is lower than the surrounding epidermis, usually resolves over a moderately long time without intervention.

Stretchback

Stretchback and thinning of the skin proximal to the scar is sometimes seen following reduction procedures, even when undermining of the surrounding scalp has been extensive.

Slot Defect

The slot defect, caused by reduction incisions that intrude anteriorly into the hairline band and posteriorly into the crown, can be avoided by shortening the reduction incision or by employing a shape variation such as the modified-S. Otherwise a Z-plasty or Frechet flap can be used to correct the slot defect.

Edema

A certain amount of edema is routinely seen over a period of days following transplantation procedures and on rare occasions may become severe. Patients should be reassured ahead of time. Edema can be forestalled by preoperative administration of corticosteroids.

Hypoesthesia

Altered sensation related to the donor area or the recipient area is not unusual. It generally resolves in a period of several months to a year. Hypoesthesia occasionally may persist for several years. Rarely it is a permanent effect.

Pain

Pain or discomfort of a minor nature may occur over a 24-hour period following transplantation. Mild analgesic drugs are usually sufficient, but occasionally a stronger medication may be necessary for a brief time. Rarely, a persistent and twinge-like pain associated with the donor area may occur and require several months to resolve.

Infection

Infection is rarely seen in association with hair transplantation or scalp reduction procedures. The routine use of perioperative (systemic) antibiotics coupled with the observance of strict sterile technique, aided by the scalp's own rich blood supply, militate against the occurrence of infection.

Cyst Formation

Cyst formation occurs, rarely, following scalp surgery and hair transplantation procedures. It can be due to an epidermal inclusion cyst, foreign body reaction, or in some cases to erratic growth direction involving a single hair. The remedy is surgical excision. Figure 13.19 shows a cyst believed to be due to an ingrown hair. It was excised uneventfully.

Nonsurgical Methods

A number of drugs in several classes have been investigated for their potential effectiveness in the treatment or prevention of androgenetic hair loss. Minoxidil, an antihypertensive, and tretinoin, a retinoid, produce a hypertrophic effect on the hair follicle. Antiandrogens act by limiting hormonal access to hair follicle end-organs, either through receptor-site blockage or through inhibition of enzymatic conversion of proandrogens to active forms. Various combinations of these drugs are also under investigation.

Minoxidil

Minoxidil is a vasodilator used as an oral medication in the control of refractory hypertension. It produces hypertrichosis as a side effect in a large number of patients. When applied to the scalp as a topical medication, it was found to interrupt or postpone the progression of baldness, particularly in young men who had just begun to show hair loss. The

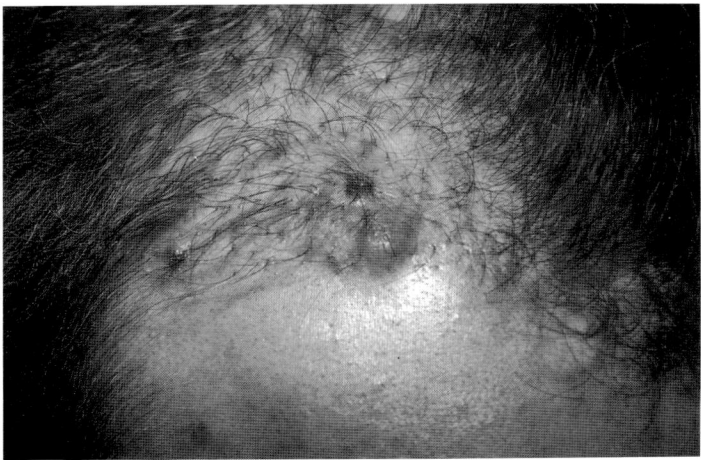

FIGURE 13.19. Cyst formed as a complication of hair transplantation.

mechanism of action of minoxidil on the hair follicle is as yet not clear, but it is known to affect various follicular cells and is believed to bring about increased hair shaft thickness and a lengthened anagen cycle.

Minoxidil continues to be the focus of an active research effort,[47] and it has been studied in combination with other drugs such as finasteride, an antiandrogen.[48,49] Certain limitations to the applicability of minoxidil should be borne in mind. First, it is effective in only a small percentage of potential candidates. Second, it must be applied, *i.e.*, rubbed into the scalp, on a daily basis. And third, any lapse in daily application will result a few months later in resumption of hair loss, with some evidence that the rate will be consistent with a catch-up phenomenon.

Retinoids

Although the mechanism is not completely understood, retinoids such as tretinoin also have the ability to stimulate hair follicles and exert a trichogenic effect[50] and have thus been studied in connection with the treatment of androgenic alopecia. Retinoids are known to affect cell membrane characteristics, and they promote epidermal cell growth, keratinization, and angiogenesis.

Antiandrogens

A number of antiandrogens have been investigated for their effectiveness in preventing hair loss. Antiandrogens exert their effects in one of two known ways: either by competing for and blocking key receptor sites or by inhibiting enzymatic conversion to an active or more active form. Compounds such as cimetidine, cyproterone acetate, and spironolactone are receptor blockers. Finasteride and certain other compounds inhibit the conversion of testosterone to the more potent dihydrotestosterone by 5-alpha reductase.

Antiandrogens have been administered systemically in females.[51] However, antiandrogen action of systemic scope is an unacceptable approach to therapy in males, for obvious reasons.

Topical preparations are under investigation, particularly in combination with minoxidil.

References

1. Price VH. Testosterone metabolism in the skin: a review of its function in androgenetic alopecia, acne vulgaris, and idiopathic hirsutism including recent studies with antiandrogens. Arch Dermatol. 1975;111:1496–1502.
2. Sawaya ME, Mendex AJ, Hsia SL. Translocation of androgen-receptor protein complex into nuclei of hair follicles and sebaceous glands from human scalp. J Invest Dermatol. 1988;90:605.
3. Kasick JM, Bergfeld WF, Steck WD, Gupta MK. Adrenal androgenic female-pattern alopecia: sex hormones and the balding woman. Cleve Clin Q. 1983;50:111–122.
4. Cotsarelis G, Sun T-T, Lavker RM. Label-retaining cells reside in the bulge area of pilosebaceous unit: implications for follicular stem

cells, hair cycle, and skin carcinogenesis. Cell. 1990;61:1329-1337.
5. Sun T-T, Cotsarelis G, Lavker RM. Hair follicular stem cells: the bulge-activation hypothesis. J Invest Dermatol. 1991;96: 77S-78S.
6. Kuster W, Happle R. The inheritance of common baldness: two B or not two B? J Am Acad Dermatol. 1984;11:921-926.
7. Hamilton JB. Male hormone stimulation is prerequisite and an incitant in common baldness. Am J Anat. 1942;71:451-480.
8. Sawaya ME, Price VH, Harris IA, Kirsner RS, Hsia SL. Human hair follicle aromatase activity in females with androgenetic alopecia. J Invest Dermatol. 1990;94:575.
9. Venning VA, and Dawber RPR. Patterned androgenic alopecia in women. J Am Acad Dermatol. 1988;18:1073-1077.
10. Hamilton JB. Patterned loss of hair in man: Types and incidence. An New York Acad Sci. 1951;53:708-727.
11. Okuda S. Clinical and experimental studies of transplantation of living hairs. Japan J Dermatol Urol. 1939;46:135-138.
12. Orentreich N. Autografts in alopecias and other selected dermatological conditions. An New York Acad Sci. 1959;83:463-478.
13. Sasagawa M. Hair transplantation. Japan J Dermatol. 1930;30:493.
14. Fujita K. Reconstruction of eyebrow. La Lepro. 1953;22:364.
15. Marritt E. Transplantation of single hairs from the scalp as eyelashes. Review of the literature and a case report. J Dermatol Surg Oncol. 1980;6:271-273.
16. Stough DB, Nelson BR, Stough DB. Incisional slit grafting. J Dermatol Surg Oncol. 1991; 17:243-253.
17. Vallis CP. Surgical treatment of receding hairline: report of a case. Plast Reconstr Surg. 1964;33:243-252.
18. Coiffman F. Use of square scalp grafts for male pattern baldness. Plast Reconstr Surg. 1977;60:228-232.
19. Brandy DA. A new instrument for the expedient production of minigrafts. 1992;18:487-492.
20. Stough DB, Schauder CS, Chu TP, Nelson BR. Linear grafting, a novel technique for hair transplantation. J Cosmetic Dermatol. 1993;6:49-52.
21. Blanchard G, Blanchard B. La rèduction de la tonsure: concept nouveau dans le traitement chirurgical de la calvitie. L'Union Mèdicale du Canada. 1976;105:618-624.
22. Blanchard G, Blanchard B. Obliteration of alopecia by hair lifting: a new concept and technique. J Nat Med Assoc. 1977;69:639-641.
23. Unger MG, Unger WP. Management of alopecia of the scalp by a combination of excisions and transplantations. J Dermatol Surg Oncol. 1978;4:670-672.
24. Bosley LL, Hope CR, Montroy RE. Male pattern reduction (MPR) for surgical reduction of male pattern baldness. Curr Ther Res. 1979;25:281-287.
25. Alt TH. Scalp reduction as an adjunct to hair transplantation, review of relevant literature, presentation of an improved technique. J Dermatol Surg Oncol. 1980;6:1011-1018.
26. Alt TH. Scalp reduction. Cosmetic Surg. 1981;1:1-19.
27. Norwood OT, Shiell RC. Scalp reductions. In: *Hair Transplant Surgery,* OT Norwood, ed. Charles C. Thomas, Springfield, 1984, pp. 160-200.
28. Fleming RW, Kabaker SS, Marritt M, Mayer TG. Panel discussion. Sixth National Symposium on Hair Replacement Surgery. Palm Springs, California, March 29, 1984.
29. Nordstrom REA. Change of direction of hair growth. J Dermatol Surg Oncol. 1983;9:156-158.
30. Marzola M. An alternative hair replacement method. In: *Hair Transplant Surgery,* 2nd ed., OT Norwood, RC Shiell, ed. Charles C. Thomas, Springfield, 1984, pp. 163-200.
31. Brandy DA. The effectiveness of occipital artery ligations as a priming procedure for extensive scalp lifting. J Dermatol Surg Oncol. 1991;17:946-949.
32. Lamont ES. A plastic surgical transformation: report of a case. West J Surg Obstet Gynecol. 1957;65:164-165.
33. Juri J. Use of parieto-occipital flaps in the surgical treatment of baldness. Plast Reconst Surg. 1975;55:456-460.
34. Elliott, RA. Lateral scalp flaps for instant results in male pattern baldness. Plast Reconst Surg. 1977;60:699-703.
35. Nataf J. Special techniques of hair transplantation by fusiform grafts and flaps of many types. J Dermatol Surg Oncol. 1979;5:620-624.
36. Ohmori K. Recent advances in the use of free flaps. An Chir Gynaecol. 1982;71:34-37.
37. Stough DB, Cates JA. Transposition flaps for the correction of baldness: a practical office procedure. J Dermatol Surg Oncol. 1980;6:286-289.
38. Stough DB, Freilich IW. Hairbearing flaps for baldness. Fac Plast Surg. 1985;2:283-285.
39. Wright MR. Psychological evaluation of a cosmetic surgical patient. In: *Cosmetic Surgery of the Skin*, WP Coleman, CW Hanke, eds. B.C. Decker Inc., Philadelphia, 1991, pp. 373-379.

40. Cotterill PC, Unger WP. Hair transplantation in females. J Dermatol Surg Oncol. 1992;18: 477–481.
41. Beeson WH. Facial analysis. In: *Aesthetic Surgery of the Aging Face*, WH Beeson, EG McCollough, eds. C.V. Mosby Company, St. Louis, 1986, pp. 1–5.
42. Frechet P. A new method for correction of the vertical scar observed following scalp reduction for extensive alopecia. J Dermatol Surg Oncol. 1990;16:640–644.
43. Schauder CS, Stough DB. Modified S pattern for scalp reduction. Am J Cosmet Surg. 1992;9:309–313.
44. Norwood OT, Shiell RC. *Hair Transplant Surgery*, 2nd ed. Charles C Thomas, Springfield, 1984, pp. 5–10.
45. Kabaker S. Experiences with parieto-occipital flaps in hair transplantation. Laryngoscope. 1978;88:73–84.
46. Fleming RW, Mayer TG. Short vs. long flaps in the treatment of male pattern baldness. Arch Otolaryngol. 1981;107:403–408.
47. Price VH, Menefee E. Quantitative estimation of hair growth I. Androgenetic alopecia in women: effect of minoxidil. J Invest Dermatol. 1990;95:683–687.
48. Diani AR, Mulholland MJ, Shull KL, Kubicek MF, Johnson GA, Schostarez HJ, Brunden MN, Buhl AE. Hair growth effects of oral administration of finasteride, a steroid 5-alpha-reductase inhibitor, alone and in combination with topical minoxidil in the balding stumptail macaque. J Clin Endocrinol Metab. 1992;74:345–350.
49. Rittmaster RS. Topical anti-androgens in the treatment of male pattern baldness. Clin Dermatol. 1988;6:122–128.
50. Bazzano GS, Terezakis N, Galen W. Topical tretinoin for hair growth promotion. JAAS. 1986:15:880–883.
51. Burke BM, Cunliffe WJ. Oral spironolactone therapy for female patients with acne, hirsutism or androgenic alopecia. Br J Dermatol. 1985;112:124–125.

14
Treatment of the Aging Hands

Robert E. Clark and Susan C. Carson

Introduction

Understanding the aging process is essential for physicians today, because an increasing proportion of the U.S. population are considered elderly. At the beginning of the twentieth century, only 4% (3 million) of the U.S. population were over age 65. Today approximately 12% (30 million) of the U.S. population are over age 65; 3 million of these are over 85. There are a significant number of cosmetic and functional dermatological problems that occur almost exclusively, or at an increased rate, in the elderly population.

The appearance of aging skin is due to a combination of intrinsic factors, or a genetic "wear-and-tear" phenomenon, and extrinsic factors, primarily sunlight. Intrinsically aged skin has a flattened dermal-epidermal junction, with loss of the normal rete ridge pattern; collagen, elastic tissue, fat, and cellularity are markedly reduced.[1] Clinically, thin, fragile skin that bruises easily is observed. Photodamage, however, accounts for most of the changes characteristic of aging skin. Microscopic examination reveals epidermal cellular atypia with loss of polarity, increased activity of melanocytes with an irregular distribution, loss of collagen, degenerated elastotic material, and a chronic inflammatory infiltrate.[2] These histologic changes are manifested by roughness, sallowness, laxity, wrinkling, mottled pigmentation, and epidermal-derived neoplasms.

Patients are eager to camouflage or reverse the appearance of aging skin and often present to the dermatologist or plastic surgeon for evaluation and treatment. There are a variety of treatments now available for improving the appearance of the aging face. Although other exposed surfaces (such as the hands, forearms, and neck) sustain similar changes due to photodamage and the intrinsic aging process, the treatment of these areas has received less attention from physicians. The same general principles used to treat the face can be applied to treatment of the aging hands; however, some modifications need to be made. The skin overlying the hands is much thinner and has fewer adnexal structures than facial skin; therefore, wound healing occurs at a much slower rate.

Wound healing is affected by intrinsic factors of aging and extrinsic factors from chronic photoaging. Extrinsic and intrinsic aging processes prolong wound healing in elderly patients, requiring the cutaneous surgeon to consider these issues and their effects on surgical procedures involving the hands.[3] The tensile strength of wounds decreases with age and is especially diminished in those individuals greater than age 70. This decrease in the tensile strength is manifested by increased rates of wound dehiscence. Clinical studies have shown that wound dehiscence increases with age. Mendoza et al.[3] found that individuals between 30 and 39 years of age had a rate of wound dehiscence of 0.9%. This increased to a wound dehiscence rate of 2.5% for individuals ages 50 to 59 and 5.5% in individuals older than 80. The cutaneous surgeon can respond to these increasing rates of wound dehiscence by placing a greater number of dermal sutures in surgical repairs and by utilizing slowly absorbing subcutaneous sutures. In addition, sutures used for approximation of the epidermis may be left in place for longer periods of time, in order to allow for additional healing and increased tensile strength prior to suture removal.

Prolonged wound healing in the elderly is thought to be secondary to decreases in cellular proliferation, wound metabolism, and collagen remodeling.[4] These profound changes in dermal structures occur gradually, resulting in a relatively avascular dermis with diminished cellularity and structural density. The amount of collagen in the dermis decreases by 1% per year throughout adult life.[5,6] Microscopically, effete collagen fibers become thickened with decreased solubility, diminished capacity for hydration, and decreased rates of collagenase digestion.[7]

Aged skin has been demonstrated to have a 35% reduction in venular cross-sectional area of the vertical capillary loops in the papillary dermis.[8] This progressively avascular change in the dermis profoundly affects those processes important for wound healing and thereby plays a vital role in prolonged wound healing.

Elastic fibers in elderly skin are also altered. These changes are most notable in skin samples from individuals older than age 50. Electron micrographic studies have revealed fragmentation of elastic fibers with cystic structures or lacunae involving the fibers, plus fuzzy, indistinct borders of these macromolecular structures.[9]

Cells of the epidermis are also noted to undergo change with aging. The basal cells in aged skin show greater variability in size, shape, and staining qualities as compared to the skin of younger individuals.[10] The keratinocyte derived from the basal cell layer shows diminished height and surface area as compared to younger skin.[11] Corneocyte adhesion is diminished in elderly skin; hence, tape-stripping injuries remove the stratum corneum, resulting in persistent inflammation secondary to diminished epidermal cell turnover time. This disruption of the epidermal barrier predisposes the elderly patient to cutaneous infection, prolonged inflammation of the skin around the surgical site, increased transepidermal movement of allergens, and increased possibility of allergic contact dermatitis.[12]

Wound healing in older individuals is also affected by underlying medical conditions, such as diabetes and peripheral vascular disease, which are more prevalent in this population. Dietary habits may result in diminished intake of nutrients, minerals, and vitamins necessary for wound healing. These factors, combined with changes due to intrinsic and extrinsic aging, result in delayed would healing, diminished final tensile strength, and increased rates of wound dehiscence, ecchymoses, tape-strip injuries, infection, and persistent contact dermatitis.

Topical Therapy

Textural changes such as roughness, sallowness, laxity, and wrinkling contribute most to the general appearance of aging skin. These qualities can be improved by several topical approaches, but accurate comparisons among methods may be difficult because of the subjective nature of the analyses. Alpha hydroxy acids are naturally occurring acids that are used in dermatology to treat a variety of conditions, including dry skin, ichthyosis, lentigines, and keratoses. Lactic acid and glycolic acid are the most common agents used and are obtained in commercial preparations in concentrations as high as 20% Pyruvic acid, an alpha keto acid, is also available. At low concentrations these acids disrupt cohesion of keratinocytes within the lower level of the stratum corneum, perhaps by interfering with the formation of ionic bonds.[13]

Because of these results, alpha hydroxy acids have been studied in photoaging. Twenty-one volunteers with photodamaged facial skin were treated with Lac-Hydrin lotion (12% ammonium lactate) twice daily. Mild to moderate improvements were observed in fine and coarse wrinkling by 8 weeks, with an overall subjective improvement in texture.[14] It is not clear whether this effect is due to a lack of corneocyte cohesion or to increased hydration from the lotion. A similar effect was seen using 5% to 10% glycolic acid twice daily for 1 year.[13] Use of these agents on hand and forearm skin would likely have similar results, although this has not been tested in a controlled setting.

Tretinoin has become the most effective and popular treatment for improving the overall appearance of aging skin. Laxity is affected first, with a generalized tightening seen in the skin after 2 to 3 days. Within 4 to 6 weeks, laxity is further improved, and there is a reduction in roughness. A rosy hue gradually replaces the sallowness seen in older patients in as few as 4 weeks. Reduction of wrinkling requires prolonged therapy; the fine wrinkles around the cheeks, forehead, and periorbital area respond first within 2 to 4 months, followed by the deeper, coarse wrinkles within 4 in 5 months. Improvement continues to occur over time, reaching a plateau at 2 to 3 years of continued therapy. At this time the results may be maintained with reduced frequency of therapy.[15]

Recommendations regarding concentration and dosing frequency of tretinoin are subject to controversy. Varying concentrations from 0.001% to 0.1% have been tested in randomized, double-blind, vehicle-controlled studies for their effects on photodamaged skin.[16-20] In general, the higher concentrations produce more significant results, and the lesser concentrations show no significant difference as compared to vehicle alone.[16] Higher concentrations have more severe side effects, however, with the retinoid reaction (redness, peeling, and irritation) occurring in 70% and 90% of patients treated with 0.05% and 0.1% tretinoin qhs, respectively, for 6 months.[15] Kligman has suggested starting with lower concentrations and gradually increasing the dose and frequency, as tolerated by the patient.[21] Others advocate starting with 0.1% tretinoin qd to bid for the quickest results, reducing the dose and frequency of application only if the patient cannot endure the side effects.[22]

Cosmetic Surgical Procedures

Procedures and treatments for the face and neck are often successful in reversing the accumulative aging effect of intrinsic and extrinsic aging factors. The changes effected by aging on the dorsa of the hands, however, prove more difficult to conceal. Alterations of the hands resulting from intrinsic and extrinsic aging include thinning of the epidermis and dermis; atrophy of subcutaneous tissues; conspicuously visible veins and tendons; wrinkling; pigmentary changes; and benign, precancerous, and cancerous lesions (see Figure 14.1A through F).

A variety of cosmetic surgical procedures are available for treatment of each of these age-revealing changes involving the hands. Benign and precancerous skin lesions are often treated with cryotherapy. Skin cancers involving the hands may require conventional surgical excision or Mohs micrographic surgery. Pigmentary changes due to solar lentigines may be treated with Retin-A, cryotherapy, chemical peeling, or laser therapy. Wrinkling and skin flaccidity with prominent veins and extensor tendons result from atrophy of fat and dermal tissue and require reconstitution of the subcutaneous fatty tissue. These have recently been approached with autologous fat transplantation.

Autologous fat transfer has been proven useful in the correction of skin defects characterized by loss of normal subcutaneous tissue. Chronic photodamage, combined with intrinsic aging, severely distracts from the appearance of the dorsa of the hands. The correction of the aged appearance of the hands has proved to be one of the more difficult problems to solve in the process of rejuvenation.[23] Autologous fat transplantation for rejuvenation of the dorsum of the hand is performed by placing freshly harvested fat into the subcutaneous compartment between the dorsal fascia and the deep dermis of the skin. The transplant is introduced into the recipient sites using a 10 ml syringe equipped with a 2 mm needle in order to prevent rupture of the lipocytes from shear forces.[24] Total implantation of each hand requires 10 to 15 ml of fat.[23] The transplanted fat is uniformly distributed over the dorsum of the hands by gentle manipulation of the skin. Typically, no dressings are required following the transplant, and patients may immediately return to near-normal activity but must avoid displacement of the graft.

The ideal donor site for autologous fat transfer for hand rejuvenation is the medial aspect of the knees.[25] Other authors feel that

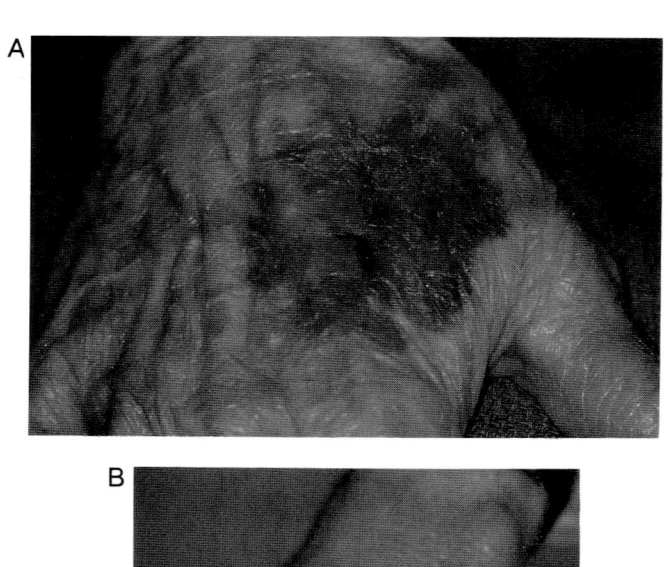
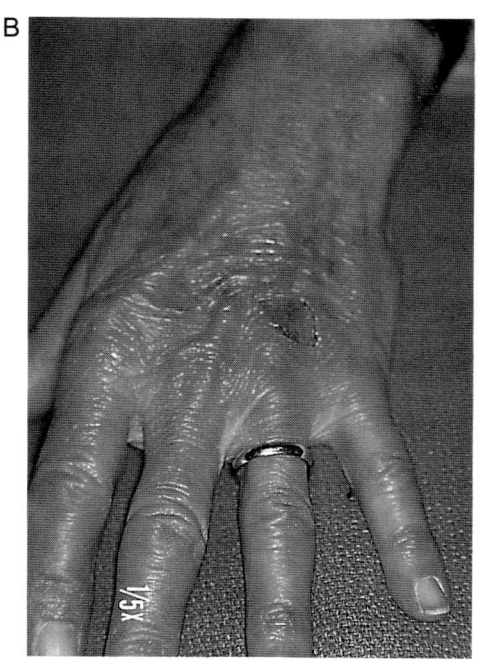
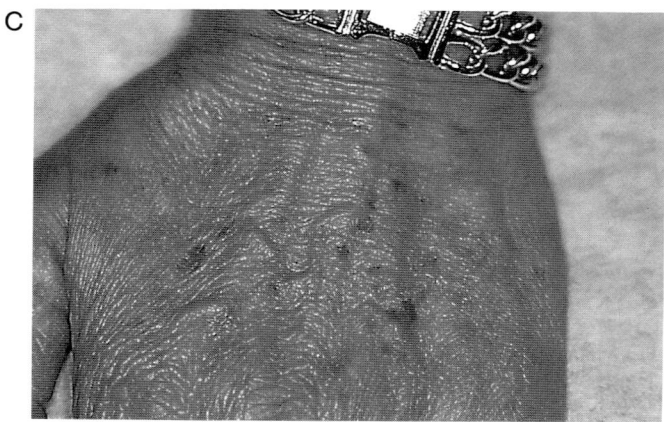

FIGURE 14.1. Examples of age-related changes in the hands. A. Actinic Purpura. B. Actinic Purpura, fine lines, lentigines, and atrophy. C. Lentigines.

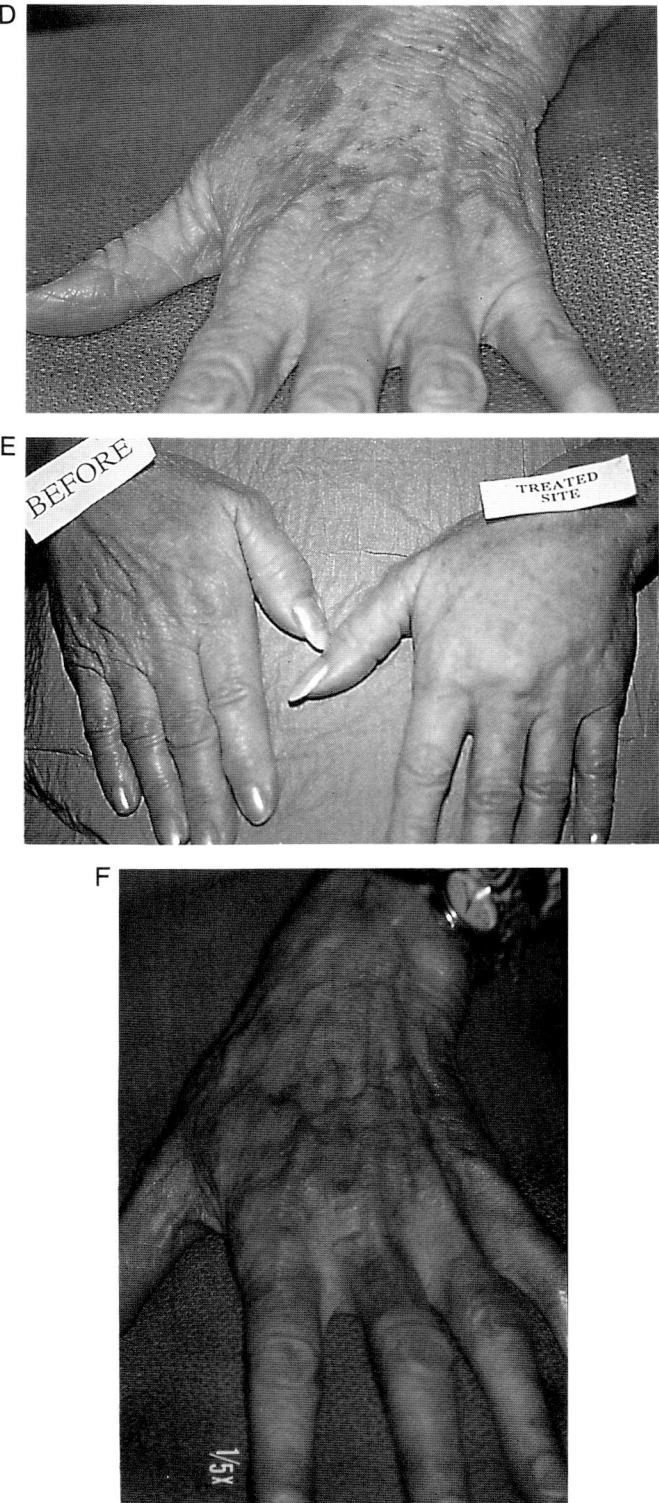

FIGURE 14.1. *Continued* D. Lentigines, atrophy, purpura, lines, and coarseness. E. Severe atrophy treated with lipotransfer. Left side: before, right side: after. (Courtesy of William Coleman, III, M.D.). F. Severe purpura, lentigines, hyperpigmentation, and atrophy.

fat tissue harvested by liposuction from a variety of donor sites works equally well.[24] The fat tissue is harvested by liposuction using a 2 to 3 mm cannula. Prior to the graft placement, the fat tissue is washed in normal saline to separate intact lipocytes from blood, plasma, free fatty acids, and cellular debris.

Aboudib et al.[23] published their experience in hand rejuvenation in 72 patients. The average age of their patients was 58 years old, with a range of 38 to 78 years old. Ten to 15 ml of fat were used to reconstitute the adipose layer of the subcutaneous compartment. No graft resorption was observed in the first 3 months of follow-up; however, moderate resorption was noted after 1 year. Resorption of the fat graft remains the key obstacle with this procedure.[26]

Three of the 72 patients experienced complications from their procedures. Two had irregularity of the fat graft, and 1 developed a postoperative infection that responded to oral antibiotics. Irregularity of the fat graft is best corrected at the time of the transplant or shortly thereafter.

Alternative approaches to rejuvenation of the dorsum of the hand could include the use of injectable collagen (Zyplast) Fibrel, or injectable-grade silicone. The use of these substances is greatly limited for this procedure, due both to the volume of substance necessary for correction and the medicolegal issues associated with their use.

Prevention

Preventive measures alone may also be extremely effective in reducing the severity of photodamage. In all the recent randomized, double-blinded, vehicle-controlled studies, the vehicle group showed significant improvement in photoaging over baseline by the end of the studies.[16,17,19,20] These individuals were encouraged to avoid the sun, wear protective clothing, use mild soaps, and wear daily sunscreen preparations.

The hairless mouse model has been used to study the effects of prevention and repair of photoaging. Mice are exposed to ultraviolet light to induce histologic changes similar to those seen in severely photodamaged human skin. When these mice are then protected from further damage by UV avoidance, a subepidermal band of new collagen is seen in the papillary dermis, which displaces the solar elastotic material to deeper areas of the dermis.[27] Treatment with tretinoin further enhances the deposition of new collagen. A similar subepidermal repair zone has been demonstrated in humans with prolonged sun avoidance.[28]

Because complete UV avoidance is impossible to achieve in the human experience, there has been much interest in the use of sunscreens to prevent photodamage and to allow for repair despite continued UV exposure. Hairless mice were irradiated to cause histologic effects of severe photodamage, then protected with the use of a broad spectrum sunscreen with a sun protection factor of 15 while continuing to receive UV exposure. Further elastosis did not occur, and there was evidence of a subepidermal repair zone, analogous to that seen in mice with complete UV avoidance.[27] Although commercial sunscreen preparations prevent damage due to UVB (280 to 320 nm) and part of the UVA spectrum (320 to 340 nm), they do not protect against long-wavelength UVA or infrared, both of which exacerbate photodamage due to UVB. However, evidence from the mouse model suggests that sunscreens do provide significant protection against photodamage and allow for natural repair processes to occur.

Idiopathic Guttate Hypomelanosis

Idiopathic guttate hypomelanosis is an extremely common pigmentary disorder characterized by depigmented macules averaging 0.5 cm in size that are located primarily on the extremities. These lesions tend to develop after age 40 and may become larger and more numerous with age. Sunlight is proposed to be a causative factor, as these are found mostly on sun-exposed areas. However, this cannot be the only explanation, as they are also seen in nonexposed sites. Genetic factors may play a role,[29] and autoimmune mechanisms have been proposed. The etiology is likely multifactorial.

In aging skin there is flattening of the dermal epidermal junction and a 10% to 55% reduction in the number of dopa-positive melanocytes.[30] The remaining melanocytes are distributed unevenly and have structural abnormalities by electron microscopy.[31] Transplanted split-thickness skin grafts from idiopathic guttate hypomelanosis lesions on nude mice repigmented within 1 month of transplantation, suggesting that there may be a systemic factor involved as well.[32]

Idiopathic guttate hypomelanosis is an asymptomatic, benign disorder that is often emotionally disturbing to the patient because of its appearance on exposed areas. Treatment of this problem is difficult.

Cryotherapy is used successfully by some, but the mechanism of action is unclear. Destruction of the lesions by liquid nitrogen may remove the malfunctioning melanocytes, thereby allowing normal keratinocytes and melanocytes to migrate from the periphery of the lesion to repigment the area, or it may inhibit a local factor that is causing the depigmentation.[31] One study was successful using a cryoprobe for 10 seconds to each lesion of idiopathic guttate hypomelanosis. Ten patients and a total of 87 lesions were treated by this method. Repigmentation began within 4 weeks and was complete by 6 to 8 weeks in 79 of 87 lesions (90.8%).[18]

Autologous exchange grafts from normal to diseased sites have been performed experimentally.[29] Of 15 patients studied, only 1 of 15 repigmented when the minigrafts were placed. However, the addition of intralesional triamcinolone 2 mg/ml caused repigmentation in 11 of the 15. Seven of 11 also had repigmentation with intralesional triamcinolone alone. Further studies were performed transferring lesional skin to normally pigmented skin, and vice versa. The normal skin grafts lost their pigmentation over 1½ years, and the depigmented areas persisted. These results suggest that an active depigmenting process is occurring locally.

Senile Lentigines

Senile lentigines, better known by patients as "liver spots" or "old age spots," are the most diagnostic change of aging seen on the hands. Clinically, they are hyperpigmented macules of varying size and shape without hyperkeratosis. Their incidence is directly related to one's age and extent of sun exposure. In elderly populations as many as 90% of individuals have senile lentigines.[33] They occur most commonly on the dorsa of the hands but can be found on the forehead, cheeks, and other sun-exposed sites.

Ephelides or freckles may be indistinguishable by clinical exam but, histologically, these two entities are very different. Ephelides have hyperpigmentation of the basal layer with a normal number of melanocytes present; there is no epidermal proliferation. In contrast, senile lentigines have basal hyperpigmentation with increased numbers of melanocytes and club-shaped budding of the rete pegs. Because lentigines represent an epidermal proliferation as well as hyperpigmentation, they are more difficult to treat by simple bleaching creams.

Bleaching agents are used extensively for hyperpigmentation disorders, such as melasma and postinflammatory hyperpigmentation, and have also been tried for ephelides and lentigines. Hydroquinone is the only agent available that is marketed for use in hyperpigmentation disorders. It is not a true "bleaching" agent, like peroxide, but instead works by inhibiting the synthesis of melanin. Concentrations of 2% to 4% are available commercially. Increased irritation is seen with increased concentrations, with little improvement in efficacy.

Reduction in hyperpigmentation is seen with prolonged use of hydroquinone for melasma and postinflammatory hyperpigmentation; less significant results are seen in the treatment of senile lentigines. Spencer[34] applied varying concentrations of hydroquinone (2%, 3%, and 5%) versus vehicle twice daily for 3 months on the dorsa of the hands of elderly Caucasians with numerous senile lentigines. Depigmentation of the lesions occurred in 28 of 41 patients treated with 2% hydroquinone and in 21 of 28 patients treated with 5% hydroquinone. However, repigmentation developed immediately after the cessation of therapy. Kligman published a formula containing 0.1% tretinoin, 5% hydroquinone, and 0.1% dexamethasone in 1975 in hopes of improving the results of hydroquinone alone for hyperpigmentation.[35]

Although his solution effectively treated ephelides, melasma, and postinflammatory hyperpigmentation, it had no effect whatsoever on 7 patients treated with senile lentigines on the dorsa of the hands.

Tretinoin is an effective therapy for the mottled hyperpigmentation seen with aging; it is also effective for improving the appearance of solar lentigines, but the effects require prolonged therapy.[2,16,18] Rafal et al.[36] recently published a double-blind, randomized controlled trial using 0.1% tretinoin versus vehicle for senile lentigines located on the face or arms, or both. After 10 months of once-daily therapy, there was statistically significant lightening seen in 71% of the tretinoin group versus 23% in the vehicle group. Thirty-two percent of the tretinoin group had complete clearing of 1 or more lesions, whereas no complete clearing was seen in the vehicle-control group. The characteristic histologic changes seen with tretinoin therapy included epidermal thickening and decreased epidermal pigmentation. Continued treatment past the 10 months caused further lightening.

Many destructive methods are used to remove senile lentigines. Because melanocytes are extremely sensitive to cold injury, cryotherapy is an effective and widely used method. Freezing is accomplished by means of a cotton tip, spray, or cryoprobe, treating just beyond the edge of the lesion.[37] Hypopigmentation is the major risk of this form of therapy, especially in dark-skinned individuals.

Senile lentigines on the dorsa of the hands can be treated by a variety of superficial chemical peeling agents. Trichloroacetic acid (TCA) in concentrations of 10% to 35% have been used to accomplish chemexfoliation of lentigines. Collins et al.[38] report excellent results in the treatment of hands using superficial, repetitive TCA chemical peels at concentrations of 20% to 25%. The chemical peel can be repeated on a 2 to 3 week basis until the desired response is achieved.[38,39] Swinehart[40] has reported the use of 50% salicylic acid ointment under occlusion for treatment of lentigines, keratoses, and actinically damaged skin on the dorsa of the hands and forearms. The salicylic acid paste was applied to the affected areas, followed by placement of a plastic wrap and then a dry gauze roll wrap.

The salicylic acid paste remains in contact with the skin for 48 hours and is then removed. Epidermal desquamation and maceration is treated by the application of an antibiotic ointment or by a synthetic dressing in order to facilitate healing. The skin is reported to heal within 4 weeks time, and it is estimated that 90% of the cutaneous lesions resolve without evidence of scarring. Signs and symptoms of salicylism may result from excessive salicylate absorption. Patients may complain of tinnitus, diminished hearing, dizziness, or headache. Increased water intake is recommended during this treatment modality in order to facilitate excretion of salicylic acid.

Alpha hydroxy acids are naturally occurring acids that can be extracted from food products. Glycolic acid from sugarcane and tartaric acid from grape wine are the most common alpha hydroxy acids utilized for chemical peeling. Solar lentigines on the dorsa of the hand have been treated with 70% glycolic acid. The peeling agent is applied using a large cotton-tip applicator followed by neutralization in 4 to 6 minutes with water or 1% sodium bicarbonate.[41] The effectiveness of the glycolic acid chemical peel can be facilitated with the use of once or twice daily-applied moisturizer containing 10% glycolic acid or a moisturizer containing 12% ammonium lactate.

Topical tretinoin can be used as a pretreatment prior to chemical peeling. Tretinoin, 0.1% cream, applied once daily, facilitates the response to the chemical peeling agent as well as reduces the time to healing.[42]

Complications following chemical peel procedures of the dorsa of the hands may include prolonged wound healing, infection and subsequent scarring, pigmentary changes, skin textural changes, milia, prolonged erythema, and pruritus. These issues should be carefully addressed with the patient prior to the chemical peeling process. Benign pigmented lesions of the epidermis have been successfully treated utilizing laser technology developed to take advantage of the concept of selective photothermolysis. This concept is utilized to target the laser energy to the melanosomes of senile lentigines. Several lasers have demonstrated efficacy in the treatment of senile lentigines, eg, Candela 510 nm pigmented lesion dye laser, copper vapor laser at 511 nm, and the argon laser at 514 nm.

The Candela pigmented lesion dye laser has been demonstrated to clear approximately 90% of senile lentigines on the hand utilizing energy levels ranging from 2.0 to 3.75 joules per square centimeter. The number of treatments required ranged from 1 to 5 treatment sessions.[43]

Dinehart and colleagues[44] report excellent results with clearing of solar lentigines with the copper vapor laser. The average power setting ranged from 160 mW to 250 mW with a beam spot size of 150 microns using a chopped beam (200 milliseconds on, 200 milliseconds off). A thin eschar develops within 3 to 4 days and separates within 2 weeks. Transient hyperpigmentation and hypopigmentation may complicate the treatment of senile lentigines with this treatment method.

The 514 nm argon laser has been shown to produce a 90% clearing of benign lentigines after only 2 treatment sessions.[45] These data include lentigines on the face, trunk, and extremities. Parameters for treatment of lentigines on the trunk and extremities include an energy density of 10 to 14 joules per square centimeter with a pulse length of 30 to 50 milliseconds.

Immediate pigment darkening of the treated lesion may be noted within the first 6 to 36 hours and requires 7 to 10 days to fade.

Adverse reactions are reportedly rare when the correct energy fluence and pulselengths are selected. Subtle, transient textural changes in the skin have been noted infrequently, as well as hypopigmentation. Electrodesiccation, curettage, and the CO_2 laser in a defocused mode are other effective destructive methods, but they have the potential for scarring.

Seborrheic Keratoses

Seborrheic keratoses are benign neoplasms of the epidermis that occur at an increased frequency with age. Although only 13% of seborrheic keratoses occur on the extremities,[46] they can be a significant cosmetic problem to the elderly patient. Removal is unnecessary for medical reasons but is often performed when the lesion is irritated or for cosmetic reasons. A wide surgical excision is never indicated, because these lesions are benign epidermal proliferations.

A variety of destructive methods have been used for removal of seborrheic keratoses. Curettage, with or without anesthesia, is the simplest method. Mohs advocated curettage followed by the application of oxidized cellulose for hemostasis.[47] No scarring was seen with this approach. Freezing the lesion first with liquid nitrogen prior to curettage has also been advocated; this method provides partial anesthesia while making the keratosis firmer and easier to remove. Cryotherapy may be used alone but often does not remove the lesion entirely. Hypopigmentation may result from this treatment method.

Superficial shave excision using either a scalpel or a Gillette blue blade removes the lesion entirely with minimal, if any, residual effect on the skin. Electrodesiccation can also be used but may result in prolonged wound healing and hypertrophic scarring. Topical acids are effective in removing keratoses if applied to the lesions directly, without damaging the surrounding normal skin. Full-strength pyruvic acid, applied for 3 to 4 minutes, causes epidermolysis.[13] The neoplasm can then be curetted gently and the area washed with water to prevent further damage by the acid. Trichloroacetic acid in concentrations of 10% to 50% can be used in a similar manner, producing a superficial frosting effect. These methods are less effective if the lesions are extremely hyperkeratotic.

Actinic Keratoses

Actinic keratoses are proliferative neoplasms directly related to chronic ultraviolet exposure. They are considered to be precancerous lesions; however, the rate of malignant transformation remains debatable. The Marks et al. study of 1,040 people followed for 12 months is the largest study to date evaluating the potential malignant transformation of actinic keratoses.[48] They observed a high spontaneous remission rate but an overall 21.8% increase in total lesions over a 12-month period. There was a 0.24% risk for each keratosis developing into a squamous cell carcinoma in this cohort of patients. Other authors have expressed concern that despite the low rate of malignant transformation rate for a given keratosis, an individual with numerous actinic keratoses may have a substantial risk of developing squamous cell carcinomas over his or her lifetime.[49] Actinic keratoses are treated not only because of this medical concern but also because they are often painful and represent a significant cosmetic problem in the elderly.

Cryotherapy is the most commonly used technique for removal of limited numbers of actinic keratoses; hypopigmentation is the major side effect. Electrodesiccation or curettage may also be used. These ablative methods have limited use, however, for the patient with multiple lesions or a concern for cosmesis.

5-fluorouracil is a commonly used topical therapy for diffuse actinic damage. This antimetabolite inhibits RNA and DNA synthesis. Topical use of 5-fluorouracil was first reported by Dillaha[10] in 1963 after others had noticed reduction of solar keratoses in patients receiving systemic 5-fluorouracil as chemotherapy for malignant neoplasms. The most striking effect seen with 5-fluorouracil is inflammation of the abnormal keratoses, with sparing of the surrounding normal skin. The conventional method advocates the use of 1% 5-fluorouracil to the affected areas twice daily for 2 to 8 weeks, depending on the body site.[50] The forearms and dorsa of the hands often require 6 to 8 weeks of therapy. Histologic resolution is not achieved; therefore, this therapy is considered to be palliative rather than curative.[50] Retreatment may be necessary within 2 years.

The major disadvantage to topical 5-fluorouracil is the brisk inflammatory response seen with its use. Many patients are reluctant to complete the treatment course because of the severe redness, vesiculation, ulceration, swelling, and pain that develop. Several investigators have altered the conventional application regimen in order to reduce these effects. Breza[51] reported the use of 1% 5-fluorouracil in combination with Triamcinolone acetonide cream. He was able to decrease inflammation without affecting the therapeutic response. A recent study changed the frequency of application of 5-fluorouracil to once or twice weekly. Although treatment was longer than the conventional method—an average of 6.7 weeks compared to 2 to 4 weeks—the response rate was equivalent.[52] Minimal erythema was the only side effect.

Multiple actinic keratoses can also be treated with tretinoin. Papa[53] suggests using 0.1% tretinoin twice daily on the forearms and dorsa of the hands for the best results. Clinically apparent as well as inapparent actinic keratoses become reddened and scaly within 1 to 2 months of therapy and then resolve with continued therapy. Hyperkeratotic lesions do not respond as well to topical therapy, and biopsies should be obtained to rule out the possibility of a squamous cell carcinoma. Although longer treatment is required with this method, there are fewer side effects than are seen with 5-fluorouracil. Tretinoin may also retard the development of new actinic keratoses.

Medical therapies for treatment of diffuse actinic keratoses are being investigated. Interferon α_{2B} causes complete clearing actinic keratoses after repeated intralesional injections, but excessive costs and severe systemic side effects preclude its widespread use.[54] Topical interferon preparations have thus far been unsuccessful in reproducing these results.[55] Topical 10% masoprocol (Actinex) has shown clinical efficacy in preliminary trials for the treatment of multiple actinic keratoses on the head and neck and has recently become commercially available.[56] To date no studies have documented histologic improvement with this therapy.

Actinic keratoses on the dorsa of the hands can be treated using several superficial chemical peeling agents. The prototypical chemical peeling agent is trichloroacetic acid. TCA chemical peels in concentrations of 10% to 35% can be used to treat solar keratoses distributed over the dorsa of the hands. Collins et al.[38] have reported the use of 20% to 25% TCA chemical peels for treatment of photodamaged skin involving the hands. These superficial chemical peels can be repeated at 2- to 3-week intervals in order to facilitate destruction of solar keratoses.[38,39]

Aronsohn[57] and Swinehart[40] have described

the use of 50% salicylic acid ointment under occlusion for the treatment of actinic keratoses on the dorsa of the hands and forearms. The resulting epidermal desquamation and maceration healed within 4 weeks with a 90% clearing of these cutaneous lesions.

References

1. Kurban RS, Bhawan J. Histologic changes in skin associated with aging. J Dermatol Surg Oncol. 1990; 16:908–914.
2. Bhawan J, Gonzalez-Serva A, Nehal K. Effects of tretinoin on photodamaged skin: a histologic study. Arch Dermatol. 1991;127:666–672.
3. Mendoza CB Jr, Postlethwait RW, Johnson WD. Veterans Administration cooperative study of surgery for duodenal ulcer II. incidence of wound disruption following operation. Arch Surg. 1970;101:396–398.
4. Goodson WH, Hunt TK. Wound healing and aging. J Invest Dermatol. 1979;73:88–91.
5. Shuster S, Black MM, McVitie E. The influence of age and sex on skin thickness, skin collagen and density. Br J Dermatol. 1975;93:639–643.
6. Andrew W, Behnke RH, Sato T. Changes with advancing age in the cell population of human dermis. Gerontologia. 1964; 10:1–19.
7. Lober CW, Fenske NA. Cutaneous aging: effect of intrinsic changes on surgical considerations. South Med J. 1991;84:1444–1446.
8. Gilchrest BA, Stoff JS, Soter NA. Chronologic aging alters the response to ultraviolet-induced inflammation in human skin. J Invest Dermatol. 1982;79:11–15.
9. Braverman IM, Fonferko E. Studies in cutaneous aging: I. The elastic fiber network. J Invest Dermatol. 1982;78:434–443.
10. Montagna W. Morphology of the aging skin: the cutaneous appendages. In: *Advances in biology of skin,* 6th ed. W Montagna, ed. Pergamon Press, Oxford, 1965, pp. 1–16.
11. Grove GL. Exfoliative cytological procedures as a nonintrusive method for dermatogerontological studies. J Invest Dermatol. 1979;73:67–69.
12. Fenske NA, Lober CW. Structural and functional changes of normal aging skin. J Am Acad Dermatol. 1986;15:571–585.
13. Van Scott EJ, Yu RJ. Alpha hydroxy acids: procedures for use in clinical practice. Cutis. 1989;43:222–228.
14. Ridge JM, Siegle RJ, Zuckerman J. Use of α-hydroxy acids in the therapy of "photoaged" skin. J Am Acad Dermatol. 1990;23:932.
15. Weiss JS, Ellis CN, Goldfarb MT, Voorhees. Tretinoin therapy: practical aspects of evaluation and treatment. J Inter Med Res. 1990; 18(Suppl3): 41C–48C.
16. Olsen EA, Katz HI, Levine N, et al. Tretinoin emollient cream: a new therapy for photodamaged skin. J Am Acad Dermatol. 1992; 26:215–224.
17. Monti M, Caputo R. Clinical efficacy and patient tolerance of topical tretinoin therapy in photoaging. J Inter Med Res. 1990;18(Suppl3): 35C–40C.
18. Weiss JS, Ellis CN, Headington JT, et al. Topical tretinoin improves photoaged skin: a double-blind vehicle-controlled study. JAMA. 1988;259:527–532.
19. Weinstein GD, Nigra TP, Pochi PE, et al. Topical tretinoin for treatment of photodamaged skin: a multicenter study. Arch Dermatol. 1991; 127:659–664.
20. Leyden JJ, Grove GL, Grove MJ, et al. Treatment of photodamaged facial skin with topical tretinoin. J Am Acad Dermatol. 1989;21:638–644.
21. Kligman AM. Guidelines for the use of topical tretinoin (retin-A) for photoaged skin. J Am Acad Dermatol. 1989;21:650–654.
22. Goldfarb MT, Ellis CN, Weiss JS, Voorhees JJ. Topical tretinoin therapy: its use in photoaged skin. J Am Acad Dermatol. 1989;21:645–650.
23. Aboudib JH, de Castro CC, Gradel J. Hand rejuvenescence by fat filling. An Plast Surg. 1992;28:559–564.
24. Matarasso HA, Aston SJ, Pitman GH. A collection device for suction-assisted lipectomy and autologous fat transplantation. An Plast Surg. 1988;20:492–493.
25. Caldeira AML, Nieves A, Arguera SP, et al. Cirurgia do rejuvenescimanto facial. Importancia do tratamento do tecido gorduroso e consideracoes sobra a lipoenxertia da face. Rev Bras Cir. 1988;78:375–392.
26. Nguyen A, Pasyk KA, Bouvier TN, Hassett CA, Argenta LC. Comparative study of survival of autologous adipose tissue taken and transplanted by different techniques. Plast Reconstr Surg. 1990;85:378–386.
27. Kligman LH. The ultraviolet-irradiated hairless mouse: a model for photoaging. J Am Acad Dermatol. 1989;21:623–631.
28. Kligman LH. Prevention and repair of photoaging: sunscreens and retinoids. Cutis. 1989; 43:458–465.
29. Falabella R. Idiopathic guttate hypomelanosis. Dermatol Clin. 1988;6:241–247.
30. Ortonne JP. Pigmentary changes of the aging skin. Br J Dermatol. 1990;122(Suppl35):21–28.

31. Polysangam T, Dee-Ananlap S, Suvanprakorn P. Treatment of idiopathic guttate hypomelanosis with liquid nitrogen: light and electron microscopic studies. J Am Acad Dermatol. 1990;23:681–684.
32. Gilhar A, Pillar T, Eidelman S, Etzioni A. Vitiligo and idiopathic guttate hypomelanosis: depigmentation of skin following engraftment onto nude mice. Arch Dermatol. 1989; 125:1363–1366.
33. Hodgson C. Senile lentigo. Arch Dermatol. 1963;87:197–207.
34. Spencer MC. Topical use of hydroquinone for depigmentation. JAMA. 1965;194:962–964.
35. Kligman AM, Willis I. A new formula for depigmenting human skin. Arch Dermatol. 1975;111:40–48.
36. Rafal ES, Griffiths CEM, Ditre CM, et al. Topical tretinoin (retinoic acid) treatment for liver spots associated with photodamage. N Engl J Med. 1989;326:368–374.
37. Humeniuk HM, Lask GP. Treatment of benign cutaneous lesions. In: *Aesthetic Dermatology,* LC Parish, GP Lask, eds. McGraw-Hill, New York, 1991, pp. 39–49.
38. Collins PS, Farber GA, Wilhelmus SM, et al. Superficial repetitive chemosurgery of the hands. Am J Cosmet Surg. 1984;1:22–24.
39. Collins PS. Trichloroacetic acid peels revisited. J Dermatol Surg Oncol. 1989;15:933–940.
40. Swinehart JM. Salicylic acid ointment peeling of the hands and forearms. Effective nonsurgical removal of pigmented lesions and actinic damage. J Dermatol Surg Oncol. 1992;18:495–498.
41. Moy L. Alpha hydroxy acid peeling for facial and nonfacial skin. Chemical peel symposium, American Academy of Dermatology meeting, San Francisco, California. Unpublished.
42. Hevia O, Nemeth AJ, Taylor JR. Tretinoin accelerates healing after trichloroacetic acid chemical peel. Arch Dermatol. 1991;127: 678–682.
43. Grekin RC, Shelton RM, Geisse JK, Frieden I. 510-nm pigmented lesion dye laser. its characteristics and clinical uses. J Dermatol Surg Oncol. 1993;19:380–387.
44. Dinehart SM, Waner M, Flock S. The copper vapor laser for treatment of cutaneous vascular and pigmented lesions. J Dermatol Surg Oncol. 1993;19:370–375.
45. McDaniel DH. Clinical usefulness of the Hexascan. Treatment of cutaneous vascular and melanocytic disorders. J Dermatol Surg Oncol. 1993;19:312–319.
46. Stern RS, Boudreaux C, Arndt KA. Diagnostic accuracy and appropriateness of care for seborrheic keratoses: a pilot study of an approach to quality assurance for cutaneous surgery. JAMA. 1991;265:74–77.
47. Mohs FE. Seborrheic keratoses: scarless removal by curettage and oxidized cellulose. JAMA. 1970;212:1956–1958.
48. Marks R, Foley P, Goodman G, et al. Spontaneous remission of solar keratoses: the case for conservative management. Br J Dermatol. 1986;115:649–655.
49. Dodson JM, DeSpain J, Hewett JE, Clark DP. Malignant potential of actinic keratoses and the controversy over treatment: a patient-oriented perspective. Arch Dermatol. 1991; 127:1029–1031.
50. Simmonds WL. Topical management of actinic keratoses with 5-fluorouracil: results of a 6 year follow-up study. Cutis. 1972;10:737–741.
51. Breza T, Taylor JR, Eaglestein WH. Noninflammatory destruction of actinic keratoses by fluorouracil. Arch Dermatol. 1976;112:1256–1258.
52. Pearlman DL. Weekly pulse dosing: effective and comfortable topical 5-fluorouracil treatment of multiple facial actinic keratoses. J Am Acad Dermatol. 1991;25:665–667.
53. Papa CM. Tretinoin therapy for precancerous skin. N J Med. 1989;86:361–365.
54. Edwards L, Levine N, Weidner M, et al. Effect of intralesional α-interferon on actinic keratoses. Arch Dermatol. 1986;122:779–782.
55. Edwards L, Levine N, Smiles KA. The effect of topical interferon α_{2B} on actinic keratoses. J Dermatol Surg Oncol. 1990;16:446–449.
56. Olsen EA, Abernethy ML, Kulp-Shorten C, et al. A double-blind, vehicle-controlled study evaluating masoprocol cream in the treatment of actinic keratoses on the head and neck. J Am Acad Dermatol. 1991;24:738–743.
57. Aronsohn RB. Hand chemosurgery. Am J Cosmet Surg. 1984;1:24–28.

15
Establishing a Dermatologic Surgicenter

Jeffrey Alan Klein

A dermatologic surgicenter is a medical facility designed and organized to facilitate optimal efficiency and safety in the surgical aspects of dermatology. "Licensed," "certified," and "accredited" are words commonly used to designate a surgicenter that has achieved a degree of official approval.

Legislation mandating certification of facilities where certain surgical procedures are performed is a virtual certainty. The criteria used to decide which surgical procedure must be performed in an accredited facility will be predicated by the mode of anesthesia. It is probable that the use of any anesthetic agent associated with potential impairment of protective airway reflexes will be permitted only in an approved facility. Dermatologic surgeons who use general anesthesia for some procedures will either have to do these procedures totally by local anesthesia or secure surgical privileges at an approved facility.

If ownership of an approved facility is a serious consideration, then its feasibility must be assessed in terms of its personal and financial costs. This assessment should include an analysis of the expected costs of consultants, real estate, tenant improvements, and the cost of maintaining the bureaucracy for continuous quality improvement. Against these considerable expenses are balanced the personal pride and marketing advantages of possessing an elegant, efficient, state-of-the-art surgical facility. Building a facility to your own specifications without the advice of an expert may lead to costly omissions and oversights.

We have survived our efforts at building a state-licensed multispecialty surgicenter in California. The following advice is given in the hope that the reader will be less naïve about the necessary investment of time and expense and more alert to the potential pitfalls of such an endeavor.

Licensure, Certification, Accreditation

There are different levels of official recognition of ambulatory surgical facilities. Among the multispecialty facilities, state licensure, Medicare certification, and American Association of Ambulatory Health Care (AAAHC) accreditation are the most widely recognized by regulators and third-party insurance carriers. The Joint Commission on Hospital Accreditation (JCHA) will also give accreditation to surgical facilities that meet certain architectural and quality-assurance criteria.

All forms of official endorsement for out-of-hospital surgical facilities have fairly similar requirements for well-documented, ongoing quality-improvement programs. Maintaining the documentation required for quality-improvement programs is quite time-consuming but is a bureaucratic necessity. It represents another level of unwelcome paperwork, but it is something that must be accepted as part of the territory of modern, high-quality, out-of-hospital surgical care.

State licensure is usually the most demanding, most expensive, and most rigorous level of official validation and endorsement of an out-of-hospital surgical facility. In California state licensure requires 6-ft-wide corridors that lead from an operating room door to 2 separate emergency exit doors, such doors being 4 ft wide. There must be separate facilities for male and female staff, including dressing rooms, locker rooms, toilet, and washing and shower facilities. Emergency back-up power supply requirements are more demanding and therefore more expensive. For example, in order to provide continuous emergency back up electricity for 12 hours, a simple battery back-up power supply might not be sufficient to meet licensure requirements; and a much more expensive diesel electric generator might be necessary to run all the heating, air conditioning, vacuum pump, general anesthetic machine, and respirator as well as lighting. In some states preexisting facilities can qualify for state licensure without having to meet the much more stringent architectural requirement of a newly constructed facility.

Medicare certification is less demanding in California than state licensure. In other states, however, state licensure and medicare certification have identical requirements. In California state licensure is necessary in order to have non-owner surgeons use the facility and still qualify for reimbursement. If a facility is merely Medicare-certified and not state-licensed, reimbursement is only possible if the surgeon is at least a partial owner of the facility.

Incentives for Accreditation

Incentives to establish a facility dedicated to dermatologic surgery include improved quality of patient care, safety, work efficiency, prestige, facility fee reimbursement by insurance companies, and professional security.

Improved patient safety is probably the most important incentive for choosing to have an approved surgicenter. Advanced dermatologic plastic surgical procedures require more sophisticated facilities, equipment, and staff training than exist in the offices of most dermatologic surgeons. It is reasonable for a patient to expect a surgeon and the surgical staff to be well trained and capable of taking care of any life-threatening emergency that might occur in the course of a surgical procedure. Most patients would be horrified by the realization that many surgical offices are not equipped nor is the staff trained to effectively prevent or manage a cardiorespiratory arrest. The requirements for an approved surgical facility eliminate many safety deficiencies common to traditional dermatology offices.

Prestige is another compensation for owning a quality surgicenter. This prestige is easily translated into both personal satisfaction and financial reward. An elegant and tastefully designed surgical facility is an important asset in marketing a cosmetically oriented surgical practice. Patients do take into account the appearance of a practice's office and surgical facility when choosing a surgeon for a cosmetic procedure.

Insurance payment for the use of an approved surgical facility is one financial incentive. Medicare and other insurance third-party payers may reimburse for facility fees in addition to the usual professional surgical fees for surgeries performed in a state-licensed or Medicare-approved facility. However, the most commonly performed dermatologic surgical procedures are relatively minor, and may not qualify for facility fee reimbursement from insurance companies. Thus, in most instances reimbursement from insurance companies is not a strong financial justification for the expense of establishing an accredited surgicenter.

Facility fee reimbursement will be paid only if the procedure is performed in a facility that has qualified by having achieved the appropriate official endorsements, such as state licensure, Medicare certification or AAAHC accreditation. If a facility is only AAAHC-accredited, then it might qualify for facility fee reimbursement for patients who have commercial health insurance coverage, but not for medicare patients. In order to qualify for facility fee reimbursement from Medicare, the facility must at least have Medicare certification.

The financial rewards of facility fee insurance reimbursement for dermatologic surgery are somewhat dubious. Reimbursement varies

15. Establishing a Dermatologic Surgicenter

as a function of time and the unpredictable nature of legislation and regulations.

A pragmatic consideration in having one's own surgicenter is achieving freedom from professional political discrimination in obtaining surgical privileges in an approved facility. In some areas of the United States it is difficult for dermatologists to obtain hospital or surgicenter surgical privileges for surgical procedures in which they have been very well trained as dermatology residents. The credentialing committees of some hospitals may harbor the prejudice that a surgical internship is an absolute prerequisite for obtaining any operation room surgical privileges, even for routine dermatolgic surgery. When a hospital credentials committee denies surgical privileges to a qualified dermatologic surgeon, the effect is to deny the dermatologic surgeon the opportunity to practice fully the profession of dermatology in the setting of hospital peer review.

There are several very real and significant disincentives for accreditation. An awareness of the significantly increased monthly operating expenses, time-consuming paper work, demands on time, and potential for stress is essential to making an informed decision about whether or not to pursue construction or ownership of a surgicenter.

Quality Improvement

From a practical point of view, a one-surgeon facility is usually small enough so that a formal quality improvement (QI) program will require relatively more paperwork than is necessary to ensure a safe clinical environment. For example, it is part of routine QI at most multiphysician surgicenters or hospitals to generate a comprehensive list of all surgical patients and then check off for each patient whether or not that patient experienced a postoperative wound infection or other complication. Clearly, such a formality is inefficient for a one-surgeon facility, where the surgeon should be aware of every clinically significant wound infection and be able to take appropriate corrective procedures. However, as soon as there are two or more surgeons using a particular facility, a formal QI program is an efficient force for minimizing the risks of substandard surgical conditions.

On the other hand, even in a one-physician office, constructing a list of all skin biopsy-proven cutaneous malignancies or severe atypia requiring further treatment or re-excision would be most helpful to avoid losing track of patients who do not return for follow-up appointments or treatment.

Most generic quality improvement programs require much more paperwork than is necessary for even an advanced dermatologic surgical practice. A very efficient and high-caliber dermatologic surgery QI program can be derived with little effort by simple modification of an existing hospital or multispecialty QI program.

It is axiomatic that the greatest risks in ambulatory surgery are those associated with the dangers of parenteral sedatives and narcotics. By avoiding the use of dangerous general anesthetic agents, including parenteral narcotics and sedatives, dermatologic surgeons eliminate the greatest risk of surgery. To the degree that a dermatologic surgical practice is limited to the use of local anesthesia only, the probability of serious morbidity or mortality is dramatically reduced. With appropriate skills and a personality that can deal with an awake patient a surgeon can accomplish virtually every dermatologic surgical procedure without resorting to parenteral narcotics or sedation. Examples of dermatologic surgical procedures that can be done totally by local anesthesia include liposuction, facelifts, dermabrasion, scalp surgery, and large excisions, flaps, and grafts.

Choice of Location

The decision of whether to acquire a surgicenter is the most crucial and requires many hours of consideration and analysis. Perhaps the next most important decision concerns choosing the location for a surgicenter. The optimal geographic location of the surgicenter will depend on the appraisal of your practice's marketing analysis.

Choosing a building will depend on availability and considerations about ownership versus leasing. The building itself may either be new or existing. An existing building may be either occupied or unoccupied.

Design Requirements

There are myriad aspects of a surgicenter that must be implemented before certification or licensure is attainable. The reality of arcane rules and irrational regulations can shatter the best laid plans of a naïve surgeon planning his or her own facility. Costly pitfalls are less of a risk with the help of appropriate consultants.

A surgicenter must meet strict design specifications. Surgicenter charts must be stored in a locked cabinet and be kept separate from medical office charts. The surgicenter must have both a "clean" and a "dirty" utility room, and staff dressing rooms. Operating rooms must have seamless floor coverings and washable walls. The number of required recovery room beds and scrub sinks is specified by the number of operating rooms, and operating rooms must have at least a minimal size.

Medicare-certified and state-licensed facilities must have a dedicated waiting room that is separate from any other waiting area; in other words, a dermatologist's routine clinic patients cannot share the same waiting room as surgicenter patients or persons who are waiting for surgicenter patients. The rationale for this rule is not entirely clear. Nevertheless, overlooking such recondite regulations can profoundly affect the efficiency and utilization of a surgicenter that shares the same building as a medical office or clinic.

Bureaucratic Requirements

Besides the architectural aspects of creating a surgicenter, the bureaucratic considerations are of critical importance. Quality improvement procedures, peer review, signed transfer agreements, written policies and procedures, maintenance agreements, and routine checks on all electrical surgical equipment are among the seemingly endless list of requirements. The documentation and organizational aspects of starting and maintaining a surgicenter must receive close attention. Receiving help from an experienced consultant is the most efficient means of establishing the required organizational structure.

Standardized Operating Room Techniques

Dermatology is a unique surgical specialty in several respects. Few dermatologists routinely admit patients to hospital or perform surgical procedures in hospital; there is no good peer review of dermatologists; and dermatology's surgical and operating room techniques are quite different from those of other surgical specialties.

Dermatologic surgery's uniqueness is most apparent in the surgical techniques aimed at minimizing the risk of wound infections. Few dermatologic surgeons routinely wear fully sterile gowns. When surgical masks are worn, it is more often to protect the surgeon than the patient.

The dogma that traditional operating room technique, with full sterile gowns, gloves, and masks, is the optimal means of avoiding wound infection is somewhat analogous to a religious conviction: Ardor of a belief is not a measure of its scientific validity. Dermatologic surgery is remarkable for the paucity of postoperative wound infections. The tradition of excellent clinical results with simple clean dermatologic surgical technique compares well with the more cumbersome and unnecessarily expensive tradition of fully sterile gown and isolated operating room.

It would be useful for academic dermatologic surgical programs to develop and publish guidelines for dermatologic surgical operating room techniques. The standard operating room techniques in almost every academic training program across the country are not well codified nor documented. As a consequence there is a conflict between traditional dermatologic surgical technique and the operating room policies and procedures of hospitals and accredited surgicenters. Most credentialing organizations will require that a surgical facility, dedicated to dermatologic surgery, accommodate traditional policies and procedures that do not conform to standard dermatologic surgical operating room technique. Until dermatologic surgeons publish a "standards of care" for dermatologic surgical operating room technique, surgicenter accrediting agencies will hold dermatologists to unnecessarily cumbersome and inefficient standards.

Choosing a Consultant

Financial feasibility is an important consideration in the process of deciding whether or not to invest time and money in acquiring a surgical facility. Criteria upon which a decision is based depend on whether the practice's income is primarily from insurance-reimbursable procedures or from cosmetic procedures.

Only a limited number of dermatologic surgical procedures qualify for facility fee reimbursement by Medicare and other third-party insurance carriers. For a practice that relies on insurance reimbursement, a financial consultant will be helpful in predicting the financial viability of surgicenter ownership. A surgicenter's profitability can be estimated by knowing the expected number of surgical cases per month that qualify for facility fee reimbursement from insurance companies, the dollar amount reimbursed for each such case, and the overhead expenses for each case. However, such projections are not infallible, because of the frequency of changes in Medicare reimbursement policy.

A cosmetic surgical practice will benefit from the intangible asset of having an elegant and prestigious facility. There are very definite financial benefits to a cosmetic surgical practice of having an approved surgical facility.

Architectural consultation is necessary to estimate the cost of design and construction or modification of the building's shell. There are very strict and demanding design requirements of these tenant improvements, including the floor plan, number and location of emergency exits, fire walls, sprinkler systems, size of operating room, number of scrub sinks, number of postanesthesia recovery beds, type of autoclave, electrical and lighting, air conditioning, plumbing, medical gases, emergency backup power supply. The cost of neglecting these requirements can be substantial. For example, after building a very expensive surgicenter, a plastic surgeon in Southern California discovered that it would not qualify for Medicare certification. Correcting the oversights cost several hundred thousand dollars and delayed completion for nearly a year.

Interior design consultants must be knowledgeable about the special regulations and requirements for surgicenters. Interior design guidance is important not only for aesthetic concerns but also for the selection of approved building materials such as floor coverings, operating room wall coverings, and lighting. Selection of these items is constrained by specific regulations dictating the type of materials that can be used in a surgicenter. The construction costs of tenant improvements can be much greater than one might expect. Good communication with an interior design consultant will help in anticipating these important budget items.

Policy and procedure manuals, which usually contain several hundred pages of written operational guidelines, are an absolute necessity for obtaining certification for an ambulatory surgical facility. Having a consultant produce a customized set of policy and procedure manuals is expensive but cost effective. The consultant should also help in the training of staff and preparation for passing the certification inspection and examination.

Other consultants can provide help in selecting expensive pieces of equipment for the office, and the operating rooms. Consultants can also provide help in obtaining financing for the project, including mortgages, as well as leases or purchases of equipment.

Caveat Emptor

Although consultants are necessary, they are not a substitute for a comprehensive understanding of the building process. Continuous and careful communication among owner, architect, consultants, general contractor, and subcontractors is an essential ingredient for the success of the construction of a surgicenter. It is almost certain that when the inevitable disaster occurs, each person will blame another for the problem. Although acquiring knowledge and insight into the complexity of the project as well as maintaining good communication is extremely time consuming, it is the surest way to avoid costly oversights. It is far easier to prevent disastrous construction mistakes than to remedy them. Although expensive construction snafus must be expected, one must strive to minimize the number of such discouraging events.

Be careful in your choice of consultants. Do not pay too much in the form of an advance or retainer fee. Check references very carefully, and do not assume that all consultants are ethical.

If possible, choose consults who are conveniently located geographically and easily accessible for meeting and conferences. The planning and construction of a surgicenter is quite time consuming. The time, effort, and expense of meeting with a consultant whose main office is far from your project would add an unnecessary degree of stress and financial strain.

Be aware that if it is in a consultant's interest for you to decide to build a surgicenter, the advice you get might not be entirely objective. You must guard against an overly optimistic assessment of the financial prospects of a proposed surgicenter.

One cannot expect consultants' estimates of costs and time to be very accurate. Relying on the good faith and efficiency of a consultant who is paid by the hour can be a very expensive mistake. One should negotiate a reasonable upper limit to the maximum fee with each consultant. All contracts should have a penalty clause to avoid or minimize delays in job performance.

Insist on a clause guaranteeing that all change orders—any changes from the architect's specifications on the architectural plans—be charged at the cost to the contractor. This will maximize the contractor's efforts to communicate with you during the initial planning stages. It will also maximize the contractor's incentive to pay attention to potential problems or potential oversights in the architectural plans.

Summary

Building an accredited or certified dermatologic surgicenter will likely require more money, time, and energy than your most pessimistic estimates. If the decision has been made to pursue this endeavor, careful selection of consultants and careful supervision of the building process and communication with contractors will minimize the risk of costly mistakes.

16
The Esthetician's Role in Skin Care

Mark Lees and Diane Young

Women are becoming more and more involved in total skin care; in the United States alone, experts estimate that by 1995, retail sales of skin care products will be $4 billion.[1] This figure includes mass merchant, department, drug, and grocery store sales but does not cover the estimated 280,000 skin care services provided every week in beauty and skin care salons. Research also indicates that more then 63 million adult women use facial moisturizers;[2] and increasing numbers are using multiple-product regimens and spa facial services. Men also seek salon skin care services, although they still account for a small percentage of the total clientele.

In the United States, there currently are an estimated 7,000 dermatologists and 30,000 salon skin care technicians, including 15,000 licensed estheticians. This means that for each dermatologist, there are 4 providers of nonmedical skin care services. Whereas patients may consult a dermatologist once every 6 months, if they are actively involved in caring for their skin, they may consult a salon skin care specialist every 4 to 6 weeks. Therefore, it is very likely that an esthetician or nonlicensed salon skin care technician will be discussing skin care with the individuals and recommending cosmetic products for use at home, whether or not the dermatologist has suggested it. Should the esthetician detect skin problems that need medical evaluation, patients often will be referred to a dermatologist. If the client is not currently under a dermatologist's care, the esthetician may recommend one.

Historical Background

Since prehistoric times men and women have used a wide variety of techniques and substances to improve and enhance their appearance. According to Gerson,[3] the essentials of skin care and the use of cosmetics were taught together with the practice of medicine in ancient times; and in medieval English universities, cosmetology and medicine were taught as combined subjects. It was not until the sixteenth century that the two were separated.

Some techniques used by dermatologists today originated with ancient skin care practitioners and were subsequently refined by the estheticians of Eastern Europe. An excellent example is chemical peeling or chemabrasion. Cleopatra used chemical peeling and sour milk (lactic acid) baths to improve and freshen her skin, and Roman women used the tartaric acid from the bottom of wine-making vessels as a chemical peel.[4] At the beginning of the twentieth century, European estheticians brought their knowledge of chemical peeling to the United States. They performed chemical peels as "nonmedical" treatments to beautify the skin. It was not until the 1960s, when Baker and Ayres developed formulas for chemical peeling, that the procedure came to the attention of the majority of dermatologists in the United States.[4]

Overview of Present-Day Esthetics

Today in the United States, dermatologists evaluate, diagnose, and medically and surgically treat diseases of the skin. Estheticians clean and beautify the skin, care for cosmetic problems, and recommend products to maintain healthy skin and correct nonmedical skin problems. In Europe, however, the esthetician is viewed as an important adjunct to medical professionals and not only provides salon skin care but also performs minor cosmetic surgical procedures such as the removal of warts and telangiectasias (couperose). In many instances European dermatologists have an esthetician on staff.

The differences between esthetics in the United States and Europe are due in part to the educational requirements for licensing. European estheticians must undergo 2 to 4 years of training in facial care, manicures, massage therapy, and electrology following high school graduation. A number of U.S. states require only a specific number of hours of skin care training, with or without a high school diploma, for licensing as an esthetician. Thirty-seven states, the Virgin Islands, and Nova Scotia (Canada) have special licenses for skin care, the requirements for which are listed in Table 16.1.[5] The remaining U.S. states include skin care as part of the regular cosmetology license (i.e., skin, hair, and nails).

Regardless of the basic requirements of an individual state, a well-qualified esthetician is trained in basic skin care; cosmetic chemistry; the use of electrical facial equipment; the extraction of comedones, milia, and other blemishes; epidermabrasion (i.e., cosmetic peeling or chemical exfoliation); and various techniques for hair removal. Some U.S. states require a special license for electrology (see Table 16.2), while others include it as part of a general cosmetology license.[5] Estheticians also are trained to recognize skin diseases that require evaluation and treatment by a dermatologist, such as precancerous and cancerous lesions, inflammatory conditions, allergic reactions, and acne rosacea.

Basic Skin Care Services

The primary functions of an esthetician are to analyze the skin and educate clients about the cosmetic care of their particular skin type and condition. Because most estheticians recognize that a person's overall health affects the skin, they also review clients' physical activity, sleep patterns, eating habits, and use of cigarettes or alcohol, and make recommendations to promote a healthy lifestyle. The esthetician may refer interested clients to a physical trainer or a nutritionist for further counseling. The importance of protecting the skin with sunscreens is emphasized, and clients with visible evidence of sun damage or fair skin are urged to have a dermatologist check them at least annually for signs of skin cancer.

The typical skin care salon provides a number of services and products (see Table 16.3). Clearly, facial treatments form the cornerstone of esthetic skin care. The basic facial provides a deep cleansing of the skin that cannot be achieved at home and also exfoliates the surface and refines the texture. For clients with very dry, dehydrated skin, special treatments and products are used for hydration. For clients with mild acne, the esthetician provides a deep cleansing facial, together with topical treatments that have an antibacterial effect; and recommends appropriate nonprescription products for use at home, such as cleansers or lotions containing ingredients such as benzoyl peroxide and noncomedogenic moisturizers and cosmetics. The Esthetician is trained to refer clients with advanced acne to a dermatologist for the appropriate medical treatment. Once the dermatologist has prescribed the necessary medications, the routine skin care and ongoing reinforcement of the dermatologist's recommendations by the esthetician can be a valuable adjunct to patient compliance. Dermatologists may perform acne surgery in their office, or they may wish to refer patients to an esthetician for more widespread extraction of less severe, noninfected lesions and comedones.

Special Skin Care for Aging Women

When providing skin care for women of any age, the esthetician determines the skin type to identify any skin problems requiring cosmetic or medical treatment, as well as to be informed of underlying medical conditions and use of prescription drugs that might affect a salon treatment. Women over age 40 often have

TABLE 16.1. Requirements of states having special skin care licenses.[5]

State	Formal education	Entrance age (yr)	Training	Exam	License period	License fee orig and exam
Alabama	10th grade	16	1200 credit unit hr or 3000 hr apprentice	Yes	Sept. 30 odd yr	$65
Alaska	N/A	N/A	350 hr	Yes	Aug. 31	$55
Arizona	10th grade	None	600 hr	Yes	Birthdate	$38
Arkansas	10th grade	16	600 hr	Yes	Dec. 31	$30
California	10th grade	17	600 hr school or 18 mo exp outside Calif.	Yes	2 yr from issuance	$32
Colorado	None	16	550 hr	Yes	March 31	$41
Delaware	NI*	NI*	300 hr	Yes	Dec. 31	$60
District of Columbia	8th grade or equiv.	16	125 hr	Yes	April 15 (biennially)	$40
Florida	None	16 or HS diploma	240 hr	Yes	June 30 (biennially)	$50
Georgia	9th grade	16	None	Yes	Biennual	$45
Hawaii	12th grade	16	550 hr in school or 1100 hr apprentice	Yes	Dec. 31 odd yr	$75
Idaho	10th grade	16½	500 hr	Yes	Dec. 31	$57
Illinois	8th grade	16	750 hr	Yes	Sept. 30 odd yr	$99
Iowa	12th grade	None	600 hr	Yes	Biennual	$55
Kansas	HS/GED	17	1000 hr in approved cosmetology school	Yes	Birth month odd/even yr	$15
Louisiana	10th grade	16	750 hr (min 3 mo)	Yes	March 1	$55
Maine	10th grade	16	750 hr (5 mo)	Yes	June 30 (biennially)	$60
Maryland	9th grade	17	300 hr or 6 mo apprentice	Yes	Oct. 31 odd yr	$91
Massachusetts	8th grade	16	300 hr skincare	Yes	Monthly	$120
Minnesota	12th or GED	None	600 hr	Yes	Dec 31-3 yr	$38
Mississippi	10th grade	17	600 hr	Yes	1 yr from issuance	$40
Nebraska	12th grade	NI*	600 hr	NI*	Sept. 30 even yr	NI*
Nevada	10th grade	18	600 hr in school	Yes	June 30 odd yr	$55
New Hampshire	12th grade	16	450 hr	Yes	June 30 odd yr	$70
New Mexico	2 yr HS	16	900 hr	Yes	Birthmonth	$45
North Dakota	12th grade	17	900 hr	Yes	Dec. 31	NI*
Ohio	8th grade	16	600 hr	Yes	Jan. 30 odd yr	$41
Oklahoma	8th grade	16	300 hr	Yes	Birthmonth	$30
Oregon	None	None	350 hr	Yes	1 yr from issuance	$35
Pennsylvania	10th grade	16	300 hr	Yes	NI*	NI*
Rhode Island	HS	18	600 hr	Yes	June 30	$15
South Carolina	10th grade	None	450 hr	Yes	March 10	$45
Tennessee	10th grade	16	750 hr	Yes	Sept. 1 (biennially)	set by contract
Texas	7th grade	16	600 hr	Yes	Birthdate	$60
Vermont	12th grade or equiv	17	550 hr	Yes	Nov. 30	$60
Virgin Islands	NI*	18	1200 hr	Yes	Dec. 31	$120
Washington	NI*	17	500 hr	Yes	Birthdate	$25
Wisconsin	HS/GED	NI*	450 hr	Yes	July 1 odd yr	$63
Nova Scotia	None	17	150 hr	Yes	1 yr	$25

*NI = Not indicated
Reproduced by permission. *Milady's 1993-1994 Guide to Cosmetic Licensing*. Milady Publishing Company, a division of Delmar Publishers Inc., Albany, New York. Copyright 1993.

clogged pores and generally have dry, sun-damaged skin. They also may have skin problems such as hirsutism related to hormonal changes associated with menopause.[6]

For the woman whose face exhibits visible signs of photodamage, the esthetician can provide light chemical exfoliation in addition to deep cleansing of the skin. The esthetician often

TABLE 16.2. Electrology licensing information at a Glance.[5]

Arkansas
Must hold a current cosmetology license and requires a separate electrology license. Arkansas State Board of Cosmetology, 1515 West 7th Street, Room 400, Little Rock, AR (501) 682-2168.

California
Must be licensed. Controlled by California Board of Barbering and Cosmetology, P.O. Box 944226, Sacramento, CA (916) 445-7061.

Connecticut
License required to practice. Controlled by Department of Health, 150 Washington Street, Hartford, CT (203) 566-1042.

Delaware
License required. Controlled by Professional Regulations Department, Division of Professional Regulation, Margaret O'Neill Building, Dover, DE (302) 739-4522.

District of Columbia
Part of cosmetology license. Controlled by Board of Cosmetology. No separate exam. Department of Consumer & Regulatory Affairs, Occupational and Professional License Administration, 614 High Street, N.W. (202) 727-7411.

Hawaii
License required. Controlled by Board of Cosmetology, Department of Commerce and Consumer Affairs, P.O. Box 3469, Honolulu, HI 96801 (808) 586-2699.

Idaho
License required. Controlled by Board of Cosmetology, 1109 Main Street, Suite 220, Boise, ID (208) 334-3233.

Indiana
License required. Must be a licensed cosmetologist. Controlled by Indiana State Board of Cosmetology Examiners, 1021 State Office Building, 100 North Senate Avenue, Indianapolis, IN (317) 232-2980.

Iowa
License required. Must be a licensed cosmetologist. Controlled by Iowa Cosmetology Board of Examiners, Lucas State Office Building, Des Moines, IA (515) 281-4422.

Kansas License required. Controlled by Kansas State Board of Cosmetology, 603 SW Topeka Blvd., Suite 100, Topeka, KS (913) 296-3155.

Louisiana
License required. Controlled by Board of Electrology, 11622 Sunbelt Court, Baton Rouge, LA (504) 336-1409.

Maine
License required. Controlled by Department of Human Service, State House, Station Ten, Augusta, ME (207) 289-5671.

Maryland
License required. Controlled by Board of Electrology, 4201 Patterson Avenue, Baltimore, MD (301) 764-4727.

Massachusetts
License required. Controlled by Board of Electrology, Room 1516, 100 Cambridge Street, Boston, MA (617) 727-3080.

Michigan
License required. Controlled by State Board of Cosmetology, 611 West Ottawa, North Tower, Lansing, MI (517) 373-0580.

Montana
License required. Controlled by Board of Cosmetologists, 111 N. Jackson, Helena, MT (406) 444-4288.

Nevada
License required. Controlled by State Board of Cosmetology, 1785 East Sahara Avenue, Las Vegas, NV (702) 486-6542.

New Mexico
License required. Controlled by State Board of Cosmetologists, Regulation and Licensing Department, P.O. Box 25101, Santa Fe, NM (505) 827-7176.

North Dakota
Licensed separately. Controlled by the Department of Health, 600 East Boulevard Avenue, Bismark, ND (701) 224-2370.

Oklahoma
License required. Controlled by Board of Medical and Licensure Supervision, P.O. Box 18254, Oklahoma City, OK (405) 848-6841.

Rhode Island
License required. Controlled by Department of Health, Board of Electrology, 3 Capitol Hill, Providence, RI (401) 277-2827.

Wisconsin
License required. Controlled by Barbering and Cosmetology Examining Board, P.O. Box 8935, Madison, WI (608) 266-1630.

Reproduced by permission. *Milady's 1993-1994 Guide to Cosmetic Licensing.* Milady Publishing Company, a division of Delmar Publishers Inc., Albany, New York. Copyright 1993.

use enzymes such as papain or an alpha hydroxy acid to digest the top layers of dead skin. They may also use green papaya to speed exfoliation. For women over 40 who commonly have dry skin, estheticians recommend "super" moisturizers containing water-binding ingredients, sunscreen, and ingredients that have a calming effect on the skin. Again, depending

TABLE 16.3. Skin care services and products provided by the typical skin care salon.

Service or product	Purpose
Services	
Skin analysis	Determine oil/water content and condition of skin
Deep cleaning facial	Thoroughly clean pores, exfoliate surface, refine skin texture
Acne facial	Deep clean pores, kill bacteria, heal skin surface
Hydrating facial or mask	Fill dry and dehydrated skin with moisture
Rapid exfoliation	Refine skin surfaces, smooth lines and wrinkles
Waxing	Temporarily remove unwanted facial or body hair
Electrolysis	Permanently remove unwanted facial or body hair
Products	
Cleanser	Thoroughly cleans the skin of dirt and pollutants, may also remove makeup
Toner/balancer/ astringent	Removes excess cleanser or debris, smooths skin, balances skin pH; may also exfoliate, reduce oiliness, etc.
Moisturizer	Hydrates and protects skin, decreases moisture loss
Masks/packs	Tightens and refines skin, makes pores look smaller; masks for clog-prone skin also exfoliate

on the client's skin type, the esthetician uses preparations containing hyaluronic acid, collagen, elastin, silicones, yeast extracts, liposomes, or other agents that provide an ongoing release of moisture-binding ingredients. The esthetician also suggests cleansers and toners that are suitable for use on dry skin.

Growth of unwanted facial hair frequently occurs in the perimenopausal period. This hair can be removed temporarily by waxing or permanently by electrolysis. However, among client using topical tretinoin, waxing is contraindicated in order to avoid damage to the skin.

Skin Care Before and After Cosmetic Surgical Procedures

Today many skin surgeons recommend pre- and postoperative skin care by a licensed esthetician for patients desiring facial cosmetic surgery. They have found that a thoroughly cleansed and hydrated skin heals better, is less red and bruised, and is less likely to become infected postoperatively.

An example of the treatment schedules suggested for various cosmetic procedures by Lees, a leader in the field of esthetics, is provided in Table 16.4.[7] According to Lees, treatments for all but collagen injections should begin 3 months before the cosmetic surgical procedure. In addition to deep pore cleansing to remove impurities in the skin and increase hydration, clients are given a skin care routine to follow at home. An added benefit is the psychological support provided by the esthetician during the preoperative period.

Postoperative skin care begins approximately

TABLE 16.4. Pre- and postoperative care schedules.[7]

Procedure	Preoperative	Postoperative
Facelift Eyelift Forehead lift	6 treatments, weekly or biweekly	• Beginning 2 to 3 weeks after surgery, or upon surgeon's recommendations.
Nose reconstruction	6 treatments, weekly or biweekly	• Beginning 3 weeks after surgery • Light (enzyme) peel soon after procedure
Surgical chemical peeling	6 treatments, weekly or biweekly	• Beginning 3 weeks after surgery • Makeup instruction to cover redness upon surgeon's recommendations.
Dermabrasion	6 to 12 treatments, weekly or biweekly, patient's skin must be clear before procedure	• May require weekly or biweekly treatments • Makeup instruction for redness or demarcation upon surgeon's recommendations
Collagen injections	Facial treatment day before procedure	Routine care

Reprinted with the permission of Dr. Mark Lees, Mark Lees Skin Care, Inc., Pensacola, Florida.

2 to 3 weeks after surgery and is designed to improve hydration and refine the pore structure of the skin. Proper home skin care is emphasized. Patients also are shown how to use camouflage makeup to cover scars, bruising, and redness during the healing process. This can be especially important if patients have young children who might be distressed by the parent's bruised face.

Client Education

Many estheticians feel that one of their most important roles is to educate clients about skin care. They are able to work one-on-one with clients to develop a home care regimen that is appropriate for their skin type and condition. In addition to skin care products that are chemically correct for a client's particular skin, the esthetician designs a regimen for the use of these products at home that will complement the client's lifestyle. Estheticians are realistic about the number of skin care products that a client will use routinely; for a busy professional, the esthetician will probably suggest a cleanser, a toner, and a moisturizer with sunscreen. If the client has more time, a night cream and an eye or neck treatment may be added. If the client's dermatologist has prescribed additional treatments, these will be incorporated in the home care regimen as well. By explaining why a particular product has been selected for the client's use, the esthetician tries to demystify skin care.

Although individuals who seek the services of an esthetician usually have decided to devote more of their time and resources to the care of their skin, they can still have difficulty adopting a new skin care regimen at home. The esthetician promotes compliance with a skin care regimen by encouraging clients to return as often as needed for deep cleansing facials. In this way a client's at-home skin care regimen can be reviewed periodically to make sure that it is still compatible with the client's lifestyle, skin type, and current skin condition. The use of any medications, sunscreens, or other products recommended by the client's dermatologist is reinforced at each visit. Clients who are having problems are urged to return to the dermatologist for further evaluation.

As the beneficial effects of improved skin care become visible, further incentive to adhere to the regimen and continue using the appropriate skin care preparations is provided. Some estheticians publish newsletters describing new services and offering special rates on regular skin care to encourage clients to return; others conduct special skin care seminars for their clients.

Respective Roles of the Dermatologist and the Esthetician

The skin treatments provided by an esthetician should not overlap those provided by a dermatologist, with the possible exception of acne care. Many dermatologists are concerned with skin problems and cosmetic disorders that have only medical or surgical solutions—for example, advanced stages of acne, broken capillaries, photodamage, skin cancers, deep wrinkles and furrows, sagging skin, and baggy eyelids. Estheticians, on the other hand, recognize that they have not had medical training and do not treat clients with problems requiring medical or surgical intervention. They provide basic skin care and individualized instruction in skin care and the use of cosmetic products.

To illustrate how the two professions can work together, a dermatologist and two estheticians were asked to examine two-dimensional color photographs of three middle-aged women and to identify any areas requiring medical treatment or esthetic care. This was done with the understanding that in actual practice, specific interventions can only be made after a thorough inspection of the subject's skin; laxity and surface texture have to be evaluated by manual examination. Subjects need to be interviewed as well to elicit information about their current skin care regimen and whether problems such as dryness, oiliness or redness are improved or aggravated by the use of certain skin care products or cosmetics. In view of the many effective alternatives for medical and cosmetic care of the skin, each dermatologist or esthetician will suggest the approaches that he or she considers best and with which he or she is most familiar.

16. The Esthetician's Role in Skin Care

Subject #1: Brunette (Figure 16.1)

Dermatologist: This subject shows all five factors of the aging face: intrinsic aging, sleep lines, gravity, expression lines, and photoaging. She would benefit from both a blepharoplasty and a rhytidectomy. In addition, her upper lip, which is turned toward the mouth and is not as large as it used to be, could be restored with some collagen injections. Collagen also could be used to soften the expression lines over the forehead, glabella, corners of the eyes, and nasolabial folds. Photoaging could be greatly improved by chemical peels, followed by an appropriate skin care program. Once all of these procedures have been accomplished, the subject should receive esthetic care including light exfoliations and product recommendations for cosmesis.

Esthetician #1: This subject exhibits significant sun damage with areas of hyperpigmentation, elastosis, telangiectasias (couperose), wrinkling, and general hypotonicity; and appears to have an oily-dry skin type. There are apparent sebaceous milia on the cheek and forehead and significant solar lentigines in front of the ear. The eyelids are severely hypotonic, the subject ought to consider upper and lower lid blepharoplasty. The neck area shows severe sun damage and elastosis, and there is severe perioral wrinkling. She should be referred for evaluation for possible cosmetic surgery which might include rhytidectomy, blepharoplasty, perioral dermabrasion, and collagen injections. Because of the extensive sun damage, she should be referred to a dermatologist for annual total body examinations to detect any cancerous or precancerous lesions. Esthetic care should ideally consist of 3 to 6 months of biweekly visits for deep cleansing, exfoliation, and extensive use of hydrating products with galvanic ionization or high frequency current. Home care should consist of: 1) cleansing with a cleansing milk or mild rinseable cleanser followed by toner; 2) use of a daily sunscreen-moisturizer incorporating a sealant ingredient such as dimethicone or petrolatum to prevent dehydration; 3) use of a night cream; 4) use of a mild exfoliator (e.g. a mild scrub cream) 2 or 3 times a week; 5) twice-daily application of an eye cream with liposomes; and 6) use of a neck cream with liposomes. The eye and neck creams would have a different emollient content than the general day or night creams.

Esthetician #2: This subject should be referred to a physician for possible cosmetic surgery, which might include blepharoplasty of the upper and lower eyelids, liposuction of the jowl and area under the chin, and collagen injections for the lines and creases at the nasal aspect of the brow line, above the upper lip, and at the corners of the mouth. Because there is sun damage, a dermatologist may consider a series of chemical peels. Esthetic care might consist of a series of 6 rapid exfoliations performed in the salon to improve the texture and surface of the skin and to lessen fine lines. For continued improvement, home care might consist of a light exfoliator and green papaya regimen. The light exfoliator loosens the layer of dead skin cells and the green papaya digests them; this makes them easily removed with cleansing and toweling.

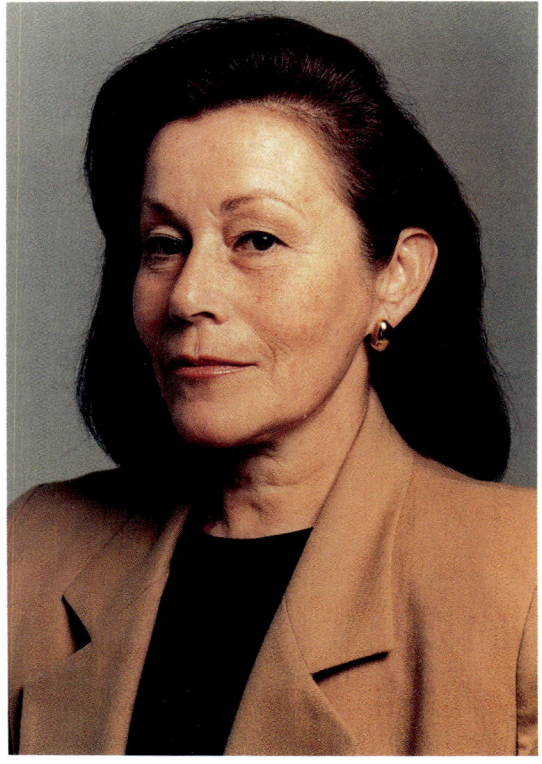

FIGURE 16.1. Subject #1: brunette. This subject shows all five factors of the aging face: intrinsic aging, sleep lines, gravity, expression lines, and photoaging.

Subject #2: Redhead (Figure 16.2)

Dermatologist: This subject appears to have had a blepharoplasty; a scar is present on the left upper eyelid. She also appears to have had a rhytidectomy, which may have loosened somewhat around the mouth. This subject mainly needs treatments for photoaging and expression lines. However, I would not suggest a trichloroacetic acid peel; her skin is very fair and there is a lot of sun damage, particularly on the neck and decollete. Collagen injections should be used to soften her features. Esthetic care following these procedures should consist of light exfoliations and product recommendations for cosmesis.

Esthetician #1: This subject exhibits typical redhead sun-damaged skin, which appears to be oil-dry. She may already have had a facelift. She has perioral wrinkling, a sebaceous filament and enlarged pores on the chin, a probable milium on the nose, and hypopigmentation or possibly a scar on the bridge of the nose. She also has mottled hyperpigmentation. Her neck exhibits the typical horseshoe pattern of poikiloderma of civatte, and the skin on her chest is very damaged. Because this subject is a redhead, she will probably have more sensitive skin in terms of treatment. She should be referred for surgical evaluation for possible lower lid blepharoplasty, collagen injections and dermabrasion, although hypopigmentation following dermabrasion might be a side effect because of her skin type. She definitely needs annual total body dermatological examinations. Esthetic recommendations would be similar to those for Subject #1 except that lotions rather than creams would be used and home care products would incorporate lighter emollients.

Esthetician #2: This subject has sun damage on the entire face, neck, and chest. She should be referred to a dermatologist for possible chemical peeling and collagen injections to improve the lines at the inner aspect of the brow line, at the corners of the mouth, and along the upper lip. A cosmetic surgeon may consider removing the fat deposit from the inner corner of her left eye. Esthetic care to improve the sun-damaged areas would consist of 6 rapid exfoliation treatments in the salon in conjunction with daily use of a light exfoliator and green papaya regimen at home. Because this subject's skin appears to be dry or dehydrated, her home care regimen should also include use of a heavy moisturizer (*i.e.*, one that is oil-based).

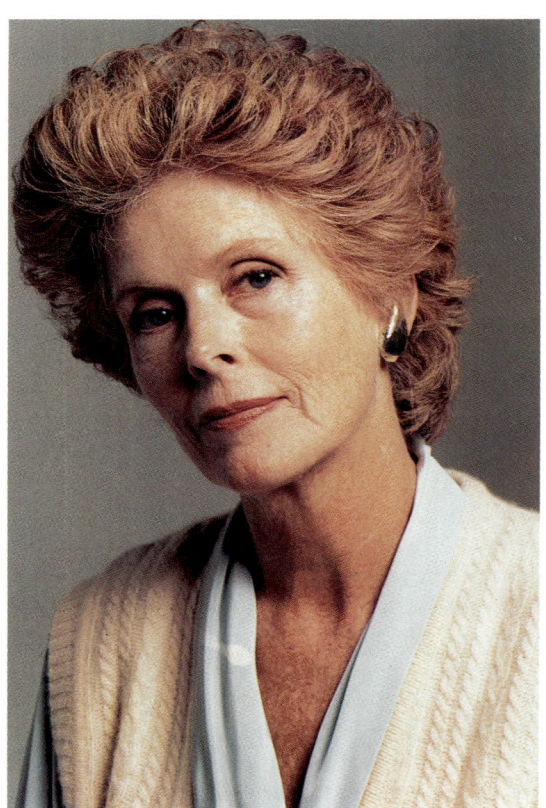

FIGURE 16.2. Subject #2: redhead. This subject exhibits typical redhead sun-damaged skin requiring treatment for photoaging and expression lines.

Subject #3: Silver Hair (Figure 16.3)

Dermatologist: Intrinsic aging in this subject is evidenced by thinning of the skin under the eye; this could best be corrected with a solid implant. However, if my other recommendations are followed, this may not be necessary. Gravity has resulted in a very small upper lip, eyelids that hang down over the eyes, and a virtually nondistinct mandibular line. This subject may benefit from a rhytidectomy, a blepharoplasty, a browlift, and collagen injections to return the upper lip to its previous position. Expression lines, the nasolabial folds, lip lines, and the chin line (a combination of both expression and gravity) need to be injected with

16. The Esthetician's Role in Skin Care

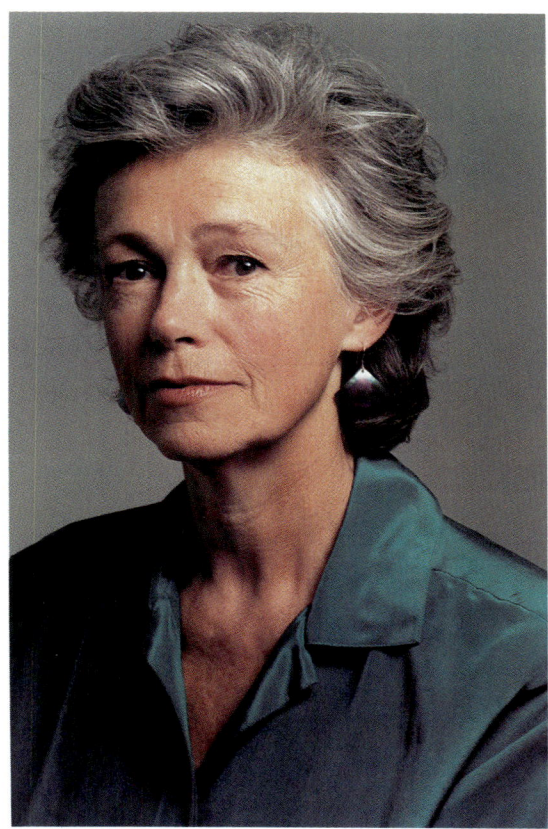

FIGURE 16.3. Subject #3: redhead. This subject's skin shows evidence of intrinsic aging.

collagen. Collagen injections also would improve the forehead. There is a good deal of photoaging, which needs to be treated. After the cosmetic surgical procedures have been completed, this subject should be seen by an esthetician for light exfoliations and to obtain the appropriate cosmetic products for her skin type.

Esthetician #1: This subject has significant sun damage with telangiectasias (couperose) and significant horizontal and vertical wrinkling, hyperpigmentation, and hypotonicity. Elastosis is present, particularly in the eye area. The eye is hooded. Her skin appears to be oil-dry. Sebaceous milia are present on the cheek and nose and possible comedones and enlarged pores complicated by sun damage are present on the chin. Sun damage on the chest and decollete is severe, with a possible actinic keratosis on the chest. There is hypopigmentation above the right eye. This subject should be referred for possible cosmetic surgery, which might include blepharoplasty, perioral dermabrasion, and possibly a forehead lift or rhytidectomy. She should be referred to a dermatologist for examination of the apparent actinic keratosis on her chest and a general checkup to be repeated annually. Esthetic care for this subject would be similar to that recommended for the other subjects; however, Subject #3 needs more emollient content, especially in the eye area. Because of the severity of this subject's telangiectasia, I would be careful with extractions; this type of sun-damaged skin tends to bruise very easily.

Esthetician #2: Referral for possible cosmetic surgery for this subject is indicated and might include blepharoplasty of the upper eyelids, liposuction of the jowl, a series of deep chemical peels of the total face and neck for sun damage, and collagen injections for the lines/creases along the upper lip, at the corners of the mouth, and under the lower lip. To continue exfoliation, the subject's daily regimen at home should incorporate a light exfoliator and green papaya. Because her skin appears to be very dry, salon care should include monthly deep hydrating facials.

Conclusion

As the above evaluations demonstrate, the salon care provided by the esthetician generally complements the care provided by the physician. More importantly, the majority of estheticians appreciate the limitations of their training and will not attempt to treat conditions requiring medical care by a dermatologist or correction by a plastic surgeon.

Identifying a Qualified Esthetician

Excellent skin care salons are not limited to the "beauty capitals," such as New York and Los Angeles; there is at least one such salon in every major city in the United States. Similarly, qualified individual estheticians can be found throughout the country. Although the minimum requirements for licensing as an esthetician in those states requiring a special license vary considerably (see Table 16.1), most estheticians have far more training and experience. Table 16.5 provides a checklist that could be used by a dermatologist to determine the qualifications of an esthetician who is being considered as part of a "skin care team."

Education

Although not all states require a high school diploma, many estheticians trained in the United States are high school graduates. A few estheticians have received cosmetology training at a junior college, some have attended a school specializing in esthetics, and others have been trained in esthetics at a school that offers general training in various areas of cosmetology. Regardless of where the esthetician has studied skin care, the curriculum should have included the use of basic electrical facial equipment. Estheticians are also trained in electrology; however, some states require a separate license for electrologists (see Table 16.2).[5]

Knowledge

The dermatologist whose patients desire an esthetician should recommend an esthetician who understands basic cosmetic chemistry and how to select products with ingredients that are appropriate for a particular skin type. The esthetician should also have a good understanding of the comedogenicity of various cosmetic ingredients. It is important that the esthetician be familiar with the different forms of acne and know how to work with the skin when the patient's dermatologist has prescribed topical tretinoin or oral isotretinoin. The esthetician should also be able to recognize common skin disorders such as actinic keratoses and precancerous and cancerous skin lesions and refer to a dermatologist for further evaluation.

Experience

A well-qualified esthetician should be experienced in the extraction of comedones and in light cosmetic peels. Some estheticians may also apply camouflage makeup, but those with a more scientific focus probably would prefer that the dermatologist or cosmetic surgeon retain a specialist in camouflage makeup to provide this service. The esthetician also should have good communications skills and a desire to educate patients in the essentials of good skin care.

Board Certification(s)

The highest credential in the field of esthetics and the international standard for education is the CIDESCO International Diploma, issued by the International Committee for Cosmetology and Esthetics. This certificate requires successful completion of a 2-day examination. An esthetician may also have the AIACA Certificate issued by the Esthetics International Association—USA. The United States' equivalent of the CIDESCO certificate is the Esthetics America Certificate, issued by the skin care education division of the National Cosmetology Association after successful completion of an examination that tests teaching as well as professional skills. State chapters of this organization are identified as "Esthetics—state name" (*e.g.*, "Esthetics—New York"). Most states require a certain number of hours of continuing education each year in order to maintain certification. Seminars are held at the annual meetings of the national organization and also are sponsored by each state chapter. Many skin care institutes also offer advanced training.

TABLE 16.5. Dermatologist's checklist when interviewing estheticians.

1. Highest level of schooling
2. Specific skin care training
   A. Where provided
   B. Number of hours: classroom/apprenticeship
   C. Training in use of electrical facial equipment
   D. Training in electrology (may require a separate license depending on state)
3. Knowledge of the following:
   A. Basic cosmetic chemistry rather than of a specific product line
   B. Comedogenicity of various cosmetic ingredients
   C. Different forms of acne
   D. How to work with patients using topical tretinoin or taking oral isotretinoin
4. Ability to recognize common skin disorders such as actinic keratoses and precancerous and cancerous skin lesions
5. Experience with the following:
   A. Extractions
   B. Cosmetic peeling (chemical exfoliation)
   C. Camouflage makeup
6. Board certification(s)
7. Continuing education activities

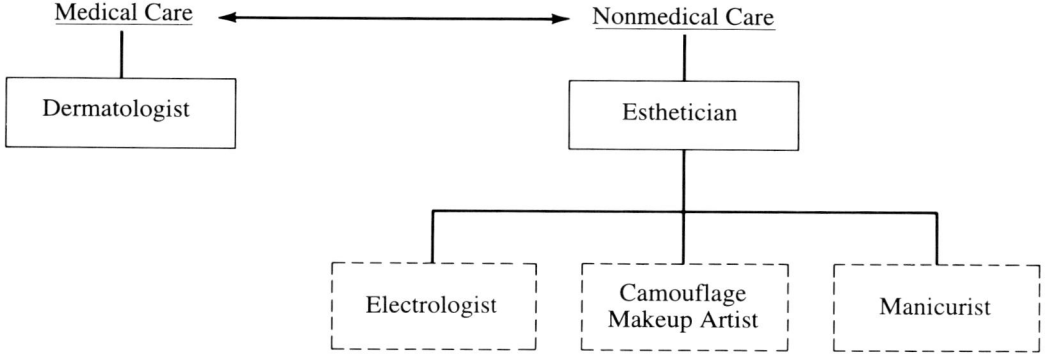

FIGURE 16.4. The skin care team.

Future Directions in Skin Care

Many dermatologists feel that they should take a more active role in coordinating each patient's total skin care program so that complete skin care is provided by a network of allied professionals. The key members of the skin care team illustrated in Figure 16.4 are the dermatologist and the esthetician. Other members might include an electrologist and an esthetician or cosmetologist who specializes in camouflage makeup. Since many women consult dermatologists for nail disorders, the network might also include a manicurist/pedicurist.

Some dermatologists have opened "skin care centers" so that the providers of dermatologic treatment and salon skin care services are at one central location. Although the dermatologist does not see the patient at each visit to the center, through the esthetician the condition of the patient's skin can be closely monitored over time. Other dermatologists and cosmetic surgeons have formed close working relationships with an experienced esthetician whose salon can provide all of the nonmedical services that patients might require.

By working as a team, the dermatologist and the esthetician can better understand the care that each provides, thereby ensuring optimal skin care results for the patient. Whether the skin care team is housed at a single facility or at separate locations, it provides an excellent support system for patients. This is especially important for those being treated for chronic skin disorders such as acne or for those undergoing cosmetic surgery. Rather than being given a vague description of any ongoing medical care by the patient, the esthetician is informed directly by the dermatologist. Consequently, esthetic care can be individualized to complement medical and surgical intervention. Moreover, the patient's compliance with both medical and nonmedical recommendations can be monitored and reinforced regularly.

Acknowledgments

Evaluations of the three photographs were provided by Melvin L. Elson, MD, The Dermatology Center, Nashville, TN; Mark Lees, PhD, Mark Lees Skin Care, Inc, Pensacola, FL; and Ms. Diane Young, Skin Care Expert and President Diane Young Anti-Aging Salon, New York, NY. Much of the information on the practice of esthetics was taken from interviews with Dr. Lee and Ms. Young. Research assistance was provided by Carol M. Sibley, Medical/Scientific Communications, Inc, Montclair, NJ.

References

1. *The Skincare Market*. Packaged facts, New York, January 1991.
2. "Cosmeceuticals"—major global growth area. Skin Inc. 1991; September: 77.
3. Gerson J. *Milady's Standard Textbook for Professional Estheticians,* 7th ed. Milady Publishing Company, Albany, 1992, pp. 24–28.
4. Elson ML. The utilization of glycolic acid in photoaging. Cosmet Dermatol. 1992;5:12–15.
5. *Milady's 1993–94 Guide to Cosmetology Licensing.* Milady Publishing Company, Albany, 1993, pp. 137, 161.
6. Byyny RL, Speroff L. *A Clinical Guide for the Care of Older Women.* Williams & Wilkins, Baltimore, 1990, p. 77.
7. *Pre & Post Operative Care.* Pamphlet from Mark Lees Skin Care, Inc., Pensacola, Florida.

17
The Psychosocial Aspects of Cosmetic Surgery

Judith Waters and George Ellis

> We restore, repair, or conceal those parts of the face which nature has taken away. Not so much that we may delight in the eye, but that we may buoy up the spirit and restore the mind of the afflicted.
>
> Gaspare Togliacozzi, 1597

While there is ample evidence to indicate that a youthful appearance leads to an increase in self-esteem and measurable improvements in social and job related outcomes, many members of the general public and the medical profession still ascribe character flaws and even psychopathology to anyone seeking surgical or other medical treatments for aging skin. In this chapter we review the psychosocial advantages of such interventions, the relevant literature relating physical appearance to personal and social outcomes, and ways of identifying patients for whom surgery may be contraindicated.

There is evidence that people throughout history have equated physical appearance with specific personality traits, intelligence, sexuality, criminal tendencies, virtue, and level of success in a variety of life endeavors. Although people have been taught that it is wrong to judge a book by its cover, they continue to do so with regularity. Thus, we love or hate, admire or distrust people, often essentially based on how they look. Since one of our deepest needs is to be considered desirable and attractive, and therefore worthy of love and admiration, it should come as no particular surprise that so many professions address the problems associated with physical appearance.

The way that we look not only influences how others treat us but also affects our own attitudes, behaviors, and accomplishments. If we look in a real mirror, not just the reflection of other people's reactions, and we are satisfied with what we see, then there is a good chance that we will deal with our daily tasks with confidence. Many physicians are still not convinced that facial defects or blemishes justify medical interventions. There is, however, sufficient evidence that defects can and do result in psychological damage more frequently than not. Since surgeons have developed extraordinary techniques that improve the chances of favorable outcomes and reduce the risks associated with any operation, it is almost unforgivable, as Margaret Mead once said to a group of family practice physicians and internists, to leave the patient without treatment. The ultimate justification for the use of any surgical procedure could be the effect that it has on the patient if it were not for the fact that people have been known to use self-destructive processes in the search for some physical ideal. Women, for example, continued to apply a lead-based makeup called "ceruse" long after it was known that the product caused cancer.

The facelift to preserve a youthful appearance has been employed by members of the theater world so frequently that, regardless of the myriad of jokes made about famous patients, it has become commonplace. Despite the fact that the entertainment industry utilizes plastic surgery to maintain the image of vitality and attractiveness, fictional accounts of plastic surgery frequently depict the patient as a "decaying dowager, spoiled heiress, and criminal fleeing the law".[1]

There are four distinct aspects involved in every cosmetic surgical procedure:

1. What the patient desires and expects.
2. What the surgeon envisions.
3. What the surgeon is actually able to accomplish given the patient's condition.
4. The final result of the surgery when the patient is fully healed.

The closer the concurrence among these four elements, the higher the level of satisfaction with the procedure; the wider the discrepancy between the patient's ideal image and the results, the greater the level of dissatisfaction. Cosmetic surgery differs from other types of operations in that the necessity for the operation is based initially on the patient's self-diagnosis or the influence of "significant others" (*e.g.*, husbands, wives, and/or employers). While there is a tendency to ascribe the desire for cosmetic surgery to the decadence of modern capitalist society, it should be known that even in communist countries before the dissolution of the Soviet Union, psysicians recognized the importance of surgical interventions.

If people have worked hard to remain healthy and have maintained their skills and mental fitness, the real question is, "Should they be judged based on the appearance of aging skin?" Perhaps, with the revelation that more than one of the previous presidents of the United States availed themselves of the skills of the cosmetic surgeon, such interventions will become widely accepted.

Improvements in Psychological Functioning

It is probable that one of the most gratifying aspects of the work of cosmetic and reconstructive surgeons is derived from the improvements in psychological functioning that result from the changes in physical appearance following surgery. In some cases there is an almost immediate and very apparent improvement in the patients' social behaviors. They may become more outgoing and less self-conscious than they were previous to surgery. Once the issue of perceived physical deformity no longer occupies so much of their thoughts, they are free to refocus their energies in other directions.

Sometimes, however, some postsurgical psychotherapy is needed, for two basic reasons. First, on occasion the result of the surgery may be even better than anticipated. Consequently, the patients may be unprepared to deal with the dramatic changes that can accompany improved physical appearance. Second, there are times when the surgical outcomes fall short of the patients' expectations. Professional expertise may be necessary to assist patients in dealing with disconfirmed expectations, especially if they were due to unrealistic hopes. While any good cosmetic surgeon must, of necessity, play the role of a "psychologist" from time to time, the advice of the professionally trained clinician or psychiatrist can prove helpful with some extreme cases.

The fact that many surgeons are amazed at the changes in personality that occur after surgery attests to the fact that even they do not always realize the depth of patients' unhappiness. Changes in physical image can, in many instances, lead to the creation (or release) of a new personality. It is important for the public to remember, however, that the scalpel is not a magic wand. More than a few patients expect to use their newly acquired faces to solve all their social problems. They think that if they only look better, all their troubles will go away.

Since the need for cosmetic surgery is primarily based on self-diagnosis, the typical scenario begins long before patients have an initial appointment with a surgeon. Sometimes the sequence starts with a trauma, such as divorce or losing one's job, or with just a casual remark by someone in a social situation that leads to the realization that one's aging facial appearance no longer reflects one's energetic and youthful inner self. When some patients contemplate cosmetic surgery, at first they experience gnawing doubts about how others will react to the idea. Clearly, no one wants to be perceived as being weak-willed or narcissistic. Of course, not everyone is worried about negative public opinion. Many potential patients don't hesitate for one minute and have no qualms at all about having a facelift or a dermatological treatment that will restore them, even minimally, to a more youthful appearance.

Case Study

Dr. Tracy Peters is a rheumatologist in a large university-based medical center in New York City.* She is widely published in her field and is currently a principal investigator on a major federal grant. She is 56 years old and has been married for 14 years to the head of her department, who is 8 years younger than she is. It is the second marriage for both of them. Recently, her husband asked for a legal separation and moved out of their house. In addition, she has noticed that he has been spending an inordinate amount of time with his assistant, a much younger woman. The situation has become so uncomfortable that Dr. Peters is thinking seriously about applying for a new position elsewhere. However, despite her reputation, she is aware of current economic conditions that favor younger (and often less expensive) job candidates. Moreover, since she does not maintain much hope for reconciliation, she is concerned about establishing a new social life. In making these life changes, Dr. Peters thinks that having a facelift and losing some weight would improve her chances both for a job and a new relationship. She has discussed the issues with a female colleague, with some trepidation, since she thinks that she should be more secure and self-confident than she feels and she is somewhat worried that her friend will not understand her fears.

But Dr. Peters is surprised to discover that her "younger" friend, Dr. Summers, is actually 58 years old and has had two facelifts, one when she was only 40 after having lost a considerable amount of weight. She also discovers that Dr. Summers earned her medical degree after she was 40 and that she, too, is very much aware of the competition for university teaching and research positions. Together they examine the credentials of several surgeons to pick the most appropriate one.

Each cosmetic surgeon's waiting room is filled with all sorts of people, including children, seeking procedures that will enhance their physical appearance. There are both men and women seeking facelifts, many primarily for the same reasons that Dr. Peters wants one. After careful consultation with three surgeons, Dr. Peters selects the one who seems to be most realistic in describing what he can do to modify her appearance. He also suggests some dermatological treatments for the fine wrinkles.

Dr. Peters decides to utilize her accumulated vacation time for the operation and for a much needed rest. The surgery not only meets her very reasonable expectations, it actually exceeds what the surgeon had predicted. Her self-esteem soars. In fairy tales, this is the point at which the transformed princess would win back the handsome prince. This is not a fairy tale. What does happen is that Dr. Peters decides to institute divorce proceedings but to remain in her job. Given her renewed confidence, she no longer feels desperate about finding a new position. People tell her how rested she looks, and she is able to return to work with new-found vigor. As frequently happens with cosmetic surgery patients, she makes other changes in her life, joining a health club, modifying her diet, and allocating time to enjoy the fruits of her labor. Whether or not there will be another romantic relationship, only time will tell.

A few years ago, this story might have taken a different turn. The patient might have evaluated her own wish for cosmetic surgery as a sign of a character disorder. Even today, think how the case study would sound if the sex of the patient were changed. We still tend to perceive a man's desire for cosmetic surgery as a sign of effeminacy or just plain weakness. Also note that we have chosen to make the surgeon a male, for the reason that the predominant number of cosmetic and reconstructive surgeons are men.

Physical Appearance and Self-Concept

In attempting to understand how attractiveness affects a person's behavior, there are two perspectives that are salient: The individual as a

---

*Note: The person's name and occupation have been changed.

social object, and the self-concept or body image view.[2] Clearly, these two perspectives interact to influence the person's level of self-esteem and his or her willingness to engage in different types of social and career related activities.

Physical attractiveness has already been shown to be one of the most compelling factors in the choices that men and women make, especially for dating and marriage. The value of an attractive appearance as a social resource is made salient very early in life. As children, most of us were exposed to fairy tales such as "Sleeping Beauty," where happy endings were associated with the physical attractiveness of the hero and heroine. "Beauty" always wed the Prince, while the ugly old witches and deformed villains were thwarted and frequently destroyed. No child was concerned with whether or not the Prince fell in love with the comatose Princess because he had come to appreciate her sense of humor, her wit, or her loving and gentle nature. We all knew better: The princess was beautiful. Nor did we concern ourselves with whether or not the princess was able to recognize all of the Prince's fine qualities by merely looking at his face when awakened by that famous kiss. In fact, children still believe that inside of every unhappy, warty frog is a prince only waiting to be released. In many children's minds, the legendary wicked dwarfs, such as Rumpelstiltskin, are malevolent because they are ugly, what is ugly is bad.[3] The same theory is applied when cosmetic surgeons and dermatologists are asked to volunteer their services to improve the appearance of prison inmates with physical deformities.

As further evidence of the importance of physical attractiveness in our society, we have the popularity of books and magazine articles on exercise and diet and the existence of countless beauty salons and health spas. Physical attractiveness is clearly considered a marketable resource, albeit a deteriorating one, that sometimes even outweighs the advantages of a large dowry.

Scientists who study authority, aggression, and prejudice have not always treated physical attractiveness as a serious subject for investigation. Cash[2] recounts his own initial reluctance to study physical appearance. For the public it seems somewhat reprehensible to acknowledge that people select friends or employees, not for their character or skills, but primarily on the basis of how they look. This value is treated in a manner very similar to marrying for money. It is considered immoral, and we just do not want to admit how often it happens. In American culture we are still led to believe that individual achievement is more important than being born beautiful or handsome or rich.

Being extremely beautiful is not always an unalloyed asset. There are any number of detractors. In fact, the stereotype of the "Beautiful People" is that they are narcissistic and shallow. The public is sometimes incredulous when informed that a particularly handsome or beautiful person has a postgraduate degree. On the other hand, research subjects usually rate attractive men and women as more intelligent than unattractive people.

Physical appearance is a very important factor in the workplace. In a study of the influence of personal appearance, skill, and age on salary for women, makeovers were done on 8 women representing 4 age groups, ranging from the late twenties through the sixties.[4] A photograph of the "before" or "after" condition was then attached to one of a set of résumés at three skill levels (secretary, editor, and financial analyst). These packages were presented to more than 300 human resources staff in 120 private employment agencies or major corporations in 3 major cities (New York, Chicago, and Los Angeles). Physical appearance did play a critical role in the hiring process on every skill level. However, the greatest difference was at the lowest skill level. The fewer the skills, the more appearance seemed to count. However, the comments of several subjects indicated that these results should be examined with care. It was pointed out that where the pool of highly trained applicants is relatively small, an unattractive candidate may be hired but will either be relegated to a "back room" to toil away out of sight or be advised, ever so subtly (since it against the law), to improve his or her appearance.

The most significant result in this study was that the older the woman in the photograph, the more important the improvement in appearance was to her economic opportunities. Since women, especially those over age 65, are at the lowest level of income in this country (less than $4,000 per year), the ability to work is of vital importance to survival. If the book is really evaluated by the cover, then it is important to make the "package" look vital, professional, and capable of doing a full day's work.

The changes that were made in the aforementioned study were cosmetic and thus would be washed off at the end of the day. Just think how much more could be gained from relatively more permanent interventions. It should be noted that the primary motivations that prompted the study were not only theoretical but practical. The author had been counseling "nontraditional" older students who were planning to return to the job market or perhaps even enter it for the first time. She was concerned about the barriers that they might face. If personnel departments reject employees based on their perceived age and appearance (used as indicators of work potential), then the accumulated experience of rejection will eventually have an impact on the person's self-esteem, even if that person had not suffered from a poor image prior to the rejections. Even if the individual is able to maintain a high level of self-confidence despite encountering discrimination, there are still some very serious objective problems. No job, no income except Social Security, no decent medical insurance except Medicare — survival is doubtful.

The problem of discrimination that older people encounter may be addressed in two ways. We can change society; or we can continue to offer the same opportunities provided to deformed prisoners to older people from all walks of life, not just to those who can afford the skill of the cosmetic surgeon or dermatologist.

There are several stereotypes about the elderly and physical attractiveness that affect how older people are perceived and treated. The first is that it is assumed that appearance is of little importance to the elderly.[5] Another commonly held attitude is that the elderly are uninterested in sexual relationships and that they are undesirable.[6] Since sexuality and attractiveness are closely related, attractiveness appears to decline with age. Older women are treated as sexually neuter long before men experience rejection.

In research studies the attractiveness stereotype has been closely associated with positive personality traits, successful social and career experiences, and preferential treatment in many situations. The situation may actually be worse than it appears in the research literature. Social desirability (saying and doing the socially acceptable thing) can confound research results, since most subjects are aware that they should not say that they value people for their physical appearance.[5,7] Despite the "fairness" value, Johnson found that attractive features are frequently correlated with perceptions of youth.[5] He stated that "Unattractive features are defined in terms associated with aging. . . . "

Real Characteristics of Attractive People

There are several important studies that attest to the value for adult men and women of being facially attractive. For example, it was reported that facially attractive men and women are not "unduly influenced by others in decision making contexts."[8] Others have found that attractive people are more assertive and eventually successful in delivering persuasive communications.[9,10] Unattractive women tend to utilize ineffective social influence styles, which include being demanding, interrupting other people, being opinionated, antagonistic, or being overly submissive.[9] It has also been demonstrated that being attractive leads to positive outcomes in a broad range of contexts, from business to legal proceedings. Until recently, however, the focus in social research has been on the value of attractiveness for young men and women with relatively little interest on how aging skin relates to personal and business outcomes for middle-aged or older people. In reality, it is probable that attractiveness as a factor becomes even more critical as one grows older. Adams suggests that in an extremely appearance-oriented culture such as contemporary American society, it may even be "psychologically devastating to be both non-youthful and unattractive."[11] Adams cites the writings of Susan Sontag, who clearly delineated differential attitudes towards signs of aging in men and women. Sontag makes the cogent argument that there is only one standard of beauty for women. In order to be considered attractive, a woman must also appear to be young. As she ages her beauty is perceived to decline. Consequently, she loses social status, and her own self-esteem falls precipitously. If a woman sees her attractiveness as a deteriorating resource, it is due to the fact that she has been socialized in the same culture that now denigrates her. She has internalized the values and standards with which she was raised.

In order to address the issue of age and physical attractiveness, Adams and Huston conducted a study of young adult and elderly subjects.[12] They were asked to evaluate middle-aged men and women (both attractive and unattractive) on a list of attributes that included sociability, self-esteem, honesty, and occupational level (professional or "blue collar"). The subjects rated the attractive men and women as having higher levels of self-esteem, higher job status, and as being more sociable than their less attractive peers. There were significant differences between the ratings of men and women for several factors. For example, facially unattractive women were evaluated lower than the attractive women, who, in turn, were rated lower than both categories of men (attractive and unattractive) with respect to occupational status and self-esteem. Unattractive women, however, were considered more honest than all three other categories. Jones and Adams conducted a study of 301 men and women ranging in age from 18 to 90 years of age.[13] In essence they found that physical attractiveness as a variable was valued by people in each age category and that the older subjects emphasized the importance of appearance more strongly than the younger subjects.

The Dorian Gray Complex

What is actually being questioned in the pursuit of youth and attractiveness is the moral fiber and even the psychological well-being of someone who wants to look younger than he or she does. Since it is probable that physical appearance is the single most important factor in face-to-face encounters, we might even call the phenomenon the "Dorian Gray Complex." In Oscar Wilde's book *The Picture of Dorian Gray*,[14] the protagonist, a handsome young man, remained young and innocent looking despite the serious social crimes he committed. His portrait, however, aged and grew uglier with each succeeding event. His picture was supposed to be a better representation of his character than his face.

The Looking Glass Self

To address the impact of the reactions of other people on a person's self perception, in 1920, C. H. Cooley developed the construct of the "Looking Glass Self."[15] In essence he said that self-concept is a reflection of how people treat the individual and of the individual's comparison of his or her own characteristics with those of others, particularly peers. Hence, given enough negative feedback, it may be virtually impossible to improve self-esteem. Without sufficient self-esteem and a sense of self-efficacy, the individual may have trouble achieving his or her goals.

The two perspectives, persons as a social object and self-concept, interact to affect the individual's psychosocial experiences and even emotional and intellectual development. Cash and Horton conducted a controlled experiment to test the hypothesis that aesthetic surgery (in this case, rhinoplasty) does produce improvements in physical appearance that lead to favorable evaluations by others.[16] The result of the study supported the hypothesis across different age categories and with both sexes.

It may be that even subtle changes in appearance can lead to increases in self esteem. A very interesting study investigated the pre- and post-operative self reports of 22 children and adolescents undergoing reconstructive surgery.[17] It found that patients rated their physical appearance as noticeably improved after surgery, while a sample of nonmedical observers noted only minor changes. The results are important because the patients reported that their self-esteem rose significantly. The patients also stated that they felt more socially adept and were better accepted than prior to the surgery. It seems that their subjective evaluation led to increased self-confidence, which eventually influenced their social relationships. The conclusion is that minor changes in appearance can and do result in major changes in self-esteem and in social outcomes.

Another study investigated the reactions of adult and children to photographs of faces taken prior to and following minor facial reconstructive surgery.[18] Although the judgments of observers under age 12 years were not affected by the surgical changes in the patients, those over age 12 rated the "after" pictures as more attractive, intelligent, and happier than the "before" pictures. Other studies have demonstrated that children as young as age 5 can distinguish between attractive and unattractive adults and children. They frequently act on their prejudices with discrimination. While the results of this previous research support the contention that patients who want to have their facial abnormalities reduced may simply be reflecting social prejudice and discrimination, it also provides evidence that people who seek such surgical interventions may not be "neurotic phantasizers."

Selection Criteria

In 1986 Wengle reviewed the literature concerning selection criteria for cosmetic surgery.[19,20] The factors he examined included personality variables, sex differences, external versus internal motivations for surgical treatment, subjective and objective assessment of the cosmetic defect, and patient satisfaction. In the past (the not too distant past), for example, plastic surgeons would diagnose aging male patients who wanted facial surgery as exhibiting symptoms of a psychological disorder, while a similar request from a female patient was considered normal. In 1991 Dull and West reported the same phenomena.[21] Wengle also assessed the question of whether surgery or psychotherapy would be a better way to deal with patients' concerns about their physical appearance.

There are several aspects to this issue that must be addressed. The first question concerns the ability and training of a surgeon to make a psychiatric diagnoses. If a surgeon does not feel competent to evaluate high-risk patients, it is always possible to refer the patient for a full battery of tests. On the other hand, it may be that the surgeon who sees pathology actually suffers from stereotypic vision. In fact, Wengle's review of the salient literature indicates that much of the material on psychopathology and cosmetic surgery actually reflects cultural norms with respect to the desire for specific surgical procedures such as facelifts.

Although the desire to improve the appearance of aging skin may be the result of external pressures and the desire to raise self-esteem in most patients, there are a few potential patients who do present significant psychological problems that should serve as a "red flag" to warn the physician against surgical intervention. Schweitzer wrote that there are patients with minimal defects who have developed into surgical "junkies," going from one procedure to another, never with any real satisfaction.[22] Schweitzer warns that schizophrenics and patients who are experiencing other personal crises should be considered as high risks. Unfortunately, Schweitzer also categorized males as being problematic with respect to the need for cosmetic surgery.

Even psychiatric evaluations may not be successful in separating appropriate from inappropriate surgical candidates. Mohl noted that there are several biases that psychiatrists have toward patients seeking cosmetic surgery.[23] He wrote that psychiatrists do not want patients to try to solve psychological problems with surgical interventions. No reasonable person, professional or otherwise, would disagree with that statement; psychopathology should be a contraindication for surgery. The difficulty arises, however, when the mere request for a surgical procedure is defined as a psychological symptom. No surgeon really wants to operate on a person who is emotionally unstable. However, if the simple desire for cosmetic surgery is defined as narcissistic and pathological, we would be left with scarcely any patients suitable for surgery. Another bias concerns the severity of the defect. The seriousness of any defect is, at least partially, a matter of subjective perception. Just because the psychiatrist is unimpressed by the severity of the defect doesn't negate the patient's distress. The next source of bias involves the judgment that candidates who can articulate their reasons for seeking cosmetic surgery clearly are better candidates than those patients who are either incapable or unwilling to express their motives. Lack of verbal facility is not a symptom. Moreover, if patients are aware of the values of some psychiatrists, it is no wonder that they are reluctant to discuss body image and self-esteem with them.

Groenman and Sauer suggest that, in fact, the majority of cosmetic surgery patients are not disturbed and are generally satisfied with the results of the treatment.[24] However, the few patients who are dissatisfied with the outcome of procedures, despite the fact that these same outcomes would be evaluated positively by disinterested and objective observers, may be exhibiting symptoms that are similar to borderline personality disorder.[25]

Thomson, Knorr, and Edgeton differentiated between the influences of internal versus external pressures when requesting cosmetic surgery.[26] They felt that responding to external considerations was less likely to lead to postoperative satisfaction than responding to the internal desire to raise self-esteem and self-acceptance. However, if self-esteem and self-acceptance are based, as Cooley suggested, on the reactions of others, then how can anyone separate the impact of each source unless the patient clearly states that the one and only reason he or she wants surgery is to please a specific person or stave off an impending divorce? Even then, it is quite likely that the individual is internally motivated, despite protestations to the contrary.

People, particularly those who are convinced that they will never need a cosmetic procedure, tend to think that an operation or treatment designed to improve one's appearance is almost immoral. In actuality, from the beginning of civilization, both men and women have devoted time, effort, and financial resources and have even experienced extreme pain in the attempt to improve how they look. Among so-called primitive tribes, for example, people have subjected themselves to such practices as scarification, tattooing, filing their teeth to sharp points, wearing rings to elongate their necks, and distending their earlobes and lips with the goal of being attractive to other members of their culture. In order to achieve the desired image, people have sought the aid of witch doctors, alchemists, magicians, cosmeticians, and, eventually, physicians and surgeons. In contemporary society the fields of cosmetic and reconstructive surgery and dermatology have provided us with methods to modify, correct, and/or restore facial features and body structures.

In the past cosmetic surgery was disrespected by members of other medical specialties and considered suitable only for people wishing to disguise their ethnic origins, entertainers, models, and rich and self-indulgent women.[27] Many cosmetic surgeons themselves were worried that their patients were already emotionally disturbed or that surgery would hasten the onset of symptoms. Being concerned about one's appearance was labeled deceitful, frivolous, narcissistic—and, for men, a clear sign of an abnormal personality structure. On the other hand, when medical staff see the physical appearance and the hygiene of hospitalized patients deteriorating, they recognize the therapeutic efficacy of cosmetic treatments.[28] As Graham and Kligman point out:[29]

The time is overdue to obtain a proper perspective of the significance in terms of human well-being. Appearance counts whether we like it or not, regardless of whether it is compatible with our democratic ideal of treating people on their own merits and not their hereditary endowments. It is important not to confuse what ought to be with what is. Medical doctors are too often insensitive to the profound influence of appearance in all walks of life, at all ages, in all endeavors, and in the sick as well as the healthy. Medical education has traditionally focused on pathological processes that cause disease and impair physical functions. By this model, blemishes and disfigurement are trivial and hardly qualify as legitimate objects for research and relief. Yet this attitude may be ruinous to the emotional growth and the social fulfillment of those with appearance problems.

Planning for the Surgery

Both physically and psychologically, there is a right time for surgery. Earlier is better than later. If a patient waits too long, the face sags too much and makeup can no longer disguise wrinkles and the signs of aging. Therefore, surgery will not achieve the maximum results. In addition, the patient who has seen positive outcomes on younger, less damaged individuals is quite likely to build up unrealistic expectations, which are destined to be unfulfilled. Although facelifts and adjunctive procedures do result in some improvement even for people in their eighties, the outcomes are better if the patients are in their forties, when the indications of aging and/or photodamage first become apparent. While some people want to wait and achieve a dramatic change in appearance for their money, the more intelligent approach is to begin with a plan for a series of minor corrections that will be scheduled on an "as needed" basis. This type of sequential program prevents the face from looking old from the start and is more gentle to the tissue than major procedures as a first line of defense. What is most important from a psychological perspective is that few observers will even be aware of the changes in appearance and the patient will not be subjected to unnecessary questions and comments.

Picking a Surgeon

Since surgeons are human beings with their own biases, it is important to find out before the initial visit, if possible, whether or not the doctor has a prejudice against cosmetic procedures. Patient–surgeon psychological rapport is essential to satisfaction with the surgery.[30]

Many patients have somewhat exaggerated images of how they will look following surgery. It is the task of the surgeon to help the patient develop realistic expectations. The primary goal of cosmetic surgery is to reduce abnormalities to a reasonable minimum given the circumstances, not to create a perfect face or to match a specific "look" that the patient may wish to imitate.

Risks and Anxieties

Cosmetic surgery, while not necessarily as intrusive as some other operations, is still an insult to the body. Although the risks are frequently less than for some other types of surgery, they should not be ignored by the surgeons. Many patients who are strongly motivated to have cosmetic surgery may still be fearful about the dangers. It is the wise physician who anticipates these anxieties and either deals with them personally or refers the patient to a therapist.

Consequences of Successful Cosmetic Surgery

It must be remembered that patients frequently seek surgery because they have experienced or they anticipate some negative changes in their lives, ranging from divorce to loss of job. They perceive these losses (real or imagined) to be related to how they look. Unfortunately, in many cases they are quite correct. Consequently, they are not basically disturbed but suffering with "problems in living," many of which will actually be improved following surgery. While some patients exhibit transient depressive reactions, others report that they had either acquired a new job, received a new promotion or merit award, or formed new close relationship and/or terminated old dysfunctional relationship.[31] Most patients do not seem to feel guilty either about the surgery or the deception about their ages. In fact, some patients say that a youthful appearance made them forget about their true chronological ages. While not all operations result in a new job or marriage, most patients state that there is a significant improvement in personal comfort, life satisfaction, ease in social situations, self-esteem, and that they engage in less self-criticism and are less self-conscious.

Although cosmetic surgery is more commonplace than it once was, there are many people who still feel uncomfortable about seeing a plastic surgeon. When the generation of baby boomers who are now showing signs of aging begin seeking surgical interventions, they will be more accepting and less embarrassed about such procedures than previous generations. That brings us to a salient point: Who pays for the operation? At the present time, insurance companies in the United States do not cover operations for strictly cosmetic purposes. In countries that have socialized medicine, such as Sweden, cosmetic surgery for deformities other than aging may be funded. Great Britain and Canada also cover cosmetic surgery in their national health care programs, but there are lengthy waiting periods. Thus, in the United States, we have a procedure that is available only to people who can afford it. As we have already noted, physical appearance and job marketability are closely associated in many, if not most, professions. In order to enhance their workplace opportunities, some people would like to avail themselves to the skills of a cosmetic or reconstructive surgeon. However, since a significant proportion of these individuals may either be out of work or in low paying jobs, they may not be able to pay for treatment. How we as a nation will deal with the issue of costs of elective surgery during the financially stressed last decade of the twentieth century is open for debate.

References

1. Brown WE. *Cosmetic Surgery*. Stein and Day, Publishers, New York, undated.
2. Cash TF. Physical appearance and mental health. In: *The Psychology of Cosmetic Treatments*, JA. Graham, AM. Kligman, eds. Praeger, New York, 1985, pp. 196–216.
3. Berscheid E, Walster EH. *Interpersonal Attraction*, 2nd ed. Addison-Wesley Publishers, Reading, 1978.
4. Waters J. Cosmetics and the job market. In: *The Psychology of Cosmetic Treatments*, JA Graham, AM Kligman, eds. Praeger, New York, 1985, pp. 113–124.
5. Johnson, DF. Appearance and the elderly. In: *The Psychology of Cosmetic Treatments*, JM Graham, AM Kligman, eds. Praeger, New York, 1985, p. 152.
6. Drew B, Waters J. Attitudes toward older men and women in three areas of functioning: physical, cognitive, and sexual. Paper presented at the First Annual Research Conference on Women, Rutgers University, New Brunswick, New Jersey, 1983.
7. Berscheid E. An overview of the psychological effects of physical attractiveness and some comments upon the psychological effects of knowledge of the effects of physical attractiveness. In: *Logical Aspects of Facial Form* (Craniofacial Growth Series), W Lucker, K Ribbens, JA McNamera, eds. University of Michigan Press, Ann Arbor, 1981.
8. Adams GR. Physical attractiveness: Toward a developmental social psychology of beauty. Human Dev. 1977;20:217–230.
9. Adams GR, Read D. Personality and social influence styles of attractive and unattractive college women. Psychol. 1983;114:151–157.
10. Chaiken S. Communicator physical attractiveness and persuasion. Personality Soc Psychol. 1979;50:492–501.
11. Adams GR. Attractiveness through the ages: implications of facial attractiveness over the life cycle. In: *The Psychology of Cosmetic Treatments*, JA Graham, AM Kligman, eds. Praeger, New York, 1985, pp. 133–151.
12. Adams GR, Huston TL. Social perception of middle-aged persons varying in physical attractiveness. Dev Psychol. 1975;11:656–658.
13. Jones RM, Adams GR. Assessing the importance of physical attractiveness across the life-span. Soc Psychol. 1982; 118:131–132.
14. Wilde O. The Picture of Dorian Grey. Heritage Press, New York, 1957.
15. Cooley CH. Human nature and the social order. Scribner, New York, 1980.
16. Cash TF, Horton CE. Aesthetic surgery: effects of rhinoplasty on the social perception of patients by others. Plast Reconstr Surg. 1983;72(4):543–548.
17. Arndt EM, Travis F, Lefebvre A, et al. Beauty and the eye of the beholder: social consequences and personal adjustments for facial patients. Br J Plast Surg. 1986;39(1):81–84.
18. Elliot M, Bull R, James D, Lansdown R. Children's and adults' reactions to photographs taken before and after facial surgery. J Maxillofac Surg. 1986;14(1):18–21.
19. Wengle HP. The psychology of cosmetic surgery: old problems in patient selection seen in a new way. Part II. An Plast Surg. 1986;16(6):487–493.
20. Wengle HP. The psychology of cosmetic surgery: a critical overview of the literature 1960–1982. Part I. An Plast Surg. 1986;16(5):435–443.
21. Dull D, West C. Accounting for cosmetic surgery: the accomplishment of gender. Soc Prob. 1991;38(1):54–70.

22. Schweitzer I. The psychiatric assessment of the patient requesting facial surgery. Australian and New Zealand J Psychiat. 1989;23(2):249-254.
23. Mohl PC. Psychiatric consultation in plastic surgery: the psychiatrist's perspective. Psychosomatics. 1984;25(6):470,474-476.
24. Groenman NH, Sauer HC. Personality characteristics of the cosmetic surgical insatiable patient. Psychother Psychosomat. 1983;40(1-4):241-245.
25. American Psychiatric Association. Diagnostic and statistical manual of mental disorders, 3rd ed. American Psychiatric Association, Washington, D.C., 1987.
26. Thomson JA, Knor NJ, Edgerton MT. Cosmetic surgery: the psychiatric perspective. Psychosomatics. 1978;19(1):7-15.
27. Kligman AM. Medical aspects of skin and its appearance. In: *The Psychology of Cosmetic Treatments*, JA Graham, AM Kligman, eds. Praeger, New York, 1985, pp. 3-25.
28. Graham JA. Overview of psychology of cosmetics. In *The Psychology of Cosmetic Treatments*, JA Graham, AM Kligman, eds. Praeger, New York, 1985, pp. 26-36.
29. Graham JA, Kligman AM. Preface. In: *The Psychology of Cosmetic* Treatments, JA Graham, AM Kligman, eds. Praeger, New York, 1985, p. vii.
30. Dicker RL, Syracuse VR. *Consultation with a Plastic Surgeon*. Nelson, Chicago, 1975.
31. Goin MK, Burgoyne RW, Goin JM, Staples FR. A prospective study of 50 female face-lift patients. Plast Reconstr Surg. 1980:65(4):436-442.

18
Surgical Vignettes

Vignette #1

Manual Dermasanding and Low Strength Trichloroacetic Acid Peeling: A Simple Technique to Improve Photodamaged Skin

David R. Harris

This vignette describes a technique we have developed over the past several years, combining silicone carbide sandpaper abrasion with low-strength trichloroacetic acid to improve actinically injured skin. We have found it to have distinct advantages over motor-driven dermabrasion or the use of deeper chemosurgical peeling solutions alone. Those of us interested in texturing procedures are acquainted with various chemosurgical peels and abrasion techniques for rejuvenation of the actinically exposed integument. These include motor driven dermabrasion, with and without the addition of trichloroacetic acid,[1,2] various peeling procedures utilizing TCA and phenol,[3,4,5] and salicylic acid applications.[6] In addition, combining topical agents to enhance the effects of chemoexfoliation has been found to have increased popularity. Improved results are reported for CO_2 and/or Jessners solution in combination with TCA[7] as well as pretreatment with retinoic and alpha hydroxy acids.[8]

However, all these strategies, regardless of efficacy, pose some disadvantages. Lower-strength TCA peeling, while quite safe, may remove only the finest of rhytids, even with repeated exposures. Deeper peeling with TCA or phenol, while far more efficacious in improving photodamaged skin, results in an increased incidence of postoperative pigmentary problems and scarring.[9] In addition, phenol can frequently cause a measure of systemic toxicity, even in monitored patients.[10]

Those of us accomplished in the use of motor-driven dermabrasion are familiar with the long-lasting improvements its use can bring to actinically injured integument. But this approach takes decided skill and experience for the procedure to be safe and uniformly pleasing. Moreover, even the most facile among us must employ extreme caution when approaching the lower lid above the orbital rim or when abrading the commissures and vermilion border. Finally, in our experience it is difficult to avoid at least some sharp lines of demarcation, especially at the orbital rim.

Our technique largely avoids these disadvantages while providing uniformly effective removal of rhytids. Called *dermasanding* rather than dermabrasion, and originally introduced to improve acne scars by Janklow and Maliner,[11] we employ the use of various grades of sterilized 3M silicone carbide "Wetordry" sandpaper to lightly abrade or "buff" the skin, removing the stratum corneum to glistening layer and bleeding points. We then enhance the result with the application of 25% TCA.

This approach takes minimal skill factor,

causes no splatter, provides uniformly pleasing results, and leaves no sharp lines of demarcation. Moreover, to date we have experienced 2 two cases of focused hypopigmentation, in more than 300 patients treated.

The Patient Population

Choosing the right candidate for dermasanding is at least as important as the effectiveness of the technique itself. Appropriate patients generally range in age from early thirties to the late fifties, with dull, lusterless skin and a measure of dyschromia. They have fine to moderately deep rhytids, forming longitudinal furrows over the upper lip with accentuation of "laugh lines" elsewhere over perioral zones. In addition, appropriate candidates may have periorbital "crow's feet" and lower lid hatchmark "sleep lines," and, perhaps, moderate to deeper glabellar folds (Figure 18.1). Patients with horizontal "worry lines" over the forehead are also helped with this procedure. An older patient with deep malar folds and sagging jowls will be less pleased with the texturing procedure alone than with a combination of texturing and lifting.

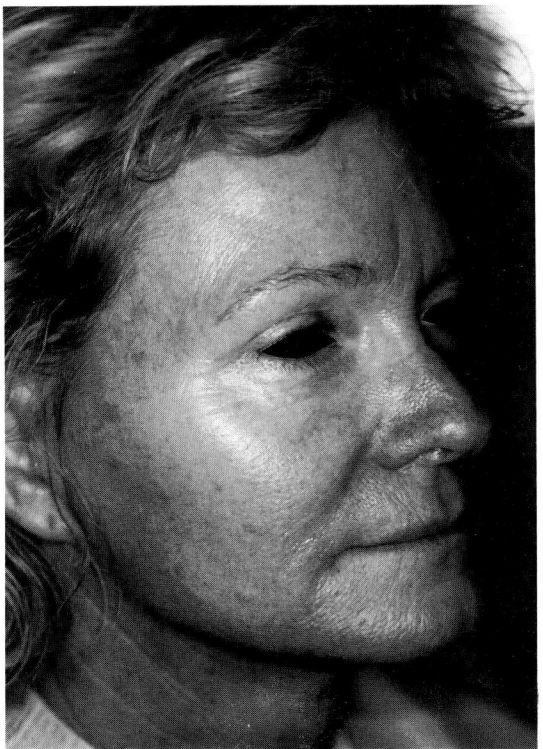

FIGURE 18.1. An appropriate candidate with moderately deep rhytids and dyschromia.

Materials

We employ various grades of 3M silicone carbide "Wetordry" sandpaper (Figure 18.2A). Fine grade #400, medium grade #220 and 320, and the courser #180 are the papers of choice (Table 18.1). The sandpaper sheets are cut into approximately 2 by 3 cm pieces, and 3 or 4 at a time are autoclaved in bull's-eye bags (Figure 18.2B). Fresh 25% TCA is the chemopeeling agent of choice.

Pretesting

Once the procedure is explained to candidates, a test site on the postauricular surface is abraded to bleeding points and painted with 25% TCA in order to evaluate the propensity for dyschromia. The results are evaluated in 7 to 8 weeks. Some erythema is universal, but the unusual patient susceptible to permanent depigmentation cannot be identified without testing. Hyperpigmentation with darker skin tones is common and can be ameliorated by pre- and postabrasion treatment with hydroquinone preparations between 4% and 8%.

The Procedure

A suitable candidate, driven by a companion to our facility, arrives premedicated with 20 mg of Valium taken 2 hours before the procedure. This is generally augmented with an IM analgesic on arrival. The skin is cleaned with an appropriate agent and defatted with either acetone/alcohol or 10% glycolic acid in an alcoholic astringent. Hair is tied and shielded. After photography each of the rhytids is marked with

18. Surgical Vignettes

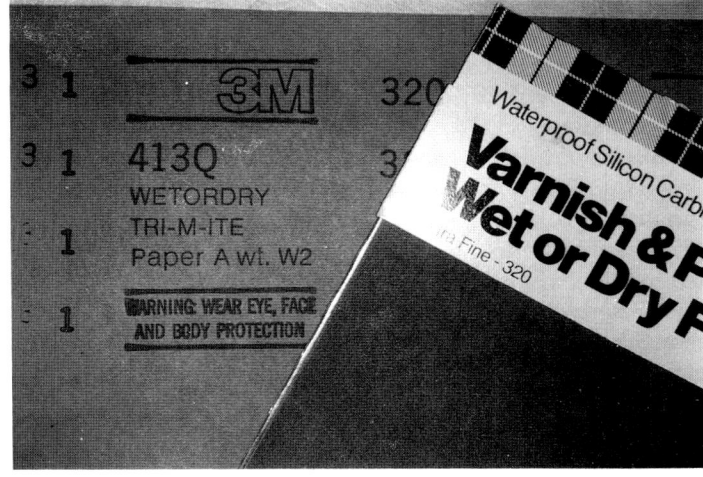

FIGURE 18.2. A. 3M silicone carbide Wetordry sandpaper is available at hardware stores. B. We cut the sheets into 2 cm by 3 cm pieces and autoclave 3 to 4 pieces together in bull's-eye bags.

TABLE 18.1. 3M silicone carbide Wetordry dermasanding.

Grade of paper	Problems best treated
Fine grade #400	Rhytids upper and lower eyelids and periorbital zones
Medium grade #200–320	Fine to medium rhytids glabella, forehead, perioral and malar
Coarse grade #180	Deeper rhytids with obvious delling when stretched

a skin marker while the patient is in a sitting position and the effects of gravity can be most efficiently observed (Figure 18.3).

With the patient in a supine position, the operator wraps a piece of the chosen grade of silicone carbide paper around 2 rolled 2-inch by 2-inch (2 by 2) coarse mesh gauze pads. The paper and gauze are dipped in water to enhance abrasiveness. (Dry paper does not work well as an abrasive tool.) While the skin is stretched, the affected area is gently abraded in a repetitive manner, both in a back-and-forth and/or circular motion (Figure 18.4A). The glistening layer is generally reached within seconds, and, depending on the grade of paper, bleeding points are appreciated within 30 to 45 seconds (Figure 18.4B).

The grade of sandpaper used will vary according to the problem and the site. Deeply etched folds over the forehead and perioral areas will best be approached using coarser grades, #180 and #220, to bleeding. Fine or even deeper lines over the eyelids and at the outer canthal folds are best treated with fine grade #400 (Figure 18.5). We find the perioral areas most amenable to medium grades, #220 or #320 (Figure 18.6). The remainder of the skin to hairline and over the mandibles is lightly sanded to glistening and fine bleeding points with a medium grade paper.

During the course of the procedure, we tend to change papers several times. A case involving full face rhytids will take 4 to 6 strips of paper of various grades. In most areas we have found that wrapping the paper around 2 pieces of rolled 2 by 2 gauze works most effectively, except with the fine rhytids at the lower lid margin, which are best approached with 1 tightly rolled gauze pad. In any event, while one is abrading in a gentle manner over the areas involved, the paper itself is causing a fine irregular pattern of epidermal debridement and scratch marks that serve to feather the edges of the abraded zones in a most effective manner.

Following the abrasion, iced compresses are applied over the entire face for about 5 minutes. Then 25% TCA is applied using 2 by 2 gauze pads (Figure 18.7). Treated areas again are covered immediately with iced compresses (Figure 18.8). Most patients experience some degree of burning with the application of TCA to dermasanded integument.

Postoperative Care

After a few minutes of icing, when discomfort has passed, the skin is lightly coated with a

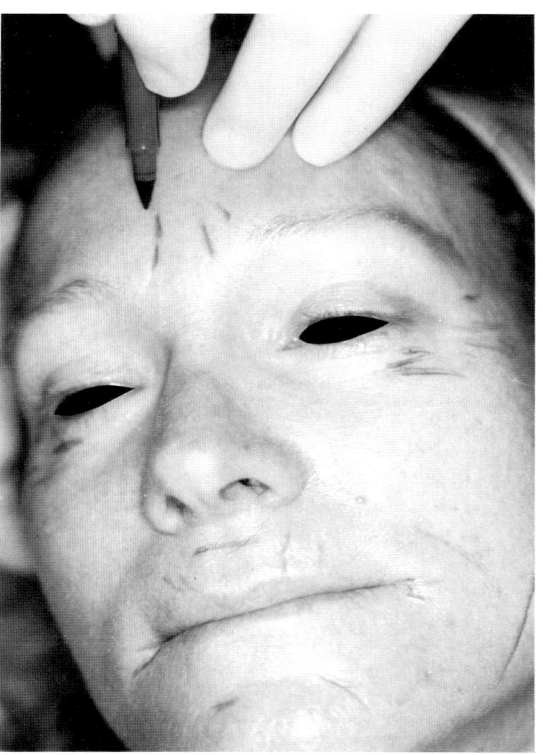

FIGURE 18.3. Before dermasanding, each of the rhytids is marked while the patient is in a sitting position.

18. Surgical Vignettes

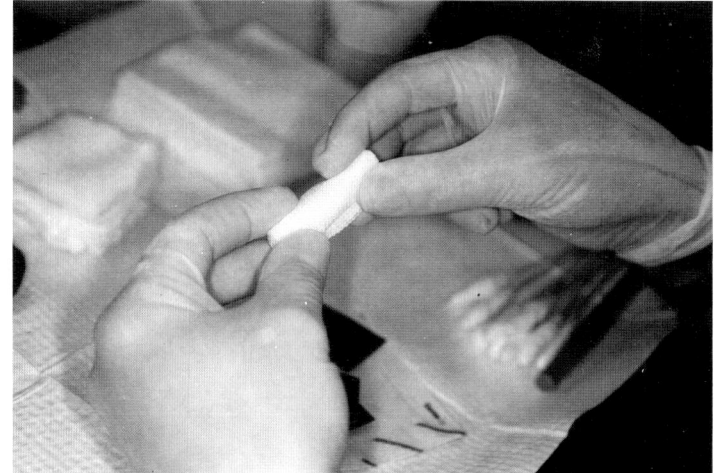

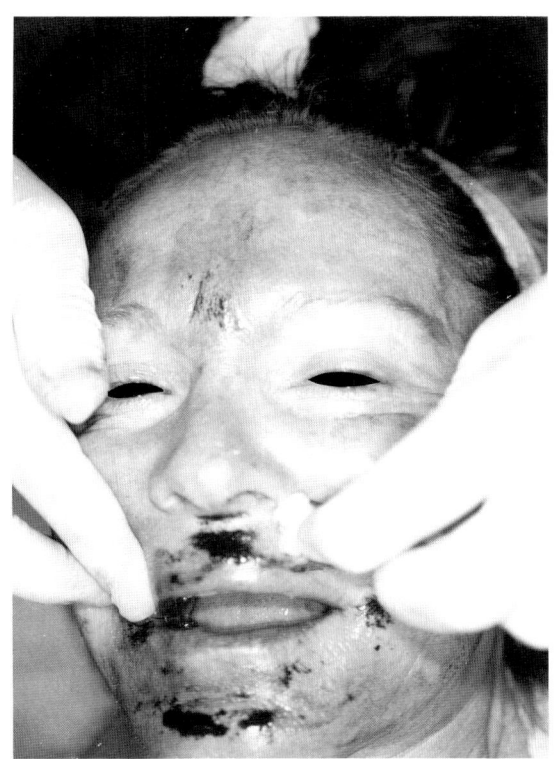

FIGURE 18.4. A. The sandpaper is folded around 2 pieces of rolled 2-inch by 2-inch gauze. B. The skin is stretched and gently abraded until the glistening layer and bleeding points are appreciated.

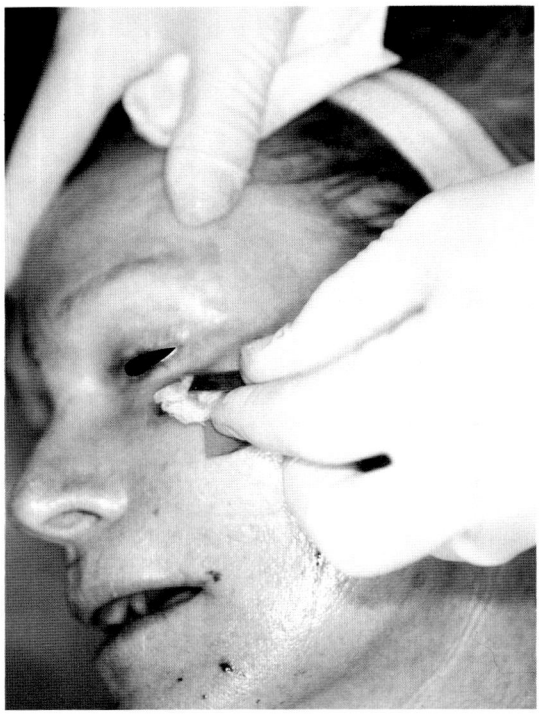

FIGURE 18.5. Fine sandpaper, grade #400, is utilized in abrading over delicate periorbital areas and at the lid margin; irregular stretch marks at the periphery ensure no sharp lines of demarcation.

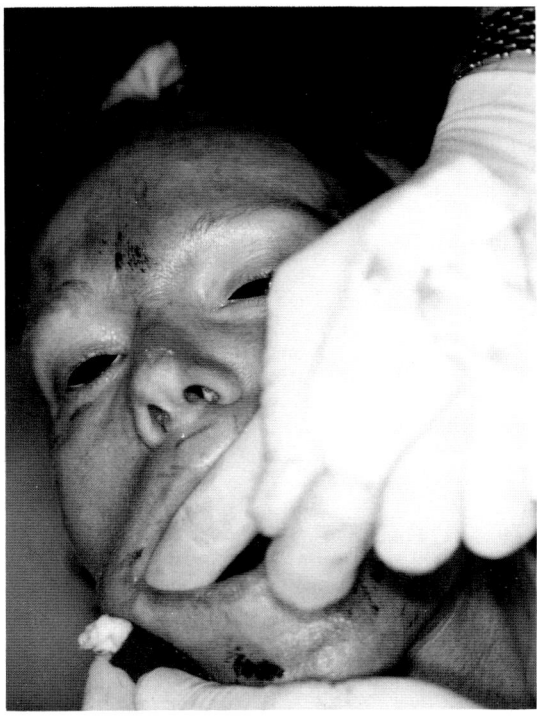

FIGURE 18.6. Medium grade #220–#320 allows the physician to abrade the stretched lips and perioral margins safely and without difficulty.

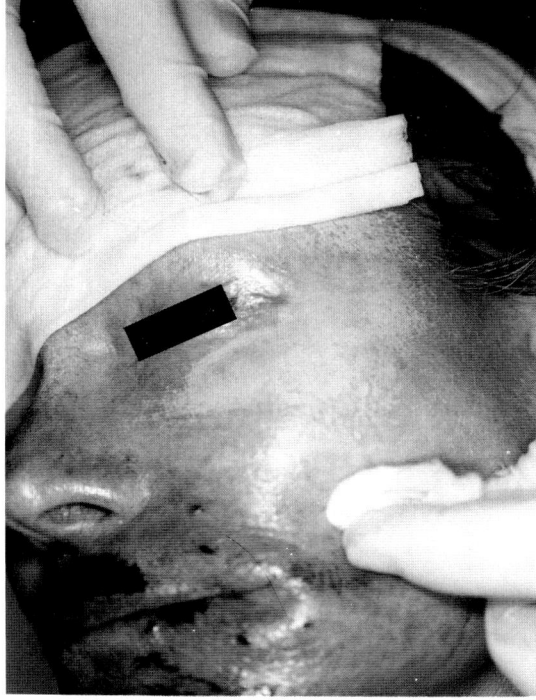

FIGURE 18.7. 25% trichloroacetic acid applied with 2-inch by 2-inch gauze pads completes the procedure.

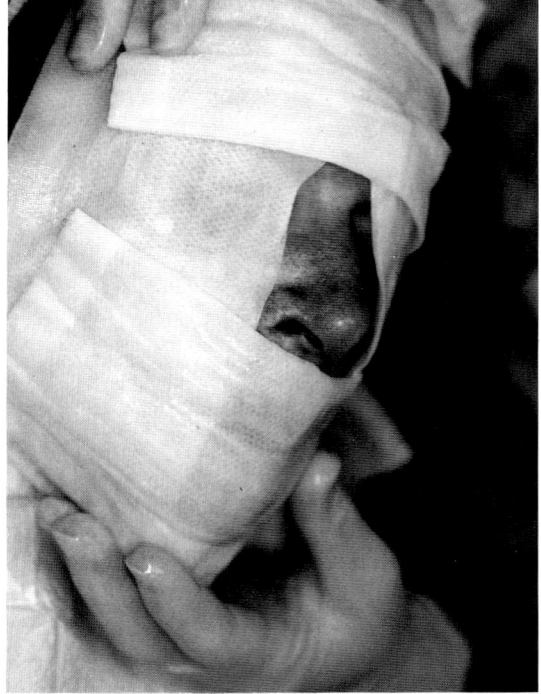

FIGURE 18.8. Iced compresses are necessary, for discomfort is common with application of the acid.

mixture of silver-sulfadiazine and Aquaphor (Figure 18.9). The patient is advised to clean the skin several times daily with a soap-free cleanser (Cetaphil, Aquanil, SFC), removing all silver-sulfadiazine before reapplying the cream. During the first 3 to 5 days, there is a generalized edema, as well as oozing at more aggressively abraded sites. After the fifth day, edema subsides, and complete shedding of a fine crust is complete at 7 to 10 days. While some note discomfort during the first few days, most patients find the silver-sulfadiazine applications quite comfortable. Infection is negligible, and crusts remain moist and flexible. Delayed healing or increased tenderness after 10 days demands immediate attention, regardless of the texturing procedure employed.

Expected Results

Following desquamation of crust, most patients note a degree of erythema at sites abraded to bleeding points. Skin that has been painted with TCA after sanding to glistening layer alone shows little change in color tone (Figure 18.10). Erythema may last anywhere from 1 to several months, but it is easily covered with makeup and fades nicely over time (Figure 18.11).

Most patients are pleased to find that 70% to 90% of their rhytids, especially in the glabella, perioral and periorbital areas, are either greatly improved or removed (Figures 18.12A and B). In addition, the skin is decidedly brighter and more lustrous (Figures 18.13A and B). We have

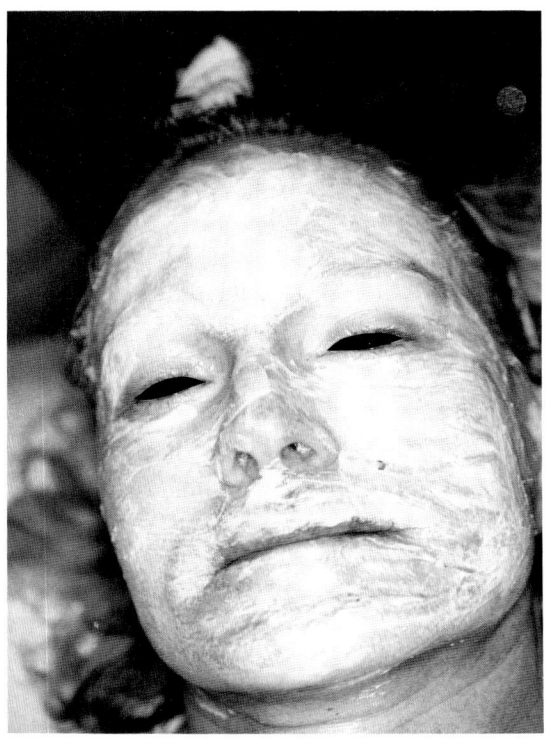

FIGURE 18.9. After icing, the skin is covered with silver-sulfadiazine cream and petrolatum. This is removed gently and fresh cream applied several times daily.

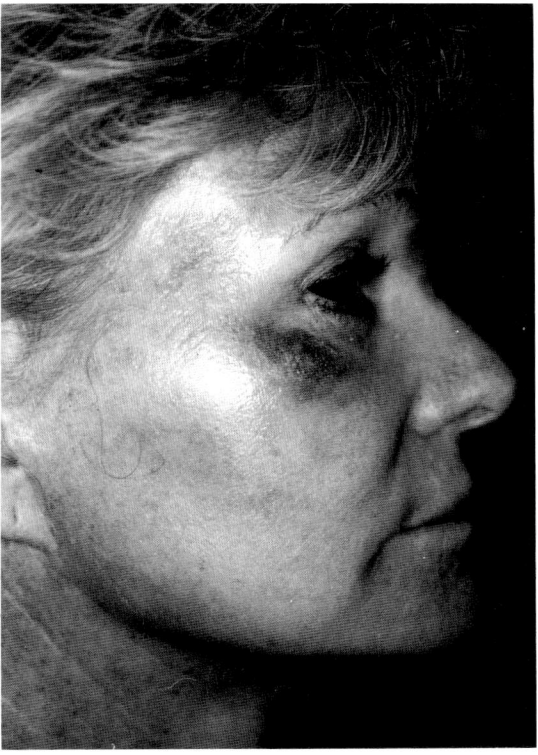

FIGURE 18.10. After desquamation of crust, erythema is appreciated in areas more vigorously abraded to bleeding points.

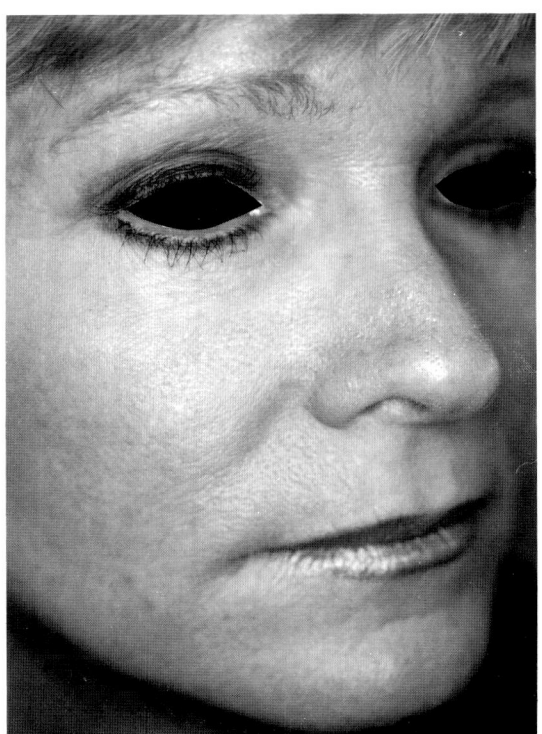

FIGURE 18.11. Erythema will fade over 30 to 120 days, leaving a uniform skin tone.

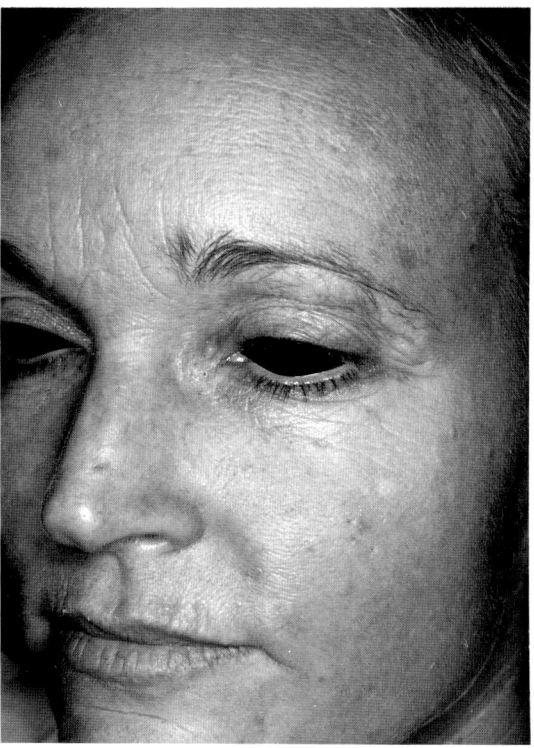
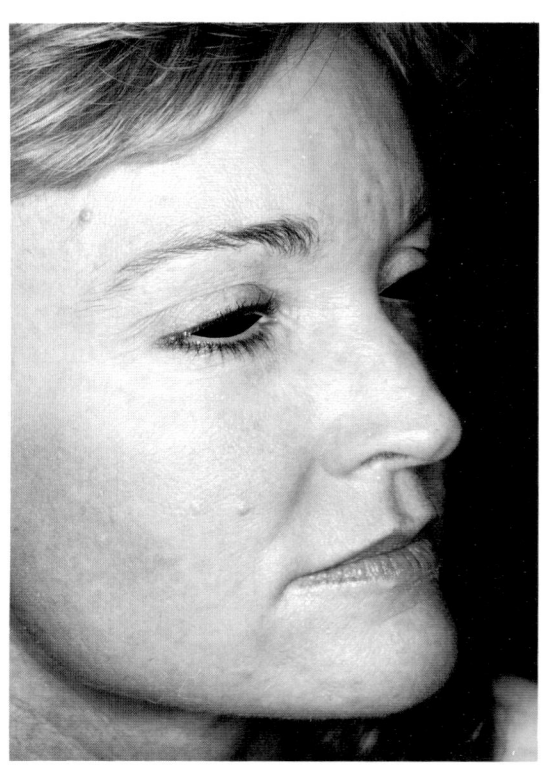

FIGURE 18.12. A. Before the procedure. B. Six weeks following the procedure. Most patients find that 70% to 90% of rhytids are improved or removed after the procedure.

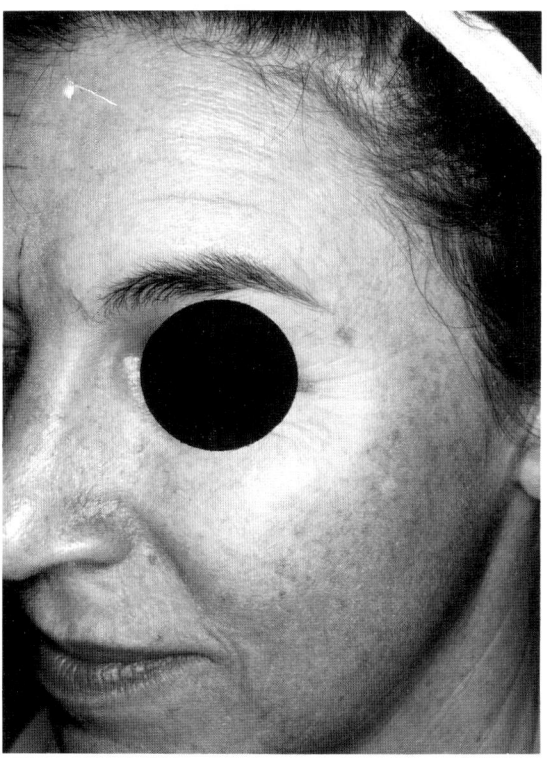 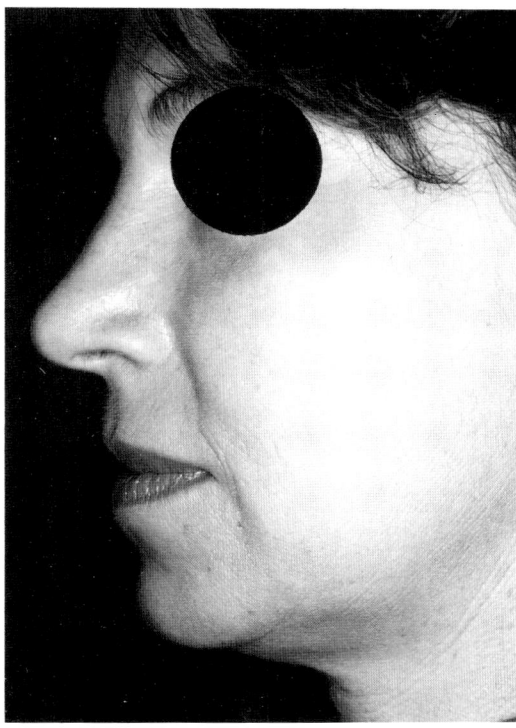

FIGURE 18.13. A. Before the procedure. B. Three months following the procedure. Dyschromia is greatly improved, with generalized lightening of the skin.

had only a handful of patients who, over a period of several months, noticed long-delayed focal hypopigmentation in a few small spots, in spite of no depigmentation at test sites.

Advantages of the Procedure

This manual abrasion technique demands little skill or experience to deliver an effective result. Moreover, there is no splatter, as is the case with motor-driven dermabrasion. A most beneficial aspect about using abrasive papers manually is that there are no sharp lines of demarcation following the procedure, and the efficacy of low-strength TCA is, of course, greatly accentuated with the removal of the stratum corneum barrier.

Finally, at future visits it is quick and easy to simply "touch up" small rhytids that were not completely removed during the initial procedure. The physician need not set aside special time for touch-ups, which can be accomplished in a matter of a minute or two during an office visit (Table 18.2).

Other uses associated with photodamaged skin include the treatment of actinic cheilitis, or leukoplakia.[12] After local anesthesia, the affected lips and vermilion are abraded with a silicone carbide paper to bleeding points and painted with 25% trichloroacetic acid. The crust separates in a matter of several days, leaving a softer, more uniform lip with obvious

TABLE 18.2. Advantages of manual dermasanding combined with light TCA peeling.

Advantages
Minimal skill and experience for uniformly pleasing results
Simple and safe to use at margins of the lips and eyelids
No splatter
No sharp lines of demarcation
Simple and fast to repeat ("touch-up" spots)
Depigmentation and scarring rare

clinical improvement. Additional uses include the treatment of all manner of scarring, including acne, surgical and traumatic.

Finally, we are asked if silicone granulomas are ever an issue with dermasanding. We have encountered absolutely no foreign bodies from silicone carbide sandpaper abrasion in more than 8 years of experience.

Vignette #2

Cosmetics vs. Cosmeceuticals: A New Rational Science

Nia K. Terezakis

We are an appearance-driven society, and cosmetics are almost programmed into our genetic and social nature. Every culture has evidence of personal adornment and cosmesis of some form. Anthropologists describe the urge to transform and improve one's body as almost akin to instinct and equally present in prehistoric times as in the twentieth century.

Although cosmetic products and procedures primarily alter the skin surface, their beneficial effects may transform the entire person. Modern cosmetics retain the same functions that ancient ones served, with the result that psychological health as well as human needs and sexual attraction are often fulfilled. The importance of the psychological benefits of cosmetics has spawned a new science as well as a new and important therapeutic technique.

The cosmetics industry has evolved over the last 50 to 60 years from an era of "secret formulas," "elusive promises," and "false hope" to an entirely new industry based on science. No longer are the cosmetic giants isolated scions, but there is an ever growing interaction and interdependence among cosmeceutical, pharmaceutical, biochemical, and medical laboratories.

New developments have been successfully translated into more effective treatments as well as preventive treatments for dry or aging skin. The problems of oily skin have also been addressed in a scientific way. Many of these new "treatment cosmetics" are serendipitous side effects of medications for diseased skin.

Because of a more educated, informed and inquiring populus, advertising hype has been challenged by healthy skepticism. Pseudoscience is being replaced by applied science.

For many years the cosmetics industry directed the basics of skin care sometimes passing on unscientific information as "facts." In the last 2 decades dermatologists have begun to reeducate the public in terms of basic skin care and preventive measures via sound therapeutic scientific developments. Thus cosmeceuticals were born.

Although aging may be predetermined by heredity and inefficient tissue metabolism, our new sciences offer hope of reversal and rejuvenation through our new therapeutics.

The cosmetics of the future are now products of the true specialists in skin care. Dermatology as a specialty has contributed a new form of cosmetics. "Educated cosmetics," "treatment cosmetics," "performance products"—call them what you may, but cosmeceuticals initiate a new era in personal adornment based on rational and scientific facts.

But let us not become so smug as to believe that we did this alone or that we can isolate ourselves in our new science. As never before the interactions of the cosmetic, pharmaceutical, and medical industries will ensure new products for the twenty-first century that not only beautify and adorn the skin but scientifically change the skin in a more positive and meaningful way.

Vignette #3

Cryosurgery

Gloria F. Graham

Cryosurgery is a versatile tool in the treatment of the aging face. Lesions of actinic keratoses that do not respond to tretinoin and/or 5-fluorouracil may be cleared with 5 to 10 seconds of freezing with a spray of liquid nitrogen using any one of several cryosurgical units. While many dermatologists prefer using a spray, probes are also available with most units, and cotton swabs continue to be used by many for treatment of benign and premalignant lesions. Cotton swabs, however, are inadequate for treating deeper lesions, especially those present in the dermis. A new technique described by Chiarello,[13] full face cryosurgical peeling, results in clearing of actinic keratoses, lentigos, seborrheic keratoses, and an overall improved cosmetic appearance to the skin (Figures 18.14, 18.15, and 18.16).

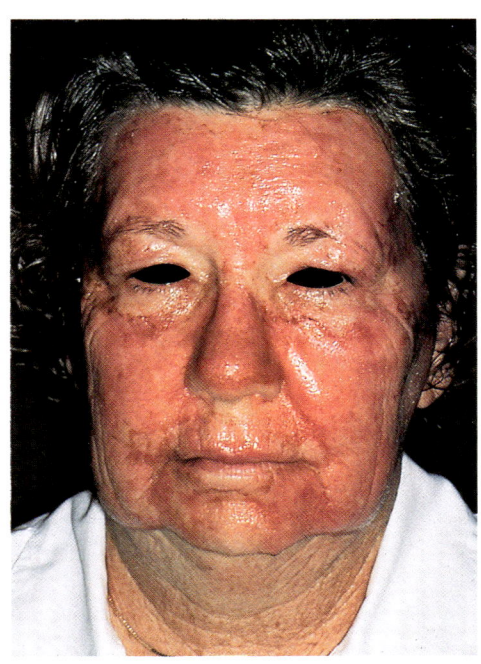

FIGURE 18.15. Four days after cryopeel. There is marked edema, erythema and weeping.

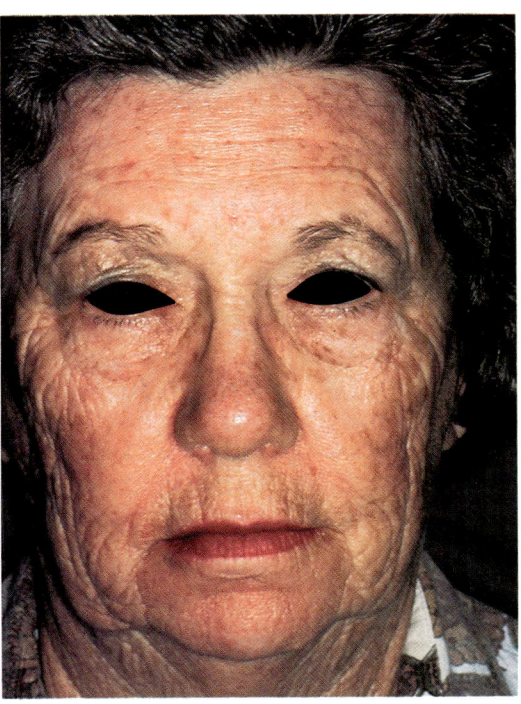

FIGURE 18.14. Sixty-eight-year-old female with multiple actinic keratoses and severe photo damage.

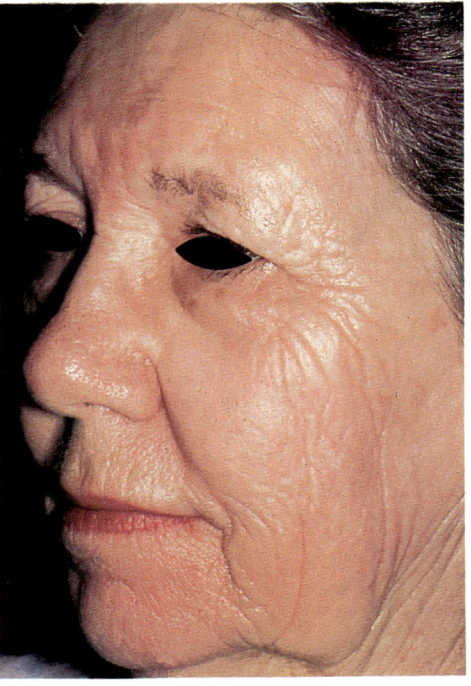

FIGURE 18.16. Seven months post cryopeel. Keratoses are gone, wrinkles improved, and the overall color and texture of the skin is better.

The cure rate of actinic keratoses reported by Lubritz and Smolewski is 98%.[14] Some thick and hypertrophic lesions may require a second freeze. Bowenoid actinic keratoses, hypertrophic, and comedonal actinic keratoses require 20 to 30 seconds of LN spray using a B tip on the CryAC unit.[15]

Lentigines that do not respond to tretinoin, hydroquinone, or alpha hydroxy acids respond well to cryosurgery, since the melanocyte is quite cold-sensitive. Freeze times vary from 7 to 10 seconds using the B tip. Levin compared laser surgery with freezing and found that freezing worked as well or better and was more cost-effective.[16]

While extensive and flatter seborrheic keratoses respond well to freezing, thicker lesions are best treated by electrodesiccation or freezing, followed by curettage. Freeze times are usually 10 to 15 seconds or longer using the B tip. Freezing should be continued until a 1 to 2 mm halo of freeze extends beyond the visible border of the tumor. Some very thick tumors may require up to 30 seconds of freezing.

Basal cell carcinoma, squamous cell carcinoma, keratoacanthoma, and lentigo maligna all yield high cure rates with cryosurgery, usually in the 96% to 99% range.[17-20] Freeze times range from 45 to 90 seconds for most tumors, with halo thaw times of 60 seconds or longer and clinical, or complete, thawing of 1½ to 5 minutes. A double freeze/thaw cycle is preferred in deeper lesions, especially those 3 mm or greater in depth, combining freezing with a shave excision of the tumor, followed by curettage, which has yielded the highest cure rate.[15] A freezing halo of normal tissue around the tumor should be about 0.5 cm or greater.

The care of the cryosurgical wound, which is nature's own biological dressing, is quite simple. Since it is wet and exudative shortly after the procedure, a dressing may be applied. However, many prefer cleansing with soap and water, leaving the wound open to the air.

Cryosurgery is a cost-effective, convenient method used by many dermatologists for treating multiple benign and malignant skin tumors. Cure rates are high and cosmetic results good when proper attention is paid to freeze times.

Vignette #4

Evaluation and Treatment of the Aging Face

Richard G. Glogau

As the much vaunted baby boomer generation moves into their fourth and fifth decades of life, it is obvious to dermatologists that there will be major problems to be addressed in the area of treatment of photoaging. The current surge of interest in chemical peeling reflects more than a changing practice profile on the part of the dermatologists who are being battered by socioeconomic changes in health care delivery. The reality is that we are seeing extensive photodamage in individuals whose fates were sealed during the Eisenhower years. One wonders whether the wide availability of sunscreens will affect this pattern in the coming decades or whether the emphasis on outdoor activities will continue to provide ever increasing populations of wrinkled, sun-damaged skin.

Almost every patient over age 30 in our practice is a candidate for some form of pharmaceutical or chemical resurfacing, not only on the basis of premature wrinkling, but many have palpable and visible keratoses just beginning. The challenge is to find just the right degree of superficial injury that will permit the normal wound healing process to reestablish a more desirable papillary dermal network of collagen and elastin and a regenerated epidermis with normal pigment and adnexae.

There are two directions for future research. We must concentrate our efforts on developing agents that alter epidermal penetration in a controlled way. By varying the degree of penetration, we can look forward to the day when we can "tune" the peel more specifically to the skin type and extent of photodamage. Retinoic acid and alpha hydroxy acids are only the initial moves in this direction.

The second area that begs more light is the biological response to injury. What are the desirable components of the inflammatory reaction that might be selectively augmented or suppressed to enhance the effectiveness of the chemical peel? We have embarrassingly little information that is clinically useful in this regard.

Vignette #5

The Ligmaject

Arnold William Klein

Keloids and hypertrophic scars are difficult surgical problems. Although there are many therapeutic modalities and dressings currently in vogue, intralesional steroids remain the mainstay of therapy. Oftentimes while attempting to inject such lesions, the operator utilizing a simple syringe cannot generate enough pressure to implant steroid in the tough collagen matrix of the scar. Furthermore, without excellent control the steroid is easily extravasated into the surrounding tissue, resulting in the most undesirable sequelae of pseudoatrophy.

Many years ago we became intrigued with the Ligmaject. It is primarily utilized for dental anesthesia and accepts the normal anesthetic carpules. Force is generated by the instrument via a spring whose action is controlled by a simple trigger (Figure 18.17). By way of cartridges prefilled by the operator with triamcinolone acetonide of various strengths (10, 20, 30, and 40 mg/cc) it became the ideal device to inject even the toughest scar. That is, one squeeze of the trigger accurately delivers 0.2 cc of the contained solution under a much greater pressure than can be generated with a simple syringe. Furthermore, there is greater control of injection, obviating the worrisome problem of pseudoatrophy. Prior to injection, a light freeze of the intended scar with liquid nitrogen makes this procedure even easier.

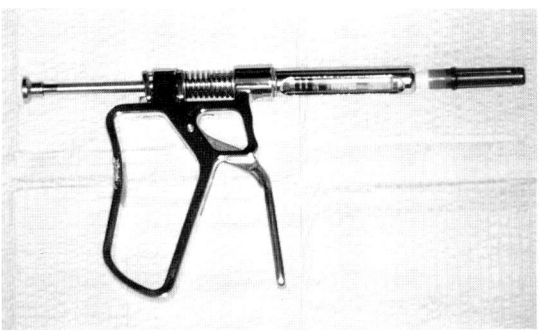

FIGURE 18.17. The Ligmaject.

Vignette #6

The Dermatologist's Role in Treating the Aging Skin

Sheldon V. Pollack

Where facial aging is concerned, one of the most evident developments in the past decade has been the increasing involvement of dermatologists in its treatment. The future is likely to yield even greater participation by dermatologic surgeons, not only as providers of established techniques but also as innovators in this flourishing field. This is not surprising, considering past significant contributions by dermatologists to the development of dermabrasion, hair transplantation, injectable dermal augmentation, laser therapy, chemical peeling, and liposuction.

The dermatologist's advantage in upcoming years will continue to be a broad-based familiarity with the histology, physiology, anatomy, and care of skin. Upon this framework we will, as in the past, build our artistic and innovative approach to cost-effective patient care. We will search for more effective ways to enhance the currently available facial rejuvenation techniques of removal, resurfacing, recontouring, and redraping, discussed so aptly in this text.

We have become aware of an increasing global interest by dermatologists in venting their artistic talents through the treatment of again skin. Fortunately, as a medical community, we have unlimited talent within our ranks and more than enough thoughtful teachers to educate not only ourselves but also interested colleagues from other surgical specialties. We must, however, endeavor to maintain our recent preeminence in facial rejuvenation within the broader context of our historical role as experts in the diagnosis and treatment of all skin disease. In this way we will maintain our advantage in a very crowded arena.

Vignette #7

Microsurgical Treatment of the Aging Face

Toshio Kobayashi

Recent experimentation with a new surgical technique involving the use of an operative microscope for accuracy in skin surface removal has proven successful in the treatment of larger facial wrinkles and age spots (lentigines). Nasolabial, glabellar, and upper lip wrinkles have been treated with a technique involving the precise removal of surrounding upper skin layers with microscissors (micropeeling) followed immediately by the direct excision of the target wrinkle. This technique is based on the premise that a wide superficial scar will form over and camouflage an underlying linear scar.[21,22]

Lentigines and other pigmentary marks can be treated using the micropeeling procedure only. Due to the absence of intense heat or cold and disuse of chemical agents, the occurrence of secondary pigmentary alteration is greatly reduced.

The operative technique is shown in Figures 18.18A, B, and C. The wrinkle is first outlined so that the area to be removed is equal to that of the redundant skin. Other lines are made about 3 mm beyond the first to mark the surrounding area for micropeeling.

After local anesthetic application, light parallel incisions, 0.7 to 1.0 mm apart, are made in the outer area with a number 11 blade. While the area is held taut with the operator's fourth and fifth fingers, each strip is grasped and pulled up with microforceps and then cut with microscissors. The peeling level should be within the upper reticular dermis. This level is important for achieving good results.

The wrinkle area is excised and intradermal sutures are made using very thin suture mate-

18. Surgical Vignettes

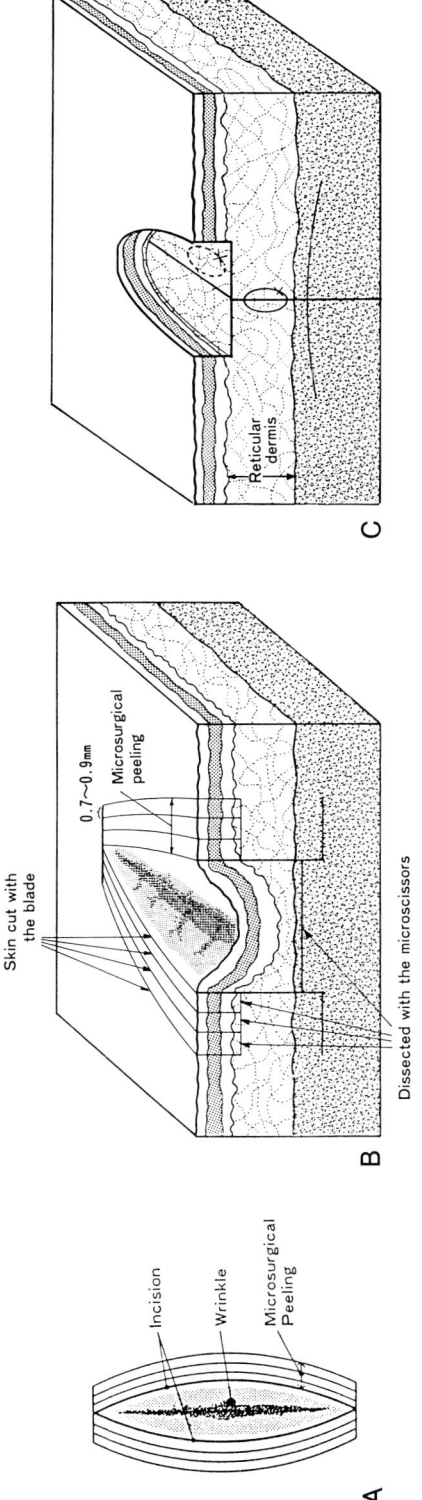

FIGURE 18.18. A. Overview of a wrinkle marked for excision and micropeeling. B. Lateral view. The surrounding skin is removed only to the depth of the upper reticular dermis, but the target wrinkle is completely excised. C. Lateral view after wrinkle removal and intradermal suturing.

rial. These are followed by superficial sutures and the application of a dressing.

Healing is complete in about a week, and postoperative redness disappears 3 or 4 months later.

Results from the removal of vertical wrinkles (glabellar and upper lip) have been found to be excellent, while those after the removal of horizontal wrinkles (as on the forehead) are less acceptable. Typical results are shown in Figures 18.19A and B as well as in Figures 18.20A and B.

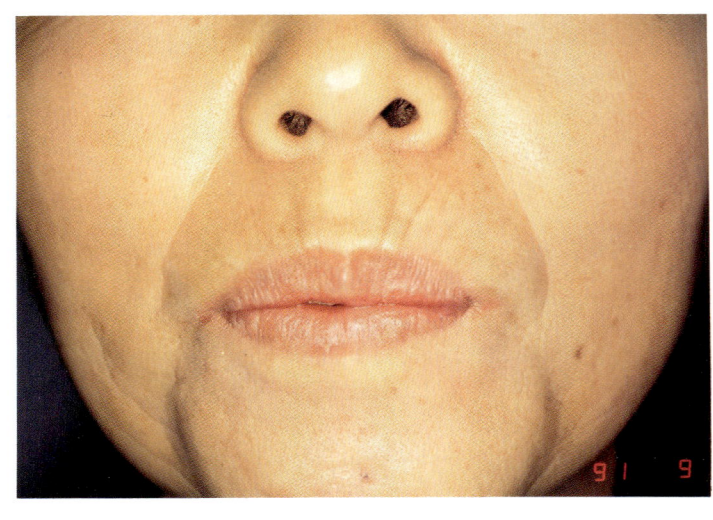

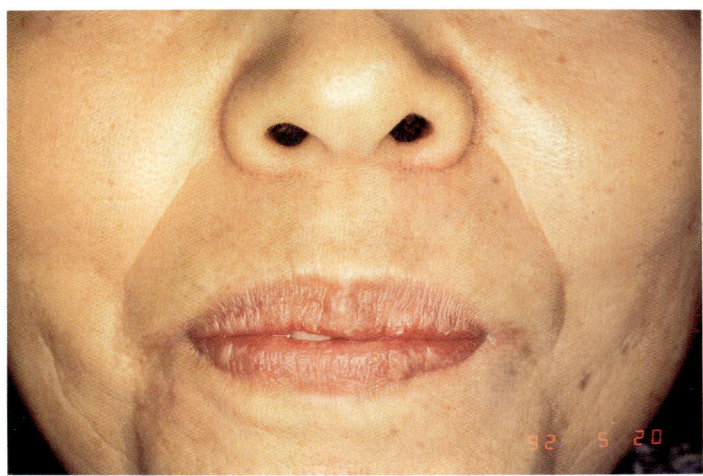

FIGURE 18.19. A. A preoperative view of a patient with upper lip wrinkles. B. The same patient 8 months after microsurgical peeling and immediate direct excision.

18. Surgical Vignettes

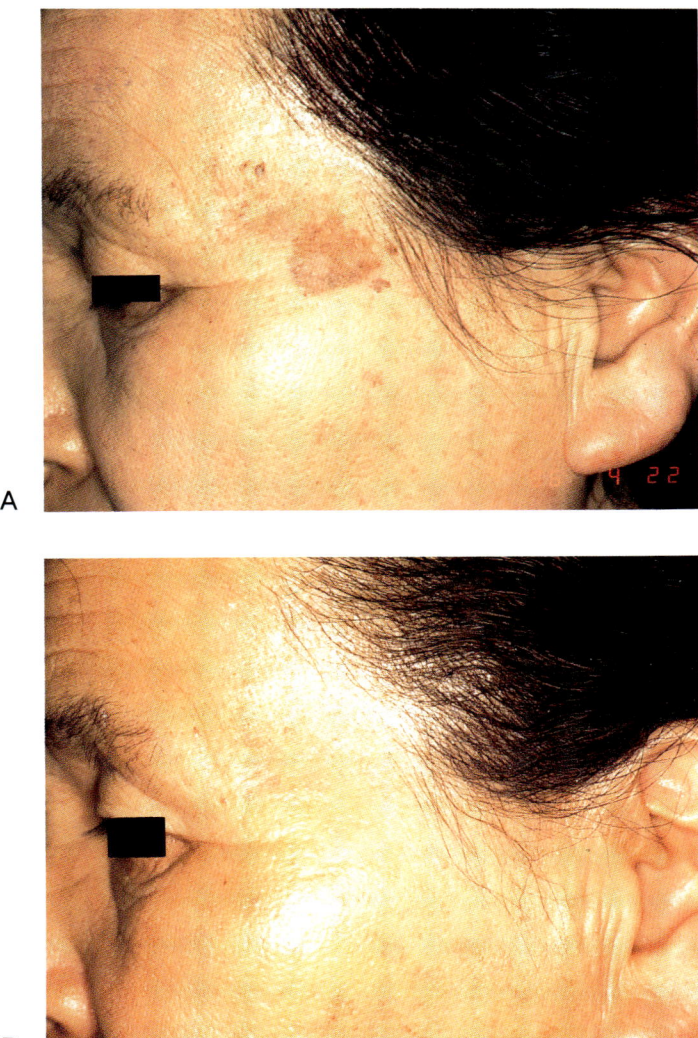

FIGURE 18.20. A. A preoperative view of a patient with senile lentigines. B. The same patient 2 years after microsurgical peeling.

Vignette #8

Vitamins: Therapy for Aging?

Wilma F. Bergfeld and
Thomas N. Helm

Aging is a complex process that involves not only chronological changes but also the effects of physical agents such as ultraviolet light on the skin. The facial changes associated with aging are often most troubling to a sense of well-being and positive self-image. Surgical modalities such as rhytidectomy and chemical peels offer gratifying improvements that are achieved over a relatively short period of time. Other agents such as tretinoin have more gradual effects.

Whether or not vitamins and micronutrients can influence the aging process is unclear and so far unproven. Nonetheless, we feel that a greater understanding of antioxidants and vitamins offers much promise as a preventive form of therapy for aging. The hypothesis that these agents can help slow aging changes will likely remain unproven for many years, because of the enormity of the scope of changes considered integral to the process of aging. The science of aging and gerontology has only recently been pursued by rigorous scientific method, in part because in past decades estimated survival was considerably less than life expectancy today and the intrinsic limitations of the human body to withstand the onslaught of time in the absence of a primary disease process was a problem besetting only a relatively small segment of society.

Vitamin therapy, especially with vitamins A, C, and E, does appear to have positive effects on a variety of physiological functions. Extrapolating some of these changes to cutaneous physiology is not unreasonable. Vitamin E helps stabilize lipid membranes[23] and decrease photoreceptor membrane shedding,[24] and it protects the endocardium of rabbits on a high-fat diet from endocardial changes when given in concert with selenium.[25] In skin models ascorbate can donate electrons to vitamin E derivatives so that vitamin E is recycled.[26] This, however, diminishes the reserve of antioxidants like ascorbate.[26] Vitamin E appears to be unable to prevent DNA breaks induced by ultraviolet B light but may prevent UVB-induced cytotoxicity by scavenging free radicals.[27] Ointment consisting of sunflower oil, beeswax sintopholin, chloramphenicol, procaine, and vitamin E is said to promote healing of burns in test animals.[28] Whether the vitamin E is helpful or not in this regard, or whether the benefits noted are simply from the occlusive effect of the ointment, remains to be shown. Low levels of vitamin E have been associated with degenerative changes of aging and impart increased risk for cataracts, cancer, and decreased immunity in addition to increased atherosclerosis.[29]

Vitamin C in conjunction with vitamin E appears to be particularly helpful. Mice pretreated with both vitamin C and vitamin E had a decrease elastogenic effect from X rays.[30] Other effects such as postburn capillary permeability are decreased by vitamin C, minimizing need for fluid replacement.[31] Other beneficial effects such as decreased bronchoconstriction and increased collagen production in skin fibroblast cultures have been ascribed to treatment with vitamin C.[32,33] Selenium has been shown to increase concentrations of IgG2 and IgG4 in children with Down syndrome.[34]

In a personal communication Dr. Sheldon Pinnell has described his studies on the photoprotective effects of topical ascorbate on laboratory animals subject to UVB exposure. His preliminary data suggest that pretreatment with topical vitamin C can decrease the number of dyskeratotic "sunburn cells."

The effects of vitamins on cancer, cataract formation, and other oxidative stresses to the body suggest that they likely have important effects on the skin as well. In addition to corrective therapies for damaged skin, preventive treatment will have a greater role in the future. It is our feeling that tretinoin is just one agent that may have a positive effect in altering the manifestations of cutaneous aging. Ensuring proper dietary intake of these agents will likely affect aging over time. Unfortunately, more than 40% of men in one study had less than two-thirds of the recommended daily allowance of vitamins A and E in their diet, and more than 40% of women had less than two-thirds of the recommended daily allowance of vitamin E.[34,35] Clearly, further work in this area and greater awareness of the effect of diet and vitamins on health and aging are required.

Vignette #9

European View of Evaluation and Treatment of the Aging Face

Eckart Hancke

The treatment of the aging face as performed by German dermatologists is predominantly conservative. There are two main reasons for this attitude: First, compulsory social and health insurances cover more than 80% of the German population, and the remainder have private insurances; people are not used to paying their doctors what they would have to for cosmetic surgical procedures that are not reimbursed by the insurance. Second, although almost everybody wants to become old and nobody wants to look old, aging is accepted as a natural process by the society. Many of our patients, consulting for example for multiple actinic keratoses and skin cancer, have to be convinced that treatment of the entire face would not only be a cosmetic procedure but an effective therapy for subclinical precancerous lesions, solar lentigines, and actinic elastosis, with considerable aesthetic improvement being a side-effect. These patients usually want to be reassured that they will be reimbursed by their insurance.

Our approach in more than 90% of the patients is an informative discussion about aging, photodamage, and their consequences; and treatment options, with pros and cons of different methods. Our preferred management of the aging photodamaged face is removal of any lesion suspicious for advanced precancer or invasive cancer as well as of thick seborrheic keratoses and pretreatment with retinoic acid. Six to 8 weeks after wound healing, a full face, medium-strength Jessner's solution and trichloroacetic acid peel is done. Because of increasing public concern regarding toxicity, phenol peels are rarely performed. Retinoic acid treatment is reinstituted after complete re-epithelialization, starting with once every other day and increasing the application frequency until a slightly pink skin appears.

Mainly young female subjects may ask for a laser treatment of wrinkles. However, their expectations are almost always very unrealistic, and we therefore refuse to use the laser for this purpose. Laser abrasion is certainly not superior to dermabrasion and is not considered by us to be appropriately used for the aging face. However, the attitude of cosmetic surgeons in Germany does not differ from that in any other country.

Vignette #10

The "How Did This Happen to Me?" Syndrome

Daniel A. Gross

In the middle of a procedure you experience that uneasy feeling that all is not going well; an internal voice informs you that you missed earlier clues that suggested that this doctor–patient relationship would be a most difficult one for all parties. Perhaps it is a short period of time after the procedure is completed that the voice relates this information to you. Perhaps it is months after what you believe was a successful procedure and you are having problems with a dissatisfied or angry patient. Your response may be the following: "Why didn't I listen to that feeling? I wish I were elsewhere." This is not an unusual situation; it is one that every physician has experienced at one time or another.

The above is not the experience of a doctor and patient who together confront one of the known surgical complications. To the contrary, this is an event in which you noted an internal feeling of discomfort or anxiety during the presurgical interaction with your patient but didn't recognize the feeling. Now, during the procedure or during the postoperative period, you realize that your conscious judgment was in error and it is too late to do anything more to improve the situation. Typically, there is a satisfactory outcome; however, this is not always the case, and the solution is realized in a courtroom. How can such situations be prevented?

We recommend that each physician become aware of those subtle feelings that we all have during each patient interaction. Your capacity to receive and properly interpret information on two levels is significant and must become part of the interaction. For example:

1. Did you note that the patient believed that this procedure would have tremendous impact upon his or her life?
2. Did the patient show no emotion or reaction upon your discussion of potential complications associated with the procedure?
3. Did the patient ask an extraordinary number of questions regarding the procedure?
4. Did the patient indicate that this procedure would require a significant sacrifice in his or her life?

Perhaps a checklist should be associated with each patient interaction. Among the questions for this list might be the following:

1. Am I communicating with the patient?
2. Does the patient truly comprehend what I am saying?
3. Am I correctly interpreting what the patient is telling me, both verbally and nonverbally?
4. Do we share the same realistic goals?
5. Am I confident that this is the right choice for the patient?
6. Am I confident that this is the right choice for the physician?
7. If the results of the surgery are less than acceptable, will I feel that I never should have done this surgery?

These questions are not totally inclusive of all significant aspects of the relationship; however, they can act as guides. If there is a concern regarding any of the above questions and/or answers, then additional consultation(s) may be necessary. Surgery is not something that can always be repeated until you get it right. Take the time to do it right the first time.

Vignette #11

The Use of Gore-Tex Combined with Other Fillers

Alejandro Camps-Fresneda

Any material used to fill wrinkles, folds, and other depressions of the skin should satisfy the following requirements. It should be safe (sterile, not unhygienic, not carcinogenic) and effective (in the sense that the results should last for as long a time as possible). At present the principal materials used for this purpose are silicone, bovine collagen, and Fibrel gel, alone or in combination to give greater support to each of them, or a combination of some of them. We suggest the application of Gore-tex thread (PTFE-2N07) in the deep dermis. This acts as a support, leveling the fold and making it possible to use a smaller quantity of the other fillers.

For the treatment of superficial wrinkles, we should use those fillers that can be applied in the upper areas of the dermis. When dealing with folds or deep wrinkles, it is more convenient to use fillers that help to repair the defect in the deeper areas; this is where Gore-tex is especially interesting.

Gore-tex is a synthetic material, long lasting and inert, presented in a plaque form, which can be cut in any way necessary, depending on the area to be filled[36,37]; or in the form of a suture thread, a form that has recently begun to be used as a filler.[38] From the chemical point of view, Gore-tex is a synthetic polymer (polytetra-fluoro-ethylene). It is one of the most inert polymers known. It does not provoke allergic reactions, it is not carcinogenic, and it does not produce foreign body reactions.[39]

The application techniques of collagen and silicone (350 CS) in microdroplets are well known. With respect to the former agent, there is the advantage that its filling effects are immediately noticeable after only one application; however, this action does not last very long. Concerning the latter agent, its action is long lasting, but several applications are necessary to be able to see its filling effects.

Gore-tex alone, implanted in the naso-genian folds, glabellar fold, and upper lip area, as well as in other zones, has an immediate effect, superior to a single application of silicone but much inferior to a single application of collagen, despite being able to place several threads in the deeper dermis in only 1 session. On the other hand, the effects of this implantation are permanent; and, in the case of the first application being insufficient to repair the defect completely, it is possible to place as many threads as are necessary in the same area. A prudent time should pass between treatments to guarantee that there are no effects of intolerance due to an incorrect application during the first treatment.

Before proceeding to insert the thread (folded twice, 4 times, or however many times may be considered necessary), the 2 ends of the fold or wrinkle to be treated should be anesthetized. Using a straight needle, the type normally used in general surgery, enter perpendicularly in the skin at 1 end of the fold until reaching the deeper dermis, where the direction of the needle is changed to continue parallel to the surface, always at the level of the deeper dermis. When the other end of the fold has been reached, the needle is brought out perpendicularly. The threads are then tensed and the treated area is gently squeezed between the thumb and index finger, always keeping the threads tensed. At this moment the assistant quickly cuts the 2 extremes of the thread and the area is released rapidly in such a way that the ends of the threads are pulled away from the epidermis and are buried deeply in the dermis. It is fundamental that if there is any doubt that an end of the thread or threads has remained near the surface, the threads must be removed and the process repeated.

Some authors[38] consider it necessary to administer oral antibiotics for some days following the intervention. But this choice depends on the individual dermatologist.

As noted previously, Gore-tex applied in the above-mentioned way can also be used as a support for other fillers, basically collagen and silicone.[40] Once the thread has been put in place and after the disappearance of the edema caused by the anesthetic and the moderate inflammation caused by the manipulation of the tissue, the results obtained are assessed. If these are insufficient, proceed to an additional filler using 1 or more of those mentioned earlier, in general using smaller quantities than would be necessary without the support of Gore-tex. Experience in the treatment of some very accentuated defects and the guarantee of a correct application of Gore-tex make it possible to combine both treatments in the same session. This consequently means fewer sessions and less cost to the patient.

Vignette #12

The "Sandwich Technique" for Filling the Nasolabial Fold

António Picoto

A deep nasolabial fold gives an impression of sadness and older age, so naturally, all the techniques available to suppress or attenuate this effect are greatly appreciated. But patients want quick results, with no pain and no need for hospitalization and withdrawal from work and social activities.

For many years we used injections of silicone with good results, but it takes time for the effect to supervene. If the folds are really deep, we normally tell the patients that they should expect 2 to 4 injections and 1 year of treatment. As is well known, silicone is difficult to inject and produces some pain. Local anesthesia distorts the anatomy; and hence, we do not use it injecting silicone.

In the last 2 years we have developed a technique that solves all these problems quoted. It has an immediate effect, is lasting, and produces no pain. So far we have had excellent results. We term this the "Sandwich Technique":

1. Take clinical photos, before and after the procedure.
2. The patient can be sedated if he or she wishes. We use Valium (R) 10 mg per os, 10 minutes before the procedure.
3. Apply EMLA® cream liberally, filling the two folds. In Caucasians it stays for 30 minutes, no occlusion needed; when the skin turns whitish, superficial anesthesia is achieved. For darker skin wait 40 minutes.
4. Inject Zyderm II using the regular technique (previous double skin testing). With Zyderm II or in severe cases, Zyplast, an immediate effect erasing the sulcus is achieved and anesthesia is now deep because of the lidocaine content of the Zyderm.
5. Next inject silicone Sebbin, 1 cc in each sulcus. As usual the silicone is injected deeply and we always do the multipuncture technique.
6. The patient is advised to apply cold compresses immediately after the procedure, and normal life is resumed immediately.

Vignette #13

Crosslinked Hyaluronic Acid (Hylan Gel) as a Soft Tissue Augmentation Material: A Preliminary Assessment

Daniel Piacquadio

Hyaluronic acid (HA) is an ubiquitous component of all mammalian connective tissue, where it forms an integral part of the intercellular matrix and creates the elastoviscous, hydrating, lubricating and stabilizing matrix in which cells are embedded.[41] Pure HA, however, even in its largest polymeric form (5×10^6 MW) cannot provide the physical properties needed for most medical applications, including soft tissue augmentation. Hyaluronic acid derivatives have therefore been developed that have enhanced rheological properties but yet maintain the desired biological properties of natural HA.[42] Hylan gel is a viscoelastic, insoluble, crosslinked derivative of the natural hyaluronan polymer. Hylan gel is obtained by a chemical crosslinking process using vinyl sulfone in which the hydroxyl groups of the polysaccharide react with each other to form an infinite network through sulfonyl-bis-ethyl crosslinks.[43] This gel is well suited for use in dermal augmentation because of its insolubility and resistance to degradation and migration. The high water content mimics the natural hydrating functions of the precursor, hyaluronic acid. Hylan gel has also been shown to be well tolerated in vivo, and it does not exhibit any known clinically significant immunologic activity, making it an excellent candidate as a soft tissue augmentation material.

A variety of materials have been used for the correction of soft tissue defects including paraffin, silicone, and collagen.[44,45,46] Paraffin and silicone cause intense foreign body reactions and are known to migrate from the site of injection.[47,48] Collagen implants have been used with great frequency and success for the correction of soft tissue defects (dermal contour deformities). It has been widely documented, however, that collagen implants are resorbed by the body,[49,50,51] necessitating regular repeated injections of the material. Collagen therapy is also associated with a low incidence of hypersensitivity reaction, and prospective patients must undergo skin testing before receiving collagen therapy.

In contrast, hylan gel is a polysaccharide, not a protein, and is produced from the natural hyaluronan polymer, which exhibits no species specificity, i.e., the chemical identity of the molecule is maintained and is the same in all species. The immunologic compatibility associated with hylan gel is most likely due to the fact that the glycosaminoglycan chain in hyaluronan remains unaltered after chemical modification that produces the gel.[52] Richter et al. have shown that purified hyaluronic acid does not possess known clinically significant humoral or cell-mediated immunologic activity.[53,54] Studies, however, have shown that other forms of HA (different source and purification methods that may not remove significant "foreign" materials, including inflammatory fractions) and other glycosaminoglycans are somewhat immunologically reactive, but no known clinical significance has ever been associated with this property.[55,56]

Hylan gel is used mainly for dermal augmentation, but also as a viscosupplementation product to replace the vitreus in retinal detachment surgery.[57] Other developmental applications of HA-based products include augmentation of the periurethral/bladder tissues for treatment of urinary incontinence, drug delivery, the management of adhesion formation, osteoarthritis, etc. Currently, hyaluronic acid is approved as a viscoelastic tool in ophthalmology for cataract replacement. It has been used in more than 1 million patients worldwide for this procedure without any significant device-related concerns.

Preclinical Studies

Hylan gel was evaluated in preclinical in vivo studies for biocompatibility and residence times selected tissues. In a 12-month in vivo feasibility and characterization study in guinea pigs, the behavior of hylan gel was compared to that of "collagen" implants. Hylan gel was found to be biologically compatible and stable in the dermal tissue. At 1 year hylan gel was detected in a majority (12 of 16) test sites. Hylan gel was observed to persist in the skin longer than the collagen controls (Zyderm and Zyplast). In contrast to the hylan gel, none of the collagen implant material was found at 1 year.[58,59,60] These findings are consistent with published reports in the literature.

In another in vivo dermal study in guinea pigs, radiolabeled hylan gel was used in order to quantitatively assess recovery of the implant. At 1, 2, and 4 weeks postimplantation, analysis of recoverable radioactivity revealed only a slight decrease in the total amount of injected radioactivity. Histological evaluation of duplicate sites confirmed the presence of gel in the dermal tissue and indicated that the biological compatibility was similar to the nonradiolabeled gel.[61,52]

Immunogenic activity of hylan gel was evaluated in an adjuvant enhanced study in rabbits. Repeated intramuscular injections of hylan gel emulsified in Freund's adjuvant failed to produce a humoral (antibody) immune response in 21 rabbits. A control group of rabbits was immunized with ovalbumin by the same procedure and was observed to develop serum antibody titers of >800 to this protein within 35 days from the start of treatment. In addition, chronic exposure of primates to hylan gel (up to 3 years) did not produce a cell-mediated immune response as measured by the standard dermal challenge test. There was no evidence of a hypersensitivity reaction to hylan gel. Serum obtained from these primates did not contain detectable levels of hylan gel antibodies.[61,52]

Human Clinical Studies

A multicenter, open study was initiated in 1991 under an FDA-approved IDE. Patients who had previous injections of tissue (skin) augmentation materials within the last year were excluded from the study. Because of the nature of the product, skin testing was not required. Scars suitable for injection were identified by their ability to be manually stretched to the point that the defect could be eliminated. Wrinkles suitable for inclusion were those that historically are known to respond well to soft tissue augmentation (*e.g.*, glabellar lines, nasolabial folds, other facial lines). Up to 4 sites per patient were injected. Hylan gel was administered at the first visit, and touch-up injections were permitted at the next 2 visits (weeks 2 and 4), if necessary. Hylan gel was administered by injection, in a manner similar to other soft tissue augmentation products, into the dermal tissue through a 30-gauge needle. Anticipated adverse reactions commonly seen with any soft tissue augmentation product, such as erythema, swelling, pain, itching, tenderness, etc., were documented. Patients were monitored closely; however, for all adverse events, be they anticipated or not. Patients who met the inclusion/exclusion criteria signed Informed Consent forms prior to entering the study and were free to withdraw at any time.

Clinical Assessment

After the initial visit, patients were evaluated at follow-up visits at weeks 2, 4, 6, and 12. A long-term follow-up visit occurred at week 18. Device performance assessment include serial clinical expert grading and photographs. At each posttreatment visit, the physician and patient separately evaluated the degree of correction for each treatment site, using a 100 mm Visual Analog Scale (0 = no correction, 100 = total correction). Patient evaluation of device performance was also noted. The values from the visual analog scale for each time point and for each site were added together and the mean value was determined. Any complications or adverse events were recorded at each follow-up visit.

Results

Preliminary results from the ongoing trial (5 investigators, 150 patients, 3-4 sites/pt.) are highlighted in Figure 18.21. In general, most patients received an initial treatment at week 0 and 1 touch-up treatment at week 2 or 4. At week 12 approximately 84% of the treatment sites show a moderate (33% or better) degree of correction (Figures 18.22A and B). Approximately 50% of these sites maintained marked or complete correction (65% or greater improvement) as compared to baseline. At week

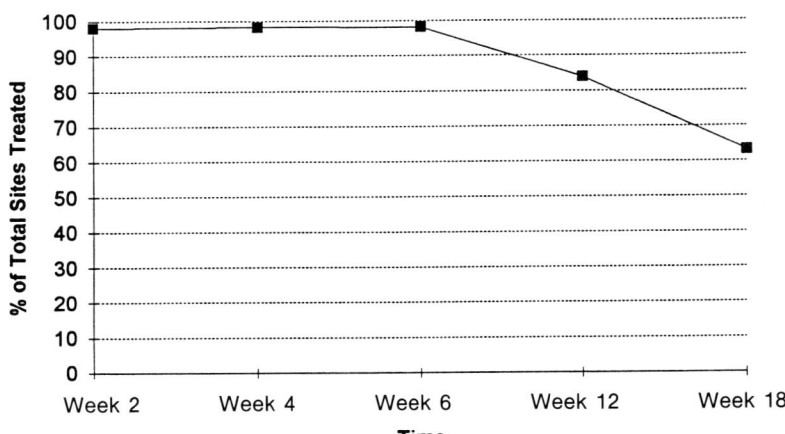

FIGURE 18.21. Treatment sites with moderate (33% or greater) degree of correction based on investigator's assessment (includes 5 multicenter clinical investigator sites).

Degree Corrected	Total Scars & Wrinkles (%)				
	Week 2	Week 4	Week 6	Week 12	Week 18
Moderate or better	98.1	98.3	98.2	83.9	63.3
Less than moderate	1.9	1.7	1.8	16.1	36.7
Total sites treated	480	467	440	367	223

18 more than 60% of the sites treated still showed a moderate or better degree of correction. Patient assessment has paralleled the physician's evaluation, but has consistently yielded higher values (Figure 18.23). At week 12 patients rated 74% of their scars and wrinkles to be improved at least moderately or better. In terms of overall level of patient satisfaction with this treatment, 80% of the patients reported moderate or higher satisfaction at week 12.

Anticipated complications were as expected and included transient and mild erythema, itching, swelling, and pain. Related or probably related device adverse reactions occurred in fewer than 2% of all treatments and included persistent erythema, acne papule formation, and ecchymotic changes, among others. No known antigenic or immunogenic responses were observed.

Summary

Preliminary results from the preclinical and human clinical studies indicate that hylan gel is a safe and efficacious soft tissue augmentation product. Skin testing prior to treatment with hylan gel was not required, thus allowing patients to be treated immediately and it minimized patient safety concerns. Clinical results suggest that hylan gel performs as well as or better than products currently available. The product may be placed in both the superficial and deep dermal tissues obviating the need for a two product approach to treat deep fold/wrinkle areas like nasolabial folds. Use of hylan gel was not associated with any clinically significant device-related adverse reactions in the studies reviewed.

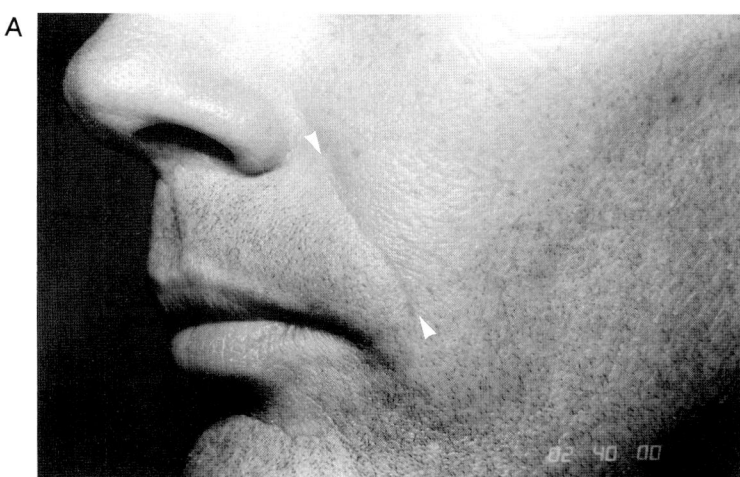

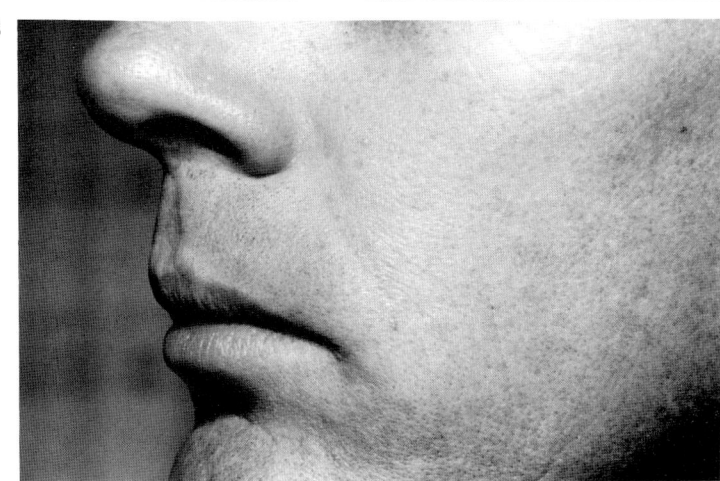

FIGURE 18.22. A. Pretreatment. Arrows note nasolabial fold wrinkle to be treated. B. Posttreatment, week 12.

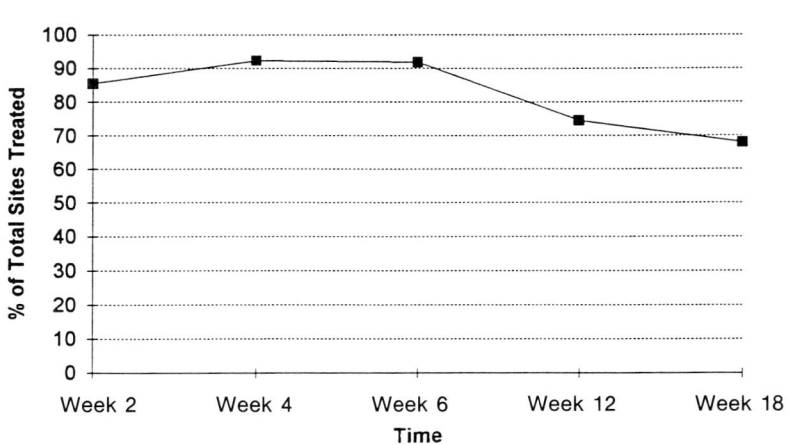

FIGURE 18.23. Treatment sites with moderate (33% or greater) degree of correction based on patient's assessment.

Degree Improved	Total Scars & Wrinkles (%)				
	Week 2	Week 4	Week 6	Week 12	Week 18
Moderate or better	85.5	92.4	91.9	74.5	68
Less than moderate	14.5	7.6	8.1	25.5	32
Total sites treated	482	471	443	369	225

Vignette #14

Surgical Correction of Neck Flaccidity in the Older Male

Arthur K. Balin

Some males who are troubled by excess skin hanging down below their chin would like to have this problem corrected but do not want to have a standard cheek neck lift (Figures 18.24 and 18.25). Patients with excess skin and fat in their upper neck can achieve considerable improvement by direct removal of the excess skin and fat.[62] This procedure is less extensive than a standard cheek neck lift and can be comfortably performed by the dermatologic surgeon under local anesthesia as an outpatient in the office surgical suite.

Standard history, physical examination, preoperative evaluation, and preoperative explanation, counseling, and consent are performed but are not further detailed in this section. An outline is drawn under the chin originating approximately 1 cm from the mandibular symphysis and extending in an eliptical fashion posteriorly to meet a transverse incision in the hyoid crease (refer to Figures 18.26 and 18.27). The posterior (inferior) margin of the transverse incision is oriented in a curvilinear fashion in the hyoid crease. No incision is made below the hyoid bone.

After the outline is drawn, but before the incisions are made, liposuction of the neck is performed by the tumescent technique. The patient is prepped for surgery and 100 to 200 cc of Klein solution[63] (0.1% lidocaine; 1:1,000,000 epinephrine; 12.5 meq $NaHCO_3$/l) is injected into the neck area. After waiting 20 minutes to allow the epinephrine to cause vasoconstriction, thereby maximizing hemostasis, liposuction surgery is performed. The initial entry is at the apex of the outline 1 cm from the mandibular symphysis. A 3 mm spatula cannula on a Toomy syringe is used. Syringe assisted liposuction is performed as described by Fournier[64] below the dermis but above the platysma in a fanlike fashion from the point of entry. Liposuction is extended laterally to the

18. Surgical Vignettes

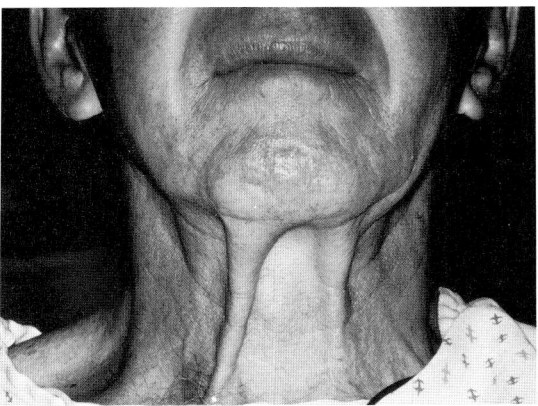

FIGURE 18.24. A 75-year-old male with a pacemaker presenting with excess submental skin and fat who did not want a facelift. Preoperative front view.

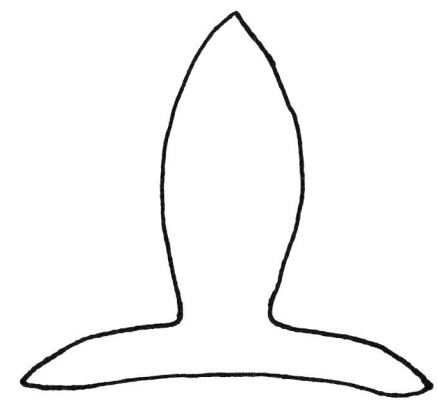

FIGURE 18.26. A diagram of submental design.

sternocleidomastiod muscle. Caution is noted in the area of the mandible because of the potential for injury to the marginal mandibular branch of the facial nerve. Approximately 30 cc of fat will be obtained in a typical case. Although crisscrossing with incisions at each side of the sternocleidomastoid muscle is used for pure neck liposuction, it has not been necessary to make these additional incisions in this procedure.

After the liposuction is completed, the tissue is incised along the previously drawn outline with a number 15 blade. The incision extends through the epidermis and dermis to the subcutaneous space, which is freely movable because of the liposuction undermining. The skin is excised and the wound is closed with buried deep dermal and subcutaneous suture of 3-0 and 4-0 vicryl as needed and cutaneous mattress and interrupted sutures of 6-0 ethilon (Figures 18.28 and 18.29).

A pressure dressing of gauze, cotton balls and elastic "French" tape is applied, followed by an elastic neck chin support. The tape dressing is removed in 4 days. The patient is encouraged to wear the neck chin support for 2

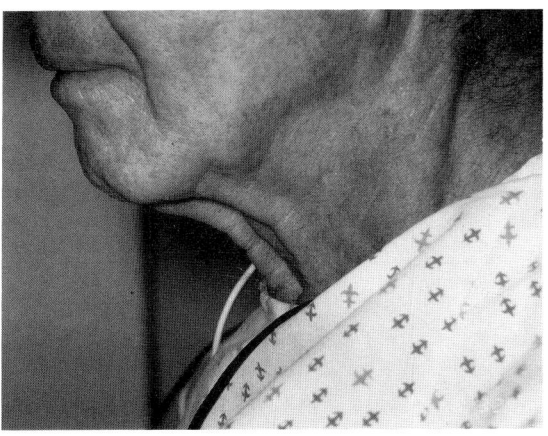

FIGURE 18.25. A 75-year-old male with a pacemaker presenting with excess submental skin and fat who did not want a facelift. Preoperative left side view.

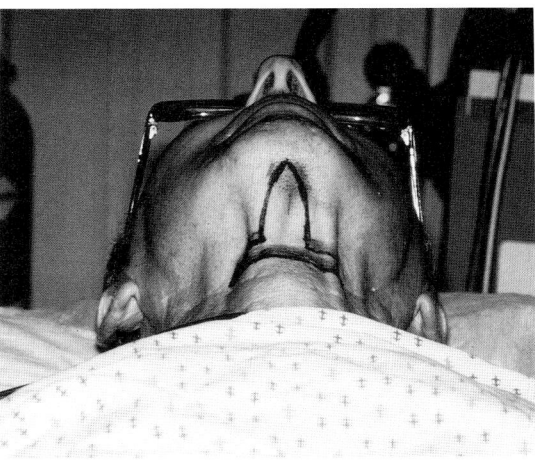

FIGURE 18.27. An outline drawn on patient prior to surgical preparation.

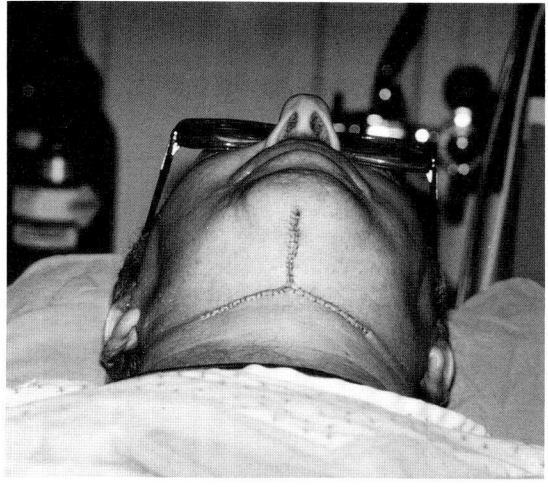

FIGURE 18.28. Immediately after surgery, prior to bandaging.

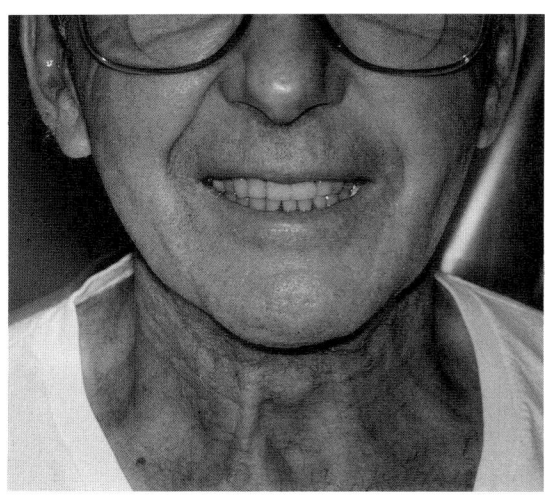

FIGURE 18.30. Two weeks postoperative. Front view.

or 3 additional weeks. Improvement is apparent as soon as the neck chin elastic support is discontinued (Figures 18.30 and 18.31). Improvement continues over the next 6 to 8 months (refer to Figures 18.32, 18.33 and 18.34). Figure 18.33 shows that the suture line is barely perceptible at 9 months.

We have not noted hypertrophic scars or vertical scar contracture in our patients. Patients have been very pleased by this procedure. Castillo[62] noted no vertical contracture but a 50% incidence of a hypertrophic vertical scar component, which was treated by intralesional triamcinolone injections.

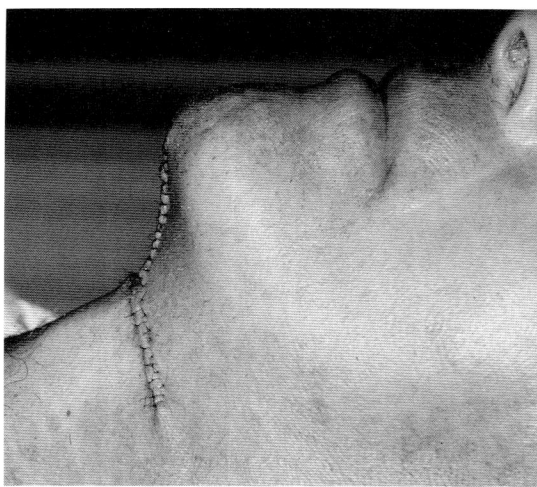

FIGURE 18.29. Immediately after surgery, prior to bandaging. Left side view.

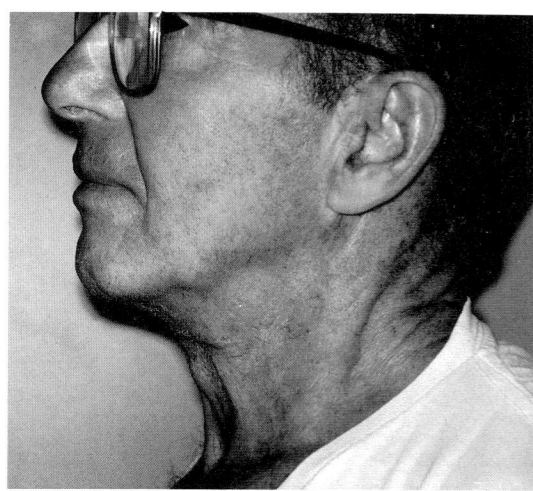

FIGURE 18.31. Two weeks postoperative. Left side view.

18. Surgical Vignettes

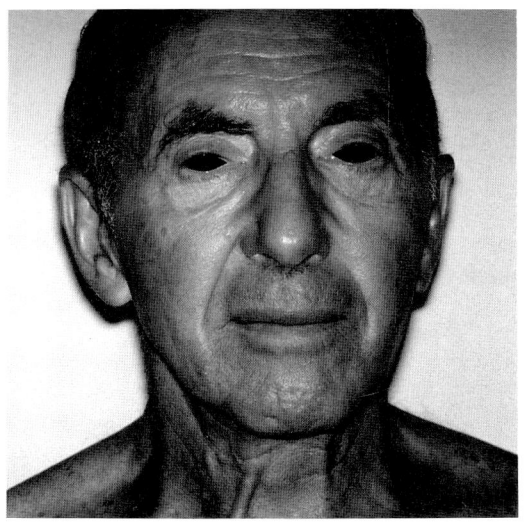

FIGURE 18.32. Nine months postoperative. Front view.

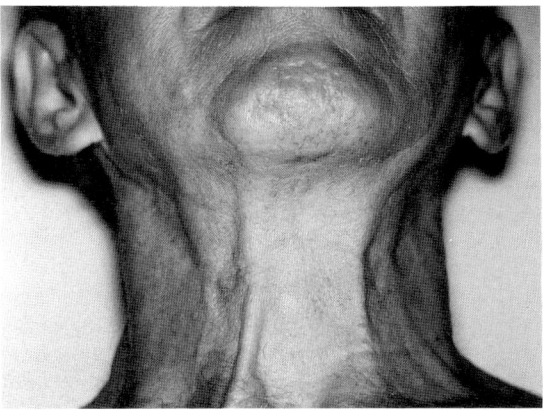

FIGURE 18.33. Nine months postoperative. Note that the surgical suture line is barely perceptible.

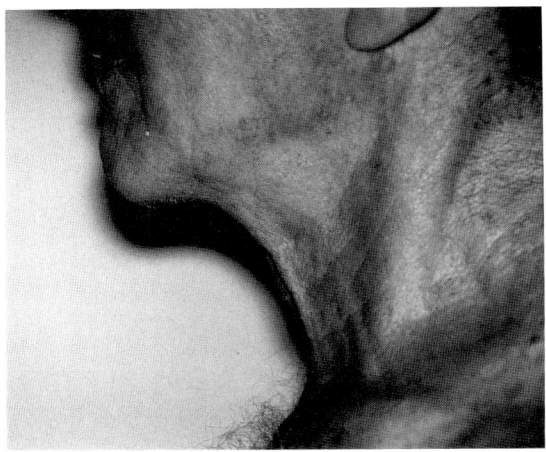

FIGURE 18.34. Nine months postoperative. Left side view.

References

1. Benedetto AV, Griffin TD, Benedetto EA, et al. Dermabrasion: therapy and prophylaxis of the photoaged face. J Am Acad Dermatol. 1992;27:439–447.
2. Stagnone JJ, Stagnone GT. A second look at chemabrasion. J Dermatol Surg Oncol. 1982;8:701–705.
3. Brodland DG, Roenigk RK. Mayo Clin Proc. 1988;63(9):887–896.
4. Resnik SS. Chemical peeling with trichloroacetic acid. J Dermatol Surg Oncol. 1984;7:549–550.
5. Collins PS. The chemical peel. Clin Dermatol. 1987;4:57–74.
6. Swinehart JM. Salicylic acid ointment peeling of hands and forearms. J Dermatol Surg Oncol. 1992;18:495–498.

7. Brody HJ. Variations and comparisons in medium depth chemical peeling. J Dermatol Surg Oncol. 1989;9:953-963.
8. Collins PS. Trichloroacetic acid peels revisited. J Dermatol Surg Oncol. 1989;9:933-940.
9. Lober CW. Chemexfoliation—indications and cautions. J Am Acad Dermatol. 1987;1:109-112.
10. Litton C, Trinidad G. Complications of chemical face peeling as evaluated by a questionnaire. Plast Reconstr Surg. 1981;6:738-744.
11. Maliner JS. Regional hand dermabrasion. Plastic and Reconstructive Surgery of the Head and Neck, the Third International Symposium, Vol. 1, Aesthet Surg. Grune and Stratton, New York, 1981, pp. 191-194.
12. Robinson JK. Actinic cheilitis: a prospective study comparing four treatment methods. Arch Otolaryngol Head Neck Surg. 1989;115(7) 848-852.
13. Chiarello SE. Cryopelling. J Dermatol Surg Oncol. 1992;18:329-332.
14. Lubritz RR. Smolewski SA. Cryosurgery cure rate of actinic keratoses. J Am Acad Dermatol. 1982;7:631.
15. Graham GF. Cryosurgery. Clin. Plast Surg. 1993;20:131-147.
16. Levin JA. Cryotherapy found cost-effective for lentigines. Skin All News. 1989;20(7):3.
17. Graham GF, Clark LC. Statistical analysis in cryosurgery of skin cancer. In: *Clinics in Dermatology: Advances in Cryosurgery*, Vol. 8, E Breitbart, E Dachow-Siwiec, eds. Elsevier, New York, 1990, p. 101.
18. Kuflik EG, Gage AA. The five-year cure rate achieved by cryosurgery for skin cancer. J Am Acad Dermatol. 1991;24:1002.
19. Holt PSA. Cryotherapy for skin cancer: Results over a 5-year period using liquid nitrogen spray. Cryosurgery. 1988;119:231.
20. Zacarian SA. Cryosurgery for cancer of the skin. In: *Cryosurgery for Skin Cancer and Cutaneous Disorders*. SA Zacarian, ed. C.V. Mosby, St. Louis, 1985, pp. 96, 199.
21. Kobayashi T. Microsurgical treatment of nevus of Ota. J Dermatol Surg Oncol. 1991:17: 936-941.
22. Kobayashi T. Microsurgical treatment of nasolabial and glabellar wrinkles. J Dermatol Surg Oncol. 1992:18:31-37.
23. Urano S, Inomori Y, Sugawarea T, Kato Y, Kitahara M, Hasegawa Y, Matsuo M, Mukai K. Vitamin E: inhibition of retinol-induced hemolysis and membrane-stabilizing behavior. J Biol Chem. 1992;267(26):18365-18370.
24. Williams DS, Roberts EA. Modification of the daily photoreceptor membrane shedding response in vitro by antioxidants. J Invest Ophthal Vis Sc. 1992;33(10):3005-3008.
25. Rozewicks L, Barcew-Wiszniewska B, Wojcicki J, Samochowiec L, Krasowska B. Protective effect of selenium and vitamin E against changes induced in heart vessels of rabbits fed chronically on a high-fat diet. Kitasato Crch Exper Med. 1991;64(4):183-192.
26. Kagan V, Witt E, Goldman R, Scita G, Packer L. Ultraviolet light-induced generation of vitamin E radicals and their recycling. A possible photosensitizing effect of vitamin E in skin. Free Rad Res Comm. 1992;16(1):51-64.
27. Sugiyama M, Tsuzuki K, Matsumoto K, Ogura R. Effect of vitamin E on cytotoxicity, DNA single strand breaks, chromosomal aberrations, and mutation in Chinese hamster V-79 cells exposed to ultraviolet-B light. Photochem Photobiol. 1992;56(1):31-34.
28. Zanoschi C, Ciobanu C, Berbuta A, Frincu D. The efficiency of some natural drugs in the treatment of burns. Revista Medico-Chirurgicala A Societatii De Medici Si Naturalisti Din Iasi. 1991;95(1-2):63-65.
29. Bendich A. Vitamin E status of US children. J Am Coll Nutr. 1992;11(4):441-444.
30. Odagiri Y, Karube T, Katayama H, Takemoto K. Modification of the clastogenic activity of X-ray and 6-mercaptopurine in mice by prefeeding with vitamins C and E. J Nutr. 1992;122(7):1553-1558.
31. Matsuda T, Tanaka H, Shimazaki S, Matsuda H, Abcarian H, Reyes H, Hanumadass M. High-dose vitamin C therapy for extensive deep dermal burns. Burns. 1992;18(2):127-131.
32. Miric M, Haxhiu MA. Effect of vitamin C on exercise-induced bronchoconstriction. Plucne Bolesti. 1991;43(1-2):94-97.
33. Geesin JC, Darr D, Kaufman R, Murad S, Pinnell SR. Ascorbic acid specifically increases type I and type III procollagen messenger RNA levels in human skin fibroblast.
34. Anneren G, Magnusson CG, Nordvall SL. Increase in serum concentrations of IgG2 and IgG4 by selenium supplementation in children with Down's syndrome. Arch Dis Child. 1990;65(12): 1353-1355.
35. Ryan AS, Craig LD, Finn SC. Nutrient intakes and dietary patterns of older Americans: a national study. J Gerontol. 1992;47(5):M145-150.
36. Lassus C. Utilisation d un tissu de reforcement pour le traitement des ridules et des vides du visage. XIV Cong National de Med Est et de Chir Derm. 25-27 September 1987, Paris France.
37. Mole B. Interet des implants prothetigues souples dans la chinirgie du rajeunement facial.

Annales de Chinergie Plastigic et Esthetigic. 1989;34(3):227–233.
38. Cisneros JL, Singla R. Correccion de pliegues faciales y relleno de labios con hilo de sutura Gore-tex. Med Estetic. 1991; July–September: 5–7.
39. Boyce B. Physical characteristyics of expanded polytetrafluoroethylene grafts. En J Stanley Biologic and Synthetic Vascular prostheses. Grune and Strattoce, New York, 1982, pp. 553–561.
40. Stegman SJ, Tromovitch TA, Glogau RG. Filling agents. Cosmet Dermatol Surg. Year Book Medical Publishers, Inc., 1990, pp. 145–184.
41. Comper W D, Laurent TC. Physiological function of connective tissue polysaccharides. Physiol Rev. 1978;58:255–315.
42. Balazs EA, Denlinger JL. Clinical uses of hyaluronan. In: *The Biology of Hyaluronan* (Ciba Foundation Symposium #143), D Evered, J Whelan, eds. John Wiley & Sons, Chichester and New York, 1989, pp. 265–280.
43. Balazs EA, Leshchiner EA. Hyaluronan, its crosslinked derivative-hylan-and their medical applications. In: *Cellulosics Utilization: Research and Rewards in Cellulosics* (Proceedings of Nisshinbo International Conference on Cellulosics Utilization in the Near Future), H Inagaki, G O Phillips, eds. Elsevier Applied Science, New York, 1989, pp. 233–241.
44. Barton JL, Cunliff WJ. Oil granuloma. In: *Textbook of Dermatology*, A Rook, DB Wilkonson, FJG Ebling, RH Champion, JL Burton, eds. Blackwell, Oxford, 1986, pp. 1870–1871.
45. Knapp TR, Kaplan EN, Daniels JR. Injectable collagen for soft tissue augmentation. Plast Reconstr Surg. 1977;60:398–405.
46. Selmanowitz VJ, Orentreich N. Medical-grade fluid silicone: a monographic review. J Dermatol Surg Oncol. 1977;3:597–611.
47. Editorial: Complications with silicones—what grade of silicone? How do we know it was silicone? Plast Reconstr Surg. 1988;61:892.
48. Matton G, Anseeuw A, DeKeyser F. The history of injectable biomaterials and the biology of collagen. Aesthet Plast Surg. 1985;9:133–140.
49. Arem A. Collagen modifications. Clin Plast Surg. 1985;12:209–220.
50. Donald PJ. Collagen grafts—here today and gone tomorrow. Otolaryngol Head Neck Surg. 1986;95:607–614.
51. Kramer FM, Churukian MM. Clinical use of injectable collagen. Arch Otolaryngol. 1984;110:93–98.
52. Larsen NE, Pollak CT, Reiner K, Leshchiner EA, and Balazs EA. Hylan gel biomaterial: dermal immunology compatibility. J Biomed Mater Res (in press).
53. Richter AW. Non-immunogenicity of purified hyaluronic acid preparations tested by passive cutaneous anaphylaxis. Int Arch All Appl Immunol. 1974;47:211–217.
54. Richter AW, Ryde EM, Zetterstrom EO. Non-immunogenicity of a purified sodium hyaluronate preparation in man. Int Arch All Appl Immunol. 1988;59:45–48.
55. Poole R, Reiner A, Roughley PJ, Champion B. Rabbit antibodies to degraded and intact glycosaminoglycans which are naturally occuring and present in arthritic rabbits. Bio Chem. 1985;260:6020–6025.
56. Fillit HM, McCarty M, Blake M. Induction of antibodies to hyaluronic acid by immunization of rabbits with encapsulated stretococci. J Exper Med. 1986;164:762–776.
57. Nussbaum JJ, Roarty J. Hylan gel and retinal detachment surgery. Invest Ophthalmol Vis Sci (Suppl). 1991;32:880 (abstract).
58. Piacquadio D. Hylan gel: a new substance for soft tissue augmentation. American Academy of Dermatology, 51st Annual Meeting, December 5–10, 1992, San Francisco, California.
59. Piacquadio D, Jarcho M, Larsen N, Balazs EA, Goltz R. Evaluation of hylan gel as a soft tissue augmentation implant material. American Society for Dermatologic Surgery, 19th Annual Clin. & Sci. Meeting, March 11–15, 1992, Scottsdale, Arizona.
60. Piacquadio D, Jarcho M, Larsen N, Balazs EA, Goltz R. Evaluation of hylan gel as a soft tissue augmentation implant material (manuscript in preparation).
61. Larsen NE, Kling MD, Balazs EA, Leshchiner EA. Hylan gel for soft tissue augmentation. Society for Biomaterials 16th Annual Meeting, May 20–23, 1990, Charleston, South Carolina. Trans Soc Biomat. 1990;XIII:302 (abstract).
62. Castillo G. Alternatives in the management of neck flaccidity for males. Am J Cosmet Surg. 1991;8:23–27.
63. Klein J A. The tumescent technique. Dermatol. Clin. 1990;8:425–437.
64. Fournier P. Liposculpture: the syringe technique. Arnette, S. A., Paris, 1991, pp. 123–140.

Index

A

Abscess formation, and soft tissue augmentation, 86
Accreditation, dermatological surgicenter, 255, 256–257
Accutane. See Isotretinoin
Acne
  and alpha hydroxy acids (AHAs), 23, 26
  and chronic radiation dermatitis, 201
  post-peel, 62
Acne rosacea, 205
Actinic cheilitis, 198
  alpha hydroxy acids (AHAs) for, 31
Actinic keratosis, 198, 251–252
  malignant transformation of, 251–252
  treatment of, 198, 252, 293–294
  types of, 198
Aging face
  divisions of, 5–6
  European view of treatment, 301
  expression lines, 4
  extrinsic aging, 16
  future view, 295
  and gravity, 3–4
  intrinsic aging, 1–2, 16
  micropeeling procedures, 296–299
  photoaging, 4–5
  relative value scale for, 6–7
  sleep lines, 2–3

Aging skin, 243–245
  definition of, 23–24
  factors in appearance of, 243
  role of dermatologist in treatment of, 296
  topical treatment of, 244–245
  and wound healing, 243–245
Alopecia, and facelift, 162
Alpha hydroxy acid (AHAs) peel, 29–30, 40, 43, 51–52
  application of solution, 30, 51
  maintenance peels, 30
  post-peel care, 52
  results of, 30
  solutions used, 30
Alpha hydroxy acids (AHAs), 22–32
  and acne-prone skin, 23, 26
  and aging skin, 24–25, 244–245
  buffering effects, 24–25
  chemical properties of, 22–23, 40
  combined with 5-fluorouracil, 29
  combined with hydroquinone, 29
  combined with retinoic acid, 29–30
  concentrations in products, 24
  derivatives of, 22
  and dry skin, 26
  effects of, 26, 43
  for lips, 31
  and oily skin, 26
  compared to retinoic acid, 27
  side effects, 26–27
  for solar lentigines, 250
  treatment approach, 25–27

  treatment of forearms/hands, 31
  uses of, 23
Androgenic alopecia, 212–214
  and heredity, 212–213
  hormonal factors, 212
  incidence of, 213
  in women, 213
Angiogenesis, and tretinoin, 18–19
Angiokeratoma of scrotum, 187
Angiosarcoma of face/scalp, 192
Anthranilates, sunscreen, 11
Antiandrogens, and hair loss prevention, 240
Anticoagulant effects, drugs related to, 179
Arsenical keratosis, 198
Asteatotic dermatitis, 208
Atypia, 17
Atypical fibroxanthoma, 192
Atypical scarring, 72
Autoimmune disease, and soft tissue augmentation, 86
Autologen method, soft tissue augmentation, 90
Autologous collagen. See Lipotransfer

B

Bacterial infection
  and chemical peeling, 55, 62
  and facelift, 162
  and hair transplantation, 239
  and soft tissue augmentation, 83–84

Baldness. *See* Hair loss; Hair restoration
Basal cell carcinoma, 192–193, 195–196
Benzophenones, sunscreen, 10
Biologic dressings, 76
Bioplastique, soft tissue augmentation, 90
Bleeding
 and facelift, 160
 and hair transplantation, 238
 retrobulbar hemorrhage, 186
Blepharoplasty, 169–186, 209
 anesthesia, 184
 complications of, 182–183, 186
 eyelid, anatomical factors, 174–178
 gender-related considerations, 170, 173
 and ideal of eye/eyelid area, 169–171
 lower lid, 171, 172–173, 182–186
 methods for lower lid, 182–185
 methods for upper lid, 180–182
 patient consent form, 180–181
 patient selection, 178–179
 postoperative care, 185
 preoperative evaluation, 179, 183
 preoperative photography, 179, 183
 preseptal approach, 185
 retroseptal approach, 184–185
 transconjunctival blepharoplasty, 184
 transcutaneous blepharoplasty, 182–184
 upper lid, 178–182
Botulinum A exotoxin, frown line elimination, 91
Bovine collagen, soft tissue augmentation, 79–88
Bowen's disease, 200
Buccal fat pads of face, liposuction for, 100

C

Cancer
 angiosarcoma of face/scalp, 192
 atypical fibroxanthoma, 192
 basal cell carcinoma, 192
 malignant melanoma, 196
 Merkel cell carcinoma, 196–197
 squamous cell carcinoma, 197
Chemical peeling, 5, 34–66
 alpha hydroxy acids (AHAs) for, 29–30, 40, 43, 51–52
 application methods, 44–45
 avoidance of complications, 56–58
 Baker and Litton formulas, 37, 41
 combined with surgery, 63
 complications of, 52–66
 consent form for, 45
 croton oil in, 37, 38, 41
 definition of, 34
 hands, 250, 252
 histological effects, 42–43
 history of, 34–39
 Jessner's formula, 38, 41–42
 methods of, 43–52
 phenol for, 35–39, 42–43, 45–48, 63–65
 preparation of skin for, 44
 resorcinol for, 40, 65–66
 results of, 30
 salicylic acid for, 66
 trichloracetic acid, 39–40, 48–51
Cherry hemangioma, 187
Chondrodermatitis nodularis helicis, 187
Chronic heliodermatitis, 17
Chronic radiation dermatitis, 200
CIDESCO International Diploma, estheticians, 270
Cinnamates, sunscreen, 10
Cobblestoning, and hair transplantation, 238–239
Collagen implants, 305
Collagen vascular disease, 87
Conjunctiva, 176–177
Contact dermatitis, 202
Contour irregularities, and facelift, 162–163
Cosmetics industry, 292
Cosmetic surgery
 choosing surgeon for, 280
 cost factors, 281
 patient selection criteria, 278–279
 and psychological functioning, 273–274
 and self-concept, 275
 and self-esteem, 277–278
 See also individual procedures
Croton oil, in chemical peel, 37, 38, 41
Crow's feet, 208–209
Cryosurgery, 293–294
 indications for, 293–294
 postsurgical care, 294
Cryotherapy, and senile lentigines, 250
Cyst formation, and hair transplantation, 239

D

Demarcation lines, and chemical peeling, 55–56, 62, 65
Dermabrasion, 4, 5, 68–78
 anesthesia for, 73
 complications of, 76–78
 contraindications for, 72
 dermabrading tools, 74
 history of, 68
 indications for, 68–70
 after isotretinoin treatment, 72
 medications after procedure, 73
 method for, 74–75
 patient selection, 70–72
 postoperative care, 75–76
 preoperative preparation, 72–73
 surgical equipment for, 73–74
Dermasanding, 283–292
 advantages of, 291
 method in, 284, 286–289
 patient selection, 284
 postoperative care, 286, 289
 results of, 289–291
 sandpaper for, 284
 test site, 284
Dermatoheliosis, meaning of, 68
Dermatological surgicenter, 255–260
 accreditation, 255, 256–257
 administrative aspects, 258
 consultants for, 259–260
 design aspects, 258
 licensure, 256
 location for, 257–258
 Medicare certification, 256
 operating room technique, 258–259
 quality improvement program, 257
Dermographism, and chemical peeling, 56

Index

Dibenzoylmethanes, sunscreen, 11
Distraction test, 183
Dorian Gray complex, 277
Dry skin
   and alpha hydroxy acids (AHAs), 26
   eczema craquelé, 208
   estheticians recommendations for, 264–265
   and tretinoin, 19
   xerosis, 208
Dysplasia, 17

E

Eczema craquelé, 208
Edema
   and chemical peeling, 46, 56, 63
   and hair transplantation, 239
Elastosis, 17
Elliott flap, 236, 238
Erythema
   and chemical peeling, 55–56, 62–63
   and dermabrasion, 76
   and soft tissue augmentation, 83
Erythroplasia of Queyrat, 200–201
Estheticians
   CIDESCO International Diploma, 270
   client education by, 266
   dry skin care, 264–265
   European versus American licensing requirements, 262, 263–264
   facials, components of, 262
   preoperative/postoperative skin care, 265–266
   products recommended by, 262, 265
   qualifications for, 270
   role of esthetician compared to dermatologist, 266–269
   skin care for aging women, 262–265
   skin care services of, 265
Esthetics, historical view, 261
Expression lines, 4, 7
Extramammary Paget's disease, 200–202
Extrinsic aging, 16

F

Face
   and aging. *See* Aging face
   liposuction of, 99–100
Facelift
   and age, 111
   anesthesia, 127–128
   complications of, 160–163
   liposuction with, 130–131, 139–140
   marking for, 125–127
   modified Webster short flap technique, 123–124
   and pain, 158, 163
   patient consultation, 111–113
   postoperative care, 158–160
   postoperative dressing, 156, 158
   postoperative instructions to patient, 115
   postoperative results (photos), 163–167
   preauricular flap, 136, 138–139, 153–156
   preoperative evaluation for, 113, 117
   preoperative instructions to patient, 116
   preoperative medication, 113
   preoperative photographs, 113, 117, 118–122
   preparation for, 117, 123
   purposes of, 110
   redraping of skin flap, 145–156
   retroauricular flap, 131–133, 146–151
   retroauricular sulcus, 156
   superficial musculoaponeurotic system (SMAS), 124–125, 141–142, 144–145
   temporal flap, 133, 135–136, 151–153
Eyelid
   conjunctiva, 176–177
   levator aponeurosis, 176
   Muller's muscle, 176
   orbicularis muscle, 175
   posterior lamella lower lid, 178
   septum orbitale, 175–176, 177
   tarsus, 176
   upper lid skin, 174–175
   See also Blepharoplasty

Fat augmentation. *See* Lipotransfer
Favre-Racouchot syndrome, 202
Fibrel, 88–89
Flap procedures in hair restoration, 215, 235–238
   Elliott flap, 236, 238
   Juri flap, 236
   Stough flap, 236
5-fluorouracil
   for actinic keratosis, 252
   combined with alpha hydroxy acids (AHAs), 29

G

Glycolic acid, 5
   See also Alpha hydroxy acids (AHAs)
Glycosaminoglycans (GAGs), 17
Gore-tex threads, 302–303
   insertion method, 303
   soft tissue augmentation, 90–91
Granuloma fissuratum, 202
Gravity, and aging face, 3–4, 7

H

Hair loss, 209–210
   androgenic alopecia, 212–214
Hair restoration, 213–240
   anesthesia, 223
   and antiandrogens, 240
   and color of hair, 221–222
   complications of, 238–239
   crown baldness, 220–221
   and curly hair, 222
   and density of hair, 222
   design principles, 217–218
   flap procedures, 215, 235–238
   goal of, 217
   graft harvesting, 223
   graft placement, 229
   graft trimming, 225–226
   hairline height determination, 218–219
   hairline shape determination, 219–220
   history of, 213–215
   incisional slit grafting, 214
   lateral canthus indicator, 219–220
   linear grafting, 215, 228
   micrografts, 214, 226, 227–228
   minigrafts, 228

Hair restoration (*continued*)
  and minoxidil, 239–240
  patient assessment for, 215–217
  postoperative care, 229
  posttransplant styling, 222–223
  preoperative antibiotics, 223
  round graft harvesting, 225
  round punch grafts, 214, 228
  scalp reduction, 215, 229–235
  strip grafting, 214–215
  strip harvesting, 223–225
  temporal area, 220
  and texture of hair, 222
  and tretinoin, 240
  tripartite-face analysis in, 218–219
  turgor, increasing in donor area, 223
  vertex region, 221
  and women, 216–217
  See also Scalp reduction
Hands
  actinic keratoses, 251–252
  chemical peeling, 250, 252
  idiopathic guttate hypomelanosis, 248–249
  lipotransfer, 104, 245, 247–248
  prevention of photoaging, 248–249
  seborrheic keratoses, 251
  senile lentigines, 249–251
  treatment with AHAs, 31
Heredity, and androgenic alopecia, 212–213
Herpes simplex
  and chemical peeling, 55, 61–62
  and dermabrasion, 72, 77
Hyaluronic acid for soft tissue augmentation, 91, 304–307
  human clinical studies, 306–307
  hylan gel, 305–306
  preclinical studies, 305
  results of, 306–307
Hydroquinone
  combined with alpha hydroxy acids (AHAs), 29
  for hyperpigmentation, 249
Hylan gel, 305–306

I

Ichthyosiform genodermatoses, and AHAs, 23
Idiopathic guttate hypomelanosis, 248–249

Incisional slit grafting, hair restoration, 214
Intrinsic aging, 1–2, 6, 16
Isotretinoin, scarring after treatment, 72

J

Juri flap, 236

K

Keloids, and ligmaject, 295
Koken atelocollagen, soft tissue augmentation, 90

L

Lactic acid. *See* Alpha hydroxy acids (AHAs)
Laser treatment, and solar lentigines, 250–251
Lentigo maligna, 202
Leukoplakia, alpha hydroxy acids (AHA) for, 31
Levator aponeurosis, 176
Licensure, dermatological surgicenter, 256
Ligmaject, 295
Linear grafting, hair restoration, 215, 228
Liposculpture. *See* Liposuction of face
Liposuction, and neck lift, 308–309
Liposuction of face
  for buccal fat pads, 100
  cervical liposuction, 130–131
  complications of, 99
  during facelift, 130–131, 139–140
  for nasolabial folds, 100
  and rhytidectomy, 100
  for sagging jowls, 100
Liposuction of neck, 93–99
  complications of, 96
  consultation with patient, 93–94
  contraindications to, 93
  with excision of excess skin, 97–98
  liposuction method, 95–96
  postoperative care, 96
  preoperative procedure, 94–95

Lipotransfer, 90, 101–108
  complications of, 108
  fat processing method, 107
  for hands, 104, 245, 247–248
  histological aspects, 102
  history of, 101
  longevity of transplantation, 108
  patient selection, 102, 105
  postoperative care, 106
  for soft tissue augmentation, 90, 106–107
  technique in, 104–106
  uses of, 102, 105
Liver spots. *See* Senile lentigines
Looking glass self-concept, 277–278

M

Malignant melanoma, 196
Medicare certification, dermatological surgicenter, 256
Mercedes reduction, scalp reduction, 234
Merkel cell carcinoma, 196–197
Micrografts, hair restoration, 214, 226, 227–228
Microlipo injection. *See* Lipotransfer
Microliposuction. *See* Liposuction of face
Micropeeling procedures, 296–299
  indications for, 296
  method in, 296, 298
  results of, 298–299
Milia
  and chemical peeling, 56, 62
  and dermabrasion, 77
Minigrafts, hair restoration, 228
Minoxidil, and hair restoration, 239–240
Modified-S reduction, scalp reduction, 233–234
Muller's muscle, 176

N

Nasolabial fold, sandwich technique, 304
Nasolabial folds, liposuction for, 100
Neck, liposuction of, 93–99

Neck lift
  case study, 308-311
  and liposuction, 308-309
  marking for, 308
  postoperative care, 309-310
Necrosis
  and facelift, 162
  and soft tissue augmentation, 84-85
Nerve damage, and facelift, 160-161

O

Oily skin, and alpha hydroxy acids (AHAs), 26
Oral commissure, 4
Orbicularis muscle, 175

P

PABA (para-amino benzoic acid), 9, 10, 14
Pain, and hair transplantation, 239
Paramedian reduction, scalp reduction, 231-233
Perleche, 202, 204
Phenol peel, 35-39, 42-43, 45-48, 63-65
  aftereffects of, 46
  application of solution, 47-48
  Baker and Litton formula, 41
  bleaching effect, 65
  chemical aspects, 39
  effectiveness of, 45
  histological aspects, 42
  ideal patient, profile of, 46
  medical clearance for, 45, 46
  pain from, 46, 47, 64-65
  phenol cardiotoxicity, 63-64
  postpeel care, 48
  preparation of skin for, 47
  systemic absorption of phenol, 46-47, 64
  tape mask, 48, 65
Photoaging, 4-5
  alpha hydroxy acids (AHAs) for, 22-32
  and chemical peeling, 34-66
  and dermabrasion, 68-78
  dermasanding, 283-292
  prevention of, 248-249
  signs of, 16-17
  tretinoin for, 17-20

Physical attractiveness, 275-277
  characteristics of attractive persons, 276
  and elderly, 276, 277
  societal importance of, 275
  and workplace, 275-276
Physician/patient relationship, 301-302
Pigmentation abnormalities
  bleaching agents, 249
  and chemical peeling, 52-54, 58-60, 65
  and dermabrasion, 71-72, 76
  fading formulas, 59
  idiopathic guttate hypomelanosis, 248-249
  senile lentigines, 249-251
Pigment removal, and tretinoin, 18-19
Poikiloderma of Civatte, 204
Portwine stain, 187-188
Posterior lamella lower lid, 178
Preauricular flap, in facelift, 136, 138-139, 153-156
Pruritus, and chemical peeling, 56
Psychological functioning, and cosmetic surgery, 273-274
Pulsed-dye laser treatment, 188
Pyruvic acid, 40, 43
  histological effects, 97

Q

Quality improvement program, dermatological surgicenter, 257

R

Resorcinol peel, 65-66
  chemical aspects, 40
  complications of, 65-66
  histological aspects, 40
Retin A. See Tretinoin
Retroauricular flap, in facelift, 131-133, 146-151
Retrobulbar hemorrhage, 186
Rhinophyma, 205
Rhytidectomy, and liposuction, 100
Rosacea, 205
Round punch grafts, hair restoration, 214

S

Sagging jowls, liposuction for, 100
Sagittal mid-line reduction, scalp reduction, 230-231
Salicylates, sunscreen, 10-11
Salicylic acid peel, 66
  actinic keratosis, 253
  complications of, 66
Scalp lifts, 234-235
Scalp reduction, 215, 229-235
  complications of, 239
  Mercedes reduction, 234
  modified-S reduction, 233-234
  paramedian reduction, 231-233
  sagittal mid-line reduction, 230-231
  and scalp laxity, 229-230
  scalp lifts, 234-235
  Z-plasty, 231
Scarring
  and chemical peeling, 54, 60-61
  and facelift, 162
  and hair transplantation, 238
  after isotretinoin treatment, 72
Scrotum, angiokeratoma of scrotum, 187
Sebaceous hyperplasia, 188, 190
Seborrheic keratosis, 190, 251
  classification of, 190
Self-concept, and cosmetic surgery, 275
Self-esteem, and cosmetic surgery, 277-278
Senile lentigines, 249-252
Senile purpura, 205
Septum orbitale, 175-176, 177
Silicone, soft tissue augmentation, 89-90
Silicone gel sheeting, and dermabrasion, 76-77
Skin care, historical view, 261
Skin dermatoses/infections
  contact dermatitis, 202
  Favre-Racouchot syndrome, 202
  granuloma fissurtum, 202
  Perleche, 202, 204
  poikiloderma of Civatte, 204
  rosacea, 205
  senile purpura, 205
  stasis dermatitis, 205
  telangiectasia, 205
  tinea pedis, 205, 208
  xerosis, 208

Skin lesions
  actinic cheilitis, 198
  actinic keratosis, 198
  angiokeratoma of scrotum, 187
  angiosarcoma of face/scalp, 192
  arsenical keratosis, 198
  asteatotic dermatitis, 208
  atypical fibroxanthoma, 192
  basal cell carcinoma, 192–193, 195
  Bowen's disease, 200
  cherry hemangioma, 187
  chondrodermatitis nodularis helicis, 187
  chronic radiation dermatitis, 200
  eczema craquelé, 208
  erythroplasia of Queyrat, 200
  extramammary Paget's disease, 200–202
  lentigo maligna, 202
  malignant melanoma, 196
  Merkel cell carcinoma, 196–197
  portwine stain, 187–188
  rhinophyma, 205
  sebaceous hyperplasia, 188, 190
  seborrheic keratosis, 190
  skin tags, 191
  solar lentigo, 192
  spider angioma, 192
  squamous cell carcinoma, 197
  venous lakes, 192
Skin tags, 191
Sleep lines, 2–3, 6, 211
Slot defect, and scalp reduction, 239
Snap test, 183
Soft tissue augmentation
  augmentation method, 81–82
  Autologen method, 90
  bioplastique, 90
  Botulinum A exotoxin as alternative to, 91
  collagen implants, 305
  Fibrel, 88–89
  future view, 91
  gore-tex threads, 90–91
  hyaluronic acid, 91, 304–307
  Koken atelocollagen, 90
  microlipo injection, 90
  pre-procedure skin testing, 80–81
  side effects, 82–88
  silicone, 89–90
  Zyderm-I, 79–82, 88
  Zyplast, 79, 81–82, 84–85, 88
Solar lentigo, 192
Spider angioma, 192
Squamous cell carcinoma, 197
Stasis dermatitis, 205
Stough flap, 236
Stretchback, and scalp reduction, 239
Strip grafting, hair restoration, 214–215, 223–225
Sun damage. *See* Photoaging
Sun protection factors (SPF) system, 11–12
Sunscreen, 5, 9–14
  anthranilates, 11
  benzophenones, 10
  cinnamates, 10
  dibenzoylmethanes, 11
  future view, 14
  lack of effective vehicles for, 12
  PABA, 9, 10, 14
  reactions to, 13–14
  salicylates, 10–11
  sunblocks, 9–10
  sun protection factors (SPF) system, 11–12
  and tretinoin use, 19–20
Superficial musculoaponeurotic system (SMAS), facelift, 124–125, 141–142, 144–145
Surgicenters. *See* Dermatological surgicenter

T

Tarsus, 176
Telangiectasia
  characteristics of, 205
  and chemical peeling, 56, 63
  and dermabrasion, 77
  treatment of, 205
Temporal flap, in facelift, 133, 135–136, 151–153
Tinea pedis, 205, 208
Toxic shock syndrome, post-peel, 62
Transconjunctival blepharoplasty, 184
Transcutaneous blepharoplasty, 182–184
Tretinoin, 5, 17–20
  and actinic keratosis, 252
  and aging skin, 245, 250
  compared to AHAs, 27
  combined with AHAs, 28
  and hair restoration, 240
  and senile lentigines, 249–250
  side effects, 19
  structural improvements from, 18–19
  treatment guidelines, 19–20, 245
Trichloroacetic acid peel, 39–40, 48–51
  application of solution, 51
  chemical aspects, 39
  concentrations used, 48, 51
  and dermasanding, 283–292
  histological aspects, 42
  post-peel care, 51
  preparation for, 51
Tripartite-face analysis, in hair restoration, 218–219
Turkey-neck deformity, 4

U

Ultraviolet light
  effects of, 4–5, 9
  immunological effects of, 12–13
  skin disorders related to, 188
  See also Sunscreen

V

Venous lakes, 192
Vitamin therapy, 300

W

Wound healing, and age, 243–245
Wrinkling
  Crow's feet, 208–209
  severe, 211
  sleep creases, 211
  See also Aging face

X

Xerosis, 208
  and AHAs, 23

Z

Z-plasty, scalp reduction, 231
Zyderm-I, 79–82, 88, 106